MANUAL OF PSYCHIATRIC THERAPEUTICS

Third Edition

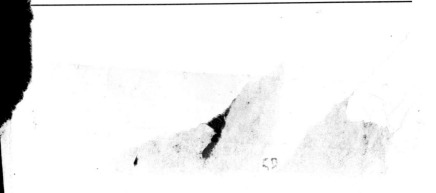

MANUAL OF PSYCHIATRIC THERAPEUTICS

Third Edition

Richard I. Shader, M.D.

Professor
Department of Pharmacology and
  Experimental Therapeutics
Department of Psychiatry
Tufts University School of Medicine
Boston, Massachusetts

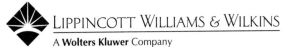

LIPPINCOTT WILLIAMS & WILKINS
A **Wolters Kluwer** Company
Philadelphia · Baltimore · New York · London
Buenos Aires · Hong Kong · Sydney · Tokyo

Acquisitions Editor: Charles W. Mitchell
Developmental Editor: Selina M. Bush
Production Editor: Christiana Sahl
Manufacturing Manager: Colin Warnock
Cover Illustrator: Christine Jenny
Compositor: Circle Graphics
Printer: R. R. Donnelley/Crawfordsville

© 2003 by Richard I. Shader
Published by Lippincott Williams & Wilkins
530 Walnut Street
Philadelphia, PA 19106 USA
LWW.com

Printed in the USA

Library of Congress Cataloging-in-Publication Data

Manual of psychiatric therapeutics / [edited by] Richard I. Shader.—3rd ed.
  p. ; cm. — (Spiral manual)
  Includes bibliographical references and index.
  ISBN 0-7817-2470-8
  1. Mental illness—Chemotherapy—Handbooks, manuals, etc. 2. Mental illness—Treatment—Handbooks, manuals, etc. I. Shader, Richard I., 1935- II. Series.
  [DNLM: 1. Mental Disorders—drug therapy. 2. Mental Disorders—therapy. 3. Psychotropic Drugs—therapeutic use. WM 402 M294 2003]
  RC483 .M26 2003
  616.89′1—dc21

                                                          2002040639

Care has been taken to confirm the accuracy of the information presented and to describe generally accepted practices. However, the authors, editor, and publisher are not responsible for errors or omissions or for any consequences from application of the information in this book and make no warranty, expressed or implied, with respect to the currency, completeness, or accuracy of the contents of the publication. Application of this information in a particular situation remains the professional responsibility of the practitioner.

The authors, editor, and publisher have exerted every effort to ensure that drug selection and dosage set forth in this text are in accordance with current recommendations and practice at the time of publication. However, in view of ongoing research, changes in government regulations, and the constant flow of information relating to drug therapy and drug reactions, the reader is urged to check the package insert for each drug for any change in indications and dosage and for added warnings and precautions. This is particularly important when the recommended agent is a new or infrequently employed drug.

Some drugs and medical devices presented in this publication have Food and Drug Administration (FDA) clearance for limited use in restricted research settings. It is the responsibility of the health care provider to ascertain the FDA status of each drug or device planned for use in their clinical practice.

10 9 8 7 6 5 4 3 2 1

To my late wife Aline for her unfaltering love and her courage in the face of daunting illness; to my children (and their spouses) and grandchildren for their unwavering love, support, and concern; to the innocent victims of disease and premeditated violence; and to all who willingly and generously try to provide assistance, care, and relief.

CONTENTS

Appendices

CONTRIBUTING AUTHORS

W. Stewart Agras, M.D.
Professor, Department of Psychiatry, Stanford University School of Medicine, Stanford, California

Jane E. Barbiasz, R.N., C.S.
Psychiatric Clinical Nurse Specialist, Department of Nursing, Lawrence Memorial Hospital of Medford, Medford, Massachusetts

Ann Marie Ciraulo, R.N.
Assistant Professor, Division of Psychiatry, Boston University School of Medicine; Clinical Research Registered Nurse, Division of Psychiatry, Boston University Medical Center, Boston, Massachusetts

Domenic A. Ciraulo, M.D.
Professor and Chairman, Department of Psychiatry, Boston University School of Medicine; Psychiatrist-in-Chief, Department of Psychiatry, Boston Medical Center, Boston, Massachusetts

Barbara J. Coffey, M.D., M.S.
Associate Professor, Department of Psychiatry, New York University; Director, Institute for the Study of Tourette's and Movement Disorders, New York University Child Study Center, New York University School of Medicine, New York, New York

James M. Ellison, M.D., M.P.H.
Associate Clinical Professor, Department of Psychiatry, Harvard Medical School, Boston, Massachusetts; Clinical Director, Geriatric Psychiatry Program, McLean Hospital, Belmont, Massachusetts

Laura J. Fochtmann, M.D.
Associate Professor, Department of Psychiatry and Behavioral Sciences; State University of New York at Stony Brook School of Medicine; Director, Electroconvulsive Therapy Service, Stony Brook University Hospital, Stony Brook, New York

Claire M. Frederick, M.D.
Clinical Instructor in Psychiatry, Harvard Medical School, Boston, Massachusetts

David J. Greenblatt, M.D.
Louis Lasagna Professor and Chairman, Department of Pharmacology and Experimental Therapeutics; Professor of Psychiatry, Medicine, and Anesthesia, Tufts University School of Medicine; Physician, Division of Clinical Pharmacology, Tufts-New England Medical Center, Boston, Massachusetts

Thomas G. Gutheil, M.D.
Professor, Department of Psychiatry, Harvard Medical School; Codirector, Program in Psychiatry and the Law, Massachusetts Mental Health Center, Boston, Massachusetts

Sandra A. Jacobson, M.D.
Assistant Professor, Department of Psychiatry, Tufts University School of Medicine; Director of the Consultation-Liaison Service, New England Medical Center, Boston, Massachusetts

Jessica R. Oesterheld, M.D.
Medical Director, TSS, Portland, Maine

David N. Osser, M.D.
Associate Professor, Department of Psychiatry, Harvard Medical School, Brockton, Massachusetts; Associate Medical Director; Director of Psychopharmacology, Taunton State Hospital, Taunton, Massachusetts

Janet E. Osterman, M.D.
Assistant Professor, Department of Psychiatry, Boston University School of Medicine; Vice Chair of Education and Training, Department of Psychiatry, Boston Medical Center, Boston, Massachusetts

Dean X. Parmelee, M.D.
Associate Dean for Academic Affairs; Professor, Departments of Psychiatry and Pediatrics, Wright State University School of Medicine, Dayton, Ohio

Robert D. Patterson, M.D.
Lecturer on Psychiatry, Department of Psychiatry, Harvard Medical School, Boston, Massachusetts; Attending Physician, Department of Psychiatry, McLean Hospital, Belmont, Massachusetts

Stephen G. Pauker, M.D., M.A.C.P., F.A.C.C.
Sara Murray Jordan Professor of Medicine, Department of Medicine, Tufts University School of Medicine; Vice Chairman for Clinical Affairs, Department of Medicine; Associate Physician-in-Chief, Department of Medicine, New England Medical Center, Boston, Massachusetts

Chester Pearlman, M.D.
Clinical Professor of Psychiatry, Boston University School of Medicine, Boston, Massachusetts

Katharine A. Phillips, M.D.
Associate Professor, Department of Psychiatry and Human Behavior, Brown Medical School; Director, Body Dysmorphic Disorder Program, Butler Hospital, Providence, Rhode Island

Ronald W. Pies, M.D.
Clinical Professor, Department of Psychiatry, Tufts University School of Medicine, Boston, Massachusetts; Lecturer on Psychiatry, Harvard Medical School, Cambridge, Massachusetts

John A. Renner, Jr., M.D.
Associate Professor, Division of Psychiatry, Boston University School of Medicine; Associate Chief of Psychiatry, Outpatient Clinic, VA Boston Health Care System, Boston, Massachusetts

Richard Saitz, M.D., M.P.H., F.A.C.P.
Associate Professor of Medicine and Epidemiology, Section of General Internal Medicine, Department of Medicine, Boston University Schools of Medicine and Public Health; Director and Attending Physician, Clinical Addiction Research and Education (CARE) Unit, Boston Medical Center, Boston, Massachusetts

Richard I. Shader, M.D.
Professor of Pharmacology and Experimental Therapeutics, Professor of Psychiatry, Tufts University School of Medicine; Program Director for Pharmacology and Experimental Therapeutics, Sackler School of Graduate Biomedical Sciences, Tufts University, Boston, Massachusetts

Aradhana Bela Sood, M.D., F.A.A.C.A.P.
Associate Professor, Department of Psychiatry; Chairman, Child and Adolescent Psychiatry, Virginia Treatment Center for Children, Virginia Commonwealth University, Medical College of Virginia, Richmond, Virginia

Judith E. Tintinalli, M.D., M.S.
Professor and Chairman, Department of Emergency Medicine, University of North Carolina at Chapel Hill; Professor and Chairman, Department of Emergency Medicine, University of North Carolina Hospitals, Chapel Hill, North Carolina

Wayne A. Ury, M.D.
Assistant Professor, Departments of Medicine and Psychiatry, New York Medical College, Valhalla, New York; Chief, Section of Palliative Medicine, Department of Medicine, St. Vincent's Hospital of New York, New York, New York

Karthik Venkatakrishnan, Ph.D.
Graduate student, Department of Pharmacology and Experimental Therapeutics, Tufts University School of Medicine, Boston, Massachusetts[1]

Lisa L. von Moltke, M.D.
Research Associate Professor, Department of Pharmacology and Experimental Therapeutics, Tufts University School of Medicine, Boston, Massachusetts

Paul H. Wender, M.D.
Distinguished Professor Emeritus of Psychiatry, University of Utah School of Medicine, Salt Lake City, Utah

Suzanne R. White, M.D.
Associate Professor, Departments of Emergency Medicine and Pediatrics, Wayne State University; Medical Director, Children's Hospital of Michigan Poison Control Center, Detroit Medical Center, Detroit, Michigan

[1]Affiliation at the time the chapter was written. Karthik Venkatakrishnan is now a Senior Research Scientist in Pharmacokinetics, Dynamics and Metabolism at Pfizer, Inc., in Groton, Connecticut.

PREFACE

The first edition of the *Manual of Psychiatric Therapeutics* was written about 20 years after the advent of modern psychopharmacology. Diagnostic systems were in flux at that time, partly because responses to specific psychopharmacologic agents were provoking some psychiatrists to rethink certain traditional descriptive and etiologic concepts. The *Diagnostic and Statistical Manual of Mental Disorders,* 4th edition, (DSM-IV) and the *International Statistical Classification of Diseases and Related Health Problems,* tenth revision, (ICD-10) are now in place, and, in many instances, treatment efficacy can be anticipated for patients who meet these descriptive and course criteria. The second edition of this manual was written in the early 1990s; it contained changes in treatment and management strategies reflecting the broad acceptance of the DSM-IV and the penetration of managed care into the lives of both treating clinicians and their patients. The new millennium has brought globalization of the pharmaceutical industry, an increasing use of practice guidelines and algorithms, an even greater impact from managed care, an increasing reliance on evidence-based medicine that is being countered by trends emphasizing effectiveness over efficacy and challenges to the use of placebo controls to support claims of efficacy, a growing use of assessments of the economic impact of disorders and of specific therapies, the greater use of quality of life assessments in the evaluation of both new and older agents, more informed patients and families who advocate for themselves, and an almost blind faith in so-called natural products (e.g., herbals and botanicals). In the face of these changes, the introduction of a third edition of this manual seemed appropriate. In addition, with the years that elapse between each edition, awareness of the benefits and limitations of electronic media is growing, especially regarding the Internet and other online resources.

Although the limitations to online publications are obvious, real time resources, such as textbooks and briefer manuals, by their very nature also have limitations. To be truly practical, manuals have to be small enough to be portable, with the pocket size being preferable. To accomplish this, they must be succinct. Manuals are temporally bound; therefore, they cannot be completely up-to-date. For more current information and new research findings, interested readers may wish to consult the *Journal of Clinical Psychopharmacology* (*JCP*) to which many of the authors of this manual regularly contribute. The tables of contents of the *JCP* can be found online at *http://www. psychopharmacology.com/*.

This edition features two new chapters (Chapter 21, "Approaches to the Psychopharmacologic Treatment of Children and Youth," and Chapter 28, "Understanding and Assessing Pain and Pain Syndromes"), and all of the chapters from the second edition have been updated, expanded, or reordered. Chapter 21 has been added because the Food and Drug Administration has added patent extension incentives to encourage the development of more information about the use of some agents in children and because more and more children are being treated with these medications, reflecting a trend that is not yet adequately supported by an understanding of the impact that some of these agents may have on their development. The chapter on attention deficit hyperactivity disorder (ADHD) (Chapter 22) has been enlarged to reflect not only the greater likelihood of treatment for this condition but also the growing number of adults who are seeking treatment for behaviors that they attribute to unrecognized and untreated residual ADHD from childhood. The chapters have been reordered to improve the flow in this edition, although the logic behind the new ordering may be questioned by some. For example, the chapter covering tic disorders (Chapter 7) is located after the chapter on obsessive-compulsive disorders (Chapter 6) because of the high incidence of overlapping comorbidity, even though some might have preferred to see the chapter on tic disorders aggregated with Chapters 21 and 22. The chapter on drug interactions (Chapter 29) has been totally revamped and expanded to reflect the fact that so many psychotherapeutic agents have a narrow therapeutic index or range. Inhibition of their metabolism can readily lead to toxicity, and induction can easily compromise efficacy. No chapter has been devoted exclusively to the elderly. Instead, appropriate material has been included where it is relevant. In this century, the aged are the modal patients for many clinicians. While special issues of dosing, receptor sensitivity, metabolism, and side effects are present, the inclusion of a separate chapter would have required more space than is appropriate for this format.

Another addition in this edition is Appendix VII. In it, Osser and Patterson provide a bibliography of treatment algorithms and guidelines that contains not only basic references and a conceptual framework but also websites that can be consulted for updated iterations (an example of how online materials can act as supplements to traditional texts). *The fact that these algorithms are presented is not an endorsement of them.* Rather, the purpose for their presence is to give readers of this manual a perspective on treatment alternatives that some clinicians or groups have found useful.

Some may still take issue with the chapters on seclusion and restraints, and new guidelines or regulations are now in place in many states, as well as at the federal level. However, whenever I am in hospitals or emergency departments that care for seriously disturbed psychiatric patients or for those suffering from toxic delirium, I find that, while seclusion, restraints, or both are in use, staff often have not thought through what they are about to do or have done, nor have they received adequate training and retraining in the proper uses and limitations of these strategies.

The indications and dosages of all drugs in this book have been recommended in the medical literature or conform to the practices of many in the general medical community. The medications described do not necessarily have specific approval from the Food and Drug Administration (FDA) for use in the diseases and dosages for which they are discussed or recommended. The package insert for each drug should be consulted for the use and dosage as approved by the FDA. Because standards for usage change, it is advisable to keep abreast of the revised recommendations, particularly those concerning new drugs. It is important to realize that, when a drug is withdrawn from the market for reasons other than safety (e.g., the manufacturer feels either that the need is no longer sufficient or that profitability has diminished significantly), the practicing community may not become aware of this. Notices of drug withdrawals eventually appear in the *Federal Register,* but they may not appear until some time (e.g., a year) after the drug has been withdrawn.

Particular attention should be paid to the so-called **"black box warnings"** whenever they appear for a given agent. These warnings are almost always added after a drug has been marketed for some time and postmarketing surveillance has revealed an adverse outcome that was not noted in premarketing trials. In most instances, this was because of the careful selection of the patients studied in the trials or the limited size of the exposed population.

Interested readers may also wish to review Appendix II for information about the FDA and herbal remedies and dietary supplements.

My hope is that the approaches and perspectives offered in this text will encourage readers to engage in the treatment of those suffering from psychiatric disorders and that they will continue to reduce the dual burdens of stigma and hopelessness that are so often felt by patients, their families, their physicians and other care providers. Some physicians may even be encouraged to do clinical and basic research in order to reduce ignorance. If reading this edition improves the care of patients or inspires or enables research, then the energy put into its creation and publication will surely have been worthwhile.

Richard I. Shader
Bourne, Massachusetts

ACKNOWLEDGMENTS

For those who have never written or edited a book, the process may seem opaque. To the author or editor, the process can be rather perplexing; rarely does a project go smoothly—snags are always encountered, and many deadlines are not met. Along the way, many people have facilitated the process of writing the *Manual of Psychiatric Therapeutics,* and I wish to single some out for special thanks.

Many people enabled both the writing and the production of this manual. I am particularly indebted to James V. Forgione, PHARM.D., of the Drug Information Center at the New England Medical Center. Whenever I had reason to question whether a particular drug or dosage form was actually available, he cheerfully used his resources to track down such facts for me. Because of the revision of the chapter covering attention deficit hyperactivity disorder and the addition of a new and extensive chapter focusing on youth, a number of colleagues were asked to review early drafts and to provide feedback. Special thanks go to Drs. Pablo Davanzo, Bruce Fogas, Joseph Horrigan, Bennett Leventhal, Andres Martin, Gabriella Weiss, and Issac Wood.

My gratitude also goes to Charley Mitchell, my Aquisitions editor at Lippincott Williams & Wilkins, for his persistance and tolerance when I required accomodations because of my wife's illness and death. There is also a tedious aspect to the final stages of book production. Christiana Sahl, my production editor at Lippincott Williams & Wilkins, brought her skills and good sense of humor to this stage and not only kept me on track but also added some fun to this task.

I also want to thank my patients, trainees, and colleagues who have taught me over the years or who have challenged me to think about human suffering; the distress and pain we cause each other; the burdens imposed by stigma, prejudice, ignorance, and bias; the importance of forgiveness, tolerance, and owning one's own behavior; respect for individual differences; and the complexities of the human condition.

MANUAL OF PSYCHIATRIC THERAPEUTICS

Third Edition

1. INTRODUCTION: A PERSPECTIVE ON CONTEMPORARY PSYCHIATRY AS A BACKGROUND TO PSYCHOPHARMACOLOGY

Richard I. Shader

Psychiatry primarily focuses on the capacity for integration of mind, brain, behavior, experience, intellect, and emotion as they relate to human growth and development and the prevention and treatment of mental disorders. An expanding body of clinical experience and research has clarified the idea that, to treat patients with psychiatric disorders, frequently an understanding not only of the patient's symptoms and complaints but also of the developmental, cultural, and present contexts in which symptoms develop, the meanings these symptoms have to the patient, the patient's relevant past experiences, and their available support systems is necessary.

The older concepts of "organic" and "functional" have polarized thinking about mental diseases (disorders) in detrimental ways and have little, if any, current value. Contemporary psychiatry places a heavy emphasis on an integrative model that combines a vulnerability–stress paradigm with a biopsychosocial perspective, including attention to neurobiologic substrates, subjective experiences, and sociocultural factors, and that assumes the following important elements:

1. Genetic predispositions underlie most, if not all, major psychiatric disorders;
2. Disturbances of the functions or faculties of the mind and brain are present in all major psychiatric disorders (e.g., cognition is impaired in dementias, affective control is impaired in bipolar disorder);
3. Protective genetic factors, mitigating interpersonal relationships, and phenotypic or temperamental variations (e.g., shyness versus extroversion, stimulus-seeking or harm–avoidance traits, fantasy proneness, eidetic imagery) shape patients' presentations and experiences;
4. Considerable variation exists in the strengths and weaknesses of adaptive capacities arising from earlier experiences, especially, but not limited to, those in childhood;
5. Individualized stressful experiences often may trigger or may expose episodes of dysfunction or underlying pathology.

Notwithstanding these considerations, the actual pathophysiologic underpinnings of most psychiatric disorders typically remain unknown. Unfortunately, these gaps in knowledge are sometimes used to bolster the arguments of those who view psychiatric disorders as arising merely from a lack of moral fiber or willpower or simply as a result of bad parenting.

Although some controversy exists about the validity and importance of psychodynamic and psychologic explanatory concepts in understanding and treating certain major mental disorders, some descriptive concepts are useful for comprehensive approaches to these disorders. A full explanation of all relevant terminology is beyond the scope of this chapter, but a brief review of selected conceptually important terms may help clinicians in their efforts on behalf of their patients.

I. Selected Explanatory Concepts

The existence of **unconscious** mental activity or storage is a basic tenet of a psychologic perspective on mental functioning—feelings, ideas, or memories of experiences not within conscious awareness or accessible by introspection exist in the human mind.

A. Repression

Repression is a process by which some feelings and memories may be actively kept from one's awareness. This is a type of selective, defensive, or self-protective "not remembering." Repression conveys more than merely not remembering: usual strategies that promote recall are not effective in

1

retrieving the repressed material, which is often related to conflictual, traumatic, embarrassing, or affect-laden experiences. An example of repression would be a failure to recognize an earlier experience of physical or sexual abuse that nevertheless unconsciously influences adult behavior and relationships (e.g., as inhibitions in normal assertiveness or in the experience of sexual pleasure). The idea that repression is self-protective bridges to other important terms and concepts.

B. Ego

The terms **self** and **ego** are often used interchangeably to refer to the awareness and sense of self or "selfness," including a continuity of one's identity over time, a coherence of one's values and aims, a basis for moral integrity, and an experience of boundaries (self versus non-self or the outside world). **Self** is actually a broader concept than **ego**. Ego commonly implies the executive functions of the self that have to do with adaptation and conflict resolution. To "survive" and function in what the self experiences as a complex and sometimes hostile or overly stressful world, the ego uses protective strategies (sometimes called defense mechanisms[1]), often unconsciously, to reduce or to contain feelings or experiences that would otherwise be overwhelming (e.g., too much uncertainty or ambiguity, too little control, or betrayal by trusted persons). This concept is reminiscent of T. S. Eliot's statement, "Humankind cannot bear very much reality." Animals, for instance, instinctively protect their young and their own bodies. People, without *consciously* choosing to do so, add to these basic behaviors a protection of the sense of intactness of self. The importance of this postulate is that some of the psychopathology seen in persons with mental disorders or reactions to physical illness may represent *unconsciously* or instinctively motivated behaviors that serve to protect the individual from knowing that his or her mind is malfunctioning—an idea that might be too disorganizing for a putatively needed sense of intactness of the self.

Supportive psychotherapy generally focuses on examining patients' coping styles to promote behavioral change; it strengthens those that are productive for the patient at the present time. Efforts may also be made to modify those that are maladaptive. Validation, compassion, acceptance, and trust are important elements.

C. Denial, Projection, Rationalization, Displacement, Transference, and Regression

These are a few of several postulated **reality-distorting** but self-guarding coping styles or defense mechanisms. Each coping style influences a patient's behavior and ability to provide an accurate history. Coping styles are potentially important in all areas of medicine but particularly in psychiatry. In the absence of clinical tests or a definitive confirmation of a psychiatric diagnosis, observing the patient, obtaining cooperation in the mental status evaluation, noting a pattern of symptoms and complaints, continuing interaction with the physician, and knowing the course and history support making a reliable and accurate diagnosis. An essentially normal physical examination combined with normal-range laboratory tests does not establish a psychiatric diagnosis, except to rule out an etiology secondary to a primary pathology outside of the brain (e.g., depression and mental slowing secondary to hypothyroidism). One should note that, although cultural and other experiential factors may influence a patient's presentation, most major psychiatric disorders continue to be remarkably similar to their earliest descriptions in religious and medical texts, as well as across disparate cultures.

1. **Denial**, which is closely related to and is often confused with **repression**, is a coping style in which the affected person experiences a minimal awareness of appropriate feelings or information that would reasonably and ordinarily be expected to be felt or known; overt behavior, however, may be incongruent (e.g., while talking about being re-

[1] The author prefers the term **coping style**.

fused life insurance, a patient tells the physician that he understands and that he is not angry, yet the doctor observes the patient's tense jaw and tight grip on the chair). Denial usually is an unconscious mechanism or process, the function of which is to circumvent distress or anxiety. In denial, one reduces the impact of serious matters through self-deception. Bad news (and occasionally good news) may then be experienced as irrelevant, nonexistent, exaggerated, or inconsequential. Denial may hide feelings, the impact of events, or the events *per se* from others or from oneself. As Johnny Mercer's popular admonition in song says, "You've got to accentuate the positive, eliminate the negative, latch on to the affirmative, don't mess with Mister In Between," denial may, in some instances, be health promoting. For example, in a patient with a recently diagnosed myocardial infarction, denial may circumvent hopelessness and a lack of will to live and may thereby contribute to recovery. When appropriate, a treating clinician may choose not to challenge a patient's denial. In contrast, denial could undermine recovery in a chronically ill cardiac patient who, as a result of denial, will not make the needed health-promoting changes in lifestyle and habits. Denial can also lead to avoiding needed help or to delays in seeking diagnosis or treatment. This can be extremely dangerous in some disorders (e.g., breast carcinoma). Denial is particularly frequent among adolescents and young adults who appear to ignore the dangers of many of their behaviors (e.g., smoking, unprotected sexual activity, disregard for speed limits when driving), although counterphobic elements may also be present for some in many of these same behaviors. Denial may be prominent in addictions (e.g., to **alcohol**, cigarettes) and substance abuse. Addicted persons often deny both the fact and the seriousness of their addiction. The frequent denial by spouses, friends, and employers that a drug abuse problem exists (see Chapters 9, 10, and 11) is a remarkable revelation of the same kind of avoidance.

2. **Projection** is the externalization onto another person of one's own feelings, thoughts, or motives that are, for some reason, not acceptable to the self or ego at the time at which they are experienced (perhaps because they are related to shame or guilt), thereby allowing the person to feel less distressed or possibly more justified. For example, a patient who is annoyed at waiting to see her physician for over an hour tells the nurse that she is sure that the doctor—who unbeknownst to the patient is dealing with an emergency—must be angry with her. Another example is the patient who should feel guilty about his neglect of his wife but who is unaware and unaccepting of his guilt feelings; instead he blames the hospital and his doctor for inadequate care.

3. **Rationalization** is the creation of a specious justification or of a false explanation for one's own or another's behavior to make the behavior seem more palatable (e.g., the same waiting patient from before assumes the doctor must be angry with her because she has not been following her diet).

4. **Displacement** may also be linked to projection. In displacement, feelings are shifted from the person who evokes them onto another, perhaps safer, person, object, or institution. For example, a patient who is unaware of her anger toward her physician instead is inappropriately caustic toward her husband later that day. Another example of displacement is the patient who shifts his or her concerns and fears about being ill to an inappropriate preoccupation with the inadequacies of his or her room or care.

5. **Transference** refers to the unconscious attribution of feelings that were originally connected to someone or something in the patient's past to a current person, institution, or even a medication in one's life (e.g., a patient may be immediately trusting, dependent, or obedient with his or her physician because he or she unconsciously sees the physician as a

positively viewed parental figure—understanding, knowledgeable, strong, and compassionate). Transference is a powerful determinant of a patient's expectations, both positive and negative, and it may contribute to compliance or noncompliance with the doctor's recommendations (see Chapter 13).

Transference may sometimes underlie perceptions of cultural or racial bias that, in turn, may interfere with access to treatment or its effectiveness. Transference brings the past into the present, typically not for defensive purposes. One must also remember that the reciprocal concept, **countertransference**, may also influence patient care (e.g., the physician perceives the patient in an altered or distorted way because of past relationships, including prior patients, in his or her own life).

6. **Regression** is the last **reality-distorting** coping style to be reviewed. Over a lifetime, new skills and mechanisms evolve to help one cope with the external world. In health, this development forms a continuum of increasingly effective styles of coping and adaptation, as survival and integration into one's family and community require growth and change. Regression represents a return, at times of extreme stress and upheaval, to earlier ways of coping. Patients typically become regressed when they feel overwhelmed or anxious about an illness or life crisis; their regressed state may color both their presentations and their abilities to participate in their own care. They behave less autonomously, and they become more dependent, passive, and helpless. Regression and helplessness may, in turn, make them feel considerable distress and anxiety. Regressed patients may also be very distrustful. Extremely regressed patients may be so childlike that they take no responsibility for getting better. Their transference expectations cause them to view physicians and other helping persons as complete and total caretakers, and they feel no need to be self-reliant. Many clinicians have difficulty tolerating regression in their patients; the recognition by the clinician and other caregivers that the regressed behavior is neither conscious nor willful may help to improve tolerance. Regression may be normative in childhood as developmental changes occur.

Some forms of expressive psychotherapy make use of the concept of regression. Through the facilitation of regression, the hope is that patients may be able to work through earlier conflicts, to rebuild their self-image, and to mature.

D. Cognitive-Behavioral Concepts

In addition to the selected psychologic concepts (e.g., regression, denial, transference) described above, an awareness of some of the principal constructs underlying certain **behavioral treatment approaches** might be useful for the concerned clinician. Specific approaches and more details are enumerated in later chapters of this manual.

1. **Exposure**. This is a concept central to all approaches derived from avoidance and stimulus–response theories. Exposure assumes that repeated systematic contact with a feared idea, image, or object in a safe and supportive environment will lead to a reduction in fear or anxiety and avoidance. The reduction in anxiety also promotes a sense of mastery and confidence. Exposure works best when the stimulus is, in reality, a nondangerous or a neutral one (conditioned stimulus) that has become associated with or is linked unconsciously to a threatening one (unconditioned stimulus) by the patient. The resulting decrement in fear or anxiety is referred to as **extinction**. In this context, anxiety is distinguished from fear by defining anxiety as a dysphoric response that is out of proportion to the danger cue (see Chapter 14).

2. **Systematic desensitization**. Repeated gradual exposure using a progressive series of imagined fear stimuli when coupled with relaxation strategies is sometimes referred to as **systematic desensitization**. Many effective uses of exposure are carried out *in vivo* (i.e., an actual

graded confrontation of the feared or anxiety-evoking stimulus that has led to avoidance). Obviously, this type of therapy is time-consuming and demanding for both the therapist and patient.

3. **Flooding**. This term is used when the exposure is controlled and safe but, at the same time, intense and inescapable. Flooding is infrequently used because little evidence exists to suggest that this approach is more effective than the graded *in vivo* exposure.

E. **Treatments Based on Social Learning Theory**
These are derived from notions of faulty modeling at formative life stages that can be corrected by **role playing** or **imitation**. Social skills training for patients with schizophrenia is an effective example of this approach (see Chapter 20).

F. **Cognitive-Behavioral Therapies**
These therapies promote a questioning of or confrontation with one's assumptions, beliefs, or doctrines with the suggestion that they may be false or distorted (see Chapters 6 and 8). Such false or distorted assumptions may significantly impair an individual's self-esteem or trust in others. Examining and challenging negative assumptions or even grandiose or self-centered ones may facilitate better coping and may promote a sense of mastery and self-efficacy. Terms such as **cognitive restructuring** are based on this concept.

G. **Operant Conditioning Theories**
Some treatments are rooted in **operant approaches** derived from the notion that behavior can be modified through **positive reinforcements** (rewards) or **punishments**. An important element in this approach is the skill of the therapist in selecting effective contingencies. **Negative reinforcement** is a confusing term that is currently used by many practicing clinicians to denote the use of an aversive experience before an undesired behavior occurs to block it (e.g., administering **disulfiram** to **alcohol-**dependent patients) rather than after the behavior to reduce or to suppress it (i.e., punishment).

II. **The Clinician–Patient Relationship**
A comprehensive understanding of a patient's illness and needs coupled with the patient's cooperation and **adherence** to the treatment plan should promote positive therapeutic outcomes. Cooperation is facilitated by a strong clinician–patient relationship. The strength of this relationship is enabled by the provision of useful information and the development of **trust**. The evolution of trust is encouraged when the clinician is successful at **therapeutic listening**. The patient must believe that the treating clinician has a genuine interest in the patient's well-being, inner experiences, and assumptions about life and the world. Trust and the provision of useful clarifications and information are among the core components of a **therapeutic** or **working alliance**.

An element of the bond of trust created between patient and clinician is rooted in the concept of **confidentiality**. Although the legal aspects may vary somewhat among jurisdictions, the core of confidentiality is the patient's right to control access to the information he or she provides to clinicians. Third-party health insurance programs, managed care plans, computerized pharmacy records, and Internet-accessible databases are among the many factors that have eroded the sense of personal privacy that many patients have customarily felt when sharing personal or painful material or genetic testing results with their caregivers. Treating clinicians must understand the applicable privacy statutes in their states, and they should be apprised of current federal guidelines and regulations. Early in treatment, establishing with patients an understanding of the limits of their privacy protection and working with them and their clinicians to find ways to share important experiences and facts are essential.

When treating children and youth (see Chapters 7, 21, and 22), multiple alliances may be needed to work with the child, the family, the school, and other involved parties and institutions. Similar issues may be involved when treating older patients who are no longer independent. Achieving an optimal therapeutic collaboration is another goal that is not easily met by current patterns of health care delivery, especially in the setting of **managed care**.

Managed care emphasizes time management and cost containment, which are often accomplished by following treatment protocols or by parsing out elements of the treatment plan to different health care personnel (e.g., prescribing clinicians, case managers, psychotherapists); inherent in this arrangement may be difficulties in maintaining confidentiality. Treatment protocols and guidelines can ensure that consideration is given to systematic and comprehensive treatment planning or diagnostic assessment. However, for some patients, protocols (with their emphasis on the modal patient) and the parsing out of their components can be antithetical to an evolving treatment alliance, to continuity of care, or to their unique features and needs.

Alliance maintenance is also essential for optimal patient care. Clinicians need to ensure that a way is always available so that patients can reach them or a previously designated surrogate during emergencies or times of heightened distress. Answering machines do not substitute for contact with a person. E-mail contact is increasing in acceptability among some people, but this route also has obvious limitations. Anticipating patients' needs and providing them with workable options in advance is important; knowing that a clinician can be reached and is willing to be reached may be sufficiently reassuring to obviate some patients' urgencies and emergencies.

Therapy protocols and manuals are an additional element that can affect the clinician–patient relationship. The recent increase in their use has had important benefits for psychotherapy research. Following outlined procedures enables standardization and the assessment of adherence by the clinician to the type of therapeutic intervention being provided. Unfortunately, although some features of this trend may be positive, a potential downside also exists; any standardization of treatment has the potential to downplay the uniqueness and unpredictability of each therapeutic encounter.

In any treatment relationship, interplay between the patient's appropriate need for **autonomy** and some amount of **paternalism** inherent in the clinician's care provider and healer role is almost always present. Although empowering patients has obvious merits, effective clinicians are always more than mere technologists or providers of information and choices. Few would dispute the value of the healing touch and a caring attitude. Emanuel and Emanuel (1992) described and advocated the so-called deliberative model of the clinician–patient relationship, a view that integrates the provision of information with clinicians' teaching, technical, and caring healer skills and promotes the self-development of patients with regard to their use of medical care. This perspective, although persuasive and appealing, can be compromised when clinicians ignore the ever-present impacts of transference and countertransference. For many psychiatric patients, careful attention must be paid to their distortions of reality, the acuteness of their distress and turmoil, and any other factors unique to their illness and circumstances.

III. Genetic Factors

After decades of research, little support exists for the notion that specific cytogenetic abnormalities are the major causal factors for the psychiatric disorders covered in subsequent chapters of this manual. Many psychiatric patients appear to be at increased risk for having more than one comorbid disorder, probably because of shared risk factors. That genes regulate a spectrum of behaviors also seems likely; practically speaking, this means that the presence of a psychiatric disorder in one member of the family may provide clues into the nature and appropriate treatment of the problems of another family member, even when their manifest problems are not identical. A multifactorial causality model has both heuristic and pragmatic value for the understanding of psychiatric disorders. It acknowledges the role of gene-related dysregulation of behavior, but it does so in the context of contributing environmental circumstances that are developmental, historical, and current, and it points the way to the beneficial application of both psychopharmacologic and psychotherapeutic treatment interventions. The bottom line of the perspective is that genetic liabilities combine with environmental risk factors to create a vulnerability or predisposition to a given disorder or disorders. This is the central theme of the vulnerability–stress and biopsychosocial models of psychiatric disorders.

IV. Additional Comments and Caveats

Epidemiologic data suggest that, in any 6-month period, between one in six and one in five adults in the United States will manifest some form of clinically significant and definable mental disturbance. Anxiety and depression are among the most common complaints mentioned by patients seeking medical attention. The annual economic burden associated with the diagnosis and treatment of mental disorders and substance abuse problems is estimated at over a quarter of a trillion dollars. Therefore, for clinicians, regardless of their specialty, to be able to recognize major psychiatric disorders and to understand basic elements of treatment is important.

Not all mental disorders and substance abuse problems reveal themselves through obvious or florid symptoms or bizarre behavior. Mental illness or a substance abuse disorder should be suspected, for example, whenever patients complain of or are observed to be having difficulty in (a) performing simple or sequential tasks or sticking to a reasonable pace of work, (b) following or understanding instructions, (c) planning their day or following through with responsibilities, (d) getting along with other people, or (e) asking others for guidance or assistance when needed.

Variations in phenotypic expression and cultural, experiential, and developmental factors contribute in some measure to the uniqueness of each human being. This uniqueness in turn contributes to difficulties in classifying forms of mental illness. Whenever a disorder does not have pathognomonic features or when a patient does not present the full expression of the disorder, individual variation may make the diagnosis less than straightforward. Patients, especially children, often suffer from more than one disorder at a time or in sequence. In an effort to establish descriptive and phenomenologic diagnostic criteria, the American Psychiatric Association issued the *Diagnostic and Statistical Manual of Mental Disorders* (DSM) in 1952. Various transmutations have culminated in the current edition, the DSM, 4th edition, 2000 (DSM-IV-2000). Readers familiar with the development of DSM-III through DSM-IV-text revision (DSM-IV-TR) iterations will recognize that many of the descriptions of diagnostic entities contained in the subsequent chapters of this manual are similar to some of the criteria sets contained in the DSM-IV-TR but that these are not always listed in the familiar tabular format. This choice is intentional—this manual is not intended to serve as a diagnostic handbook. Moreover, DSM-IV-TR and the widely used *International Statistical Classification of Diseases and Related Health Problems*, tenth edition, (ICD-10) do not always use identical criteria. Therefore, emphasizing a perspective about psychiatric illness that will probably remain viable and practical even with changing and variable diagnostic concepts and criteria seems sensible.

This manual cannot substitute for a textbook or reference book on psychiatry. An attempt has been made instead to highlight specific disorders, treatments, and management strategies that are likely to be seen by a broad spectrum of clinicians in various practice settings and to illustrate some of the challenges facing those who work with psychiatric patients. Problems of the mind disquiet not only the affected persons but also those who care for them. For example, clinicians all too often fail to recognize depression, anxiety, and stress-related symptoms in their patients not only because they may need to deny these states in themselves but also because they are confused about what is pathologic and amenable to treatment. Progress in the neurosciences and in related and complementary disciplines continues to bring further clarity to the understanding both of self-protective mechanisms and of mental illness *per se*. To foster these efforts, the community of clinicians and others who are interested in psychiatric disorders and patients must do all that they can to reduce, and ultimately to remove, the stigma associated with having a psychiatric illness or a family member who suffers from a mental disorder. This is even more important than in many other areas of medicine, because the mentally ill generally cannot be advocates for themselves because of their symptoms, disabilities, and self-protective distortions. Fortunately, many advocacy groups that add and provide a much needed voice for the support of vulnerable patients and their families now exist.

ADDITIONAL READING

Alexander FM. *The use of the self.* New York: EP Dutton, 1932.

Bibring E. The development and problems of the theory of the instincts. *Int J Psychoan* 1941;22:102–131.

Department of Health and Human Services. Standards for the privacy of individually identifiable health information: final rules. *Federal Register* 2000;65:82461–82510. Available at: http://www.hhs.gov/ocr/regtext.html.

Dobson KS. *Handbook of cognitive-behavioral therapies,* 2nd ed. New York: Guilford Press, 2000.

Ellenberger HF. *The discovery of the unconscious: the history and evolution of dynamic psychiatry.* New York: Basic Books, 1970.

Emanuel EJ, Emanuel LL. Four models of the physician-patient relationship. *JAMA* 1992;267:2221–2226.

Fellous JM. Neuromodulatory basis of emotion. *The Scientist* 1999;5:283–294.

Freud A. *The ego and the mechanisms of defense.* New York: International University Press, 1946.

Hartmann H. *Ego psychology and the problem of adaptation.* New York: International University Press, 1958.

Lazarus RS. The costs and benefits of denial. In: Dohrenwend BS, Dohrenwend BP, eds. *Stressful life events and their contexts.* New York: Prodist, 1981:131–156.

Nestler EJ, Hyman SE, Malenka RC. *Molecular neuropharmacology: a foundation for clinical neuroscience.* New York: McGraw-Hill, 2001.

White RW. *Ego and reality in psychoanalytic theory.* New York: International University Press, 1963.

2. THE MENTAL STATUS EXAMINATION

Richard I. Shader

A mental status examination (MSE), sometimes called the mental status schedule or the psychiatric examination, is an integral part of a comprehensive medical examination. Adolph Meyer championed the use of the MSE in the United States during the first third of the last century. This chapter reviews the MSE as it is conducted in adults and older adolescents. Assessing younger children requires modifications of the MSE that are beyond the scope of this chapter, although some ways to adapt the MSE to children and youths are discussed in Chapter 21. In any initial clinical interview, the clinician usually has several goals, including understanding why the patient is seeking help (or why someone else has asked the physician to see and evaluate the patient), creating rapport and laying the groundwork for working together (i.e., establishing a therapeutic relationship), and developing a diagnosis and treatment plan and presenting these conclusions to the patient. Whenever a clinician suspects some alteration in a patient's level of consciousness; the individual's awareness of his or her environment; his or her orientation to time, place, or person; or some other aspect of cognitive or emotional functioning, an MSE, which is a cross-sectional picture of a patient's functioning, should be included in the initial interview and should be administered again if the patient's condition changes. Moreover, a complete evaluation includes taking a pertinent personal and family history, with special emphasis on recent and relevant life changes and on stresses, assets and adaptive strengths, and social networks and support systems. When something has changed, developing a clear picture of what has changed is important. This means asking about its onset and duration, any precipitants, the context in which the shift occurred, and what might be reinforcing or maintaining any new symptoms or findings. In other words, what has happened, why did it happen, why now, and why to this particular patient?

Just as clinicians may omit selected parts of a physical examination, they may infer some aspects of mental and cognitive performance. However, omissions may lead to clinician errors. For example, one physician omitted testing for orientation because the patient had correctly said, "I'm glad to see you, Dr. Smith, I know you are busy today." This patient had a mild delirium and said to the nurse after Dr. Smith left the room, "They picked a good one to play his part . . . he really looks like a doctor." This anecdote also highlights the importance of interviewing other informants. When parts of the MSE are omitted, this fact should be recorded.

Optimal circumstances for conducting an MSE include comfortable, well-lit, but not overly bright, surroundings that enable open discussion. The clinician needs to be comfortable and familiar enough with the task to encourage trust and confidence in the doctor–patient relationship. Obviously, the context in which the clinician is called on to see the patient may be far from ideal. Having privacy and establishing rapport may be difficult in a busy emergency department or on an open ward, even when curtains are available and closed. Nevertheless, the clinician must try to demonstrate concern, compassion, empathy, and sensitivity. Eye contact and an optimal distance between the patient and interviewer are important. Note-taking may be necessary to ensure accurate recording of findings, but the clinician's style of note-taking should not be obtrusive—it should be done in a way that does not interfere with the flow of the interaction. The clinician must also be free to observe and to record the nonverbal responses and behaviors of the patient (e.g., blushing, tearfulness). Making notes on a prepared document or checklist is sometimes helpful.

The clinician must be sensitive to the patient's feelings and reactions; this is best accomplished by having opportunities to practice conducting MSEs. Tolerating silence also needs to be mastered, as does the art of encouraging responses to both direct and open-ended questioning. Taking a detailed sexual history or asking about homicidal or suicidal thoughts (see Chapter 17) may feel awkward during an initial visit, but tactful inquiry, particularly about suicide, may be central to what needs to be understood about the patient at the time of the assessment (e.g., in the depressed patient). Going into the vicissitudes and techniques of interviewing is beyond the scope of this chapter. However, a rapid-fire style or an abruptly given series of questions may discourage spontaneous responses from the patient and thus should be avoided. These issues are raised to heighten students' awareness of the importance of developing interview skills.

In the sections that follow, elements of the MSE, along with possible facilitating questions, are reviewed. These are meant to be illustrative only, and they are not exhaustive in scope. The order of the elements of the MSE given below does not imply a sequence that must be followed. The interviewing clinician should adopt a sequence that encourages the flow of information and that is responsive to the patient's affect and condition. Appendix III contains a prototypical outline for the MSE.

I. Demography, Appearance, Behavior, and Attitude

Even though a receptionist, triage nurse, or referring physician may already have recorded pertinent information about the patient, redocumenting the patient's name, age, gender, education, and marital status and collecting data about children, siblings, and parents can have value. Data on race and religion may also be helpful. Is English the patient's primary language? If not, this should be recorded. Discrepancies from any previously recorded data should be explored. The clinician should also ascertain whether the patient can **read** and write and can **hear** adequately. Does the patient require eyeglasses or a hearing aid? This should be recorded.

A. Appearance and Level of Consciousness

What is the patient's physical build (e.g., short, thin)? Does the patient have any obvious physical limitations, disabilities, or abnormalities? Does he or she have any visible scars, asymmetries, or disfigurements? Are the patient's grooming, personal hygiene, and style of dress appropriate? Depression, for example, may reveal itself in lack of self-care. What is the patient's level of alertness and/or consciousness? Scales that delineate levels from alert to comatose are useful for standardization. Does the patient seem drowsy? Has anyone noted that the patient becomes less alert or cooperative when the room is dark or when evening begins (sometimes called sundowning)?

B. Motor Status and Behavior

Posture (e.g., slumping in the chair, waxy flexibility) and gait (e.g., ataxic, broad-based, festinating) should be described. Noting the patient's facial expression (e.g., tension, fearfulness, gaze aversion, tearfulness) is important. Is the facial expression consistent with the patient's affect? Are the pupils constricted or dilated? Difficulty sitting still (e.g., hyperactivity, agitation, akathisia), mannerisms or rituals, repetitive or involuntary movements (e.g., chorea, tremor, tics, tardive dyskinesia), nail biting, arms hugging the body, and echopraxia are also important to note and describe. Is any overt evidence of impaired coordination or any observable nystagmus present? This section of the MSE must be complemented by a thorough neurologic examination to clarify any suspicious findings and to provide a documented baseline.

C. Interpersonal Behavior and Attitude

The style of the interaction with the clinician (e.g., cooperativeness, indifference, guardedness, suspiciousness, embarrassment, assaultiveness, seductiveness) should also be recorded.

II. The Chief Complaint

The clinician should record verbatim the patient's explanation of why he or she is seeing the doctor or why he or she is in the clinic or hospital. Early questions such as "How can I help you?", "What has been troubling you?", or "What led you to come in for help?" may be useful. For example, one patient responded to the question "What brought you into the emergency department?" with "My own two feet, stupid!" Such a response may tell the clinician a lot about what to expect in the forthcoming discussion; in this situation, the patient was being sarcastically angry rather than showing concrete thinking. A medical student and a resident had asked him this question before he was seen by the attending. This example also illustrates the idea that the interviewer should phrase questions with care. For the elderly or with very young patients, having an informant may be essential. Some approaches to the MSE are exemplified in section V. As a general rule, a separate inquiry and recording of the chief complaint has value. Providing time for patients to offer their chief complaints and any other concerns before responding in a way that narrows the scope of inquiry is important. If only one complaint is given (e.g., "I'm having nervous attacks."), saying something like, "That must be upsetting to you and in a few moments I'm going to ask more about them, but before I do, has anything else been bothering you?" or "Are there any other concerns you'd like to bring up?", may be useful

III. Characteristics of Speech (Talk)

This descriptive dimension combines elements that are also listed in sections I.B and V. It is listed separately here to emphasize the importance of speech as a window to the individual's overall thought processes and emotional state. The following are some key elements of speech that should be assessed.

A. Descriptors

1. **Volume, tone, and quality**. Is speech loud or soft? Does the patient sigh at key points?
2. **Articulation and enunciation**. Abnormalities are numerous, and they include stuttering; stammering; slurring; staccato speech (as in multiple sclerosis); cerebellar or explosive speech (loud and sudden with slurring); clipped speech; lisping; and other forms of dysfluency, dysarthria, or dysphemia. Describing accents that may reflect regional or national differences is also important. Is English this person's primary language? Enunciation can be tested by the use of selected phrases (e.g., "Methodist Episcopal," "liquid linoleum").
3. **Rate and coherence**. Is speech coherent or incoherent? Is the patient overly talkative (as in mania), or is the rate of speech retarded (as in some depressions)? Speech can be characterized by its **tempo** (i.e., the rate of patterned rhythmic speech), its coherence or logical connectedness, and its continuity (i.e., uninterrupted connectedness).
4. **Initiation**. Does the patient have a problem initiating a stream of speech (as in Parkinson disease), or is a long latency to speech onset present?

B. Patterns and Styles

1. **Loose associations**. This term describes a pattern of disconnected speech (and thought) in which sentences or a string of ideas seem either unrelated or only loosely connected. The apparent lack of continuity may worsen as the patient, who is usually suffering from schizophrenia, continues to talk.
2. **Word salad**. This term is used to describe incoherent speech in which the associative continuity within the stream of spoken words is lost or inapparent. **Neologisms** (self-invented words) are often heard in word salad. This pattern, although not frequent, is found more often in schizophrenia than in other psychiatric disorders. It is replicated in Wernicke aphasia. Word salad differs from **verbigeration** (oral stereotypy), which refers to the repetition of meaningless phrases.
3. **Blocking**. In blocking, the flow of speech stops suddenly without apparent connection to either the thought content of the moment or the interchange between the patient and the listener.
4. **Circumstantiality**. Although the patient exhibiting circumstantiality eventually gets to the point, excessive, unnecessary, or irrelevant detail is included, and the message lacks incisiveness. Circumstantiality may be used to mask memory impairment in dementia (see Chapter 5).
5. **Tangentiality**. This term is used to describe responses that are "off the mark" but that are usually related to the question in some way and are oblique to the central idea. Tangential responses are more coherent than the repeated derailments seen in loose associations. Sometimes, tangential responses feel as if they are an evasive tactic.
6. **Perseveration**. This consists of the involuntary repetition of words or phrases. It may interfere with the patient's efforts to answer or make a

point. The term **palilalia** is sometimes used to describe this pattern of perseveration; **palilalia** is not uncommon in Tourette disorder (see Chapter 7). **Palilalia** is not the same as **echolalia**, in which the repetition is an involuntary parrot-like restating of words or phrases just heard from another speaker; **echolalia** is found more commonly in patients with schizophrenia.

7. **Flight of ideas**. This increased rate or pressure of speech, often with frequent or abrupt changes in topic, may result in fragmentation of speech. The patient may seem distracted but he or she is not easily interrupted; he or she may also produce **clang** associations (i.e., sound determines the connection to subsequent words), rhyming, or punning. The original goal of a particular thought is usually lost during the process.

8. **Mutism**. The patient with mutism seems to be engaged with the questioner, but no response is forthcoming. In some instances, the mutism is voluntary, perhaps stemming from terror; more often, it is the result of stubbornness or negativism, hence the use of the term **elective mutism**.

IV. Cognitive Status

A. Attention and Concentration

Is the patient connecting with the interviewer (i.e., paying adequate attention)? How distracted or preoccupied does the patient seem to be? Many approaches can be used to establish impairments in attention and concentration. When one is selecting tests, choosing those that give additional information relevant to other sections of the MSE is also possible. For example, asking the patient to spell the name of the **city** in which he or she lives tests orientation, as well as attention, spelling, and memory. Then asking the patient to spell the **city** name backwards tests concentration and elements of memory. When a word other than the **city** is used, choosing a five-letter word is reasonable for testing purposes. Patients can also be asked to listen to and then repeat sequences of numbers. The ability to retain and repeat seven digits forward (the length of a standard telephone number) is common; achieving six digits is probably modal; and being able to repeat no more than five digits suggests impairment of attention. The advantage of using numbers is the ability to standardize performance. With the **city** task, the length of the word becomes a factor in the test. Patients can be asked to name in sequence the days of the week or the months of the year and then to reverse the direction (i.e., say them backward).

Another commonly used method is to have patients subtract 7 from 100 and then to subtract 7 from each subsequent answer, continuing the task serially—hence the name "**serial 7s**." With older patients, performing the first two subtractions for them may make the task less anxiety provoking. **Serial 3s** are sometimes used to make the task simpler. Assessing arithmetic ability while one is testing attention and concentration can also be useful. The patient can be asked to multiply 3 by 7, to add 3 and 7, to divide 21 by 7, and so forth. Obviously, this area of testing can be made into a task with graded degrees of difficulty. If a patient fails on the more standard tasks, the interviewer should simplify the tasks to distinguish impairments in attention from defects in memory, spelling, or calculation.

B. Orientation

The goal is to establish whether the patient is oriented to time, place, person, and self (in this context, person refers to others). Disorientation to self is rare, except in psychotic states where the patient identifies himself or herself as royalty, a deity, or someone else (e.g., schizophrenia, bipolar disorder). Some patients may both give their correct name and also say that they are a deity, a form of double orientation for self. Beginning this section by asking if the patient remembers the interviewer's name may be helpful for the interviewer. When the patient does not remember the interviewer's name, one should restate the name and should then ask the patient to repeat it. Again, this procedure tests a number of dimensions. The patient can then be asked to give his or her full name, followed by "Do you have a nickname?" or "What do you prefer to be called?" Next, the interviewer may ask,

"Do you know where you are?" Here, determining various spatial levels (e.g., in a hospital, in which city, in which state, in which country) is possible. Another question should be "Have you been keeping track of time?" The patient may have been asleep or unconscious and may not know the hour; the examiner then shifts to the day of the week, date, month, season, or year (e.g., "Do you know today's date?" or "Today is what day of the week?"). When the patient gives an incorrect response, the interviewer should supply the correct one and should then repeat the question later. This process adds data to the testing of registration, recall, and retention.

C. Memory

Scientific understanding of memory processes continues to increase. Many current models exist, each with its own definitions and terms (e.g., fluid, logical). When significant memory impairment is suspected, referral to a neuropsychologist should be considered to obtain more objective and more sophisticated answers. Getting to that point is the goal of memory assessment in the MSE. Perhaps the most appropriate initial step is reflection on what the patient has revealed through his or her responses to earlier questions and the way the history was given. Next, one can probe for memory problems through questions such as "How far did you go in school?" Direct questioning, as in the following, is mandatory: "Have you noticed any problems with your memory [or with remembering things]?" For the MSE, the effort is to establish whether information gets in (registration), whether it can be repeated (very short term or immediate recall), and whether it can be restated after a specific amount of time (delayed recall). The delay interval for the MSE is usually 5 minutes, and more complete testing also elicits recall after 30 minutes. The usual test consists of naming three to five unrelated words (e.g., vine, table, purple, fence, mirror) to the patient and then going through the process just described.

More remote memory (i.e., a period of a week or a month ago, or longer) should also be assessed. Here the point is to determine something that both the interviewer and the patient know happened. For instance, asking the patient what he or she ate or was served for breakfast is of little value unless the answer can be verified.

Remembering that motivation influences performance in many elements of the MSE is important. Lack of motivation may particularly obfuscate memory assessment in depressed elderly persons.

Testing visual memory separately has value. Can the patient copy simple figures or shapes, such as a triangle touching a circle or three parallel swerving or sine wave-like lines, and later (e.g., after 5 minutes) reproduce them? This is usually a good point in the examination to see whether the patient can draw a clock and insert the hands at a specified time (e.g., 8:20 or 2:45); this form of testing may also reveal apraxias or visual field problems.

D. Language and Communication Ability

By this point in the assessment, the clinician should have already learned a great deal about the patient's use of language; vocabulary, which is usually highly correlated with intelligence; and ability to communicate. Testing a few additional areas may help to complete this assessment. Can the patient name selected objects that the interviewer presents (e.g., a key, a spoon, a wooden pencil, a plastic pen, a notepad)? Reasoning and categorization ability can also be assessed through this task. Objects that are used can be chosen so that they can be sorted (e.g., pen and pencil = writing instruments; pen, pencil, and notepad = written communication devices; key and spoon = metal objects). When this has been done, the patient can then be asked, "What do these things have in common?" The patient can also be asked to tell a story that incorporates the objects or to describe a picture on the wall or what can be seen from the window. This activity can also be helpful for checking the patient's ability to spell (e.g., ask the patient to spell "notepad"). From the tasks and activities evaluated so far and from the subsequent assessment of judgment and ability to think abstractly, making a reasonable estimate of the patient's functional intelligence should be possible.

E. Judgment and Abstraction

The goal of this section is to assess a patient's ability to cope with everyday matters, to make generalizations, and to form opinions. When possible, questions should be free of cultural bias. Unfortunately, sociocultural background, education, and prior exposure to the ideas influence much of what is tested in this area. In listening to the patient's responses, one is looking for patterns (e.g., consistently concrete, literal, personalized, or bizarre responses). Some impressions of the patient's mental assets and abilities may have already been gleaned from earlier responses (e.g., from object naming and sorting [see section IV.D]). Formally developed tests are also available. Some potential probes are discussed in the following.

1. **Reasoning**. One may test reasoning skills by asking "What would you do if you found a stamped and addressed envelope on the street?" or "What would you do if you were the first person to notice a fire in this building?"

2. **Similarities and differences**. Another check involves queries like "How are a dwarf and a child different from one another?" or "In what way are an orange and an apple alike?" (both are fruit or food), "A horse and an airplane?" (both are forms of transportation), "A radio and a newspaper?" (both are forms of communication), and "A fly and a tree?" (both are alive).

3. **Proverb interpretation**. The interviewer asks the patient to restate the meaning of common sayings. This is usually begun by asking, "Do you know this saying?" If the patient does not know the proverb, trying several more is useful. In addition to disorders such as schizophrenia, many factors, including the patient's general level of intelligence and sociocultural background, can influence his or her interpretation of the proverb. Table 2.1 contains a sampling of common proverbs.

   Answers to these proverbs are then categorized as *concrete, subjective, personalized, bizarre,* or *well conceptualized.* The author also uses the proverb "The tongue is the enemy of the neck," as it tends to be less familiar to patients; it may elicit bizarre or highly idiosyncratic responses from psychotic patients.

V. Content of Thought

The previously elicited chief complaint (see section II) may guide this area of inquiry. The goal here is to see what is on the patient's mind. For example, is anything preoccupying, troubling, or frightening the patient?

A. Delusions

In response to general and open-ended questions about life, family, work, play, and relationships, the patient may reveal delusions, which are false beliefs that are not corrected by an appeal to reason or by contradictory evidence. Delusions are inconsistent with the facts, if they are all known. The clinician should not challenge the patient's beliefs but rather should explore them so that they can be differentiated from superstitions or ideas supported

---

TABLE 2.1. SOME PROVERBS THAT APPEAR TO BE RELATIVELY FREE OF BIAS

"The bigger they are, the harder they fall."
"What goes around comes around."
"Don't judge a book by its cover."
"Two wrongs don't make a right."
"Don't count your chickens before they are hatched."
"You don't realize what water is worth until the well has run dry."
"A stitch in time saves nine."
"A bird in the hand is worth two in the bush."
"People who live in glass houses shouldn't throw stones."
"The grass is always greener on the other side of the street."

by a subculture and that are consistent with the patient's social and educational background. When delusional material does not emerge spontaneously and some form of distorted thinking can be reasonably suspected, selective probes, such as the following, may be used:

"Do you have the sense that people like you?"
"Do you ever feel singled out?"
"Do you ever feel that anyone has it in for you or that you are being watched?"
"Do you have experiences that you don't think you could easily explain to others?"
"Do you ever feel someone else is controlling your mind or your thoughts?"
"Do you feel that you are in special touch with heaven or God?"
"Do you feel that you have special powers or that you are destined for a special role or job?"

Kendler et al. proposed a useful way to describe delusions in terms of delusional involvement (cognitive and emotional) and content (disorganization, bizarreness, encapsulation). To what degree does the patient challenge the false belief by wondering if it is his or her imagination? To what degree does the delusion preoccupy the patient? Is it encapsulated, or does it spill into the patient's other thoughts and alter activities? How much does the content depart from customary consensual reality? Is the delusion logical, consistent, and systematized?

B. Hallucinations

A patient may spontaneously mention false sensory experiences, or the clinician may infer them from the patient's responses to cues that are not seen or heard by others. Hallucinations may be auditory, visual, tactile, gustatory, or olfactory. The presence of the latter four should raise suspicion of a toxic state, a mental disorder due to an altered metabolic state (e.g., anticholinergic overactivity or exposure to organic solvents), or a degenerative neurologic disease or space-occupying lesion (e.g., partial complex seizures) that is present in the brain. The location of auditory hallucinations in space may be important. In toxic metabolic states, the patient usually describes the auditory hallucinations as coming from a location that is within reason (e.g., from inside a closet). In schizophrenia, the location tends to be more unusual (e.g., from radar or from the patient's shoulder). Knowing when, where, and under what circumstances hallucinations occur (e.g., only with the use of alcohol or drugs) is also useful. Do they occur only when the patient is just waking or falling asleep? Only when the patient is feeling lonely or is actually alone? Are they consistent (congruent) with the patient's mood (e.g., when feeling depressed, the patient hears a voice saying he or she has sinned and deserves punishment)? This same question also applies to delusions. Some general probes include the following:

"Are you sensitive to sound or noise? To light?"
"Do you daydream?"
"Do your daydreams ever seem real?"
"Do you have a strong imagination?"
"Have you ever felt as if you were outside your own body and could watch yourself?"
"Do you ever hear a voice speaking to you when no one is actually there?"
"Do you ever experience odors or smells that you don't think others notice?"
"Have you ever seen things crawling on your skin or on the floor or walls when others claim not to see them?"
"If these questions don't seem to apply to what you have experienced, can you tell me what would be a better way of describing your experience?"
"Do such experiences seem natural to you? Are they frightening? Are they ever comforting or reassuring?"

C. Other Forms of Disordered Thought

Many types of thought content (and related feelings) may trouble and preoccupy people, including suicidal and homicidal thoughts, sexual impulses, ruminations, obsessions, illness fears, depersonalization, and so on. To the extent that they are consistent with specific disorders, these types are discussed in the subsequent chapters dealing with those symptoms, problems, or disorders.

VI. Affect and Mood

A. Affect

Affect refers to the patient's observable feeling tone that accompanies behavior, communication (i.e., both during silence and when thoughts are being expressed), or reactions to life events. A patient's affect influences others. In that sense, affect is "in the eye of the beholder." Not all clinicians watch and listen carefully enough to be attuned to shifts in or subtle expressions of affect. Numerous words have been used to characterize affect, including anxious, blunted, bright, broad, constricted, expansive, flat, full range, inappropriate, labile, sad, and sluggish. Affect can be harmonious (congruent or consonant) with behavior and ideation (e.g., a manic patient expresses grandiose ideas and appears expansive and too upbeat), inappropriate to the thought content (e.g., the person laughs nervously during the communication of a sad story), or isolated (e.g., the patient does not show sadness while telling a sad story).

B. Mood

Mood refers to what the patient describes about his or her own feeling state. Mood may be communicated spontaneously (e.g., "I feel great today, Doctor"), or the clinician may have to ask questions (e.g., "How are your spirits today, Mr. Smith?"). Mood tends to be more sustained than affect (i.e., prevailing mood). Again, noticing and documenting congruence or its absence among behavior, ideation, and stated mood is important. As with affect, numerous words with subtle shifts in emphasis can describe the mood (e.g., blue, depressed, despondent, low, sad). Other common descriptors include angry, anxious, bland, fearful, flat, irritable, nervous, and restless. Mood is said to be subjective, whereas affect, because it is observed, is considered more objective. This distinction may have limited value. Elderly persons and some adolescents may deny low moods, believing they have to "bear up."

VII. Insight

Understanding whether the patient has insight is a central element of the MSE. For a clinician to establish an alliance with a patient who denies or who does not recognize something is wrong is difficult. The patient who can reasonably reflect on his or her illness and life situation is a better partner at all steps of the diagnostic, treatment, and rehabilitation process. Simple probes are as follows: "What view do you have about your troubles?" "How do you understand what is going on with you?" Lack of insight is common in schizophrenia. As suggested in Chapter 1, this alteration may be self-protective.

ADDITIONAL READING

Andreasen NC. Thought, language, and communication disorders. I. Clinical assessment, definition of terms, and evaluation of reliability. *Arch Gen Psychiatry* 1979; 36:1315–1321.

Apell KE, Strecker EA. *Practical examination of personality and behavior disorders.* New York: Macmillan, 1936.

Kendler KS, Glazer WM, Morgenstern H. Dimensions of delusional experience. *Am J Psychiatry* 1983;140:466–469.

Small SM. *Outline for psychiatric examination.* East Hanover, NJ: Sandoz Pharmaceuticals Corporation, 1984.

Wells FL, Ruesch J. *Mental examiners' handbook.* New York: Psychological Corp., 1945.

3. MEDICAL EVALUATION OF PSYCHIATRIC PATIENTS AND THE ACUTE TREATMENT OF PSYCHOTROPIC DRUG OVERDOSE

Richard I. Shader
Judith E. Tintinalli
Suzanne R. White

The incidence of medical problems in psychiatric patients depends on their age and the presence of comorbid conditions. In addition, the likelihood of occurrence of specific disorders can vary with the psychiatric setting in which the patient is seen. Acute medical problems can coexist with psychiatric problems, thereby compounding the difficulty of making a correct diagnosis. For example, in patients with preexisting psychotic disorders or dementia, identifying a superimposed delirium can be difficult (see Chapters 5 and 12). Substance abuse, especially of **alcohol**, **cocaine**, or **heroin**, coexists in patients with psychiatric disorders, and signs of intoxication, overdose, and/or withdrawal must be distinguished from the features of psychiatric illness (see Chapters 9 through 12). Violent patients or patients who self-mutilate are subject to injuries. As psychiatric patients age, disorders common to an aging population, such as diabetes mellitus, coronary artery disease, cerebrovascular disease, and renal insufficiency, should be expected. The adverse effects and drug interactions of prescribed psychoactive drugs or herbal medications should be considered in the medical evaluation of elderly psychiatric patients. Finally, medical problems may have gone undetected during prepsychiatric admission screening, or they can develop during psychiatric hospitalization. The goal of this chapter is to provide a framework for the recognition, diagnosis, treatment, and appropriate referral, when necessary, for psychiatric patients with acute medical problems.

I. Prepsychiatric Admission Medical Evaluation

The accuracy and completeness of the medical evaluation of psychiatric patients seen in emergency departments or ambulatory settings are variable. Standards for pretransfer evaluation should be developed between the transferring medical facility and the accepting psychiatric facility. Medical evaluation should include documentation of the following:

1. Vital signs and drug allergies;
2. Medical history, including gynecologic and reproductive history for women;
3. General physical examination;
4. Screening neurologic examination, including mental status (see Chapter 2) and evaluation for focal findings;
5. Results of any laboratory and imaging studies;
6. Description of any acute treatment;
7. Listing of current medications and dosage;
8. Discharge instructions, including recommendations for the type and interval of, as well as need for, follow-up medical care.

Experience has taught that history alone has a greater than 90% sensitivity for the detection of acute medical conditions in psychiatric patients. Consequently, the medical screening evaluation for psychiatric patients is generally quite basic. Pelvic or rectal examinations are not done unless directed by a chief complaint relative to these body systems. Most studies support the use of clinical judgment in the selection of laboratory or imaging studies, and most of the time, these studies are not needed for medical evaluation. No clinical evidence suggests that routine toxicology testing is needed for medical evaluation because most patients provide accurate self-reports of substance abuse.

II. Acute Medical Conditions in the Psychiatric Setting

The psychiatric facility should be prepared to identify medical emergencies and to provide **basic life support** (BLS) until a more experienced team arrives.

Both physicians and nurses in the psychiatric setting should know how to activate the local **Emergency Medical Services (EMS) system** and should be well informed about its treatment capabilities. Protocols should be in place to determine which conditions can be treated in-house through consultation and which conditions should instead be transferred to an appropriately staffed medical facility for further stabilization and evaluation. Options for transfer to another facility for emergency and elective conditions should be outlined and delineated in a transfer protocol procedures manual.

For those settings in which the psychiatric facility is located within a general hospital, all clinical staff should be familiar with the procedures for activating the in-house cardiac arrest team and should know how to obtain in-house emergency medical or surgical consultation.

III. **Treatment of Acute Medical Conditions in the Psychiatric Setting**

A complete list of acute medical conditions and their evaluation, treatment, and disposition is beyond the scope of this manual. However, contemporary advances have resulted in a number of time-limited treatments for acute conditions, such as acute myocardial infarction (AMI) and acute stroke. Identifying acute medical conditions as soon as possible is important. A general categorization of selected acute symptoms includes the following:

- Cardiac arrest
- Alterations in vital signs
- Altered mental status or coma
- Shortness of breath
- Chest pain
- Abdominal pain
- Hearing or visual loss
- Acute neurologic signs or headache
- Fever
- Acute injury

A. **Cardiac Arrest**

The acute management of a cardiac arrest is the same whether it occurs in the home, community, or hospital setting. The **American Heart Association** has delineated the following response steps as the **Chain of Survival**:

1. Activate the EMS system (call 911).
2. Begin **cardiopulmonary resuscitation (CPR)**.
3. Assess cardiac rhythm and **defibrillate**.

The best survival after a cardiac arrest is seen in the group of patients with a witnessed arrest, bystander **CPR**, and immediate **defibrillation**. Psychiatric facilities should attempt to meet these goals by developing a simple and straightforward system that includes health care provider–administered **CPR** and immediate **defibrillation**.

Instructions for **CPR** can be found readily at *http://www.learncpr.org/* and for **advanced cardiac life support** (ACLS) at *http://www.cpr-ecc.org/*. In the absence of a **portable external defibrillator** (see discussion below), psychiatric facilities should have a plan for managing cardiac arrest that includes up-to-date training for staff in the application of bystander **CPR**. At a minimum, they should be able to do the following:

- Determine unresponsiveness and call for help;
- Open the airway (use head tilt or jaw thrust);
- Give two slow breaths if the patient is found to be breathless;
- Determine pulse status, and, when a pulse is present, continue rescue breathing at 10 to 12 breaths per min;
- Perform chest compressions when no pulse is elicited, and continue rescue breathing (15 compressions and then two breaths for one rescuer; 5 compressions and then one breath for two rescuers).

A number of options exist for acute airway management, including bag-mask ventilation, an esophageal obturator airway, a laryngeal mask airway, and endotracheal intubation. The simplest method for a psychiatric setting might well be the use of bag-mask ventilation. This method can be used until personnel with more experience at airway stabilization arrive. Wall-mounted containers with a bag and mask can be placed at key areas for easy access in an emergency. Posters describing the application of the chest or abdominal thrust for removal of upper airway foreign body obstruction may be similarly posted.

Another consideration in psychiatric facilities is the installation of **automatic external defibrillators (AEDs)**. These devices are now commonly found in airports, shopping malls, and even gambling casinos. Directions for its use are clearly presented on the device itself, and nonmedical personnel have been effectively trained in its application.

Basic **CPR** and the use of **AEDs** should be available. **ACLS steps**, such as definitive airway management and advanced pharmacologic care, are not likely to be available in some psychiatric settings, and these patients should be deferred to the local **EMS system** or an in-house cardiac arrest team.

B. **Alterations in Vital Signs**

Giving general parameters for abnormal vital signs is difficult, but the presence of symptoms *and* abnormal vital signs usually suggests the need for emergency evaluation. Parameters for abnormal vital signs include fever (above 38°C [100.4°F]), hypotension (systolic blood pressure <100 mm Hg), hypertension (systolic blood pressure >160 mm Hg, diastolic blood pressure >90 mm Hg), tachycardia (pulse rate [PR] >120 beats per min [bpm]), bradycardia (PR <60 bpm), and hypoxia (oxygen saturation at room air <90%). Severe pain has been suggested as the fifth vital sign. The value of vital signs as triage variables in themselves has been questioned; usually the presence of other serious signs and symptoms, rather than an isolated determination of vital signs, raises the question of an acute medical condition.

C. **Alterations in Mental Status or Coma**

The Glasgow Coma Scale (GCS) can be used as a rough parameter of abnormal mental status for adults. A normal GCS rating is 15. Table 3.1 provides the elements of the GCS.

Although the GCS was developed for trauma evaluation, using it serially provides one objective way of describing a change in the level of consciousness as one aspect of mental status. Loss of attention, hallucinations, disorientation, and decreased arousal are other signs of altered mental status. The differential diagnosis of altered mental status is complex, including central nervous system (CNS) hemorrhage, infarction, space-occupying lesions, infections, and toxic-metabolic conditions. Although preparations should be

TABLE 3.1. GLASGOW COMA SCALE

Eye opening	Motor response
4 Spontaneous	6 Follows commands
3 To speech	5 Localizes pain
2 To pain	4 Withdrawal to pain
1 No response	3 Decorticate flexion
	2 Decerebrate extension
Verbal response	1 No response
5 Alert and oriented	
4 Disoriented conversation	
3 Speaking but nonsensical	
2 Moans or unintelligible sounds	
1 No response	

The Glasgow Coma Scale is available for download at *http://www.trauma.org/*.

made to transfer the patient for medical evaluation, the following steps can be taken:

- Obtain vital signs and maintain airway and oxygen saturation at more than 90% with supplemental oxygen;
- Establish intravenous (i.v.) access;
- Determine a bedside glucose; if less than 60, administer 25 g glucose i.v.;
- Administer 2 mg of **naloxone** i.v. when a narcotic overdose is a possibility.

D. Shortness of Breath

The differential diagnosis of shortness of breath is broad. Distinguishing cardiac causes from pulmonary causes is often extremely difficult. About one-third of patients with AMI complain of shortness of breath as the most prominent symptom. One should begin by obtaining an oxygen saturation level. If this is less than 90% on room air, supplemental oxygen can be given at 2 L per min, unless the patient has known chronic obstructive pulmonary disease. Auscultation of the chest can be helpful to distinguish rales, wheezes, or decreased breath sounds if present. Chest x-ray (CXR) is necessary to determine conditions such as pneumonia, effusion, pneumothorax, or hemothorax; CXR should be negative in patients with bronchitis or asthma. For known asthma patients, standing orders for the administration of nebulized **albuterol** can be developed. The dose of **albuterol** (5 mg in 5 mL of saline) is administered in a nebulized solution; another approach consists of administering four puffs from a **metered dose inhaler** every 20 min. Additionally, while preparations are made to transfer the patient for more thorough medical evaluation, the following can be done:

- Obtain vital signs and maintain oxygen saturation at more than 90% with supplemental oxygen unless patient has known chronic obstructive pulmonary disease;
- Establish i.v. access, if possible;
- Obtain an immediate CXR and electrocardiogram (ECG). *Make sure copies of both are provided if the patient is transferred to another unit or facility for care.*

E. Chest Pain

Signs and symptoms of coronary artery disease as a cause of chest pain can occur at any time in adulthood. Although risk factors, such as hypercholesterolemia, hypertension, diabetes, or smoking, are associated with coronary artery disease, their presence or absence does not assist in making the diagnosis of acute coronary ischemia or AMI in the individual. About one-third of patients, most often women or patients with diabetes mellitus, with an AMI have atypical signs, such as weakness or shortness of breath. In addition, patients without chest pain who develop an AMI have about a twofold greater in-hospital mortality rate. Furthermore, differentiating musculoskeletal causes of chest pain from other severe disorders besides acute coronary ischemia or AMI can be difficult; these include pulmonary embolism, myocarditis, pericarditis, and aortic dissection. Patients with chest pain, acute weakness, or shortness of breath deserve serious attention whether these symptoms are believed to be typical or atypical of cardiac ischemia or not. Contemporary time-dependent treatment modalities include thrombolytics, angioplasty, beta-blockers, platelet inhibitors, and anticoagulants. Their use is beyond the scope of this chapter.

While preparations are made to transfer the patient for medical evaluation, the following can be done:

- Provide supplemental oxygen and i.v. access, if possible;
- Administer aspirin (160 to 325 mg chewable);
- Obtain a stat CXR and ECG, if possible;
- Arrange for EMS transport using advanced life support;
- Make additional copies of the CXR and ECG to accompany the patient.

F. Abdominal Pain and Gastrointestinal Bleeding

Improved diagnostic and imaging techniques allow the clinician to make accurate and more rapid diagnoses for abdominal pain. A useful general rule is that abdominal pain persisting for 6 hours or more or abdominal pain accompanied by nausea, vomiting, or diarrhea should receive emergency evaluation. Patients with prior abdominal surgery who develop acute abdominal complaints should be viewed as having a suspected small bowel obstruction until proven otherwise. Upper or lower gastrointestinal (GI) bleeding always requires emergency evaluation, unless the patient describes only small streaks of blood in the vomitus or stool. In such patients, elective ambulatory evaluation can be considered. Causes of acute abdominal pain stratified by age are listed in Table 3.2. Transfer orders should include the following:

- Nothing by mouth (eating will complicate condition if operative intervention becomes necessary; certain studies such as gallbladder ultrasound require 6 hours of fasting to visualize the gallbladder properly);
- Intravenous access, if possible;
- Supplemental oxygen;
- Transport using advanced life support.

G. Hearing or Visual Loss

Acute hearing loss can result from simple causes, such as cerumen impaction, or from serious disorders. Visual loss can be from neurologic or ophthalmic causes. Neurologic causes include stroke, migraine, and ocular problems (e.g., retinal detachment, acute glaucoma).

H. Acute Neurologic Signs and Headache

The American Heart Association and the National Institute of Neurological Disorders emphasize the following signs of stroke in their public education programs:

- Alteration in consciousness;
- Intense headache or any headache associated with a decreased level of consciousness, neurologic deficit, and severe neck or facial pain;
- Aphasia (incoherent speech or difficulty understanding speech);
- Facial weakness or asymmetry;
- Incoordination, weakness, paralysis, or sensory loss in one or more limbs;
- Visual loss;
- Dysarthria (slurred or indistinct speech);
- Intense vertigo, double vision, unilateral hearing loss, nausea, vomiting, photophobia, or phonophobia.

TABLE 3.2. LIKELY CAUSES OF ACUTE ABDOMINAL PAIN BY AGE COHORT

Final Diagnosis	Under 50 Yr of Age (%)	Greater Than or Equal to 50 Yr of Age (%)
Biliary tract disease	21	6
Nonspecific abdominal pain	16	40
Appendicitis	15	32
Bowel obstruction	12	2
Pancreatitis	7	2
Diverticular disease	6	<0.1
Cancer	4	<0.1
Hernia	3	<0.1
Vascular	2	<0.1
Acute gynecologic disease	<0.1	4
Other	13	13

From Gallagher J. Acute abdominal pain. In: Tintinalli J, Kelen G, Stapczynski S, eds. *Emergency medicine: a comprehensive study guide.* New York: McGraw-Hill, 2000:497–515, with permission.

Some clinicians believe that thrombolytic therapy is indicated only if it can be initiated in the first 2 to 3 hours after an acute ischemic stroke. Evaluation of possible acute stroke includes imaging modalities, such as computed tomography and magnetic resonance imaging, and often requires neurologic consultation. Differential diagnosis of acute severe headache includes a hypertensive emergency, a subarachnoid or intracerebral hemorrhage, or meningitis. Transfer to an emergency medical facility is warranted for any of these acute signs or symptoms. Strict criteria for the management of hypertension in acute stroke have not been defined, and caution is recommended. Conservative guidelines for acute hypertension treatment in acute stroke include treatment only if the systolic blood pressure exceeds 220 mm Hg or if the diastolic blood pressure exceeds 130 mm Hg. Overly aggressive lowering of blood pressure is believed to expand the ischemic stroke penumbra and to convert transitional ischemic areas to infarcted areas.

Transfer orders should include the following:

- Supplemental oxygen and monitoring of vital signs;
- Intravenous access, if possible;
- Nothing by mouth to avoid potential aspiration;
- ECG and CXR, if possible; send copies with transfer.

I. Fever

The development of fever should prompt an investigation for the common infectious disorders.

1. **Respiratory tract infections**. Upper respiratory tract and pharyngeal infections and bronchitis are common causes of fever, and these are usually easily diagnosable by signs and symptoms.

   Clinical signs and symptoms of fever, cough and sore throat, myalgias, and its epidemic nature usually lead to the diagnosis of influenza, although rapid viral diagnostic testing may be increasingly available. Influenza vaccine is the best method to prevent outbreaks and morbidity. The course of the disease is reduced if treatment is begun within 48 hours of symptom onset. Treatment through inhalation is with **zanamivir**, two puffs twice a day for 5 days. However, this treatment plan requires some manual dexterity. Oral treatment choices include **oseltamivir**, which is effective against both influenza A and B (75 mg orally [p.o.] twice a day for 5 days).

   Pneumonia is readily diagnosed by CXR. Outpatient treatment is with **azithromycin** (standard **azithromycin** dose-pak [500 mg p.o. on day 1, then 250 mg p.o. on days 2 to 5]) or **levofloxacin** (500 mg per day p.o.). Hospital admission should be considered if the patient appears toxic or hypoxic (oxygen saturation <90%) or if he or she has significant comorbidities, such as diabetes mellitus or steroid administration.

2. **Urinary tract infections**. Cystitis (lower urinary tract infection [UTI]) is characterized by urinary frequency, urgency, suprapubic pain, and hematuria. Pyelonephritis usually manifests as fever and flank pain. Lower UTI symptoms may not be present. A urinalysis and urine culture should be obtained. Cystitis can be treated with 3 to 7 days of **trimethoprim-sulfamethoxazole** (also Bactrim DS or Septra DS; 1 tablet p.o. twice a day) or **ciprofloxacin** (500 mg p.o. twice a day). Pyelonephritis is termed uncomplicated in young or middle-aged otherwise healthy individuals, and it is generally treated with **ciprofloxacin** (500 mg p.o. twice a day for 10 to 14 days). Pyelonephritis is termed complicated in the elderly, in those with renal insufficiency or structural kidney abnormalities, in those who are immunocompromised or toxic, and in those with renal calculi or sickle cell disease. Complicated pyelonephritis requires inpatient treatment.

   Prostatitis may be evidenced by lower abdominal or rectal pain, back pain, and fever. Signs of cystitis are often not present. Treatment usually consists of 2 to 4 weeks of **ciprofloxacin** (500 mg p.o. twice a day). Any patient with prostatitis who appears toxic requires inpatient treatment.

3. **Meningitis**. Bacterial meningitis is an uncommon disorder, but its serious morbidity requires early diagnosis and treatment. In adults, computed tomography is often performed before lumbar puncture, and antibiotics should be given as soon as the diagnosis is suspected. Treatment is generally with **ceftriaxone** (2 g i.v.); when the presence of resistant *Streptococcus pneumoniae* is suspected, **vancomycin** (15 mg per kg i.v.) is also added. **Ampicillin** (2 g i.v.) can be added when *Listeria* is suspected. To cover all diagnostic possibilities, some emergency department clinicians recommend the use of **acyclovir** (10 mg per kg i.v.) to treat potential herpes simplex encephalitis as well. Steroids are not recommended.

Meningococcal prophylaxis should be given to close contacts. Regimens include **ciprofloxacin** (500 mg p.o.) and **rifampin** (600 mg p.o.), twice a day for 4 days, or **ceftriaxone** (250 mg intramuscularly [i.m.]) as a single dose.

Aseptic or viral meningitis is the most common CNS infection in the United States. It is most commonly due to enterovirus or echovirus. Symptoms include fever, headache, vomiting, eye pain, nausea, photophobia, and myalgia. The diagnosis is made by lumbar puncture. Antibiotics are withheld unless bacterial meningitis is being considered.

4. **Cellulitis**. Cellulitis is another common infection that is characterized by fever and localized erythema, edema, and tenderness. It is most common in the lower extremities and in those patients with venous or arterial insufficiency. If the patient is nontoxic, treatment with oral **cephalexin** (500 mg, four times a day) for 10 to 14 days is usually sufficient.

5. **Acute injury**. The spectrum of acute injury care is beyond the scope of this manual, but a few principles can be described here. Any injury resulting in persistent pain, loss or limitation of function, or inability to bear weight or walk unaided requires emergency evaluation.

Head injuries resulting in change in mental status or loss of consciousness, however brief, need emergency medical evaluation. Cervical spine immobilization should be provided until EMS personnel arrive. Temporary methods for cervical spine immobilization can be as simple as rolled towels or blankets placed on opposite sides of the head and securely taped to the stretcher or bed to prevent head and neck movement.

Lacerations in which the epidermis is gaping generally require suturing. Lacerations around important functional areas, such as the face, eyes, and joints, require emergency evaluation. The appeal of synthetic glues is great, but their application is limited to small nongaping lacerations that are not near the eyes and that are not subject to skin tension. Most lacerations will require suturing or stapling. After suturing, instructions should be provided for the timing of suture removal. Staples require a separate instrument, a staple remover; if the institution does not have these in stock, the patient may have to be returned to the emergency facility for staple removal.

Distal limb injuries, such as those involving the arms, hands, legs, or feet, require emergency evaluation and possibly radiography if attempted function causes pain. Punctures to the hands or feet should be medically evaluated to determine if radiographs or antibiotics are needed and to evaluate the need for **tetanus toxoid**.

IV. **Abuse and Assault**

Victims of violent acts, such as robbery or unprovoked assault by strangers, or accidents probably comprise the largest group of individuals who experience the emotional impact of trauma; their experiences, unfortunately, have not been systematically studied. Data are emerging about some forms of abuse and assault, particularly in the following three distinct epidemiologic groups: children, domestic partners, and the elderly or impaired. Although signs and symptoms of abuse and assault in these three groups are obtained when medical histories are taken, corroboration by physical evaluation and imaging studies is often essential. This is yet another reason for why a medical examination is complimentary to psychiatric evaluation.

A. Children and Youths

1. **Sexual abuse** is often suspected when the child complains of symptoms referable to the genitourinary tract, such as vaginal discharge or bleeding, dysuria, urethral discharge, or symptoms of urinary tract infection (see Chapter 27). Other symptoms include inappropriate sexually oriented behavior, nightmares, regressive behaviors, or bedwetting. Frequently, sexual abuse is suspected at a time remote from the actual episodes. When seen acutely, children need evaluation for acute genitourinary tract injury. Children with any suspicion of sexual abuse should be referred to pediatricians trained in this area because familiarity with the prepubertal genital examination and the legal process of evidence collection is necessary. Teaching or children's hospitals are the best sources for these services.

2. **Physical abuse** of children often presents with a constellation of the following signs: injuries incompatible with the alleged mechanism; multiple bruises, abrasions, bites, or lacerations of different ages or in disparate locations; cigarette or scalding burns; twisting (spiral) fractures of long bones; intracranial or retinal hemorrhage in infants; or facial injuries in older children. To identify a systematic pattern of injuries when abuse is suspected, radiographs of long bones, ribs, clavicles, fingers, toes, pelvis, and the skull (skeletal survey) are usually obtained. Social Services or the hospital child abuse team should be notified if one has suspicion of abuse, and the child can be hospitalized and placed in protective custody as mandated by law or when otherwise appropriate.

B. Adults

1. **Sexual assault** (see Chapter 27). Incidents of acute sexual assault are usually reported to the police, and part of the emergency department evaluation includes crisis intervention and referral for counseling services. However, many patients prefer to put the acute episode behind them, and they do not seek counseling. It may be weeks, months, or years later that unresolved issues with the assault present with symptoms such as nonspecific anxiety, depression, hyperventilation, concerns about sexually transmitted diseases or human immunodeficiency virus, pelvic pain, nightmares, relationship difficulties, or sleep disturbances. In addition, issues may surface in adulthood for those who have experienced sexual assault as children or who have grown up in households with an alcoholic or abusive parent. Consequently, psychiatric assessment of adults should always include questions about past or current sexual or physical assault or abuse, especially in those with symptoms for which no organic cause can be identified.

2. **Domestic partner violence**. Victims of partner violence rarely present with a chief complaint of "partner violence." Patients usually present to the emergency department with acute injuries, and an astute health care team should be aware of the patterns of partner violence and of the situational response to an acute battering episode. Health care professionals at every level of the health care delivery system—from emergency care to primary care to consultative services—should be alert to the signs and symptoms of partner violence so that they can identify the syndrome and can encourage counseling at every patient encounter.

   A number of the following signs and symptoms should raise suspicion of partner violence:

   1. Pregnant women with an unexplained pattern of injury, especially to the abdomen;
   2. Injuries to the face, head, and neck with an unexplained pattern of injury;

3. Any injury that is inconsistent with the alleged mechanism;
4. Injuries suggesting a posture defensive to blows, such as forearm bruises or fractures;
5. Multiple injuries in various stages of healing;
6. Any substantial delay between the time of acute injury and of presenting for treatment;
7. Noncompliance with important follow-up care, such as for fracture or dental care;
8. Visits to multiple care providers or emergency departments for injuries.

Other signs and symptoms include depression and suicidal behavior, pelvic pain, or repetitive visits for complaints for which no clear basis can be found.

The partner's behavior during the encounter can also be a clue. Excessively caring behavior and an insistence to remain with the patient throughout the interview are two suspicious signs.

Unfortunately, a common response by a battering victim is the denial of abuse. The high frequency of denial has led clinicians to see denial as a feature of the partner abuse syndrome. Reasons for denial include the victim-patient's concern that violence will escalate if the battering is acknowledged, fears for the safety of any children or other family members, the victim's economic dependence on the partner, and/or a basic affection for the partner and a belief that these behaviors can and will spontaneously change. When suspicion is high, alternatives for safety, even hospital admission, should be explored. The patient should always be asked if children have been battered and if the patient has concerns about the children's safety. Child Protective Services or the Child Abuse Team should be notified if any concerns about the welfare of the children are present. *Keep in mind that the expected victim response is to deny battering and to return to the battering environment.* As more is learned about battering victims, the fact that numerous offers for help must be extended before victims are able to free themselves from their situation has become clear. For any individual health care encounter, predicting if the patient is close to, or far from, problem resolution is not possible. Therefore, continued persistence and encouragement to seek care at every encounter are important; the cumulative effect of such urgings will be important.

3. **The elderly and impaired**. Abuse in the elderly and impaired is difficult to determine, in part because of the complex psychosocial dynamic and also because the victim may be unable to corroborate the suspicions. The same principles that apply to the identification of child or adult abuse apply to the diagnosis of elder or impaired abuse. Reasons for the difficulty in arriving at an unequivocal diagnosis of abuse in the elderly or impaired include the following:

1. Any behavioral signs and symptoms associated with elder abuse, such as depression, confusion, withdrawal, anxiety, or helplessness, may be a part of progressive dementia (see Chapter 5);
2. Mentally retarded persons or patients who are psychotic may not be able to communicate effectively;
3. Physical deterioration in the elderly may lead to frequent falls, resulting in multiple fractures and bruises of different ages;
4. Skin fragility associated with aging can result in dramatic epidermal tears from trivial injury;
5. Determining whether injuries are a consequence of battering or are secondary to agitated or violent behavior in a demented or psychotic patient can be difficult;
6. Falls and injuries may be consequent to alcohol abuse or the misuse of prescribed sedative or anxiolytic agents, which can mimic or mask battering;

7. The caretakers or health care professionals responsible for care may not be aware of techniques to handle behavioral problems; they are just doing the best they can.

C. Treatment

Acute medical problems should be treated promptly. Specialists in geriatric psychiatric care or in the care of mentally retarded adults or children should be consulted. Often admission to specialized units can result in changes in medication to improve behavior. Social workers can arrange for a more appropriate environment, either in the patient's own home, a living-assisted community, or an institution.

V. Acute Overdose

In 2000 in the continental United States, an estimated 601,776 drug-related emergency department visits occurred. That clinicians have at least some familiarity with the care of a patient after an acute overdose is essential. The United States Department of Health and Human Service's Substance Abuse and Mental Health Administration maintains a useful website (*http://www.samsha.gov*) for data on emergency department visits due to drug ingestions; their toll-free number is 1-800-729-6686.

A. General Approach

The ABCs (Airway, Breathing, and Circulation) of resuscitation and stabilization take precedence over all other aspects of drug overdose management. In the patient with altered mental status, cervical spine protection and treatment with **oxygen**, **naloxone**, **glucose**, and **thiamine** are important aspects of early care. Next, the patient should be completely disrobed to allow a careful physical examination. This may uncover occult trauma or may suggest a specific toxic syndrome (i.e., **anticholinergic**, **opioid**) or toxidrome. A core temperature should be obtained. When hyperthermia is noted, aggressive evaporative cooling (mist and fan) should be carried out.

Once the patient is stabilized, attempts should be made to obtain a complete history. For example, information from family, friends, or EMS personnel may assist with exact substance identification, the time of ingestion, current medication use, allergies, past medical events, and the circumstances surrounding the exposure. Attention can then be directed toward patient decontamination, laboratory evaluation, enhancement of drug elimination, and, occasionally, the administration of specific antidotes.

No less important than the initial treatment of the poisoned patient is the continuing provision of supportive care and appropriate disposition. In general, after the diagnosis and initial treatment is established, appropriate disposition may include transfer to a medical unit, observation, and patient and family education in poison prevention. Exposure to some intoxicants (e.g., monoamine oxidase inhibitors [MAOIs]) requires prolonged medical observation. Definitive therapy includes appropriate referral for follow-up care.

Although general management guidelines such as those discussed below should be readily available, *a Regional Poison Control Center should be contacted early in the treatment of any poisoning or overdose. Within the United States, the closest center can be reached by calling 1-800-222-1222; in California, call 1-800-876-4766.*

1. **External decontamination. Ocular or skin exposure** to chemicals should be treated with immediate water irrigation, which should be carried out by staff wearing adequate skin and respiratory protection.

2. **GI tract decontamination.**

   a. **Gastric emptying.** As the time following an ingestion lengthens, the value of measures used to empty the stomach decreases. Recovering significant amounts of toxin 1 hour or more after the ingestion is unusual. **Gastric emptying** is contraindicated after the ingestion of **caustic** substances or **hydrocarbons**.

   b. **Induced emesis.** In health care facilities, the use of syrup of ipecac is no longer recommended, and it may in fact delay the administration of charcoal. Other historic methods of stimulating emesis (**apomorphine, lobeline, zinc sulfate, copper sulfate, potassium antimony tartrate, sodium chloride, powdered mustard,** mechanical means) are *never indicated, and they are potentially hazardous.*

c. **Gastric lavage**. This procedure is time consuming and uncomfortable for the patient, and it may cause morbidity. Recovery of intact pills or large particles of undissolved poison is unlikely. Clinical studies do not show an improved outcome with this method of decontamination, and no indication for a role for routine use in poisoning exists. It may be considered for the patient who has ingested a life-threatening amount of a toxic substance within 1 hour of the presentation to the clinician, if he or she has not already vomited. Contraindications include an unprotected airway or the ingestion of **corrosive substances** or **hydrocarbons.**

When gastric lavage is used, **the following procedure can be followed. An unresponsive patient** should have **endotracheal intubation** before gastric lavage to prevent reflux and aspiration of gastric contents. (*Note: The endotracheal tube cuff should be briefly deflated during the actual passage of the orogastric tube to reduce the risk of esophageal laceration at the site of the cuff.*) **A conscious adult patient** is placed first in the left lateral decubitus position. The lubricated tip of a French orogastric tube (size 36 or 40) is placed into the posterior pharynx. With the placement of a bite block between the patient's posterior molars, the tube is easily advanced into the stomach. If the left lateral head-down position does not result in a prompt return of gastric contents, auscultation of the stomach while 50 mL of air is injected into the proximal end of the tube verifies that the distal end is in the stomach. Gastric **lavage** is performed by repeated injection and withdrawal of 250 to 300 mL of **water** or isotonic **saline** until the lavage fluid is clear. Hypertonic **saline** should not be used.

These instructions do not apply to the pediatric patient.

d. **Activated charcoal** (e.g., **activated charcoal USP, Norit-A, Superchar, Actidose**). This charcoal can adsorb and can prevent absorption of significant quantities of a wide variety of substances, including many psychotropic agents. Studies in volunteers show that **activated charcoal** is most effective when given within 1 hour of ingestion. Its administration should be considered after the recent ingestion of a potentially toxic amount of a substance that is known to adsorb to charcoal. Substances that do not adsorb well to **activated charcoal** include some metals, hydrocarbons, alcohols, and pesticides. One half to 1 g per kg of **activated charcoal** suspended in **water** (frequent stirring is important) is given by mouth or is administered through an orogastric or nasogastric tube. The first dose of **activated charcoal** is often given with **sorbitol**, although cathartics have not been shown to be beneficial. Additional doses of **activated charcoal** may be considered for certain situations (see below).

e. **Whole bowel irrigation (Golytely)**. Balanced polyethylene glycol solutions are isoosmotic. These solutions allow for mechanical cleansing of the gut without the risk of fluid or electrolyte imbalance. Potential indications for whole bowel irrigation include the ingestion of (a) massive amounts of a toxic substance, (b) metals (e.g., lithium, iron) because they do not adsorb to **activated charcoal**, (c) sustained-release preparations, (d) wrapped packages of **cocaine** or **heroin**, (e) large pills or foreign bodies, and (f) concretions. The dose of polyethylene glycol solution is 2 L per h until the rectal effluent is clear in adults. For children, 40 mL per kg per h is used.

3. Enhanced elimination of intoxicants

  a. Multidose charcoal. Serial doses of **activated charcoal** can be used to enhance drug elimination. Consider this method for significant intoxications with **carbamazepine, dapsone, phenobarbital, quinine,** or **theophylline.** Limited studies in volunteers suggest a possible role for the use of multidose charcoal in poisonings from **amitriptyline, dextropropoxyphene, digitoxin, digoxin, disopyramide, nadolol, phenylbutazone, phenytoin, piroxicam, salicylates,** and **sotalol.**

  b. Urinary alkalinization. Drugs that are weak acids tend to ionize in solution. Trapping the drug in its ionized form in the renal tubule can enhance the renal excretion of a few drugs. This requires manipulation of the urinary pH through the administration of i.v. **sodium bicarbonate.** By this method, the reabsorption of **salicylates, phenobarbital,** and **chlorpropamide** is reduced. The technique of urinary alkalinization should not be confused with the antiquated practice of forced diuresis, which relied on the administration of high volumes of fluid to maintain high urinary flow rates and which was fraught with hazardous side effects, such as cerebral and pulmonary edema. The most important therapeutic manipulation is now known to be that of urinary pH and not of the volume of urinary output. To institute urinary alkalinization, an indwelling Foley catheter is inserted, and urine outputs and pH are measured hourly. **Sodium bicarbonate** can be given either by bolus or by infusion to achieve a urinary pH of 7.5. A general approach involves the administration of sodium bicarbonate, 1 to 2 mEq per kg, by bolus, followed by a dose of 100 to 150 mEq per L added to each L of i.v. fluids (dextrose 5% water solution [D5W]) that is infused at approximately 1.5 times the maintenance fluid rate. (*Note: For daily [24-h] maintenance fluid requirements, the rates are 100 mL per kg for the first 10 kg of body weight, 50 mL per kg for the second 10 kg, and 20 mL per kg for each additional kg of body weight.*) Close monitoring of volume status and serum electrolytes, especially potassium and calcium, is necessary. Patients with congestive heart failure, cerebral edema, renal failure, or hypernatremia may not be candidates for this therapy. (*Note: Acidification of the urine to "ion trap" weakly basic drugs, such as phencyclidine and amphetamines, was conducted historically; because rhabdomyolysis often complicates such intoxications, urinary acidification places the patient at an unacceptable risk for myoglobinuric renal failure, and thus it is no longer used.*)

  c. Peritoneal dialysis. This method of enhanced elimination is not used unless hemodialysis is unavailable.

  d. Hemodialysis. The physical characteristics of the intoxicant determine whether it will be amenable to dialysis. The substance must be able to cross the dialysis membrane freely, and it should have a molecular weight below 500 Da, high water solubility, low protein binding, and a small volume of distribution (less than 1 L per kg). Although hemodialysis has been recommended for a wide variety of intoxications, clear benefits outweigh the risk for only a small number of substances. Examples include **salicylates, phenobarbital, methanol, ethylene glycol, lithium,** and **certain metals. Renal failure** in a patient who has ingested a drug for which the kidney is a major organ for elimination is another potential indication for hemodialysis. Hemodialysis can also be used for the treatment of a refractory acid–base imbalance, an electrolyte disturbance, or a volume-overload state.

  e. Charcoal hemoperfusion. This technique interposes a cartridge filled with **activated charcoal** or **resin beads** into the dialysis circuit. These beads are able to adsorb drugs with a low volume of distribution, even if they are lipid soluble or are highly protein bound. Few well-studied indications for its use are available, but it has been applied in the setting of **theophylline** or **carbamazepine** toxicity or overdosing. Complications related to hemoperfusion include thrombocytopenia, leukopenia, reduced glucose and calcium levels, and hemorrhage secondary to heparinization.

B. Identification, Evaluation, and Treatment of Intoxication from Specific Psychotropic Agents

    1. Conventional antipsychotic agents. Phenothiazines and butyrophenones accounted for 6,825 reported poisonings in the United States in 2000. These agents are pharmacologically complex, and they impact muscarinic, α-adrenergic, histaminergic, and dopaminergic receptors, as well as cardiac potassium and sodium channels. Toxicity may be seen after acute overdose or as an idiosyncratic reaction related to therapeutic use.

        a. Manifestations of acute overdose

            (1) Central nervous system effects. Aliphatic and piperidine phenothiazines (e.g., **chlorpromazine, thioridazine, mesoridazine**) tend to sedate more than do the higher potency piperazine phenothiazines, thioxanthenes, and butyrophenones (e.g., **fluphenazine, perphenazine, trifluoperazine, thiothixene,** and **haloperidol**) due to the greater antihistaminic and antimuscarinic effects of the former. However, any of these agents can cause coma and unresponsiveness after the ingestion of large amounts. Agitation, delirium, muscular rigidity, spasm, twitching, hyperreflexia, tremor, or seizures can also occur.

            (2) Cardiovascular effects. Hypotension results primarily from α_1-adrenergic receptor blockade and vasodilation. A reflex tachycardia that is compounded by the antimuscarinic effects of these agents may result. Sodium channel blockade may cause QRS prolongation on ECG. Potassium channel blockade, which manifests as QTc prolongation, is a serious complication that may lead to ventricular dysrhythmias, such as *torsade de pointes*. QTc prolongation is most commonly associated with **thioridazine** and **mesoridazine** overdose, and it may have a delayed onset after an acute overdose.

            (3) Autonomic nervous system effects. Thermoregulatory impairment may cause hypothermia or hyperthermia. Antimuscarinic effects may manifest as hyperthermia, absence of sweating, dry mucous membranes, tachycardia, ileus, and urinary retention. Mydriasis is an expected finding as a result of the muscarinic blockade, but, because these agents cause concomitant potent α-adrenergic receptor antagonism, the pupillary size generally is from pinpoint to midrange.

        b. Treatment of acute overdose

            (1) Gastric lavage followed by the administration of **activated charcoal** should be considered soon after significant ingestions (see above).

            (2) ECG monitoring should be continuous **for all patients** because of the possibility of cardiac dysrhythmias. QRS widening beyond 100 ms should be treated with i.v. sodium bicarbonate, 1 to 2 mEq per kg bolus. *Torsade de pointes* should be treated with magnesium, 2 g i.v. bolus; i.v. potassium supplementation; **isoproterenol;** and transcutaneous or transvenous pacing. All class Ia (e.g., **quinidine, disopyramide, procainamide**), Ic (e.g., **flecainide, encainide**), and III (e.g., **bretylium, amiodarone, sotalol**) antidysrhythmics should be avoided.

            (3) Hypotension is treated with volume expansion with **crystalloids.** A bolus of isotonic **saline** (250 to 500 mL) is administered over 30 minutes or less, as long as cardiac function is normal. When hypotension is refractory to a fluid bolus, the administration of vasopressors are indicated (e.g., direct-acting α-adrenergic receptor agonists, such as **norepinephrine** and **metaraminol**, are the pressors of choice). Catechol-amines having β-adrenergic receptor activity (e.g., **isopro-terenol, epinephrine**) can theoretically cause a further **fall** in blood pressure, and they may also further increase the heart rate.

(4) **Seizures** should be treated with i.v. benzodiazepines (e.g., **lorazepam** [1 mg]), followed by barbiturates, if necessary. **Phenytoin** is not effective in controlling drug-induced seizures. **Flumazenil** and **physostigmine** should be avoided. Many causes of seizures exist, and different etiologies may coexist in poisoned patients. Therefore, all patients with seizures should be evaluated for metabolic, toxic, infectious, or structural causes. Treatment is indicated when seizures are repetitive or in-tractable or when they are associated with deteriorating vital signs. Emergency medical consultation is indicated for any pa-tient with seizures.

(5) **Hypothermia and hyperthermia** are treated symptomati-cally. The core temperature should be monitored, usually with rectal thermometer or urinary bladder probe. The initial treat-ment of mild **hypothermia** (32.2°C to 35°C [90°F to 95°F]) con-sists of the administration of heated humidified **oxygen** and passive external rewarming with heated blankets. The special warming devices or temperature-controlled water baths needed to heat i.v. fluids are beyond the scope of care expected in psy-chiatric settings. For patients with core temperatures below 35°C (95°F), transfer to an appropriate medical setting is es-sential. Other serious causes of hypothermia should be ruled out (e.g., hypoglycemia, thiamine deficiency, endocrinopathy). When evaluating patients with **hyperthermia**, sepsis and neuroleptic malignant syndrome (NMS) must be considered in the differential diagnosis. Hyperthermic patients should be transferred to an appropriate medical setting. Mild hyperther-mia may be treated with **cooling blankets, cool moist tow-els**, or **antipyretics**. Drug-induced hyperthermia, however, usually is unresponsive to these measures; it requires aggres-sive evaporative cooling measures via mist and fan.

Forced diuresis or extracorporeal elimination have no role in the treatment of acute overdose.

c. **Idiosyncratic toxicities from antipsychotic agents**

(1) **Acute dystonias**. Although dopaminergic receptor antagonism accounts for many of the therapeutic effects of antipsychotic agents, it is also responsible for causing unwanted extrapyrami-dal reactions. Because of their antidopaminergic properties, an-tipsychotic agents are often associated with a variety of motor disorders involving acute involuntary muscle movements and spasms. Although any muscle group in the body can be involved, the most common manifestations are oculogyric crisis, trismus, torticollis, facial grimacing, and retrocollis. Rarely, rigidity, laryngospasm, dysphagia, dysphonia, or opisthotonus may occur.

Treatment consists of **diphenhydramine** (50 mg i.m. or i.v.) or **benztropine** (2 mg i.m. or i.v.). Improvement generally occurs within seconds or within 15 to 30 minutes. These doses can be repeated in 30 minutes. Refractory dystonias may be treated with benzodiazepines (e.g., **lorazepam** [1 mg i.v.]). Even if the antipsychotic agent is discontinued, oral treatment with either **diphenhydramine** or **benztropine** should be continued for the next 3 to 7 days as dystonias can recur.

(2) **Neuroleptic malignant syndrome.** NMS is a rare, life-threatening syndrome that can occur with a variety of antipsychotic agents, including **phenothiazines**, **butyrophenones**, **substituted benzamides**, and **thioxanthenes**, at any time during treatment. **MAOIs** and **lithium** can also cause significant hyperthermia. NMS has most often been reported in association with the initiation of medication or with rapid dose escalation.

Common signs and symptoms include **hyperthermia, muscular rigidity**, an **altered level of consciousness**, and **autonomic instability.** Body temperatures can exceed 40°C (104°F). Muscular rigidity can be localized, as in oculogyric crisis; generalized; or associated with opisthotonus. Mutism, disorientation, agitation, stupor, or coma can result. Diaphoresis, tachycardia, labile hypertension, or hypotension characterizes autonomic instability.

Historically, the mortality rate for NMS was 30%; with the advent of the intensive care unit, mortality should not be expected. The complications are primarily pulmonary and renal. Deaths usually result from a failure to recognize the syndrome or from inadequate or delayed treatment and supportive therapy.

The differential diagnosis for NMS includes sepsis, CNS infection, seizures, thyrotoxicosis, tetanus, **strychnine** toxicity, **lithium** toxicity, lethal catatonia, abrupt discontinuation of **clozapine**, heat stroke, cocaine toxicity, ecstasy (methylene-dioxymethamphetamine [MDMA]) or other stimulant intoxication, salicylate toxicity, MAOI toxicity, anticholinergic toxicity, delirium tremens, sedative-hypnotic withdrawal, stiff man syndrome, and toxic serotonin syndrome.[1]

Treatment for suspected NMS is as follows. The causative agent(s) should be discontinued, and the patient should be moved to an intensive care unit as soon as possible. Cooling should be initiated to reduce the hyperthermia, and airway and cardiovascular support should be provided as needed. Benzodiazepines can be given for muscular rigidity. For intubated patients, refractory rigidity can be treated with short-acting neuromuscular blocking agents (e.g., **vecuronium** [10 mg]) or with **dantrolene sodium**, which also acts particularly in skeletal muscle (the initial dose of **dantrolene** is 1 mg per kg i.v. repeated every 5 minutes as necessary to a total dose of 10 mg per kg). The disadvantages of **dantrolene** include its high pH, which may lead to tissue necrosis with extravasation and hepatotoxicity, which is common. **Bromocriptine**, a centrally acting dopamine agonist that is available in an oral form, should be started as soon as possible to reverse the central antidopaminergic effects of the antipsychotic agent (the starting dose is 5 mg p.o.; then 2.5 to 10 mg four times a day until the symptoms resolve).

As the comments on differential diagnosis noted, catatonia must be distinguished from NMS. Because affective disorders have a notable incidence among patients with NMS and because catatonia can also be comorbid with affective disorders, distinguishing between catatonia and NMS is of considerable importance. Catatonia may respond promptly to benzodiazepines, and, when necessary, electroconvulsive therapy (see Chapter 24) may be beneficial. Although **bromocriptine** may help in

[1] Toxic serotonin syndrome is now the preferred term.

NMS, it can precipitate manic symptomatology in patients with affective disorders. *For these reasons, calling the NMSIS Hotline (1-800-NMS-TEMP [667-8367]; 315-428-9010 from outside the United States) may be prudent and clinically beneficial. This will give the caller access to a consultation with a psychiatrist who has extensive experience in both the treatment and differential diagnosis of NMS.*

2. **Atypical antipsychotic agents.** These (**clozapine, quetiapine, olanzapine, risperidone,** and **ziprasidone**) are more selective for limbic than for extrapyramidal sites, and they also possess greater selectivity for dopamine-1 (D_1) than for D_2 receptors. In general, overdose results in less severe toxicity than with conventional antipsychotic agents, and extrapyramidal effects are less common. **Clozapine** and **olanzapine** have greater antimuscarinic and antihistaminic properties than do **quetiapine, risperidone,** or **ziprasidone,** and they are more likely to cause anticholinergic toxicity and sedation in an overdose. Seizures may also occur. All of these agents antagonize α_1-adrenergic receptors, and they may cause hypotension and miosis. Conduction disturbances and QT prolongation can also occur.

   Treatment is supportive. Gastric decontamination should be considered, as outlined above. Continuous ECG monitoring is warranted. Hypotension should be treated with **crystalloids**; in refractory patients, **crystalloids** are followed by α-adrenergic receptor agonists that act as vasopressors (e.g., **norepinephrine**).

3. **Tricyclic antidepressants (TCAs) and other heterocyclic antidepressants**

   a. **Epidemiology.** In the United States, TCAs accounted for 13,848 poisonings in 2000, and they were the second largest category of drugs causing death. The agents that were most commonly implicated were **amitriptyline, doxepin, imipramine,** and **nortriptyline.** As with antipsychotic agents, these drugs are pharmacologically complex; they also harbor even greater toxicity in overdose. Their pharmacologic properties include the blockade of sodium and potassium channels and of α_1-adrenergic, muscarinic, histaminergic, and γ-aminobutyric acid A receptors. The reuptake of biogenic amines, including **serotonin** and **norepinephrine,** also occurs.

   b. **Manifestations.** Signs of overdose most commonly include CNS depression, seizures, hypotension, and cardiac dysrhythmias.

      (1) **Central nervous system effects.** The rapid onset of sedation, coma, and respiratory depression is most commonly seen. Myoclonic jerking is noted in up to 50% of patients and may be mistaken for tonic-clonic seizures. When seizures occur, they usually are brief and isolated, except for when **amoxapine** or **maprotiline** is the index drug; in these patients, seizures may be protracted. Agitation, delirium, and hallucinations are less common than are CNS depression and seizures.

      (2) **Cardiac effects.** Cardiac dysrhythmias due to TCAs are potentially fatal; they most commonly result from sodium channel blockade. QRS widening on the ECG (greater than 100 ms) indicates significant sodium channel blockade, and it is a predictor of seizures and cardiac dysrhythmias. Dysrhythmias are rate dependent (i.e., sodium channel blockade is more likely to occur in patients with tachycardia). Therefore, patients with tachycardia are not considered medically stable after a TCA overdose. QT interval prolongation stemming from potassium channel blockade may also be seen.

      (3) **Hypotension.** Hypotension resulting from α-adrenergic receptor antagonism is common. In severe toxicity, hypotension

may also result from myocardial depression related to sodium channel blockade.

   (4) **Anticholinergic effects**. These are inconsistently observed; they may be masked by other drug effects. When present, antimuscarinic toxicity manifests as delirium, tachycardia, urinary retention, paralytic ileus, mydriasis, absent sweating, dry mucous membranes, and hyperpyrexia.

 c. **Treatment**
   (1) **Gastric decontamination**, as discussed above (see section V.A.2), should be considered as soon as the patient's airway is secured.
   (2) **Continuous ECG monitoring** is mandatory.
   (3) **Alkalinization of the serum** by **hyperventilation** of the intubated patient and **sodium bicarbonate** administration is the initial treatment of choice for dysrhythmias, hypotension, or QRS widening greater than 100 ms. **Sodium bicarbonate** is given as a bolus of 1 to 2 mEq per kg, followed by repeat boluses or an infusion to maintain the blood pH at 7.5.
   (4) **Hypotension** is best treated initially with a **crystalloid** bolus, followed by **sodium bicarbonate**, if it is persistent. When hypotension is unresponsive to fluids, α-adrenergic receptor agonist vasopressors (e.g., **norepinephrine**) may be indicated. Avoid vasopressors with β-adrenergic receptor effects, as they may further accelerate heart rate.
   (5) **Seizures** are treated initially with benzodiazepines (e.g., **lorazepam** [1 to 2 mg i.v.]). In patients who are not hypotensive, barbiturates may be given for seizures refractory to benzodiazepines. **Phenytoin** is not an effective agent for seizure control. Noting that **sodium bicarbonate** does not have an impact on seizures is important; it may, however, be administered in an effort to protect the myocardium against the acidosis that may occur with protracted seizures, as acidosis enhances the binding of TCAs to sodium channels.
   Physostigmine, flumazenil, procainamide, disopyramide, quinidine, and α-adrenergic receptor antagonists are **contraindicated** in the treatment of TCA overdoses. These agents may increase QRS widening, QT interval prolongation, or conduction disturbances.

4. **Monoamine oxidase inhibitors**
 a. **Epidemiology.** MAOIs, such as **phenelzine, tranylcypromine, isocarboxazid, selegiline**, and **moclobemide** (although **moclobemide** is not available in the United States, it is available in Canada and some other countries), may be highly toxic in overdose. Fatal poisoning has occurred with as little as three to four times the therapeutic dose of **tranylcypromine** and with five to six times the therapeutic dose of **phenelzine**. In recent years, the clinical use of MAOIs has started to increase. As a result, overdoses have been seen more frequently. In 2000, 360 poisonings related to MAOIs were recorded in the United States. Many drugs can precipitate life-threatening drug interactions, when they are given to a patient taking MAOIs (see Tables 3.3 and 3.4 and Chapter 29 for drugs to be avoided).
 b. **Manifestations after overdose.** Clinical signs and symptoms do not appear immediately after ingestion. The latent period can be as long as 12 hours. Signs of CNS and neuromuscular excitation then appear; these include confusion, agitation, delirium, diaphoresis, tachycardia, hyperreflexia, muscular rigidity, and seizures. Malignant hyperpyrexia is the usual terminal event. After the hyperadrenergic period, the clinical picture may unpredictably

TABLE 3.3. SOME INDIRECT-ACTING AND DIRECT-ACTING SYMPATHOMIMETIC AGENTS AND MONOAMINE OXIDASE INHIBITORS

Avoid	Use with Caution
Amphetamines, dextroamphetamine	Norepinephrine
Other anorexiants (diet pills)	Epinephrine
Cough and cold preparations	Isoproterenol
Pseudoephedrine	Caffeine
Ephedrine	Guarana ("natural" caffeine)
Phenylpropanolamine	Theobromine (tea, chocolate)
Ephedra (Ma huang)	Theophylline
Methyldopa	Phenylephrine
Reserpine	Methoxamine
Guanethidine	Albuterol
Methylphenidate	Terbutaline
Pemoline	Clonidine, guanfacine
Bretylium	
Dopamine	
Metaraminol	

TABLE 3.4. SOME DRUGS TO AVOID OR TO USE WITH EXTREME CAUTION IN PATIENTS TAKING MONOAMINE OXIDASE INHIBITORS

Agent	Effect
Opioids	Prolonged sedation
Codeine	Serotonin excess or toxic serotonin
Meperidine	syndrome
Dextromethorphan	
Tramadol	
Antidepressants	Serotonin excess or toxic serotonin
Lithium	syndrome
Cyclic antidepressants	
Selective serotonin reuptake inhibitors	
Trazodone	
Nefazodone	
Bupropion	
Mirtazapine	
St. John's wort	
Levodopa	
Central nervous system stimulants	Adrenergic crisis
Theophylline, theobromine	
Caffeine, guarana	
Cocaine, ephedra	
Phenylcyclidine	
Tryptophan	
Hypoglycemic agents or insulin	Potentiation of hypoglycemia
Barbiturates, ketamine	Prolonged sedation
β-Adrenergic receptor antagonists	Increased blood pressure
Phenothiazines	Hyperthermia

progress to one of catecholamine depletion with hypotension, bradycardia, and coma.

   c. **Treatment**. Management should begin immediately, preferably before the patient becomes symptomatic. Attention to the airway, cardiac monitoring, the establishment of i.v. access, gastric decontamination, and admission to a monitored setting are required. Pharmacologic treatment involves the use of titratable short-acting agents. Recommended therapeutic agents are as follows:

   1. For **hypertension**—nitroprusside or **phentolamine**;
   2. For **tachyarrhythmias**—benzodiazepines, esmolol, adenosine (for supraventricular tachycardias), and **lidocaine** (when ventricular);
   3. For **agitation**—benzodiazepines, short-acting neuromuscular blocking agents;
   4. For **hyperthermia**—aggressive cooling;
   5. For **hypotension**—direct-acting vasopressors (e.g., **norepinephrine**);
   6. For **seizures**—benzodiazepines, barbiturates (*note:* barbiturates may have prolonged effects);
   7. For **serotonergic symptoms**, reduce dosage or stop and follow recommendations in section IV.B.5.c.(2).

5. **Selective serotonin reuptake inhibitors (SSRIs) and other reuptake inhibitors**
   a. **Epidemiology and manifestations**. Although overdosing with SSRIs is comparatively common (e.g., 36,672 cases were reported in 2000), fatality is rare. Representative drugs include **citalopram, fluoxetine, fluvoxamine, paroxetine,** and **sertraline**. The most common symptoms seen in overdose are sinus tachycardia, drowsiness, tremor, vomiting, and rarely seizures. **Venlafaxine** is a somewhat less selective inhibitor of biogenic amine reuptake, and it manifests greater toxicity in overdose. **Venlafaxine** is much more likely to cause seizures, serotonergic symptoms, hypertension, and tachycardia after overdose compared with the SSRIs. The sustained-release formulation (**venlafaxine XR**) currently is more commonly used; this may further complicate management.
   b. **Treatment**. After an overdose, care is supportive. Gastric decontamination may be considered as discussed above (see section V.A.2). Cardiac monitoring should be instituted, and seizure precautions should be maintained. A high index of suspicion for coingestants should be maintained. A minimum period of 6 hours of cardiac monitoring is indicated for SSRIs after overdose. Those symptomatic at 6 hours should be admitted. At least a 24 hour period of monitoring is necessary after the ingestion of **venlafaxine XR**.
   c. **Toxic serotonin syndrome**. Certain symptoms and signs have been recognized collectively as the toxic **serotonin** syndrome. Occurring only rarely after an overdose and more commonly when two or more proserotonergic agents are coingested, the clinical presentation is similar to NMS; it consists of mental status changes, autonomic dysfunction, and neuromuscular hyperexcitability. Common symptoms include mydriasis, nystagmus, anxiety, CNS depression, salivation, sweating, tachycardia, hypertension, diarrhea, piloerection, ankle clonus, rigidity, shivering, teeth chattering, and ataxia.

   Any combination of the following agents may precipitate the toxic **serotonin** syndrome: MAOIs, SSRIs, **dextromethorphan**, TCAs, **bupropion, meperidine, amphetamines, trazodone, nefazodone, risperidone, tramadol**, St. John's wort, **buspirone, tryptophan, lithium**, sibutramine, or **MDMA**.

   (1) **Clinical features** that differentiate toxic **serotonin** syndrome from NMS are (a) rapid onset after the administration of

an offending serotonergic agent, (b) lack of involvement of a dopamine antagonist, (c) greater likelihood of hyperreflexia and/or myoclonus in the lower extremities that is out of proportion to the upper extremities, (d) an increased incidence of diarrhea, and (e) improvement within 24 hours after onset and discontinuation of the proserotonergic agents.

(2) **Treatment** is supportive and is similar to that for NMS with the following exceptions: dopamine agonists are not likely to be effective and the use of **cyproheptadine** (a 5-hydroxytryptamine 1A [5-HT$_{1A}$] receptor antagonist) may be considered. The initial dose of **cyproheptadine** is 4 to 8 mg p.o.

6. **Other antidepressants**

   a. **Trazodone**. This agent acts through serotonin reuptake inhibition and α-adrenergic receptor antagonism. Overdoses are relatively common, with 12,656 cases reported in 2000 in the United States. After overdose, a mild toxicity, typically manifesting as CNS depression, is generally seen. Orthostatic hypotension, miosis, and priapism may occur from local α-adrenergic receptor antagonism. Hypotension is best treated with **crystalloid** bolus; for patients unresponsive to volume expansion, an α-adrenergic receptor agonist vasopressor (e.g., **norepinephrine**) is added. Very rarely, conduction disturbances are described on ECG.

   b. **Bupropion**. In overdoses, this widely used biogenic amine uptake inhibitor has a toxicity profile similar to that of an SSRI. Common symptoms include sinus tachycardia, lethargy, and tremor. One unique feature of **bupropion** overdose is a greater propensity for generalized seizures (seen in >20% of overdoses), the onset of which may occur more than 6 hours after ingestion. Of note is the fact that most ingestions of **bupropion** now involve sustained-release formulations and therefore warrant prolonged monitoring.

   c. **St. John's wort**. This agent is an over-the-counter herbal preparation that is commonly used to self-treat depression. Although its mechanism of action is still unknown, two of its putatively active components, hyperforin and hypericin, appear to be proserotonergic. Toxicity in overdose is rare; however, several patients have had seizures, and serotonergic symptoms have been reported. Its side effects include GI upset, photosensitization, fatigue, anxiety, and tremor.

   St. John's wort should not be combined with other serotonergic drugs (see V.B.5.c. above); herbal stimulants, such as **Ma huang (ephedra)**; or cold preparations. Treatment is supportive. **St. John's wort** is an inducer of the gut transport protein p-glycoprotein or MDR1. When taken at therapeutic dosages or in overdoses, it may increase the presystemic extraction of other agents (e.g., **digoxin** or **indinavir** [see Chapter 29]).

   d. **Mirtazapine**. Mirtazapine (Remeron) is a new antidepressant with noradrenergic and serotonergic effects. Through antagonism of the α_2-adrenergic receptors, it promotes the release of **norepinephrine** and **serotonin**. It also antagonizes 5-HT$_2$ and 5-HT$_3$ receptors, allowing released **serotonin** to exert its effects on 5-HT$_1$ receptors more fully. Clinical data following a significant overdose with **mirtazapine** are limited. **Mirtazapine** appears to enhance the CNS depression caused by other agents in overdose. Other findings include tachycardia, confusion, agitation, and nonspecific ECG changes. Potentially, serious interactions with MAOI or a toxic **serotonin** syndrome could occur with the use of **mirtazapine**. Management is supportive, and it should include cardiac monitoring.

7. **Lithium carbonate or citrate**

   a. **Epidemiology**. In 2000, 4,663 poisonings related to **lithium** occurred in the United States. **Lithium** toxicity can develop slowly during maintenance therapy or after acute overdose. Some factors that may lead to insidious **lithium** toxicity include (a) a failure to monitor plasma concentrations; (b) coadministration of diuretics, angiotensin-converting enzyme inhibitors, or nonsteroidal anti-inflammatory drugs; (c) dietary sodium restriction; (d) aging and reduced glomerular filtration; and (e) dehydration. Serum **lithium** concentrations of greater than 1.5 mEq per L may be associated with toxicity, although levels after acute ingestion correlate very poorly with symptoms. Severe toxicity, especially in those on chronic therapy, may be seen at relatively low serum levels (approximately 2.5 mEq per L).

   b. **Manifestations**. Early signs of **lithium** toxicity include nausea, tremor, drowsiness, thirst, behavioral changes, and muscle irritability. More severe poisoning produces coarse tremor, dysarthria, muscle fasciculations, twitching, rigidity, clonus, hyperreflexia, seizures, hyperpyrexia, obtundation, seizures, and coma.

   c. **Treatment**
      (1) **Gastric decontamination** may be considered for recent significant ingestions. **Lithium** does not adsorb to **activated charcoal**, but **activated charcoal** may still be given if coingestants are a possibility. **Whole bowel irrigation** is indicated for recent large ingestions or after overdose with sustained-released products (see section V.A.2.e).

      (2) **Cardiac monitoring** is indicated. T wave flattening, U waves, bradycardia, conduction blocks, and ventricular dysrhythmias may be seen.

      (3) **Restoration of sodium and water balance** should begin with gentle hydration with normal **saline**.

      (4) **Hemodialysis** is highly effective because of **lithium's** lack of protein binding and its small volume of distribution. Indications for hemodialysis include severe neurotoxicity, moderate neurotoxicity and serum levels that do not decline by at least 20% in 6 hours, renal failure, and a serum **lithium** level greater than 4 mEq per L, even if the patient is asymptomatic.

      Rebound increases in serum levels may occur after hemodialysis. Neurologic recovery may lag behind declining serum levels due to slow equilibration between the intraneuronal and/or intracellular **lithium** concentrations and the plasma.

8. **Anticholinergic agents**. Anticholinergic agent exposure is extremely common in the United States, with 194,000 cases reported in 1998. Several agents already discussed—TCAs, phenothiazines, and some atypical antipsychotic agents—can cause antimuscarinic findings in overdose. Anticholinergic toxicity may also occur after drug overdose or as a side effect of medications used to combat motion sickness (e.g., **scopolamine, meclizine**), GI spasm (e.g., **dicyclomine, propantheline**), diarrhea (e.g., **diphenoxylate** and/or **atropine**), bladder instability (e.g., **oxybutynin, tolterodine**), skeletal muscle spasm (e.g., **cyclobenzaprine, orphenadrine**), asthma (e.g., **ipratropium**), parkinsonism (e.g., **benztropine, trihexyphenidyl, amantadine**), colds and allergies (e.g., **diphenhydramine, chlorpheniramine, hydroxyzine, cyproheptadine, loratadine, fexofenadine, cetirizine**), seizures (e.g., **carbamazepine**), or cardiac dysrhythmias (e.g., **procainamide, quinidine**). Recent outbreaks of anticholinergic toxicity have been encountered in both intentional abuse (e.g., Jimson weed, **scopolamine**-adulterated **heroin**) and malicious administration (e.g., **scopolamine**-tainted alcoholic beverages). The major morbidity and mortality associated with anticholinergic drug toxicity stem from hyperthermia and rhabdomyolysis caused by agitation and ineffective heat dissipation. Even patients taking these medications therapeutically may become ill under conditions of heat stress.

Peripheral antimuscarinic signs include dry skin and mucous membranes, thirst, blurred vision, mydriasis, tachycardia, hypertension, rash or flushing, hyperthermia, absent bowel sounds, and urinary retention. Central antimuscarinic receptor antagonism causes lethargy, anxiety, confusion, hallucination, coma, seizures, ataxia, and respiratory and circulatory collapse. The classic presentation can be remembered as **"hot as a hare, blind as a bat, red as a beet, dry as a bone, and mad as a hatter."** Any ECG finding other than sinus tachycardia suggests either a massive exposure to anticholinergic agents or the presence of other cardiotoxic substances.

Treatment of anticholinergic toxicity is based on supportive care and basic life support, establishment of an i.v. line, and cardiac monitoring. **Physical restraint** may be needed for the delirious patient (see Chapter 26). Once an airway is established, gastric decontamination may be considered as outlined above (see section V.A.2). Hyperthermia should be aggressively treated with **evaporative cooling** methods. Sedation should be carried out with benzodiazepines. **Physostigmine** (a tertiary ammonium compound) achieves **anticholinesterase** inhibition and reverses both central and peripheral anticholinergic effects because it crosses the blood–brain barrier. Unfortunately, **physostigmine** may be as dangerous as it is beneficial. Its use may aggravate seizures and arrhythmias and may potentiate the toxicity of TCAs. Indications for its use include peripheral refractory seizures or hemodynamically unstable tachydysrhythmias that are unresponsive to conventional therapy. In general, **physostigmine** is a **last resort** medication. Initial doses range from 0.5 to 2 mg i.v. given over 5 to 10 minutes. Before its use, (a) a baseline ECG showing no conduction disturbances or axis deviation should be obtained; (b) the patient should have no history of exposure to other toxins with potential cardiac effect; (c) peripheral and central signs of antimuscarinic toxicity should be present; and (d) bronchospastic disease, vagotonic symptoms (especially bradycardia), intestinal and/or bladder obstruction, severe peripheral vascular disease (gangrene), diabetes mellitus, cardiovascular disease, and recent coadministration of **succinylcholine** should be excluded. Having **atropine** at the bedside as a precaution is important. Patients with mild anticholinergic poisoning should be observed for at least 6 to 8 hours; moderate to severe poisoning cases should be admitted to the critical care unit. Monitoring of creatine phosphokinase, transaminases, renal function, and coagulation studies is warranted.

9. **CNS stimulants**. Catecholamines are key neurotransmitters in the sympathetic nervous system. **Epinephrine, norepinephrine**, and **dopamine** are involved in the innervation of the skin, eyes, heart, lungs, GI tract, and exocrine glands. α-Adrenergic and β-adrenergic receptors are classified into certain subtypes as follows: α_1 **receptors** are primarily peripheral, postsynaptic, and excitatory to smooth muscle and exocrine glands; α_2 **receptors** are primarily central, presynaptic, and inhibitory, causing a decrease in catecholamine release; β_1 **receptors** are primarily cardiovascular and excitatory; and β_2 **receptors** primarily affect smooth muscle relaxation, insulin release, and gluconeogenesis. Receptor cloning suggests that this family of receptors is more complex; nevertheless, this limited classification system still has heuristic and clinical value. Most synthetic sympathomimetic agents are structurally similar to natural catecholamines. Predictably, the sympathomimetic toxidrome includes manifestations of CNS excitation, seizures, hypertension, tachycardia, hyperthermia, nausea, vomiting, diarrhea, and diaphoresis.

a. **Cocaine** produces its excitatory response by blocking the presynaptic reuptake of **norepinephrine, serotonin**, and **dopamine** and by stimulating their presynaptic release. Intoxication with **cocaine** is therefore characterized by excessive stimulation of the sympathetic nervous system. In the United States, 5,000 cases of primary cocaine toxicity were reported to poison centers in 2000.

(1) **Manifestations**. These include agitation and hyperactivity, tachycardia, hypertension, sweating, increased respirations, seizures, hyperthermia, acute psychosis, and occasionally chest pain.

(2) **Treatment**. After initial stabilization and assessment for rapidly treatable causes of altered mental status, hyperthermia must be aggressively treated with **evaporative cooling** measures. Continuous core temperature monitoring should be used. Seizures should be treated with **benzodiazepines** or **barbiturates**. **Phenytoin** has no clear role in the management of drug-induced seizures. Benzodiazepines may be needed to control extreme agitation, and they have been shown to be safe in **cocaine** intoxication. Their use may also suffice for hypertension and tachycardia because they attenuate both the cardiac and central nervous system toxicity of cocaine when given in sedative dosages. For the management of hypertension unresponsive to sedation, β-adrenergic receptor antagonists should be avoided because unopposed α-adrenergic receptor-mediated vasoconstriction could result in increased blood pressure or coronary artery vasoconstriction. Hypertension could be managed with an α-adrenergic receptor antagonist (e.g., **phentolamine**) or with other direct-acting vasodilators (e.g., **nitrates**, **hydralazine**, or **nitroprusside**). Dosage titration for sodium **nitroprusside**, starting at 0.5 μg per kg per min, is used with the goal of reducing the mean arterial pressure by 30%. Administering maximally titratable agents in the treatment of **cocaine**-induced cardiovascular toxicity is generally desirable because the clinical picture is often dynamic. Myocardial ischemia should initially be managed with **oxygen**, **aspirin**, benzodiazepines, and vasodilators (e.g., **nitrates**, **phentolamine**). Dysrhythmias should be treated with benzodiazepines and **sodium bicarbonate** (if a wide QRS complex is present). Many tachydysrhythmias will terminate spontaneously with drug metabolism. Those associated with hypotension require cardioversion. For suspected ventricular dysrhythmias, either **lidocaine** or **magnesium** is a reasonable antidysrhythmic choice. **Bretylium** could theoretically accentuate catecholamine release, so it should not be used.

(3) **Complications**. Myocardial infarction and ischemia, myocarditis, congestive heart failure, and ventricular and atrial arrhythmias have been reported. ECG findings of QT prolongation and QRS widening may occur. Bronchospasm, pneumonia, pneumothorax, pneumomediastinum, ischemic and hemorrhagic cerebrovascular accidents, rhabdomyolysis, renal failure, thrombophlebitis, abscess formation, hepatotoxicity, mesenteric ischemia, human immunodeficiency virus infection, and osteomyelitis are other complications.

b. **Methylenedioxymethamphetamine (MDMA, ecstasy)**

(1) **Manifestations**. This illicit drug is currently one of the most widely abused drugs in the United States. Like other amphetamines, MDMA displaces biogenic amines from storage vesicles, ultimately inducing serotonin, norepinephrine, or dopamine efflux. However, MDMA stimulates a greater release of serotonin than of dopamine, which may explain its greater psychoactive effect compared with that of other unsubstituted amphetamines. Other actions occur through a false neurotransmitter effect, the prevention of monoamine reuptake, and

monoamine oxidase (MAO)-A and MAO-B inhibition. A commonly ingested dose is 75 to 100 mg. Higher doses may cause muscle spasms, involuntary bruxism, nausea, vomiting, dehydration, urinary retention, diaphoresis, restlessness, autonomic fluctuations, and hallucinations. Postrecreational "let down" effects include confusion, depression, sleep disturbance, anxiety, and paranoia; these effects may persist for weeks. Severe MDMA toxicity is not necessarily dose dependent, and it may occur after the ingestion of a single tablet. Serious complications include hyperthermia; the toxic serotonin syndrome (see section V.B.5), which is characterized by mental status changes, neuromuscular overactivity, autonomic instability, and diarrhea; hyponatremia; hypoglycemia; hepatic necrosis; renal failure; seizures; and intracranial hemorrhage.

(2) **General treatment.** Unless a large recent ingestion is suspected, gastric decontamination has a limited role. Mortality correlates best with the degree of hyperthermia, and therefore aggressive **cooling** is indicated. Cardiac monitoring is also indicated. Other treatment follows the same principles as those for cocaine toxicity (see section V.B.9.a.(2)). Although **dantrolene** has been advocated for MDMA-intoxicated patients with temperatures above 41°C (105.8°F), others have found it to be of no benefit when the thermoregulatory mechanisms are overwhelmed. In the setting of catecholamine depletion from end-stage amphetamine toxicity, hypotension may be more responsive to direct-acting vasopressors (e.g., **norepinephrine**) than to **dopamine**. Treatment of hyponatremia related to MDMA toxicity depends on the determination of extracellular fluid volume status via physical examination, the measurement of central venous pressure or pulmonary capillary wedge pressure, and the assessment of urine electrolytes and osmolarity. In the absence of dehydration plus a history of excessive water intake, fluid restriction may be indicated. The use of hypertonic **saline**, **mannitol**, or loop diuretics may be considered for more severe cases. Forced acid diuresis, which historically was advocated to enhance the elimination of basic amphetamines, is no longer recommended.

(3) **Disposition and clinical relapse.** With the advent of long-acting preparations and particularly potent substances such as **methamphetamine**, medical observation for at least 24 hours is often warranted. Patients with only mild symptoms usually can be discharged after about 6 hours; they should be provided with appointments for follow-up psychiatric and medical care. Follow-up care is essential because withdrawal symptoms, such as depression, increased appetite, nausea, diarrhea, cramps, restlessness, and headache, may occur within 2 or 3 days after the abrupt cessation of **MDMA**, **cocaine**, or **amphetamines**.

c. **Hallucinogens** include synthetic and naturally occurring compounds that can be divided into the following two groups: **agents** that cause true hallucinations (i.e., perceptions of things that do not exist) and **psychedelic agents** that cause altered perceptions (i.e., distorted images of things that do exist). With the latter, however, the person having the altered perception may have some degree of awareness that the perception is not real. **PCP** (phencyclidine), **lysergic acid diethylamide** (LSD), **mescaline**, certain **mushrooms**, **jimsonweed**, and **amphetamine analogues** may all produce alterations of reality. Most patients who use hallucinogens do not seek medical attention, which is evidenced by the relatively low number of cases reported to poison centers in 2000 (e.g., lysergic acid diethylamide, 1,024; mescaline, 229; PCP, 555).

(1) **Manifestations**. These include agitation (this may be extreme in **PCP** intoxication), hypertension, nystagmus, seizures, hyperthermia, rhabdomyolysis, tachycardia, coma, hallucinations, and acute psychosis.

(2) **Treatment**. Initiate the ABCs. Treat agitation with **benzodiazepines**. When necessary, initiate rapid cooling through evaporative methods. If coingestants are suspected, **gastric decontamination** may be considered. Although acidification of the urine to enhance **PCP** elimination has been described historically, the amount cleared is small because the drug is 90% hepatically metabolized and is somewhat "acid trapped" in the stomach. The potential for myoglobinuric renal failure and worsening of systemic acidosis makes the use of acidification an unwarranted therapy. Nasogastric suction with multidose activated **charcoal** may be more beneficial.

Most patients with hallucinogen exposure require only a quiet environment and possibly sedation with benzodiazepines. They can generally be discharged after a period of observation, once their mental status normalizes. Patients with cardiovascular complications, seizures, severe agitation, renal dysfunction, or hyperpyrexia should be admitted to a medical unit.

d. **Alcohol (ethanol)** is the most commonly abused drug in our society. In 2000, 36,869 exposures were reported to poison centers. **Alcohol's** CNS depressant properties are primarily mediated by agonist activity at γ-aminobutyric acid A receptors. **Alcohol** overdose produces glycogen depletion (hypoglycemia), nausea, vomiting, dehydration, and CNS and respiratory depression. Most fatalities occur at levels greater than 400 mg per dL. **Thiamine** deficiency is common due to diminished absorption (see Chapter 12 for a detailed overview of the recognition and treatment of alcohol intoxication and withdrawal states).

e. **Opioid** intoxication is common, with 12,227 cases reported in the United States in 2000. Fatalities related to **heroin** have recently increased, based on the increased purity of the substance, the lowered cost, and the increasing age of the abusing population. Emergency department visits for complications from or overdoses with **oxycodone** and **hydrocodone** have more than doubled in the last several years. The clinical triad of **narcotic** overdose is characterized by CNS depression, pinpoint pupils, and hypoventilation (see Chapter 10). Response to **naloxone** during the initial stabilization of any patient presenting with CNS depression may quickly confirm the involvement of **opioids**. Prescription narcotics used in combination with **aspirin**, **acetaminophen**, **carisoprodol**, **caffeine**, or other substances may contribute to the clinical presentation.

(1) **Manifestations. Acute opioid overdosage** produces shallow or absent respirations, cyanosis, pupillary miosis, and unresponsiveness. Evidence of a fresh venipuncture wound or "tracks" due to repeated i.v. injections may be present; however, most heroin abusers insufflate the drug. Massive overdose may be associated with bradycardia or hypotension.

"Heroin pulmonary edema" can follow opioid use, even in a conscious person. It is noncardiogenic in nature, and it results from increased pulmonary vascular permeability. Cardiac function is usually normal, and hemodynamic abnormalities are generally absent.

(2) **Treatment. Assisted ventilation is begun** as soon as the patient reaches the treatment area. When **naloxone** is readily available, **tracheal intubation** is generally unnecessary. If

any delay in administering **naloxone** occurs, **tracheal intubation** should be performed.

Naloxone is a specific narcotic antagonist at CNS receptor sites. It quickly reverses coma and respiratory depression secondary to overdose with oral or i.v. **narcotics**. The usual dosage requirement is 0.4 to 2 mg for adults and 0.01 mg per kg in children. Continuous infusions of **naloxone** at two-thirds of the dose required per hour may be given to prompt awakening if resedation occurs. Continuous infusions or repeat boluses are often necessary, because most narcotics have a longer duration of action than **naloxone**. This is especially true for **methadone**; its effects may last for days. In general, infusions are titrated to achieve the desired clinical response. Higher doses of **naloxone** (2 to 10 mg) may be required initially to reverse the CNS depressant effects of **pentazocine** (Talwin) or the respiratory depression of **propoxyphene** (Darvon). **Emergence from opioid overdosage** is characterized by agitation and combativeness. Patients may harm themselves and medical staff. Therefore, if possible, **physical restraints** should be applied *before* **naloxone** is administered (see Chapter 26).

(a) **Decontamination.** For oral **opioid** ingestions, gastric decontamination as outlined above may be considered (see section V.A.2).

(b) **Pulmonary edema.** This is treated with oxygen and positive-pressure ventilation. Unless evidence of concomitant left ventricular failure or intravascular volume overload is found, the usual approaches to treatment (e.g., **diuretics, nitrates, afterload reduction**) are of no value, and they should be avoided.

(c) **Supportive care and disposition.** Supportive care is directed toward any residual symptoms that are not reversed by **naloxone**. Hypotension may require **crystalloid** infusions. For mixed ingestions, a search for the coingested product may direct the treatment toward more specific supportive measures. In general, once initial stabilization has been achieved, patients should be admitted and observed for the appearance of any recurrence of **narcotic** overdose symptoms or for the onset of symptoms of **narcotic** withdrawal. Serious complications from narcotic use include infections (e.g., abscess formation, endocarditis, pneumonia, tetanus), hepatic or GI dysfunction, and neuropathies.

f. **Benzodiazepines** are among the most widely used drugs in the world, but, when they are taken alone, they rarely produce serious poisoning. The class includes a number of antianxiety, anticonvulsant, and hypnotic agents (see also Chapters 9, 14, and 15).

(1) **Epidemiology.** In 2000, 49,849 benzodiazepine overdoses were reported to poison centers. Fatal overdose with any **benzodiazepine** taken alone is quite rare. As with other sedative-hypnotics, the therapeutic concentration ranges are wide, and they reflect individual differences in metabolism, accumulation, and tolerance. Benzodiazepine levels are not useful in the management of an acute overdose.

(2) **Manifestations.** Patients can present with muscle weakness, hypotonia, ataxia, dysarthria, and somnolence. Coma, respiratory depression, hypotension, and hypothermia may occur after very large ingestions or after i.v. administration.

(3) **Treatment**. Measures other than supportive care are seldom necessary. Forced diuresis and hemodialysis are not indicated. Gastric decontamination as discussed above may be considered.

Flumazenil (Romazicon) is a competitive **benzodiazepine** receptor antagonist that rapidly reverses benzodiazepine effects. Although **flumazenil** should elicit no effects when taken in the absence of benzodiazepines or related agents, its use in the presence of benzodiazepines can be associated with undesired effects, including agitation, anxiety, nausea, hypotension, dysrhythmias, increased intracranial pressure, and seizures. The incidence of seizures in high-risk overdose patients (i.e., those with jerking movements or abnormal vital signs) is 16%. **Flumazenil** use should be avoided in chronic benzodiazepine users; patients with a known seizure disorder; and patients who have ingested other drugs, especially TCAs. **Flumazenil** may be given at a dose of 0.1 mg over 1 minute, up to 1 mg. Because CNS depression related to benzodiazepine overdose is rarely life threatening, most cases can be managed with supportive care only.

g. **Barbiturates** are still commonly implicated drugs in deliberate self-poisoning.

(1) **Epidemiology**. In 2000, 4,484 cases of barbiturate toxicity were reported to American poison centers. Because of refinements in the principles of supportive care, the case fatality rate in **barbiturate** poisoning has recently fallen to the range of 1% or less. **Short-acting barbiturates**, such as **secobarbital** and **pentobarbital**, are the most frequently fatal after ingestion. **Long-acting barbiturates** (e.g., **phenobarbital**) have a somewhat wider margin of safety, but this varies based on individual tolerance. In general, serum **phenobarbital** concentrations of 100 to 120 µg per mL indicate severe intoxication, even in the tolerant patient. By contrast, the usual therapeutic plasma concentration for **phenobarbital** ranges from 15 to 40 µg per mL.

(2) **Manifestations**. The symptoms of poisoning are similar for all types of **barbiturates**. Drowsiness, nystagmus, ataxia, dysarthria, and somnolence occur in the early stages of poisoning or in mild cases. The larger the dose, the more profound the level of general CNS depression is. Deep coma, areflexia, muscle hypotonicity, apnea, hypotension, and hypothermia occur in the most serious cases. Barbiturates are known to form concretions when many pills are taken in a short period of time.

(3) **Treatment**. For **short-acting barbiturate poisoning**, treatment is usually limited to supportive care. Urinary alkalinization is of no value. **Secobarbital** and **pentobarbital** are poorly dialyzable.

Urinary alkalinization significantly enhances the excretion of **phenobarbital**. Multiple-dose activated **charcoal** therapy can also be considered. **Phenobarbital** is removed by **hemodialysis**, although this is reserved for patients with levels greater than 100 to 120 µg per mL, those who are hemodynamically unstable, or those who cannot tolerate a prolonged coma.

h. **Glutethimide** is no longer marketed in the United States. Nevertheless, 13 poisonings were reported in the United States in 2000. Because it is dangerous and because it may be ingested by persons who have obtained it elsewhere, a discussion of it is included here.

(1) **Epidemiology and pharmacology**. Because **glutethimide** is lipid soluble and it has a large volume of distribution, the plasma concentrations do not correlate well with the depth of coma. The usual therapeutic plasma concentration for **glutethimide** ranges from 5 to 15 µg per mL. However, nearly all individuals with moderate or severe intoxication have plasma concentrations greater than 20 µg per mL. Levels greater

than 40 or 50 μg per mL are almost always associated with deep coma. Single doses of 10 g or more (10 to 20 times the usual hypnotic dose) generally produce serious poisoning. A hydroxylated polar metabolite of **glutethimide** may contribute to its CNS depression.

(2) **Manifestations**. **Glutethimide** produces dose-dependent CNS depression like the **barbiturates**. **Glutethimide** has anticholinergic properties, and it frequently produces tachycardia, paralytic ileus, and mydriasis. Cardiovascular depression (hypotension, pulmonary edema) is also common in **glutethimide** poisoning. Similar to the **barbiturates**, **glutethimide** is known to form concretions.

(3) **Treatment**. Management should be supportive in nearly all cases. Treatment of hypotension by intravascular volume expansion should be done cautiously because of the hazard of pulmonary edema.

i. **Methaqualone**, a drug that has been considered illicit in the United States since 1984, was transiently, but extremely, popular as a drug of abuse and suicide.

   (1) **Epidemiology**. Most experience with **methaqualone** overdose comes from Europe, where a combination hypnotic preparation (**Mandrax**) containing **methaqualone** (250 mg) and **diphenhydramine** (25 mg) in each pill has been available.

   (2) **Manifestations**. In Mandrax poisoning, anticholinergic symptoms can be prominent. These include mydriasis, tachycardia, muscular rigidity, twitching, hyperreflexia, and seizures. **Overdose with methaqualone** alone usually produces **barbiturate**-like CNS depression. However, excitatory phenomena with a paradoxical increase in muscle tone with hyperreflexia, myoclonus, and seizure-like activity may be seen. Pulmonary edema may occur. Thrombocytopenia and coagulopathy are described in 20% of cases.

   (3) **Treatment**. Care is supportive. Gastric decontamination may be considered. Benzodiazepines may be used to control neuromuscular hyperexcitability. Vitamin K or fresh frozen plasma may be indicated to control any overdose emergent bleeding. Hemoperfusion has been used in severe overdoses or in patients whose levels are 100 to 150 μg per mL.

j. **Ethchlorvynol** (Placidyl) can produce serious intoxication. Fortunately, it is no longer manufactured in the United States. It is an uncommon agent of self-poisoning; only 48 cases were reported in 2000.

   (1) **Epidemiology**. Single ingestions of 15 g and plasma concentrations greater than 100 μg per mL are associated with severe intoxication.

   (2) **Manifestations**. Intravenous injection, a common method of abuse, results in noncardiogenic pulmonary edema. Other findings include prolonged coma, hypothermia, hypotension, and respiratory depression. The characteristic odor of **ethchlorvynol** detected in body fluids of intoxicated patients can be recognized by comparing it with the odor of a freshly opened **ethchlorvynol** capsule.

   (3) **Treatment**. Consider gastric decontamination in oral overdose. **Oxygen** and positive end-expiratory pressure ventilation may be required for pulmonary edema. **Ibuprofen** may reduce **ethchlorvynol**-induced pulmonary toxicity. **Activated charcoal** hemoperfusion has been used in cases of severe toxicity, but the indications are controversial.

k. **Meprobamate** (Miltown, Equanil)

   (1) **Epidemiology**. In 2000, 140 poisonings were reported. The elderly population is the primary user of this sedative-hypnotic.

(2) **Manifestations**. Symptoms after overdose resemble **barbiturate**-like intoxication, with all degrees of CNS depression described. In addition, the drug is maximally concentrated in the myocardium, and it may cause severe hypotension. **Meprobamate** may also form concretions after an overdose.

(3) **Treatment**. Gastric decontamination, including whole bowel irrigation, may be considered. Care is mostly supportive. Forced diuresis will enhance renal elimination, but it may also predispose the patient to pulmonary edema. The early use of vasopressors and inotropic agents to combat hypotension is advised to avoid fluid overload. Indications for hemoperfusion include cardiovascular instability or levels greater than 100 μg per mL.

l. **Carisoprodol** (Soma)

(1) **Epidemiology**. **Carisoprodol** is a centrally acting muscle relaxant that is metabolized to **meprobamate**; it has emerged as a significant drug of abuse. In 2000, 6,125 poisonings were reported. Certain formulations contain added salicylates or **codeine**. **Carisoprodol** is commonly abused together with **acetaminophen** combined with **codeine** or with **propoxyphene** or **hydrocodone**. The latter combination results in a "high" that is similar to that achieved by **heroin** abuse.

(2) **Manifestations**. Both CNS stimulation and depression can occur. Fatalities from respiratory depression with aspiration have been described. Tachycardia, hypotension, nystagmus, intermittent agitation, seizures, and prolonged coma have been reported.

(3) **Treatment**. Care is supportive. Gastric decontamination can be considered. **Flumazenil** *should be avoided*. Extracorporeal elimination has not been reported. Examination for toxic **acetaminophen** and salicylate levels is warranted.

m. **Chloral hydrate** overdosage is not common at the present time; only 226 cases were reported in 2000. An overdose with **chloral hydrate** can be severe, and its manifestations may sometimes be confused with **opioid** overdose.

(1) **Manifestations**. Signs include hypotension, ventricular arrhythmias, respiratory depression, noncardiogenic pulmonary edema, and miosis. Deep coma can develop rapidly (i.e., within 30 minutes).

(2) **Treatment**. Management usually consists of the administration of **activated charcoal**. For more severe situations, **airway support**, **gastric decontamination**, and **naloxone** (2 mg i.v.) may be necessary. Hypotension is treated with **crystalloid** therapy. When no response occurs, the administration of **norepinephrine** is indicated. Other catecholamine vasopressors should be avoided because they may be prodysrhythmic. Premature ventricular contractions, ventricular tachycardia, and *torsade de pointes* have all been observed. When premature ventricular contractions and ventricular tachycardia are unresponsive to **lidocaine** (1 mg per kg i.v.), **propranolol** may be helpful (1 mg i.v., to a total of 5 mg). For *torsade de pointes,* **isoproterenol, atropine**, **magnesium sulfate**, or **ventricular pacing** may be required. Respiratory complications are treated with supportive measures. Although **flumazenil** (Romazicon) has been reported to improve **chloral hydrate**-induced respiratory depression, hypotension, and miosis, its use has also been shown to cause ventricular tachycardia. **Flumazenil** use for the routine treatment of overdose with **chloral hydrate** is not recommended at the present time.

C. **Identification, Evaluation, and Treatment of Intoxication from Other Agents**

1. **Acetaminophen**. *This agent is responsible for more pharmaceutical-related deaths than is any other substance. In 2000, 108,066 poisonings were reported in the United States.*
   a. **Manifestations**. Soon after ingestion, the patient may exhibit mild GI symptoms, or, more commonly, he or she will be asymptomatic. Within 24 hours, subclinical evidence of hepatic injury occurs as transaminase levels become elevated. Untreated patients or those who present beyond 8 hours of ingestion may go on to develop fulminant hepatic or renal failure within 72 to 96 hours.
   Because of the lack of early clinical signs of toxicity, performing an acetaminophen level on all patients with intentional drug overdose is imperative. In the setting of acute ingestion (where the exact time of ingestion is known), this level may be plotted on the Rumack-Matthews nomogram to determine the patient's risk for hepatotoxicity. In other situations, empiric antidotal treatment is indicated.
   b. **Treatment**. *N*-acetylcysteine (**Mucomyst**) is a very effective antidote to **acetaminophen**-induced toxicity. The dose is 140 mg per kg p.o. as a loading dose, followed by 70 mg per kg every 4 hours for 17 additional doses. *N*-acetylcysteine should be started as soon as possible after acute acetaminophen ingestion, but it should not be withheld in those presenting late. *N*-acetylcysteine is indicated in those patients who have chronically overused acetaminophen, staggered their ingestion, presented with an unknown time of ingestion, or ingested extended-release formulations or in those who have been nutritionally deprived due to alcohol.
2. **Salicylates**. Salicylate overdose is common; it accounted for 25,394 reports to poison centers in 2000. Toxicity may be acute or chronic in nature. Neurons are most seriously impacted by the ability of salicylates to uncouple oxidative phosphorylation. Central manifestations of toxicity include hyperpnea, agitation, seizures, lethargy, coma, tinnitus, and hyperpyrexia. Other findings include noncardiogenic pulmonary edema, renal failure, nausea, vomiting, acid-base disturbances, and rarely cardiac dysrhythmias. Irreversible neurologic injury may occur if patients are not aggressively managed.
   a. **Treatment**. Continuous cardiac monitoring and pulse oximetry is indicated. Gastric decontamination, as outlined above in section V.A.2, may be considered. Multidose **activated charcoal** may be administered. Careful hydration should be instituted, along with glucose supplementation and urinary alkalinization. Alkalinization is generally accomplished by administering **sodium bicarbonate**, 1 to 2 mEq per kg i.v., followed by an infusion of 100 to 150 mEq **sodium bicarbonate** per L of D5W at 1.5 times the maintenance fluid rate (see section V.A.3.b) to achieve a target urine pH of 7.5. **Potassium** supplementation is generally required to accomplish urinary alkalinization. Salicylate level, urine pH, electrolytes, glucose, and arterial blood gas should be monitored every 1 to 2 hours, which generally requires placing the patient in an intensive care unit setting.
   Hemodialysis effectively enhances the elimination of salicylates, and thus it is indicated for patients with seizures or other neurologic symptoms, renal failure or oliguria, pulmonary edema, intractable acidosis, inability to alkalinize the urine, levels greater than 90 mg per dL in acute overdose and greater than 60 mg per dL with chronic toxicity, or clinical deterioration despite full medical support.
3. **Toxic alcohols**. Toxic alcohol ingestion is common, with 2,737 **methanol**, 4,884 **ethylene glycol**, and 18,870 **isopropanol** exposures reported in 2000. Even small doses (single swallows) of **methanol** and **ethylene glycol**, usually as radiator coolant or antifreeze, may cause toxicity. A latent period before the development of symptoms is characteristic for both **eth-**

ylene glycol and **methanol** toxicity, especially when **ethanol** has been coingested. Because early treatment improves prognosis, therapy should begin immediately based on clinical suspicion of exposure to **ethylene glycol** or **methanol**. This should involve the rapid correction of acidosis with **sodium bicarbonate**, cofactor administration, and **alcohol** dehydrogenase antagonism with either **ethanol** or **4-methylpyrazole** (see below). Because the presence of acidosis in the setting of exposure to either substance indicates toxic metabolite accumulation, immediate consultation for hemodialysis should be made, even before laboratory confirmation of toxic **ethylene glycol** or **methanol** levels.

a. Methanol (wood **alcohol**) is a common solvent that is oxidatively metabolized by the liver to formic acid. It can cause blindness and irreversible neurologic injury. The presence of **methanol** and its major toxic metabolite, formic acid, results in a characteristic "double-gap" (both anion and osmolal gap) acidosis. The so-called blind staggers of **methanol** intoxication are a characteristic, but late, finding.

(1) Manifestations. In addition to visual disturbances, these include CNS depression, tachypnea, abdominal pain, nausea and vomiting, clammy skin, seizures, and metabolic acidosis. Impaired vision ranging from blurred vision to blindness may also be present, as may hyperemia of the optic disk and papilledema.

(2) Treatment. Initiate the **ABCs** and general supportive care, including i.v. administration of 50% **dextrose** in water, **naloxone**, and **thiamine**. Correction of the metabolic acidosis is achieved with **sodium bicarbonate** (1 mEq per kg). Intravenous **alcohol (ethanol)** administration, using a loading dose of 10 mL per kg of 10% **alcohol** and then a continuous drip of 1.5 mL per kg per hour of 10% **alcohol**, competitively inhibits the production of formic acid because of **alcohol's** higher affinity for the enzyme alcohol dehydrogenase. An alternative competitive inhibitor is **4-methylpyrazole (Antizol)**. **Folic acid** (as **leucovorin**) may be given at a dose of 1 mg per kg every 4 hours. Hemodialysis should be initiated when the **methanol** level is greater than 25 mg per dL or when acidosis, visual disturbances, or renal failure is present.

b. Ethylene glycol, which is usually ingested as radiator coolant, antifreeze, or windshield washer fluid, also requires **alcohol** dehydrogenase for its metabolism. Multiple toxic organic acids, including oxalic acid, glyoxylic acid, and glycolic acid, are formed. Characteristically, these acids may cause renal tubular necrosis and renal failure, but multiple organ systems may be affected.

(1) Manifestations. Inebriation is seen within 2 to 12 hours of ingestion, after which cardiopulmonary symptoms such as tachycardia, hypertension, and pulmonary edema develop. Hypocalcemia and myositis are common during this stage. At 24 to 72 hours, renal failure occurs in two-thirds of untreated patients. Delayed cranial neuropathy may be seen.

(2) Treatment. Care is similar to that for **methanol** poisoning. In addition, **thiamine**, 100 mg, and **pyridoxine**, 50 mg, are given every 6 hours, theoretically to enhance the formation of nontoxic metabolites.

c. Isopropanol (**isopropyl alcohol**, rubbing **alcohol**). Intoxication may be suspected based on apparent inebriation in which the odor of acetone, rather than ethanol, is detected on the breath.

(1) Manifestations. The patient may complain of headache or dizziness and may exhibit neuromuscular incoordination, confusion, and nystagmus. Severe ingestions may result in deep coma that is prolonged compared with that seen with ethanol. Respiratory depression or failure may occur. **Isopropanol** is a GI irritant; therefore, hematemesis or GI bleeding may be seen. Hypotension portends a poor prognosis.

(2) **Treatment.** Unlike with **methanol** and **ethylene glycol**, **alcohol** dehydrogenase antagonism with **ethanol** or **4-methylpyrazole** is not indicated in treatment of isopropranol. Hypotension should be managed with fluids and vasopressors as needed. When the patient remains hypotensive or has further vital sign deterioration despite these measures, dialysis is indicated. Some authors also recommend dialysis for **isopropyl alcohol** serum levels greater than 400 mg per dL. Coma itself is not an indication for dialysis, but it may necessitate the use of mechanical ventilation. Care is otherwise supportive, including rewarming, the administration of **thiamine**, evaluation for hypoglycemia, and monitoring for GI bleeding.

4. **Pesticides.** Anticholinesterase inhibition is usually caused by the **organophosphate insecticides**; less frequently, poisonings involve the **carbamate insecticides**. Poison centers received reports of 11,874 organophosphate and 3,754 carbamate exposures in 2000.

a. **Bond formation. Organophosphates** form a covalent, spontaneously irreversible bond with acetylcholinesterase, thus producing a cholinergic crisis. This bond, however, is pharmacologically reversible if **pralidoxime** is given before pesticide binding to acetylcholinesterase becomes irreversible (i.e., usually within 24 to 36 hours). **Carbamates** also bond to cholinesterase enzymes, but this bonding is spontaneously reversible within 6 to 8 hours.

b. **Manifestations.** These include stimulation of both muscarinic and nicotinic receptors. **Peripheral muscarinic symptoms** produce the symptom complex remembered by the mnemonic **DUMBBELS** as follows: *d*iarrhea, *u*rination, *m*iosis, *b*radycardia, *b*ronchorrhea, *e*mesis, *l*acrimation, and *s*alivation. Other effects may include hypotension or hypertension. **Nicotinic symptoms** include fasciculations, cramps, weakness, paralysis, cyanosis, and respiratory arrest. Tachycardia and hypertension may be seen early, as a result of initial stimulation of the autonomic ganglia.

   ECG findings may show almost any abnormality, from asystole to sinus tachycardia. In general, sinus tachycardia predominates initially as a result of nicotinic autonomic ganglion excitation. Later, parasympathetic tone predominates, causing sinus bradycardia and conduction delays and blocks. QT prolongation may occur.

c. **Laboratory findings.** These should establish low levels of **cholinesterase activity** in both the plasma (**pseudocholinesterase**) and red blood cells (**true cholinesterase**). **Red blood cell cholinesterase** is believed to be more accurately and more closely related to the severity of the toxicity, although **plasma cholinesterase** levels generally are more readily available.

d. **Treatment**

   (1) **Decontamination** should begin with removing all clothing from the patient, and the skin should be scrubbed by personnel wearing protective clothing and gloves to prevent contamination of their own skin. **Gastric lavage** and **activated charcoal** are indicated.

   (2) **Supportive measures** should focus on airway management and control, because copious secretions, bronchospasm, respiratory muscle paralysis, and vomiting may be present.

   (3) **Cardiac monitoring and i.v. access are mandatory**.

   (4) **Atropine** competitively antagonizes **acetylcholine's** actions at the muscarinic receptors, thereby reversing parasympathetic

overstimulation. Initial doses should be 1 to 2 mg i.v. in adults and 0.05 mg per kg in children. Doses may be repeated as needed every 10 to 15 minutes. The therapeutic end point is the drying of pulmonary secretions.

   (5) **Pralidoxime chloride** reactivates cholinesterases if it is given within 24 to 36 hours of exposure. This ameliorates toxicity occurring at both muscarinic and nicotinic sites, and it reverses the neuromuscular findings. Patients who require **atropine** therapy generally also require **pralidoxime**. A typical regimen for adults consists of an initial dose of 1 to 2 g i.v. over 15 to 30 minutes; subsequent doses are given 1 to 2 hours after the first dose and then every 6 to 8 hours as needed. Some authorities recommend that, to achieve therapeutic concentrations, about 500 mg per h needs to be infused until sustained improvement is noted.

  e. Disposition. Asymptomatic patients may require prolonged observation if they have been exposed to lipid-soluble agents (e.g., **chlorfenthion** or **fenthion**) or to those that require conversion to the active pesticide. All symptomatic patients should be admitted to a medical unit, and appropriate antidotes should be administered. Although clinical relapse is rare if the initial treatment is appropriate, months may be required for red blood cell cholinesterase to return to normal levels. Headaches, memory impairment, confusion, depression, and peripheral neuropathies commonly persist for some time in patients with significant exposures.

D. Mixed Drug Overdose

This is almost as common as poisoning with single drugs. Diagnosis, treatment, and prognostication are somewhat more complicated than for a single-drug overdose. Clinicians dealing with psychotropic drug overdose must always consider the possibility that more than one drug is involved. **Acetaminophen** is the most common coingestant, so serum levels of acetaminophen should be obtained in all patients with intentional overdose. Some of the more common "cocktails" follow.

  1. Alcohol and sedative-hypnotics are a dangerous combination because they cause CNS depression that is at least additive (see Chapters 10 through 12). Evidence suggests that chronic **alcohol** use can retard the metabolism of other CNS depressants (e.g., **chloral hydrate**).

  2. Phenothiazines and TCAs are coprescribed, and, in other countries, they are sometimes marketed in fixed combinations. Anticholinergic manifestations are prominent in poisoning with these mixtures. The mixtures used dictate the treatment. Because phenothiazines and TCAs often have common unwanted effects (e.g., prolonged cardiac conduction, anticholinergic effects), the toxicities from the combinations are often additive.

E. Withdrawal Toxidromes

The abrupt cessation of many substances can cause a complex group of symptoms that mimics a psychiatric emergency. **Alcohol, barbiturates, benzodiazepines, γ-hydroxybutyrate or its analogues, cocaine, amphetamines**, and **opioids** are but a few. Chapters 9, 10, 12, and 14 should be consulted for further details on the withdrawal syndromes associated with **alcohol, opioids**, and **sedative-hypnotics**. The manifestations of withdrawal are varied, including diarrhea, hypertension, mydriasis, tachycardia, insomnia, hyperthermia, lacrimation, hallucination, cramps, yawning, piloerection, depression, anxiety, and seizures. The agent involved largely dictates the treatment, but supportive measures include i.v. access, cardiac monitoring, hyperthermia control, and hypertension control. Seizures may generally be treated with i.v. **lorazepam** (usually 1 mg, but up to 4 mg may be required). Observation with close medical follow-up may be all that is needed for patients who present with mild withdrawal symptoms. For patients with dysrhythmias, hallucinations, hyperthermia, seizures, or symptomatic hypertension, hospitalization in a medical unit is generally required.

F. Clinical Relapse

Although not a **toxidrome** *per se*, clinical relapse refers to a phenomenon in the course of overdose treatment in which clinical worsening follows a period of improvement. It has been reported with almost every psychotropic drug. **Glutethimide, meprobamate, lithium,** and **TCAs** are the most commonly implicated drugs. **Glutethimide** and **meprobamate** use has significantly decreased, as noted above, in the last several decades.

1. **Etiology.** *The etiology of the clinical relapse phenomenon is not clear.* At least three mechanisms are theoretically possible.

   a. **The parent drug and its active metabolites** are initially "tied up" in the enterohepatic circulation, but they are subsequently released into the systemic circulation.

   b. **A portion of the ingested agent is initially unabsorbed** from the GI tract due to poor splanchnic circulation, and concretions are formed. When hypotension is treated and splanchnic blood flow is restored, the remaining quantity is rapidly absorbed.

   c. **Highly lipid-soluble drugs** (e.g., **glutethimide**, short-acting **barbiturates**) are initially distributed into lipid storage sites other than the brain. At a later time, after adequate cardiac output is restored and blood flow to these sites increases, the drug reappears in the systemic circulation.

2. **Manifestations.** The signs and symptoms of relapse include worsening of neurologic, hemodynamic, and respiratory status. Serum concentrations of the drug may rise. Deterioration usually follows a period of clinical improvement ranging from a few hours to a few days after drug ingestion.

3. **Treatment.** Management consists of continued supportive care. The possibility of relapse underscores the need for continued close monitoring after clinical improvement occurs.

ADDITIONAL READING

American Academy of Clinical Toxicology, European Association of Poison Control Centers. Position statements: ipecac syrup, gastric lavage, single-dose activated charcoal, whole bowel irrigation, cathartics. *Clin Toxicol* 1997;35:699–762.

American Academy of Clinical Toxicology, European Association of Poison Control Centers. Position statement and practice guidelines on the use of multi-dose activated charcoal in the treatment of acute poisoning. *Clin Toxicol* 1999;37:731–751.

American College of Emergency Physicians. Policy statement: management of elder abuse and neglect. *Ann Emerg Med* 1998;31:149–150.

American Heart Association. *BLS for healthcare providers.* Dallas: American Heart Association, 2001.

American Medical Association. *Diagnostic and treatment guidelines on domestic violence.* Chicago: American Medical Association, 1992.

Berkowitz CA. Child abuse and neglect. In: Tintinalli J, Kelen G, Stapczynski S, eds. *Emergency medicine, a comprehensive study guide,* 5th ed. New York: McGraw-Hill, 2000:1949–1952.

Canto JG, Shlipak MG, Rogers WJ. Prevalence, clinical characteristics, and mortality among patients with myocardial infarction presenting without chest pain. *JAMA* 2000;283:3223–3229.

Centers for Disease Control and Prevention. Influenza activity, United States, 2000–2001 season. *MMWR Morb Mortal Wkly Rep* 2000;49:1085–1087.

Centers for Disease Control and Prevention. Recommendations and reports, prevention and control of influenza. *MMWR Morb Mortal Wkly Rep* 2000;49(RR-03):1–46. Available at http://www.cdc.gov/mmwr/PDF/rr/rr4903/pdf. Accessed November, 2002.

Eisenberg MS, Mengert T. Cardiac resuscitation. *N Engl J Med* 2001;344:1304–1313.

Feldhaus KA. Female and male sexual assault. In: Tintinalli J, Kelen G, Stapczynski S, eds. *Emergency medicine, a comprehensive study guide,* 5th ed. New York: McGraw-Hill, 2000:1953–1955.

Gallagher J. Acute abdominal pain. In: Tintinalli J, Kelen G, Stapczynski S, eds. *Emergency medicine, a comprehensive study guide,* 5th ed. New York: McGraw-Hill, 2000:497–515.

Litovitz TL, Klein-Schwartz W, White SR, et al. 2000 Annual report of the American Association of Poison Control Centers Toxic Exposure Surveillance System. *Am J Emerg Med* 2001;19:337–395.

Mills KC. Tricyclic antidepressants, newer antidepressants and serotonin syndrome, monoamine oxidase inhibitors. In: Tintinalli J, Kelen G, Stapczynski S, eds. *Emergency medicine, a comprehensive study guide,* 5th ed. New York: McGraw-Hill, 2000:1063–1085.

Muelleman RA, Lenaghan PA, Pakisser PA. Battered women: injury location and types. *Ann Emerg Med* 1996;28:486–492.

Olshaker JS, Browne B, Jerrard DA, et al. Medical clearance and screening of psychiatric patients in the emergency department. *Acad Emerg Med* 1997;4:124–128.

Olson KR. *Poisoning & drug overdose,* 3rd ed. Stamford, CT: Appleton & Lange, 1999.

Salber P, Taliaferro EH. Domestic violence. In: Tintinalli J, Kelen G, Stapczynski S, eds. *Emergency medicine, a comprehensive study guide,* 5th ed. New York: McGraw-Hill, 2000:1956–1960.

Taliaferro EH, Salber PR. Abuse in the elderly and impaired. In: Tintinalli J, Kelen G, Stapczynski S, eds. *Emergency medicine, a comprehensive study guide,* 5th ed. New York: McGraw-Hill, 2000:1960–1962.

Valenzuela TD, Nichol G, Clark LL, et al. Outcomes of rapid defibrillation by security officers after cardiac arrest in casinos. *N Engl J Med* 2000;343:1206–1209.

White SR. Nonbenzodiazepine sedative-hypnotics. In: Tintinalli JE, Ruiz E, Krome RL, eds. *Emergency medicine, a comprehensive study guide,* 4th ed. New York: McGraw-Hill, 1994:761–764.

4. DISSOCIATIVE, SOMATOFORM, AND PARANOID DISORDERS

Richard I. Shader
Katharine A. Phillips

This chapter reviews a group of disorders that are among the more interesting and challenging disorders that clinicians encounter. In addition, dissociative disorders should be considered in the differential diagnosis of patients with dementia, delirium, confusion, and amnesia (see Chapter 5). In some ways, this cluster of disorders is prototypical of what would have in the past been considered the "nonorganic" forms of mental disturbance. The paranoias are included here because of some overlapping features. Patients with obsessive-compulsive disorder may also show features similar to those of several somatoform disorders (i.e., body dysmorphic disorder and hypochondriasis). Because of the severity of obsessive-compulsive disorder and the availability of treatments approved for this specific diagnosis, obsessive-compulsive disorder is discussed separately in Chapter 6.

I. Dissociative and Somatoform Disorders

For many of the following disorders, patients' complaints or behaviors may suggest physical illness, dysfunction, or impairment. For some of these disorders to follow or to occur during the course of a physical illness or after an injury (e.g., seizure disorders, head injury) is not unusual. They may occur as distinct disorders, in conjunction with each other, or as partial features of other disorders. Unconscious coping styles (see Chapter 1) and conscious motivation and behavior may be factors in their development.

Clinicians are often frustrated or even angered by these patients because generally they do not respond to reassurance when the workup does not reveal a serious underlying physical disorder; the patients may respond by "doctor shopping." A clinician who receives requests for records from another clinician or facility may find that contacting the new doctor to review concerns and impressions is worthwhile. When clinicians do not compare notes consistently, a few patients may consume unwarranted amounts of clinician time and health care dollars, and they may be exposed to unnecessary tests, medical treatment, or surgery.

A. Dissociative Disorders

These conditions involve alterations or disturbances in memory, consciousness, and identity. Some may have a sudden onset and they may be temporary; others may be gradual in onset and chronic in course. When these disorders have a sudden onset and a brief duration, some clinicians prefer to use the terms **acute stress reaction** and **brief reactive dissociative disorder** to describe **dissociative fugue** and **dissociative amnesia**.

1. **Dissociative amnesia** involves the selective exclusion of important personal information or experiences from the memory, usually after a stressful or traumatic experience. The lost memories may not be retrieved for hours; in rare instances, they may remain unrecovered for a lifetime. The extent of the anterograde memory loss, which is sudden in onset, in dissociative amnesia is too extensive to be dismissed as mere forgetting. A single episode of dissociative amnesia is most common, but, if repeated experiences of extreme stress or trauma occur, multiple episodes are possible. The precipitating stress or trauma is usually quite severe (e.g., a threat to one's life, combat, injury, or being the perpetrator or victim of an unacceptable act).

The recovery of memory may be spontaneous, or it may be aided by hypnosis (see Chapter 23) or the use of intravenous **amobarbital**. (*Note: Although procedures for the **amobarbital** interview were widely known and taught in the post-World War II era, this diagnostic method is rarely used today.*) Once memory is recovered, the return of what was excluded from the individual's consciousness is generally complete; by contrast, the memory loss from a concussion is usually retrograde and the recovery is gradual. However, for dissociative amnesia to follow an injury, including a head injury, or a seizure disorder is not unusual. Posttraumatic stress disorder with concomitant dissociative amnesia may develop as a sequela of certain stressful traumatic experiences (see Chapter 14).

2. **Dissociative fugue** and **dissociative amnesia** are sometimes considered forms of what used to be called dissociative hysteria. Dissociative fugue is also sudden in onset, and it involves an inability to recall one's identity, rather than memory loss for a period of time. Unplanned travel, usually to a distant location where the affected person is not likely to be recognized or known, occurs; and a new identity, either partial or complete, is assumed. The travel is purposeful; it does not appear to be aimless wandering. The loss of knowledge of one's real identity and past almost invariably includes a loss of knowledge of one's birthplace and birth date. As with dissociative amnesia, dissociative fugue may occur after an acute stress. **Alcohol** consumption or substance abuse at the time of onset is common.

Dissociative fugue is rare. Its prevalence rate in the United States is under 0.3%. Nevertheless, most large urban emergency or psychiatric departments can recount a few such cases. As with dissociative amnesia, hypnosis or intravenous **amobarbital** may prove helpful. Supportive discussion and psychotherapy that encourages remembering usually lead to a gradual recovery of the patient's true identity and the events preceding the onset of the fugue. Concomitant central nervous system pathology (e.g., seizure disorder) may also be present. Some persons who appear to have dissociative fugue may actually be malingering or lying for obvious secondary gain (e.g., after embezzlement); in contrast, dissociative fugue and other dissociative disorders are generally thought to arise from unconscious reality-distorting coping mechanisms.

Dissociative fugue may overlap with certain culturally syntonic states, such as *amok* among Pacific Island peoples, *pibloktoq* or "Arctic hysteria" among Greenland Eskimos, or *grisi siknis* among the Miskito Indians of Nicaragua.

3. **Dissociative identity disorder (DID; formerly called multiple personality disorder)** involves the coping strategy of developing two or more distinct personalities unconsciously, each of which usually has a distinct name, as a way of "living with" overwhelming circumstances. Typically, this dissociative adaptation develops in the aftermath of intrafamilial childhood sexual or physical abuse. Whether thinking of such patients as defensively forming additional personalities or, alternatively, seeing them as having an incompletely or inadequately formed personality (i.e., one that permits different aspects of an unintegrated and unregulated personality to emerge) is more accurate remains unresolved. Most DID patients are not forthcoming about their various personalities, which are sometimes called **alters**, even when they are aware of them. The various personalities tend to be distinctive and to dominate or control the patient's behavior when they are operant. Some patients experience a sense of struggle for dominance among their alters. A shifting importance to the role of each personality over time and of the time spent in each alter may be seen. Each personality may have its own set of relationships.

Personalities may emerge during religious or magic-related rites. Some clinicians believe these latter patients should be in a distinct diagnostic category (i.e., **trance** or **possession disorder**). For one personality to be "good" and highly moral and for at least one other to be willful, irresponsible, mischievous, sexual, carefree, or "bad" is not uncommon. The formation of multiple personalities is likely a way of emotionally managing betrayal by a trusted parent or parental figure. One personality remains unstained by the events from childhood; another part perpetuates or justifies them as follows: "I wasn't betrayed; I like the immoral life."

Pediatricians, emergency department clinicians, and others involved in the acute care of victims of sexual and physical abuse should make appropriate referrals to try to prevent the development of DID (see Chapter 27). Clinicians who learn of childhood sexual and physical abuse from their adult patients should be alert to the possibility of DID. Treatment of DID is complex; it is best undertaken by a specialist in DID, so referral is indicated.

4. **Depersonalization disorder** is another dissociative disorder. **Depersonalization** as a symptom refers to an altered sense of self. One may feel unreal, like an automaton; as if in a dream or detached or estranged from one's body or its mental representations or from one's surroundings; or as if one is outside of oneself and is looking in, observing one's own mental processes or body. **Derealization** refers to a change in one's relationship to or awareness of one's environment that creates a feeling of unreality or estrangement. To describe depersonalization, one might say, "I feel strange." When describing derealization, one might say, "My world or my surroundings feel strange."

Depersonalization and derealization may be transient phenomena; however, they also can occur together. Both symptoms may be noted by patients who are taking particular medications or drugs (e.g., tricyclic antidepressants, medications with antihistaminic properties, **lysergic acid diethylamide** [LSD]), many of which alter the serotonergic systems. Patients who are extremely anxious or depressed may report depersonalization. Childhood trauma appears to be an additional risk factor. Some authors note the co-occurrence of depersonalization with obsessive-compulsive and panic-like symptoms, which suggests a linkage to perturbations in serotonergic activity. Some support for this hypothesis derives both from the reduction in depersonalization experiences that some patients have with proserotonergic agents and from the production of depersonalization experiences by the 5-hydroxytryptamine $(HT)_{2c}$ agonist **m-chlorophenylpiperazine**. Limited data from imaging studies suggest that depersonalization represents a dissociation of perceptions; functional abnormalities have been noted in sequential hierarchical areas of the sensory cortex and in areas responsible for an integrated body schema.

Depersonalization disorder is diagnosed when depersonalization or derealization persists or recurs episodically, it does not occur exclusively during the course of another mental disorder, and it is not due to use of a substance. In depersonalization disorder, reality testing is intact; therefore, depersonalization disorder is not a delusional state. In addition to the descriptions of feelings noted above, patients with depersonalization disorder may complain of difficulty feeling their own emotions, or they may see others as lifeless, less dimensional, or "cardboard-like." Body parts, particularly limbs, may feel distorted in size or shape. Most patients are distressed by these experiences.

Typically, clinicians are alerted to this disorder by the difficulty the patients have in describing what they have been feeling and how they resort to metaphor to try to explain it. Generally, no readily apparent experience-linked or stress-linked etiology or precipitant is present in depersonalization disorder. In the authors' experience, it occurs in susceptible people at times of transition (physiologic, psychic, or environmental), and it is associated with impaired arousal.

Treatment for depersonalization disorder is based on anecdotal and case reports. One pattern emerges from these reports—a suggestion that medications that increase synaptic dopamine (e.g., amphetamines, **methylphenidate**, monoamine oxidase inhibitors, **bupropion**) may be beneficial. Another treatment approach involves the use of proserotonergic agents (e.g., **clomipramine**, selective serotonin reuptake inhibitors [SSRIs]) combined with a benzodiazepine (e.g., **clonazepam**). This latter strategy is supported by several small sample nonblinded studies, case reports, and unverified testimonials on the World Wide Web (Internet). The co-occurrence of obsessive-compulsive symptomatology with depersonalization may suggest a positive response to proserotonergic agents. Because no criteria for when and how to treat depersonalization disorder are universally accepted, a conservative approach is recommended. Medication trials may be considered for patients who are distressed or impaired by their symptoms, but only when the symptoms persist. When appropriate, patients may need to be informed that their condition is not a customary indication (see Appendix I) for these medications. A good step for risk management is obtaining and documenting a second opinion.

5. **Acute amnesia or memory impairment from drugs and alcohol**
    a. **Pathologic intoxication with alcohol,** which is sometimes called the syndrome of alcohol idiosyncratic intoxication or *mania à potu,* may also be a cause of amnesia; it is discussed here for perspective. Some of these cases may actually be cases of dissociative disorder. The amnesia is manifested as an anterograde loss of episodic memory and not as a loss of information in long-term storage. Affected people (usually males), who may have an idiosyncratic sensitivity to **alcohol**, behave in a disinhibited manner that typically involves senseless violent acts after drinking small amounts of **alcohol**, amounts that are usually so little that the person does not appear to others to be intoxicated. (*Note: In some instances, patients may merely be using their consumption of **alcohol** as an excuse for unacceptable behavior.*) Such outbursts are generally followed by a period of extended sleep that again is out of proportion to the amount of **alcohol** ingested and by amnesia for the events.

    When a patient is in this state, anyone who is trying to help should approach the patient in a calm, nonchallenging way, as confrontation usually escalates the patient's potential for violence. Because the state will pass, the safest route may be no intervention. Nevertheless, small parenteral doses of benzodiazepines (e.g., **diazepam, lorazepam, midazolam**) may be used for sedation. Once a predisposition for pathologic intoxication with alcohol is recognized, prevention by abstinence is the best treatment (see Chapter 11 for a brief perspective on alcoholism).

    b. **Drug-induced amnesia** or the impairment of registration and retention of memory without accompanying violence or excessive sleep can be seen after the ingestion or parenteral use of **alcohol, scopolamine**, and many benzodiazepines (e.g., **diazepam, lorazepam, triazolam, midazolam**). Usually, the individual has a memory gap for some hours after drug administration. New experiences and new learning may not be retained. This form of memory impairment may be dose related, and sensitivity to it varies among patients. Repression does not seem to be involved in these drug-induced amnesic states. Because of their potential for amnesic effects, the use of oral benzodiazepines is not recommended to reduce the anxiety associated with learning speeches, studying for examinations, or other similar situations.

B. **Somatoform Disorders**
    1. **Conversion disorder** is considered a form of somatoform disorder in which the unconsciously motivated dysfunction or impairment involves the voluntary muscle or sensory nervous systems. Patients present with impairments, usually of acute onset (e.g., "I woke up and couldn't move my right hand"), which on physical examination do not conform to the expected patterns of muscle groups or dermatomes or to known

pathophysiologic mechanisms (e.g., glove or stocking pattern anesthesia may be present). Conversion disorder involves motor impairment (e.g., gait disturbance or ataxia, tremor, paralysis or weakness, swallowing, or aphonia) or sensory impairment (anesthesia, usually in the form of numbness; hyperesthesia in the form of burning sensations in the head or abdomen; blindness or diminished visual fields [tunnel vision]; or deafness). Episodic seizures or vomiting may also be encountered.

With conversion disorder, in addition to the lack of correspondence to known bodily dysfunctions, information obtained from the patient (or others when necessary) should reveal a temporal connection between the onset or exacerbation and some stressful experience or heightened emotional state. The impairment unconsciously allows avoidance, gets the patient "off the hook," or sanctions access to support or care. Once the patient's history is understood, seeing that the patient's symptoms have meaning and derive from unconscious motivations (e.g., a fear of being aggressive) and produce some form of gain for the patient (e.g., control of others) should be possible. However, the reader should note that the motivations involved often reflect complex needs and concerns and that the underlying unconscious factors and their significance or meaning may not be readily apparent without extensive exploration. Alternatively, one can see the dysfunction in conversion disorder as a nonverbal communication that should be understandable once the message is decoded.

Treatment is directed at symptom removal, and it is most likely to succeed when the disorder is of recent onset. Because conversion disorder may occur in response to some distressing physical illness, treatment of the underlying disorder, when possible, is usually the first step. As with the dissociative disorders, hypnosis (see Chapter 23) or intravenous **amobarbital** or benzodiazepines may be helpful (at the present time, these drugs are used only infrequently in the United States). As in other somatoform disorders, an effort should be made to redirect the patient's attention and focus away from the impairment and to shift them toward the events and issues that provoked it. If an identifiable stressor is involved, the patient may need help in resolving or mastering it. Any reinforcing factors should be identified and reduced or eliminated. This process may be particularly problematic in treating the somatoform disorders, because the very tests (e.g., electromyogram, computed tomography, magnetic resonance imaging) needed to rule out or establish contributing physical factors may spur the patient on to find another clinician with an even more sophisticated test.

2. **Somatization disorder** is the current diagnostic term for many patients that were previously said to be suffering from hysteria or, more recently, from Briquet syndrome. (*Note: Somatization disorder should be differentiated from the overarching term somatoform disorders, of which somatization disorder is one diagnosis.*) Occurring more frequently in females, this disorder is estimated to have a prevalence in the general population of 0.5% to 2%; some studies suggest that male family members may have higher than expected frequencies of antisocial personality disorder and substance-related disorders. Onset generally is in the late teens to 20s; and, by the age of 30, these patients believe they are sickly. By 30 years of age, they have visited multiple clinicians and other health-related practitioners, such as chiropractors and naturopaths. Patients with somatization disorder are often quite distressed, and they have chronic or recurrent complaints involving multiple organ systems. Typically, at least 13 complaints are noted when the clinician sequentially reviews the organ systems. Table 4.1 lists some common complaints of patients with somatization disorder.

Patients with somatization disorder are particularly difficult to treat. Because of their multiple complaints, their poor or incomplete response to reassurance, and their resistance to accepting emotional and stress-

TABLE 4.1. COMMON COMPLAINTS OF PATIENTS WITH SOMATIZATION DISORDER

System	Symptom
Cardiopulmonary	Shortness of breath in absence of exertion
Gastrointestinal	Vomiting
Nervous	Pain in extremities
	Difficulty swallowing
	Amnesia
Reproductive or sexual	Painful menstruation
	Burning sensation in sexual organs or rectum other than during sexual intercourse

related factors as contributory, many clinicians consider these patients to be "impossible." The frustration and anger experienced by the doctor usually are not well masked, and they may further reinforce the patient's prior pattern of "doctor shopping." An important element of treatment is conservative support and reassurance with a minimum of other interventions. Studies have suggested that psychiatric referral can reduce the total health care costs for these patients, especially if the psychiatrist can gain the confidence of the patient and can establish a working alliance that acknowledges the seriousness of the concerns while shifting the dialogue away from the patient's health to his or her relationships, job, or life. In addition, regular visits (as opposed to only when symptoms occur or increase) to a supportive primary care clinician who adequately attends to the patient's physical health status without pursuing unnecessary diagnostic procedures or treatments may be helpful. Unfortunately, many of these patients may have already undergone an excessive number of expensive tests or have managed to obtain unnecessary surgeries (e.g., laparoscopy).

Pharmacologic treatment is not indicated for somatization disorder unless the patient has concomitant anxiety or depression; medication use is then directed at these comorbid conditions.

3. **Hypochondriasis** refers to a belief, either an unsubstantiated fear or a false belief, that one has a serious physical disease that is based on misinterpretation of bodily symptoms. Such unsubstantiated fears are usually associated with symptoms of anxiety, and they may be associated with depression. Particularly when depression is present (see Chapter 18), the false beliefs may be of delusional proportions. Onset is usually gradual, and it occurs most commonly in early adulthood. Once present, hypochondriacal preoccupations typically persist. This contrasts with the episode-related exacerbations of fear of illness that may wax and wane in patients with depression. Some clinicians believe that patients with hypochondriasis suffer more from their illness concerns than do depressed patients. An acute onset of hypochondriasis may be seen after the death of a loved one (see Chapter 16). Some hypochondriacal patients are self-preoccupied and invested in the sick role; others (i.e., those with hypochondriacal symptoms more similar to the symptoms of obsessive-compulsive disorder) generally are not. Patients with hypochondriasis appear to be overinterpreting and magnifying bodily sensations as representing disease, and some appear motivated by a need to persuade the clinician that their complaints are genuine and serious. Focusing on the body is a habit for these patients. Many have low self-esteem, feel incomplete, and believe that their emotional needs are not being met.

Emerging research findings indicate that SSRIs and cognitive-behavioral therapy may be effective for hypochondriasis. Psychoeducation is an important adjunct. When underlying anxiety or depression is present and appears primary, treatment should be directed toward these underlying disorders or symptoms. The overall treatment goal is to reduce the dysfunction and disability that ensue from hypochondriasis and to minimize the effects on the patient's family and others. Sometimes these patients respond to efforts to provide them with a better understanding of how the body works and to reassurance that most symptoms are transient and that they do not portend serious disease. The clinician must remember, however, that hypochondriacal patients have the same probability as others of developing a serious illness. In addition, hypochondriacal patients are extremely apt to believe they are not being taken seriously. Any tests should be carefully scheduled because delays and postponements feed the patient's insecurity. Patients should also be enlisted in formally tracking their pain or dysfunction. Charts that identify the timing and character of symptoms may be useful, and they may assist the clinician and the patient in discovering temporally related stress factors (e.g., the death of a close relative). History taking should also include eliciting whether other relatives or key persons in the patient's life have had similar symptoms. Clinicians who undertake the treatment of hypochondriacal patients must recognize that short-term interventions often will not work.

For many patients, the balance struck by the clinician over time when providing psychoeducation, reassurance, support, concern, limited testing, and clarification is the key to helping these patients overcome their impaired self-concept and feelings of being damaged or incomplete.

4. **Body dysmorphic disorder (BDD)** was previously known as dysmorphophobia. These patients are preoccupied with a nonexistent or minimal appearance flaw (e.g., a blemish, hair loss, the shape of their ears or nose, facial asymmetry) to the point where their appearance concerns cause significant distress or impair functioning. Nearly all patients perform repetitive and time-consuming appearance-related behaviors, such as mirror checking, excessive grooming, skin picking, or reassurance seeking. Patients with BDD often are initially seen by dermatologists and plastic surgeons; however, such treatment does not appear to be effective. Patients with the delusional form of BDD are completely convinced that their view of their appearance "defect" is accurate (i.e., they have an encapsulated or circumscribed false belief of delusional proportions that typically occurs in the absence of an obvious precipitant or other evidence of psychosis). These patients are diagnosed with delusional disorder, somatic type (formerly known as monosymptomatic hypochondriacal psychosis); they may also receive a diagnosis of BDD.

   a. **Onset and course**. Most patients with BDD date the onset of their preoccupations to early adolescence, a time when appearance is often a paramount concern. Others date the onset to childhood or the 20s or 30s. If BDD is left untreated, it can be a chronic condition, although exacerbations while under stress are common.

   b. **Pharmacotherapy**. A medication may be useful in the treatment of patients with BDD. Once this disorder has been identified and the patient accepts that a medication may alleviate his or her preoccupation, distress, or difficulty functioning (this is not always an easy step for the clinician to get the patient to take), a carefully monitored medication trial may prove beneficial.

      (1) **Proserotonergic agents**. Considerable evidence from case reports and series, small sample clinical trials, and controlled studies indicates that proserotonergic antidepressants, such as **clomipramine and SSRIs (e.g., fluoxetine and fluvoxamine**), are beneficial in BDD. Adding **buspirone** to an SSRI has been shown to benefit some patients. Although fixed-dose studies have not been published, higher SSRI doses and longer trials

(e.g., 12 weeks) than those that are typically used for depression appear to be required to achieve efficacy (see Chapter 18). Of note, SSRIs alone have been shown to be as effective for delusional patients as they are for nondelusional patients with BDD.

Patience is required on the part of both the treating clinician and the patient because improvement may not be noted for 6 to 8 weeks. No empirically based guidelines for maintenance or continuation therapy exist. Treating for at least 1 year beyond the attainment of maximal improvement seems reasonable.

(2) **Antipsychotic agents.** Some clinicians (including the editor) have had occasional success with **pimozide**, an infrequently used, nonstandard antipsychotic agent with a dopamine-2 (D_2) receptor antagonist, a serotonin ($5\text{-}HT_{2a}$) receptor antagonist, and T-type calcium channel blocking properties (see Chapter 7, section IX.B.2.b.(2), and Chapter 20). Although this drug is marketed as a second-line treatment for the phonic and motor tics of patients with Tourette disorder, **pimozide** has been found to be effective in some patients in a small number of anecdotal and case-based reports. (*Note:* Some case reports also indicate a lack of efficacy for **pimozide** in BDD.) A positive response to use of **olanzapine** has been reported in one patient. An unanswered question is whether the combination of an SSRI with a conventional antipsychotic agent, the nonstandard antipsychotic agent **pimozide**, or an atypical antipsychotic agent may be effective, especially for delusional patients.

c. **Cognitive behavior therapy.** This approach may also be beneficial for some patients with BDD. This treatment generally consists of cognitive restructuring, exposure (e.g., to avoided social situations), and response prevention (i.e., avoidance of repetitive behaviors, such as reassurance seeking).

II. The Paranoias
A. Paranoia
Paranoia is a complex multifaceted symptom. The term derives from the Greek **para** (beside) and **nous** (mind). As with delirium (see Chapter 5), paranoia has at times been considered synonymous with insanity. Many people, particularly when they feel disappointed and under stress, have brief experiences of paranoia—a feeling that somehow they have been singled out for victimization. Paranoia exists on a descriptive continuum that includes transient feelings that most adults and many children experience, more enduring traits that do not dominate the personality, clear symptoms in several forms of psychotic disorder (e.g., bipolar disorder, schizophrenia), and a personality disorder in which paranoid thinking controls relationships and interferes with functioning. Paranoia should not be used to refer to mistrust or suspiciousness that is based on a lack of adequate cues or information, one's past experiences, or the learned (or culture-bound) expectations of one's family or group.

The central features of all paranoid states or conditions are excessive self-referential thinking (everything is linked to "me"), self-consciousness, and concerns with distrust or mistrust and about one's autonomy. For these features to be coupled with exaggerated sensitivity to rebuff and humiliation is common. The patient rejects or avoids responsibility for events, often blaming other people or fate. Underlying feelings of inadequacy or an unusual degree of concern with powerlessness or power may be present. Combativeness, irritability, and aggressiveness are frequently present—the patient seems to believe that the best defense is a good offense. Other paranoid people are quiet and remote, and they isolate themselves. Alternatively or sometimes concomitantly, they may exaggerate their self-sufficiency to defend against feelings of vulnerability and easily threatened autonomy. Resentment, litigiousness, and suspicion are common.

People subjected to sensory deprivation or separated from familiar surroundings or persons often become transiently paranoid (e.g., visually or hearing-impaired people; migrant workers; immigrants and refugees; prisoners, especially those kept in isolation; and people with delirium and dementia, particularly when they are transferred to an unfamiliar setting). In other people, the onset is gradual, with paranoid traits emerging during adolescence or early adulthood. Drug-induced or toxin-induced and stress-related paranoias rarely occur in childhood, but they may appear at any age thereafter.

One way to understand paranoia is to see the ego as protecting the self (see Chapter 1) through denial and projection. Feelings of vulnerability related to fear; powerlessness; or feelings of inadequacy, inferiority, or distrust may be dealt with in this manner. These distortions may then be elaborated by some into ideas or even delusions of reference (e.g., "I am noticed" may mean "I am not as insignificant or as alone as I feel" or "They are noticing what I would rather not have others observe"). Delusions of persecution, jealousy, or grandiosity may be present. Grandiosity typically presents in two forms. In one, the individual has a sense of being chosen and invested with special powers; in the other, the person has a false belief that he or she is rich or famous.

B. Delusional Disorder

This condition is diagnosed when persistent nonbizarre delusions that are not related to a known toxic or metabolic underlying condition exist. Delusional disorder has historically been considered a form of paranoia. The delusions are usually persecutory, they include seemingly plausible feelings of being conspired against or cheated, and they are not determined by the current or prevailing mood (i.e., they are not affect-congruent or affect-consonant). Other types of delusional disorder may involve nonpersecutory delusions as discussed below. Delusions that are keyed into prevailing mood suggest a mood disorder with psychotic features (see Chapters 18 and 19). Auditory hallucinations may be present in delusional disorder, but they should not be prominent and no other significant evidence of thought disorder should be present. The *Diagnostic and Statistical Manual of Mental Disorders,* 4th edition (DSM-IV), indicates that delusional disorder may be further subclassified according to the predominant delusional theme and content (i.e., **erotomanic, grandiose, jealous, persecutory, somatic,** and **mixed** and **unspecified** types). Some overlap may be present among delusional disorder (somatic type), obsessive-compulsive disorder, and hypochondriasis.

C. Delusional Disorder, Somatic Type

As was discussed above, delusional BDD is also one type of delusional disorder, somatic type. Other forms of the somatic variant of delusional disorder include the belief that one emits a foul body odor (i.e., olfactory reference syndrome) and delusions of infestation (i.e., a belief that one's body is infested with bugs or some other type of crawling organism—also known as parasitosis, dermatozoonosis, or Ekbom syndrome). Although tactile hallucinations may be a component of parasitosis, the fixed belief is what is central to this disorder. Thus, delusions of infestation differ from the tactile hallucinations experienced by patients with **alcohol** withdrawal or **cocaine** intoxication (formication) or from the visual hallucinations of bugs crawling on the skin that are experienced by those with toxicity secondary to anticholinergic agents.

D. Erotomania

Sometimes known as de Clérambault syndrome or *psychose passionnelle,* erotomania involves a delusional belief that one is loved by a public or prominent figure (typically a politician, entertainer, or disk jockey) who is constrained from revealing his or her love. Typically, the individual also has a sense that the public figure is indirectly communicating with the patient (e.g., "He is telling me he loves me from the titles of the songs he chooses to play"). The patient frequently contacts the loved person by telephone or letter; the intensity of this contact may vary from an annoying nuisance to frank harassment. Erotomania occurs far more frequently in women than in men. In DSM-IV, such patients are classified as having delusional disorder, erotomanic type. The relationship between erotomania and obsessive love, which is typically seen in young men, is unclear (see Chapter 6).

E. Treatment Considerations in Paranoid Disorders

1. **General considerations.** Treatment for paranoia is as complex as the concept itself. Because the paranoid symptomatology becomes manifest in situations of both literal and figurative isolation, addressing this dimension is part of any first step. The clinician's initial approach should be one of tempered concern and understanding. Paranoia does not usually yield to confrontation. Interest, tolerance, and impartiality may help to establish an initial connection with these patients, who are often distrustful, suspicious, and guarded. Helping patients to understand that they are overinterpreting experiences because they are feeling isolated may be beneficial. Practical steps, such as providing better eyeglasses or a hearing aid, improving lighting, and increasing stimulation and contact with other people, should be considered, particularly with elderly patients who are showing paranoid features of recent onset. When more intensive psychotherapy is possible, trying to move the patient toward a recognition that self-protective mechanisms and low self-esteem are present and that depression may be the cause contributes to improvement in a few patients.

2. **Pharmacotherapy.** Based on limited, case-based, or anecdotal experiences, a carefully monitored trial of an atypical antipsychotic agent (e.g., **risperidone**) or **pimozide**, either alone or in combination with an antidepressant and in conjunction with psychotherapy may be beneficial to some patients with paranoid or erotomanic features. A Chilean group found no useful clinical benefits from **pimozide** in a 6-week trial of patients with erotomania. Conventional antipsychotic agents have not been as consistently effective for erotomania, although the evidence is limited to individual case studies. Although no placebo-controlled studies specifically on the use of low doses of atypical antipsychotic agents (e.g., **risperidone, olanzapine**) or mood stabilizing anticonvulsants (e.g., **divalproex sodium, gabapentin**) for delusional disorder have been published, preliminary evidence suggests that these agents may reduce paranoid ideation in some patients with disorders of personality (see Chapter 13). A well-monitored clinical trial may be considered.

   When the paranoia is part of a mood disorder (e.g., hypomania or mania), **lithium, divalproex sodium,** or **carbamazepine** may be useful (see Chapter 19), as may both conventional and atypical antipsychotic agents (e.g., when schizophrenia or schizoaffective disorder is present [see Chapter 20]); more specifically, **risperidone** appears to be beneficial.

   Clomipramine and other antidepressants, as well as **pimozide** and other antipsychotic agents, have been noted in case reports to be beneficial for patients with olfactory reference syndrome. **Pimozide, haloperidol,** and **risperidone** have been reported to be helpful for parasitosis. As was previously discussed, the delusional variant of BDD has been shown to respond to an SSRI alone.

   Paranoia leads to altered relationships; the preformed distrust of the clinician by the patient likely will complicate any form of medical care.

ADDITIONAL READING

Allen JJ, Movius HL 2nd. The objective assessment of amnesia in dissociative identity disorder using event-related potential. *Int J Psychophysiol* 2000;38:21–41.

Barr LC, Goodman WK, Price LH. Acute exacerbation of body dysmorphic disorder during tryptophan depletion. *Am J Psychiatry* 1992;149:1406–1407.

Barsky AJ, Wyshak G, Klerman GL. Psychiatric comorbidity in DSM-III-R hypochondriasis. *Arch Gen Psychiatry* 1992;49:101–108.

Burton N, Lane RC. The relational treatment of dissociative identity disorder. *Clin Psychol Rev* 2001;21:301–320.

Daie N, Witztum E. Short-term strategic treatment in traumatic conversion reactions. *Am J Psychother* 1991;45:335–347.

Ellason JW, Ross CA. Two-year follow-up of inpatients with dissociative identity disorder. *Am J Psychiatry* 1997;154:832–839.

Fallon BA, Feinstein S. Hypochondriasis. In: Phillips KA, ed. *Somatiform and factitious disorders*. Washington, D.C.: American Psychiatric Publications, 2001. Review of Psychiatry series, Vol. 20.

Gellenberg AJ. Pimozide. *Biol Ther Psychiatry Newslett* 1991;14:42–43.

Goldberg D, Gask L, O'Dowd T. The treatment of somatization: teaching techniques of reattribution. *J Psychosom Res* 1989;33:689–695.

Grant J. Successful treatment of nondelusional body dysmorphic disorder with olanzapine: a case report. *J Clin Psychiatry* 2001;62:297–298.

Hacking I. *Rewriting the soul: multiple personality and the science of memory*. Princeton, NJ: Princeton University Press, 1995.

Holder-Perkins V, Wise TN. Somatization disorder. In: Phillips KA, ed. *Somatiform and factitious disorders*. Washington, D.C.: American Psychiatric Publications, 2001:1–26. Review of Psychiatry series, Vol. 20.

Hollander E, Allen A, Kwon J, et al. Clomipramine vs desipramine crossover trial in body dysmorphic disorder: selective efficacy of a serotonin reuptake inhibitor in imagined ugliness. *Arch Gen Psychiatry* 1999;56:1033–1039.

Hollander E, Liebowitz MR, DeCaria C, et al. Treatment of depersonalization with serotonin reuptake blockers. *J Clin Psychopharmacol* 1990;10:200–206.

Kellner R. Somatization. *J Nerv Ment Dis* 1990;178:150–160.

Kelly BD, Kennedy N, Shanley D. Delusion and desire: erotomania revisited. *Acta Psych Scand* 2000;102:74–75.

Kitamura H. A case of delusional disorder that responded to treatment with risperidone. *Psychiatry Clin Neurosci* 1997;51:337.

Kluft RP. Treatment of multiple personality disorder: a study of 33 cases. *Psychiatr Clin North Am* 1984;7:9–29.

Maldonado JR, Spiegel D. Conversion disorder. In: Phillips KA, ed. *Somatiform and factitious disorders*. Washington, D.C.: American Psychiatric Publications, 2001: 95–128. Review of Psychiatry series, Vol. 20.

Menuck MN. Differentiating paranoia and legitimate fears. *Am J Psychiatry* 1992;148: 140–141.

Merskey H, Piper A Jr. The treatment of dissociative identity disorder. *Am J Psychiatry* 1998;155:1462–1463.

Munro A, Chmara J. Monosymptomatic hypochondriacal psychosis: a checklist based on 50 cases of the disorder. *Can J Psychiatry* 1982;27:374–376.

Munro A, Mok H. An overview of the treatment of paranoia/delusional disorder. *Can J Psychiatry* 1995;40:616–622.

Phillips KA. Body dysmorphic disorder. In: Phillips KA, ed. *Somatiform and factitious disorders*. Washington, D.C.: American Psychiatric Publications, 2001:67–94. Review of Psychiatry series, Vol. 20.

Phillips KA. Pharmacologic treatment of body dysmorphic disorder: a review of empirical data and a proposed treatment algorithm. *Psychiatric Clin North Am Ann Drug Ther* 2000;7:59–82.

Phillips KA, Albertini RS, Rasmussen SA. A randomized placebo-controlled trial of fluoxetine in body dysmorphic disorder. *Arch Gen Psychiatry* 2002;59:381–388.

Phillips KA, Dwight MM, McElroy SL, et al. Efficacy and safety of fluvoxamine in body dysmorphic disorder. *J Clin Psychiatry* 1998;59:165–171.

Phillips KA, McElroy SL, Keck PE, Jr, et al. Body dysmorphic disorder: 30 cases of imagined ugliness. *Am J Psychiatry* 1993;150:302–308.

Piper A Jr. *Hoax and reality: the bizarre world of multiple personality disorder*. Northvale, NJ: Jason Aronson, 1997.

Pope HG Jr, Olivia PS, Hudson JI, et al. Attitudes toward DSM-IV dissociative disorders diagnoses among board-certified American psychiatrists. *Am J Psychiatry* 1999;156:321–323.

Rosen JC. Cognitive behavior therapy for body dysmorphic disorder. In: Caballo VE, ed. *International handbook of cognitive and behavioural treatments for psychological disorders.* Oxford, England: Pergamon/Elsevier Science Ltd, 1998:363–391.

Rosen JC, Reiter J, Orosan P. Cognitive-behavioral body image therapy for body dysmorphic disorder. *J Consult Clin Psychol* 1995;63:265–269.

Ross CA. *Multiple personality disorder: diagnosis, clinical features and treatment.* New York: John Wiley & Sons, 1989.

Safer DL, Wenegrat B, Roth WT. Risperidone in the treatment of delusional parasitosis: a case report. *J Clin Psychopharmacol* 1997;17:131–132.

Saxena S, Winograd A, Dunkin JJ, et al. A retrospective review of clinical characteristics and treatment response in body dysmorphic disorder versus obsessive-compulsive disorder. *J Clin Psychiatry* 2001;62:67–72.

Shader RI, Scharfman EL. Depersonalization disorder (or depersonalization neurosis). In: Karasu TB, ed. *Treatments of psychiatric disorders: a task force report of the American Psychiatric Association.* Washington, D.C.: American Psychiatric Press, 1989:2217–2222.

Shiwach RS, Sheikha S. Delusional disorder in a boy with phenylketonuria and amine metabolites in the cerebrospinal fluid after treatment with neuroleptics. *J Adolesc Health* 1998;22:244–246.

Silva H, Jerez S, Ramirez A, et al. Effects of pimozide on the psychopathology of delusional disorder. *Progr Neuro-Psychopharmacol Biol Psychiatry* 1998;22:331–340.

Simeon D, Gross S, Guralnik O, et al. Feeling unreal: 30 cases of DSM-III-R depersonalization disorder. *Am J Psychiatry* 1997;154:1107–1113.

Simeon D, Guralnik O, Hazlett EA, et al. Feeling unreal: a PET study of depersonalization disorder. *Am J Psychiatry* 2000;157:1782–1788.

Simeon D, Hollander E, Stein DJ, et al. Induction of depersonalization by the serotonin agonist m-CPP. *Psychiatry Res* 1995;138:161–164.

Simeon D, Stein DJ, Hollander E. Treatment of depersonalization disorder with clomipramine. *Biol Psychiatry* 1998;44:302–303.

Singer SF. "Les psychoses passionnelles" reconsidered: a review of de Clérambault's cases and syndrome with respect to mood disorders. *J Psychiatr Neurosci* 1991;16:81–90.

Smith RC. Somatization in primary care. *Clin Obstet Gynecol* 1998;31:902–914.

Steinberg M, Rounsaville B, Cicchetti D. Detection of dissociative disorders in psychiatric patients by a screening instrument and a structured diagnostic interview. *Am J Psychiatry* 1991;148:1050–1054.

Sultana A, McMonagle T. Pimozide for schizophrenia or related psychoses. *Cochrane Database Sys Rev* 2000;3:CD001949.

Ungvari GS, Hollokoi RI. Successful treatment of litigious paranoia with pimozide. *Can J Psychiatry* 1993;38:4–8.

Veale D. Cognitive behavior therapy for body dysmorphic disorder. In: Castle DJ, Phillips KA, eds. *Disorders of body image.* Hampshire, England: Wrightson Biomedical, 2001:121–138.

Veale D, Boocock A, Gournay K, et al. Body dysmorphic disorder: a survey of 50 cases. *Br J Psychiatry* 1996;169:196–201.

Veale D, Gournay K, Dryden W, et al. Body dysmorphic disorder: a cognitive behavioral model and pilot randomized controlled trial. *Behav Res Ther* 1996;34:717–729.

Wada T, Kawakatsu S, Nadaoka T, et al. Clomipramine treatment of delusional disorder, somatic type. *Int Clin Psychopharmacol* 1999;14:181–183.

Wiener A. The Dissociative Experiences scale. *Am J Psychiatry* 1992;149:143–144.

Wise TN. The somatizing patient. *Ann Clin Psychiatry* 1992;4:9–17.

5. DELIRIUM AND DEMENTIA

Sandra A. Jacobson
Richard I. Shader

Historically, two dysfunctional states, **delirium** and **dementia**, were considered pure or prototypical "organic" disorders. In the 17th century, **dementia** was synonymous with madness or "insanity" of all origins; now, it primarily refers to a pathologic process that is often progressive and that, carried to its end point, leaves the patient literally "without mind." Intellect, personality, and cognitive abilities deteriorate. Attendant psychiatric and behavioral dysfunction becomes prominent, and self-care ultimately becomes impossible. Estimates suggest that between 2.8 and 6.8 million people in the United States have dementia.

Delirium literally refers to being "off-track," a term that is derived from the Latin *lira*, meaning "rows" or "furrows." In delirium, reduced awareness and altered attention are of recent and usually rapid onset. Consciousness ranges between normal wakefulness and stupor; dramatic fluctuations may be seen in the course of a day.

The decision to review delirium and dementia at this point in the manual is based on the goal of giving those who might be reading the chapters consecutively a perspective on differential diagnosis. The scales contained in Appendices IV, V, and VI may be helpful aids when screening for delirium or dementia.

I. Delirium

A. Diagnosis and General Observations

Delirium is a syndrome of disturbed consciousness, attention, and cognition or perception that develops acutely and fluctuates during the course of the day. Delirium is always is attributable to a medical disorder. Delirious patients are often confused and intermittently agitated, and they experience delusions, as well as hallucinations (often visual). Delirium is common in hospitalized patients, and it is associated with high morbidity from events such as falls and self-extubation. Mortality rates are also high, secondary in part to noncompliance but mostly attributable to associated disease. The presence of delirium predicts a longer hospital stay, cognitive decline after hospitalization, and a loss of independent living in the community. The most important fact about delirium, however, is that it always signals the presence of an underlying medical or surgical condition and, in some cases, a life-threatening one. Table 5.1 contains some of the more frequently encountered causes of delirium.

Delirium is part of the differential diagnosis for the cognitively impaired patient, and the need to determine the etiology drives much of the diagnostic workup for cognitive dysfunction. The initial evaluation includes a history and physical examination; the latter includes both neurologic and mental status assessments. The clinician-administered Mini Mental State Examination is a useful indicator of global cognitive dysfunction, which is disturbed in delirium, as it is in dementia (see Appendix V). *The presence of a disturbance of consciousness with prominent attentional difficulties distinguishes delirium from dementia.* An electroencephalogram can be useful in patients who are difficult to assess. The electroencephalogram is an extremely sensitive indicator of functional changes in delirium.

At this stage of the evaluation, a syndromal diagnosis is made (e.g., delirium; dementia; or single-domain impairment, such as amnestic disorder), and a differential diagnosis of etiology is formulated. Laboratory examination then helps to identify the etiology.

The standard laboratory workup for a delirious patient includes hematology (complete blood count with differential, platelet count, sedimentation rate), albumin, blood urea nitrogen, creatinine, electrolytes, glucose, liver and thyroid function tests, drug levels or toxic screen, urinalysis, electrocardiogram, and

TABLE 5.1. SELECTED ETIOLOGIES OF DELIRIUM

Cardiac dysrhythmia
Congestive heart failure
Constipation
Dehydration
Electrolyte imbalance (e.g., calcium, magnesium, potassium, sodium)
Encephalitis or meningitis
Glucose dysregulation
Hepatic insufficiency
Hypertension (severe)
Hypoxia
Intracranial bleeding
Medications (e.g., opioids, anticholinergics, sedative-hypnotics, lithium)
Myocardial infarction
Nutritional deficiency, including vitamin deficiency
Pneumonia
Renal insufficiency
Sepsis
Urinary tract infection
Withdrawal from alcohol or other central nervous system sedatives

chest x-ray. The chest x-ray, electrocardiogram, and urinalysis are particularly important for elderly delirious patients. Depending on the findings from this initial evaluation and the particular presentation of the patient, further laboratory evaluation may be performed, including computed tomography or magnetic resonance imaging of the brain, lumbar puncture, electroencephalogram, arterial blood gases, cardiac enzymes, or blood cultures.

B. Treatment

Definitive treatment of the cause of delirium (e.g., correction of hyponatremia, treatment of infection) always takes precedence over symptomatic treatment. Definitive treatment is specific to the cause(s) of delirium, and thus it is not discussed further here.

Environmental interventions are useful in most cases of delirium. These include close observation; consistent staffing; orienting cues, such as a clock and calendar; familiar personal effects, such as photos; and visits from family and friends. The patient usually appreciates reassurance, even if he or she does not have good recall of specific information or explanations.

Symptomatic treatment with a pharmacologic agent is not always required, but, when it is (e.g., for control of agitation or psychosis), a conventional high-potency antipsychotic agent, such as **haloperidol**, is currently the drug of choice. This approach is appropriate for all delirious patients, except for those undergoing alcohol or sedative withdrawal (see below) and those with significant hepatic impairment. Patients posing a danger to self or others are best treated with parenteral preparations, preferably intravenous (i.v.), but oral dosing can be used. For the nonelderly patient, dosing guidelines are as follows: **haloperidol**, 2 mg i.v. for mild agitation, 5 mg i.v. for moderate agitation, and 10 mg i.v. for severe agitation. For elderly patients, smaller doses are used as follows: 0.25 to 0.5 mg i.v. for mild agitation, 1 mg i.v. for moderate agitation, and 2 mg i.v. for severe agitation. The dose can be repeated or doubled every 30 to 60 minutes until the patient is calm. Most patients respond to one or two doses. When bolus doses of **haloperidol** reach the range of 5 to 10 mg, consideration should be given to the adjunctive use of a benzodiazepine, such as **lorazepam**. As an alternative, an infusion of **haloperidol**, starting at 1 mg per h, may be used, with titration to response. Rates as high as 15 to 25 mg per h of **haloperidol** have been documented in younger patients. When i.v. **haloperidol** therapy is used, the QTc interval must be monitored, because the use of i.v. **haloperidol** can be associated with prolongation of the QTc interval and a *torsade de pointes* pattern of ventricular tachycardia. Prolongation of the QTc interval beyond 25% of baseline or to greater than 450 ms may predict the development of *torsade de pointes*. When this is observed, **haloperidol** use should be discontinued. **Droperidol**, which is faster acting and more sedating, has been recommended as an alternative to **haloperidol**. However, **droperidol** has recently been shown to have a more significant effect on QTc prolongation. **Droperidol** is no longer available in some countries.

When behavioral control has been achieved, the patient requires a continuation of the **haloperidol** to prevent the reemergence of symptoms. Exact dosing is guided by frequent clinical assessments. A commonly used regimen for a nongeriatric patient is 1 mg i.v. every 8 hours; for a geriatric patient, the dose is 0.25 mg i.v. every 8 hours. When the symptoms begin to clear, the **haloperidol** is tapered over 3 to 5 days.

Atypical antipsychotic agents are in use for the treatment of delirium in some centers, although neither United States Food and Drug Administration approval nor controlled studies for this indication exist. The requirement for gradual dosage titration with all atypical antipsychotic agents limits their usefulness in delirium. Recently, intramuscular forms of **olanzapine** and **ziprasidone** have been approved, but the place of these formulations in delirium treatment is still unclear.

The cholinesterase inhibitor **donepezil** is in use for the symptomatic treatment of delirium in many hospital settings. Data from controlled studies are not available. Anecdotal experience suggests that **donepezil** (5 mg per d orally [p.o.]) can be effective and well tolerated but that it may not be as immediately effective as **haloperidol**. Because of the long half-life of **donepezil** (more than or equal to 72 hours), some clinicians prefer the shorter-acting cholinesterase inhibitors **rivastigmine** and **galantamine**.

For critically ill patients, such as those on ventilators or intraaortic balloon pumps in whom agitation poses a medical hazard, and for terminally ill cancer patients, more aggressive treatment of agitation may be needed. One highly effective regimen is a combination of **haloperidol, lorazepam,** and **hydromorphone** that is administered i.v.

For patients with alcohol or sedative withdrawal delirium, benzodiazepines may be used to prevent the development of severe withdrawal symptoms (see Chapter 12). An assessment tool, such as the Clinical Institute Withdrawal Assessment for Alcohol Scale, can be useful in this context; a score of 10 or more indicates that treatment with a benzodiazepine is likely to be useful. The scale can be readministered serially (see Additional Reading). For elderly patients and for those with hepatic impairment, **lorazepam** is currently the drug of first choice because it is not significantly metabolized by the liver and because it can be given intramuscularly (i.m.) if needed. Other patients may benefit from **diazepam**. In general, for withdrawal prophylaxis, **lorazepam**, 0.5 mg three times a day to 1 mg four times a day, is given p.o., i.m., or i.v. When mild to moderate withdrawal symptoms are already present, **lorazepam**, 2 mg four times a day (or more, to control symptoms), is given i.m. or i.v.; **haloperidol**, 0.5 to 2 mg every 6 to 12 hours i.m. or i.v., may be added for persistent hallucinations. The risk in using an antipsychotic agent in this context is in its potential for lowering the seizure threshold.

Delirium tremens (DTs) can be so severe as to be fatal (see Chapter 12). DTs are characterized by extreme autonomic activity (e.g., fever, tachycardia, tachypnea, hypertension, tremor, diaphoresis, anxiety, insomnia) and delirium. Severe DTs represent a medical emergency that is best treated in a monitored setting with a continuous i.v. infusion or bolus dosing of **lorazepam**. Bolus dosing is usually initiated with 1 to 2 mg i.v. doses given every 10 minutes until the patient is calm; this is followed by 1 to 3 mg i.v. boluses given every 1 to 3 hours. These patients also require rehydration; correction of glucose, magnesium, and phosphate imbalances; supplementation with thiamine and multiple vitamins; and other supportive measures. Severely psychotic or agitated patients with DTs may also be treated with **haloperidol** (usual dosage is 0.5 to 2 mg i.v. every 4 hours).

II. Dementia

A. Diagnosis and General Considerations

Identifying the etiology of dementia is imperative because the specific treatment depends on the cause. Diagnostic criteria have been formulated for Alzheimer disease (AD) (McKhann et al., 1984), vascular dementia (Roman et al., 1993), and dementia with Lewy bodies (McKeith et al., 1996) and have been proposed for frontotemporal dementia and **alcohol**-related dementia (see Additional Reading).

The course of dementias varies, but typically progressive deterioration is seen in patients with AD; in vascular dementia, the deterioration is usually step-wise, with periods of stability between periods of decline. Vascular dementia comprises about 10% to 50% of all dementia patients (partially depending on the geographic location), whereas vascular pathology is found in about one-fourth of all dementias, either as a primary or contributing factor.

Dementias can be categorized as cortical or subcortical, depending on whether deficits derive from pathology involving mainly the cerebral cortex or structures deep to the cortex. Cortical dementia, which prominently affects functions such as memory encoding, naming, and face recognition, is exemplified by AD. Subcortical dementia, which prominently affects memory retrieval, motor function, and mood, is exemplified by the acquired immunodeficiency syndrome dementia complex. Table 5.2 lists the likely causes of dementia categorized by typical age at onset.

A detailed history is the best source of information relevant to etiology. Laboratory investigation, mainly to rule out reversible causes of dementia,

TABLE 5.2. CAUSES OF DEMENTIA AND LIKELY AGES AT ONSET

Less than 50 Yr	50–70 Yr	Over 70 Yr
Infection	Depression (with cognitive dysfunction)	Alzheimer disease
Alcoholism	Drug toxicity (OTC or prescription)	Drug toxicity (OTC or prescription)
Head trauma	Vascular	Vascular
Normal pressure hydrocephalus	Basal ganglia diseases (Parkinson disease)	Metabolic imbalance
Nutritional	Hypoxemia	Hypoxemia
Endocrinopathies	Space-occupying lesions	
Pick disease	Cancer or anticancer agents	
Collagen-vascular disease	Nutritional	
Multiple sclerosis and other white matter dementias	Non-Alzheimer neurodegenerative disease (olivopontocerebellar, progressive supranuclear palsy, amyotrophic lateral sclerosis, Lewy body dementia)	
Basal ganglia diseases (Huntington and Wilson diseases)	Familial Alzheimer disease	
Prion diseases[a] (Creutzfeldt-Jakob, Scrapie, familial fatal insomnia)		

[a]A prion is an infectious protein structure without nucleic acid that produces spongiform encephalopathy, gliosis, and senile plaques; prion diseases behave much like disorders with autosomal dominant inheritance patterns, producing rapidly progressing dementia, ataxia, tremor, and rigidity.
Abbreviation: OTC, over the counter.
From Taylor MA. *The fundamentals of clinical neuropsychiatry.* New York: Oxford University Press, 1999:352, with permission.

is also helpful. Minimally, the laboratory workup should include a complete blood count, chemistries, liver function tests, thyroid function tests (thyroid-stimulating hormone), vitamin B_{12} and folate levels, serum total homocysteine, and serology for syphilis.

Neuroimaging study, preferably magnetic resonance imaging, is required for the differential diagnosis of vascular dementia. If the etiologic diagnosis of dementia remains unclear, neuropsychologic testing should be performed. Genotyping for apolipoprotein E may help to increase the specificity of diagnosis in the patient who meets the clinical diagnostic criteria for AD. Other tests, such as single photon emission computed tomography, functional magnetic resonance imaging, positron emission tomography, lumbar puncture, human immunodeficiency virus testing, and heavy metal screening, should be considered in cases where the etiology of dementia remains unclear, particularly in younger patients.

B. Definitive Treatment

1. **Acquired immunodeficiency syndrome dementia complex (human immunodeficiency virus encephalopathy).** No specific treatment for this entity exists, but the antiretroviral therapies currently in use clearly can be associated with improvement in cognitive function that is sometimes marked and immediate. These agents may also prevent the development of secondary mania, furthering their neuroprotective effect.

2. **Alzheimer disease.** Currently, the following three types of treatment are available for AD: "cognition enhancers," antioxidants, and drugs that are associated with a reduced risk of developing AD. The currently available cognition enhancers of choice are the cholinesterase inhibitors **donepezil** (a noncompetitive inhibitor), **galantamine** (a competitive and reversible inhibitor and allosteric nicotinic receptor agonist), and **rivastigmine** (a pseudo-irreversible inhibitor that is metabolized by the same enzyme it inhibits—cholinesterase), each having shown evidence of cognitive and functional improvement in some patients with mild to moderate AD. These drugs may have disease-modifying effects, as well as symptomatic effects. Moreover, they can be associated with a reduction in the behavioral disturbances associated with AD, particularly in later stages of the disease. In the early stages of AD, these drugs are used for cognition enhancement; in the later stages of AD, they enhance behavioral control. In current practice, treatment with cholinesterase inhibitors is initiated as soon as possible after the diagnosis of probable AD is established, and their use is continued throughout the disease progression.

   Donepezil is started at 5 mg per day (usually every night [qhs]) and is titrated to the target dose of 10 mg per day at 4 to 6 weeks. **Rivastigmine** is started at 1.5 mg twice a day and is increased by 1.5 mg twice a day every 2 weeks to the target dose of 6 mg twice a day. **Galantamine** is started at 4 mg twice a day (with meals) and is increased to 8 mg twice a day after 4 weeks. After another 4 weeks, it can be increased to 12 mg twice a day. These drugs are usually well tolerated when titrated slowly; the cholinergic side effects, such as nausea, diarrhea, and insomnia, typically are transient. The effects of cholinesterase inhibitors are usually apparent by 12 weeks.

   Assessing the value of cholinesterase inhibitors in individual patients may be difficult. However, long-term studies clearly indicate that, in the aggregate, patients do benefit; the differences between treated and untreated (control) patients become even more apparent as the duration of therapy increases. Because disease progression is not linear, particularly in the middle stages of AD, discontinuing treatment based on rate or extent of deterioration is generally unwise. Although no evidence indicates that cholinesterase inhibitors alter the underlying dementing process in AD, preclinical data suggest that cholinergic enhancement decreases the production of plaque amyloid, and clinical trial data suggest that patients on cholinesterase inhibitors do better than those who have never been given cholinesterase inhibitors or than those started later in the course of their illness.

Limited evidence suggests that an herbal extract of **ginkgo biloba** (40 mg p.o., three times a day) may be effective in slowing disease progression. In some AD and vascular dementia patients, it may improve cognition. The effects of this extract are not as robust as those from the cholinesterase inhibitors, however, and the extract may be less convenient because of the need for three times a day dosing. In addition, case reports have associated **ginkgo** with episodes of serious bleeding (hematoma and intracranial hemorrhage), and concerns about product purity and potency may exist because **ginkgo biloba** is a dietary supplement not currently regulated by the United States Food and Drug Administration.

The antioxidant **vitamin E** (2,000 IU daily) and the monoamine oxidase inhibitor **selegiline** (10 mg p.o. daily) have been found to slow the rate of progression of AD in patients with moderate dementia. (*Note:* No additional benefit has been found from combined therapy.) Because vitamin E has fewer drug interactions and a more benign side effect profile than selegiline, vitamin E (1,000 IU p.o. twice a day) is recommended for all AD patients, *except* in those with vitamin K deficiency.

Nonsteroidal antiinflammatory drugs may theoretically affect the pathogenesis of AD by controlling the inflammatory response to amyloid and by suppressing or delaying amyloid deposition. To be clinically effective in AD prevention, however, sustained exposure to these drugs is needed, and this exposure must predate disease onset by several years.

To date, the most promising risk reduction efforts have been directed toward decreasing the production or deposition of β-amyloid protein. β-hydroxy-β-methylglutaryl coenzyme A (HMG-CoA) reductase inhibitors (i.e., "statins") that are thought to block β-amyloid protein production are currently under study in AD.

Epidemiologic evidence suggests that the long-term use of **estrogen** also reduces the risk of developing AD. Among postmenopausal women, estrogen may reduce the risk to as low as one-third that of the control group. No prospective studies have as yet corroborated this finding. That estrogen exposure must take place during a "critical period" for effective risk reduction appears likely. In addition, whether estrogen alternatives (e.g., selective estrogen receptor modifiers, such as raloxifene) will convey the same advantage is not clear.

A vaccine for AD containing a synthetic form of β-amyloid protein is currently being tested.

3. **Vascular dementia**. Treatment of vascular dementia involves the reduction of stroke risk, the enhancement of cerebral perfusion, and the treatment of associated neuropsychiatric symptoms. Stroke risk may be substantially reduced by antiplatelet agents, such as **aspirin** (81 to 325 mg per day). For those unable to tolerate aspirin because of gastrointestinal bleeding or those who have evidence of continued ischemia on aspirin therapy, the antiplatelet agent **clopidogrel** is used. Aggrenox (a proprietary combination agent of **aspirin** and extended-release **dipyridamole**) confers greater protection against stroke than **aspirin** alone for those who have had a transient ischemic attack or an ischemic stroke in the past, but it is no better in lowering mortality in this population. It is also more expensive than **aspirin**.

For patients with vascular dementia secondary to large-vessel disease ("multiinfarct" dementia), systolic blood pressure should be lowered to the range of 135 to 150 mm Hg, where cerebral blood flow and cognitive performance are optimized. HMG-CoA reductase inhibitors such as **atorvastatin** and **simvastatin** are known to reduce cholesterol levels significantly, and they clearly lower stroke risk. Embolism secondary to atrial fibrillation is controlled with either **warfarin** or **aspirin**, and embolism after myocardial infarction is prevented with **warfarin** (when its use is not contraindicated because of risk of falls or intracranial hemorrhage). Embolism from complicated carotid plaques may be prevented by endarterectomy.

Improvement in cerebral perfusion is correlated with an improvement in cognitive and global functioning. Many of the interventions designed to lower stroke risk (e.g., lowering lipid levels) are also associated with improved perfusion. Treatment with **pentoxifylline** (400 mg p.o. three times a day) has been found to result in improved cognitive and global functioning and to slow the progression of the disease in patients with multiinfarct dementia. **Estrogen** use is associated with increased cerebral perfusion in postmenopausal women. In addition, because cigarette smoking has complex effects that are known to promote ischemia, smoking cessation is associated with improved cerebral blood flow and improved cognition.

A recent study suggests that **galantamine** may have benefit in patients with mixed vascular and AD clinical presentations.

    4. Lewy body dementia. This is a progressive dementia with cognitive and motor symptoms that are characteristic of both AD and Parkinson disease. Psychiatric symptoms are prominent, including vivid visual hallucinations, delusions, and depression. Unusual features include dramatic fluctuations in symptoms, repeated falls, and frequent transient episodes of loss of consciousness. Lewy body dementia patients may benefit even more than AD patients from treatment with cholinesterase inhibitors, such as **donepezil**, **galantamine**, or **rivastigmine**, when used as described above for AD. In responders, not only cognitive but also motor and behavioral improvements are seen. Patients with Lewy body dementia are very sensitive to the extrapyramidal effects of conventional antipsychotic agents, so conventional antipsychotic agents should be avoided in this population.

C. Treatment of Psychiatric and Behavioral Syndromes

Individuals with dementia often come to clinical attention not because of cognitive difficulties but because of behavioral and psychiatric problems related to the declining brain function. These may include significant anxiety, psychosis, depression, aggression, and agitation. Although improvement may be observed with treatment of the core neurotransmitter deficits, symptomatic treatment is often necessary. Behavioral interventions for wandering include door alarms, exits demarcated by octagonally shaped *STOP* signs, and, in some situations, by simply clearing a safe circular path for walking. Behavioral interventions for agitation include the insulation of the patient during times of high activity in the milieu and the appropriate management of bath time and other activities that are stressful to the patient.

    1. Benzodiazepines and other anxiolytic agents. Patients with dementia with acute anxiety may benefit from the short-term use of **lorazepam** (0.5 mg p.o. twice a day). For longer term treatment, **buspirone** at doses ranging from 5 mg p.o. twice a day to 20 mg p.o. three times a day or a low dose of a selective serotonin reuptake inhibitor (SSRI) may be useful. For those with insomnia, short-term intermittent use of **zolpidem** or **zaleplon** (5 to 10 mg at bedtime) may be helpful. An emerging treatment for dementia-related anxiety is the use of the anticonvulsant **gabapentin** at a dose of 100 to 300 mg three times a day. **Gabapentin** has recently become available in an oral solution (250 mg per mL), which could make even smaller doses feasible for the "old-old" patient. **Gabapentin** should be avoided or used with caution in patients with renal impairment.

    2. Antipsychotic agents. Delusions, hallucinations, and thought disorganization in patients with dementia can be treated with a higher potency antipsychotic agent. For this indication, the optimal dose of **haloperidol** is 2 to 3 mg daily (divided doses) and of **risperidone** is 1 mg daily (usually divided twice a day). For intermittent psychotic agitation, such as "sundowning," antipsychotic agents can be given 1 to 2 hours before the time of the usual behavioral disturbance to take advantage of any sedative properties the specific agent may have. The use of conventional antipsychotic agents to treat nonpsychotic behavioral disturbances in dementia is controversial, but atypical agents are increasingly used at low doses for longer durations for their mood-stabilizing effects. The risk of tardive dyskinesia with conventional antipsychotic agents is in the range of 30% per year in older patients. Conventional antipsychotic agents and **risperidone** should be avoided, if possible, in patients with Lewy body dementia.

3. **Antidepressants**. Major and minor forms of depression are common among patients with dementia, and, in general, they are treated in the same way as those in nondemented patients, except that lower drug doses and lower target plasma levels may be effective. Behavioral disturbances, such as extreme irritability or refusal of care, may be manifestations of depression, and they can improve significantly with treatment. In general, nonsedating antidepressants with minimal or no anticholinergic effects, such as the **SSRIs**, **venlafaxine**, and **bupropion**, are preferred. **Mirtazapine**, on the other hand, can be very useful in elderly patients with dementia who have insomnia and anorexia, particularly at lower doses (7.5 to 15 mg qhs).

4. **Other agents**. Persistent agitation in the patient with dementia can be treated with **trazodone** at a standing dose ranging from 12.5 mg twice a day to 100 mg three times a day. **Trazodone** can also be used *as needed,* because it has a relatively rapid onset of action. Alternatively, a mood-stabilizing anticonvulsant, such as **valproate** or **gabapentin**, can be used (see Appendix VII for two algorithms for the treatment of agitation in patients with dementia). Despite numerous contraindications and warnings about the use of β-adrenergic receptor antagonists in elderly patients, **propranolol** and **pindolol** are both used to treat agitation and aggression in patients with dementia. **Propranolol** is started at 10 mg twice a day, and the dose is increased every 3 to 7 days as tolerated until it is clinically effective. **Pindolol** may be less likely to induce hypotension and bradycardia, and it may have a faster onset of action. In geriatric patients, **pindolol** is started at 5 mg daily, and the dose is increased very slowly, by 5 mg every 3 to 4 weeks, to a maximum daily dose of 40 to 60 mg. For patients resistant to these treatments, **estrogen**, 0.625 mg daily, may be useful for both men and women.

ACKNOWLEDGMENT

The authors thank Drs. Kenneth L. Davis and Dilip V. Jeste for their suggestions and thoughtful critique of this chapter.

ADDITIONAL READING

Birkhäuser MH, Strnad J, Kämpf C, et al. Oestrogens and Alzheimer's disease. *Int J Geriatr Psychiatry* 2000;15:600–609.

De Deyn PP, Rabheruk K, Rasmussen A, et al. A randomized trail of risperidone, placebo, and haloperidol for behavioral symptoms of dementia. *Neurology* 1999; 53:946–955.

Jacobson S, Schreibman B. Behavioral and pharmacologic treatment of delirium. *Am Fam Physician* 1997;56:2005–2012.

Jacobson SA. Delirium in the elderly. *Psychiatr Clin North Am* 1997;20:91–110.

Katz IR, Jeste DV, Mintzer JE, et al. Comparison of risperidone and placebo for psychosis and behavioral disturbances associated with dementia: a randomized, double-blind trial. *J Clin Psychiatry* 1999;60:107–115.

The Lund and Manchester Groups. Clinical and neuropathological criteria for frontotemporal dementia. *J Neurol Neurosurg Psychiatry* 1994;57:416–418.

Matthews HP, Korbey J, Wilkinson DG, et al. Donepezil in Alzheimer's disease: eighteen month results from Southampton memory clinic. *Int J Geriatr Psychiatry* 2000;15: 713–720.

McKeith IG, Galasko D, Kosaka K, et al. Consensus guidelines for the clinical and pathologic diagnosis of dementia with Lewy bodies (DLB): report of the consortium on DLB international workshop. *Neurology* 1996;47:1113–1124.

McKhann G, Drachman D, Folstein M, et al. Clinical diagnosis of Alzheimer's disease: report of the NINCDS-ADRDA work group under the auspices of Department of Health and Human Services task force on Alzheimer's disease. *Neurology* 1984; 34:939–944.

Oslin D, Atkinson RM, Smith DM, et al. Alcohol related dementia: proposed clinical criteria. *Int J Geriatr Psychiatry* 1998;13:203–212.

Roman GC, Tatemichi TK, Erkinjuntti T, et al. Vascular dementia: diagnostic criteria for research studies. *Neurology* 1993;43:250–260.

6. OBSESSIONS AND COMPULSIONS AND OBSESSIVE-COMPULSIVE DISORDER

Richard I. Shader

As with dissociative experiences and paranoid or suspicious ideation (see Chapter 4), obsessive thoughts and compulsive behaviors are experienced by a broad range of people; as transient symptoms and behaviors, obsessions and compulsions occur in most older children and adults. As enduring traits or as a style of functioning (i.e., obsessive-compulsive personality disorder [OCPD]), such patterns are quite familiar. Obsessions and compulsions in the form of obsessive-compulsive disorder (OCD) may occur in 2% to 3% of the general adult population; a smaller number of children and youth—about 1%—also have OCD (see Chapter 21). Westphal, who also coined the term agoraphobia (see Chapter 14), first described OCD in the late 19th century. In Europe, the term **anancastic reactions** is sometimes used to describe patients who feel compelled to think or to act in ways inconsistent with their will or reason.

OCD can be crippling to many patients; it can also be burdensome to their families. Imagine the disruptive effects on family life that are generated by someone who must frequently wash his or her hands or who spends hours trapped by a checking routine.

I. Obsessions and Compulsions: Definitions and Concepts
A. Obsessive Thinking

Obsessive thinking involves the recurrence of undesired or disquieting thoughts, images, or impulses that cannot be dismissed at will (i.e., usually a sense of struggle is present). The affected person knows that the intrusive thoughts originate from within, as opposed to being inserted from the outside as in some patients who have schizophrenia, but he or she typically finds them unacceptable and tries to resist or control them. This effort differentiates "obsessives" from "depressives" (see Chapter 18) and "paranoids" (see Chapter 4), who accept their thoughts and ruminations (i.e., repetitive thoughts that are more volitional and less ego dystonic than obsessional thinking) and who do not try to control them. Not all obsessive thoughts are intrusive or ego alien from the start. Some examples are a young man's obsessive thoughts of love for a particular woman who may or may not know that she is the object of desire or that of preoccupations with song fragments or nonsense words. Typically, however, these thoughts become more intrusive if they truly are obsessional thoughts and not transiently preoccupying concerns or ruminations.

Examples of obsessive thinking include recurrent feelings that one has to return home to check the lock on the door or that one is going to say something inappropriate in public. Obsessive thoughts are often experienced as senseless or untrue, which is a contrast to most delusional thoughts. Six of the following somewhat interrelated themes tend to be dominant: morality or religion; aggression; contamination or dirt; health and illness; orderliness or a need for symmetry; and sex, particularly shameful or degrading acts. These themes may be remembered by the mnemonic **MACHOS**. All these themes involve harm to oneself or others. Concerns about contamination by dirt, germs, or chemicals are by far the most common.

Obsessions are not simply overvalued ideas. Rarely does an obsessional person focus on just one issue or theme, and most of the time, as noted earlier, such thoughts are experienced as intrusive. Obsessions, therefore, stand in contrast to the isolated preoccupation with thinness (often referred to as being "obsessed" with thinness) that is not resisted by the patient with anorexia nervosa (see Chapter 8). Of interest is the fact that, for young women with anorexia nervosa to show a pattern of overdoing other things as well, such as studying or exercise, is not uncommon. A similar contrast can be drawn to the transsexual, who is described by some as being "obsessed" with feeling like a woman trapped inside a man's body. These conditions seem more like the fixed body image distortions of the patient with body dysmorphic disorder and delusional disorder, somatic type, (see Chapter 4) than like obsessional preoccupations.

B. Compulsive Acts

These involve repetitive, seemingly purposeful actions and behaviors carried out in a stereotyped manner that often appears to others to be ritual. The four common domains for these actions, which are referred to as the *4 Cs*, are as follows: (a) *C*leaning, especially handwashing or cleaning one's environment; (b) *C*hecking, or concerns with safety; (c) *C*lothing, or dressing in a particular sequence or the methodical laying out of clothes; and (d) *C*ounting, often in patterns or aloud. Many readers will remember the following verse: "the man from St. Ives with his seven wives and their seven sacks containing seven cats with their seven kits"—kits, cats, sacks, wives—counting can be fun except to a compulsive counter. Counting may be both an obsession and a compulsion (i.e., the mental act of counting is an obsession; counting softly aloud—under one's breath—is a compulsion). Compulsions are urges; rituals are the observable or external actions or behaviors, although they may be hidden or covert, such as in counting under one's breath. Compulsive acts have in common the theme of incompleteness—avoiding harm by doing more. Examples that physicians may recognize include rereading laboratory reports and calling a pharmacy back to see if a prescription was filled out correctly. Compulsive face picking, a combination of cleaning and checking, is typically seen in adolescents and younger adults, particularly in young women.

II. Obsessive-Compulsive Personality Disorder

As was noted earlier, occasional transient obsessional thinking and infrequent or rare compulsive actions are not unusual in many children and adults. On the other hand, when these features are more prominent and they are characteristic of a person's style of dealing with life, the term OCPD applies. These patients often have a degree of compulsive perfectionism or orderliness that is maladaptive and that gets in their way because things have to be done so correctly that they do not get completed. Although this degree of perfectionism or orderliness may have been adaptive or previously pleasing to parents or teachers, the pattern now is self-defeating. Even so, these traits are still not unacceptable to the patient with OCPD.

Other traits of patients with OCPD include rigidity and inflexibility, valuing work over leisure activities, frugality, excessive conscientiousness, indecisiveness, obstinacy, preoccupation with unimportant or trivial levels of detail, hoarding or saving unimportant objects, and a stultifying morality that can verge on or meld into bigotry. Sometimes, these traits lead to manifest behavior that is inordinately slow. Obviously, not all patients have all these traits. When the patterns are less full blown, the patients may seem, at times, to function well; they are punctual, precise, dependable, and conscientious. Indeed these traits, when not excessive, may be seen as virtues or strengths that bolster the self-esteem. Patients with OCPD save money, appear stable in mood, and complete what they start. "If I may refer to an old friend for whom punctuality was no less a predicate than existence. . . ."[1]

OCPD patients frequently have ups and downs in their symptoms over time. Exacerbations of dysfunctional symptoms and behaviors during and after periods of stress are common. Most patients with OCPD, however, do not go on to develop OCD. Although early studies did suggest that up to 50% of OCD patients had also had preexisting OCPD, many believe that a lower figure of 5% to 10% is more appropriate. Patients with OCPD, if they do decompensate, are more likely to shift into a mood disorder than to move into OCD.

III. Obsessive-Compulsive Disorder

A. Definitions and Concepts

OCD refers to a condition in which patients are plagued by obsessions or compulsions or both. Their obsessions and compulsions, as described earlier,

---

[1] Tom Stoppard describing Bertrand Russell; *Jumpers*. New York: Grove Press, 1972:25.

are distressing, and they often interfere with relationships, work, and leisure activities. Attempts to contain and control these thoughts and behaviors are usually unsuccessful, and the failed effort itself usually produces increased anxiety.

The etiology of OCD is not known. Genetic factors may be involved. Concordance for OCD is more common in monozygotic twins than is nonconcordance; concordance is not common in dizygotic twins. The rate of OCD in the parents of OCD patients is 5% to 7%, more than double the 2% to 3% rate that is estimated for the general adult population. Overrepresentation of obsessive and compulsive symptoms and traits, often enough to fulfill the criteria for a diagnosis of OCD, is observed in male children and adolescents with Tourette disorder (see Chapter 7). Whether genetic determinants exist for this comorbidity (25% to 35% of male patients with Tourette disorder also meet the criteria for concomitant OCD) is not fully understood; some data suggest a common gene such that boys get Tourette disorder, and girls get OCD.

Neuroanatomic findings in OCD are varied. Some areas, however, seem consistently implicated, but no pattern of involvement is always present. Imaging studies reveal changes in the orbitofrontal cortex, caudate nuclei, thalamus, cingulate gyri, and parietal lobes.

The modal onset for OCD is earlier in males (between the ages of 6 and 15) than it is in females (between the ages of 20 to 29). A sudden onset can occur in adolescence, even with no prior history of symptoms or traits. One-third of OCD patients have an onset of the disorder before the age of 15 years. When OCD has its onset in childhood, it usually is seen between 3 and 15 years of age; boys have an earlier onset than girls. Onset after the age of 40 years is infrequent (less than 10%). That the age of onset is bimodal and that earlier onset is associated with more severe disease seems likely. Approximately 40% of adults place their onset of symptoms in childhood. Typical preonset stresses include pregnancy and childbirth, family deaths, and sexual failures, but 70% have no identifiable stressor that they can associate with the onset. Trichotillomania (compulsive hair pulling) has its onset in adolescence or young adulthood, and it occurs more commonly in women than in men.

OCD has a variable course. Some patients have an intermittent course, whereas others have a chronic course in which the severity waxes and wanes, even with an acute onset. Most patients will not improve spontaneously; fewer than 10% of patients have spontaneous remissions lasting more than 1 year. Severity ranges from mild annoyance to complete incapacitation. Many patients hide their disorder because their obsessions seem so silly, nasty, or horrific and because their ritualistic behavior appears so bizarre that they fear embarrassment, humiliation, or stigmatization should they be discovered. However, even with treatment-related decrements in the manifestations of OCD, about half still have enough dysfunction to qualify for an OCD diagnosis at 40 years after initial diagnosis. Early onset, particularly in males, tends to be linked to a reduction in degree of improvement.

Some patients have mostly obsessional symptoms, and others have mostly compulsions; the latter group tends to do more poorly. Furthermore, patients with more magical, stereotyped, odd, or bizarre obsessive thoughts tend to have poorer outcomes. Two useful scales for assessing OCD patients are the Yale-Brown Obsessive-Compulsive Scale and the Maudsley Obsessive-Compulsive Inventory.

B. Treatment and a Biologic Perspective

Treatment currently emphasizes specific psychopharmacologic and behavioral modalities, with psychosurgery being reserved for an exceedingly small number of severely ill patients who are unresponsive to medications and behavior therapy.

    1. Pharmacotherapy. **Clomipramine** and all the selective serotonin reuptake inhibitors (SSRIs) marketed in the United States (with the exception of **citalopram**) are approved by the United States Food and Drug Administration for the treatment of OCD (Table 6.1). **Citalopram** has shown efficacy in published trials, but it is not currently approved

TABLE 6.1. CURRENT MEDICATIONS FOR THE TREATMENT OF OBSESSIVE-COMPULSIVE DISORDER

Drug	Trade Name	Starting Dose (mg)	Range (mg)	Modal Dose (mg)
Clomipramine[a]	Anafranil	25	150–250	150
Fluoxetine[b]	Prozac	20	10–80	60
Fluvoxamine[c]	Luvox	50	25–300	200
Paroxetine[d]	Paxil	10	10–60	40
Sertraline[e]	Zoloft	25	25–200	125
Citalopram[f]	Celexa	20	10–60	60

[a]For ages ≥ 10 yr, may be dosed at 3.0 mg/kg/d up to 200 mg/d.
[b]Not approved by United States Food and Drug Administration for children; in the author's experience, some adult patients may tolerate **fluoxetine** better if it is started at 5 mg/d (dissolving the capsule in water or apple juice). Also available as an oral solution of 20 mg/5 mL. Literature exists to support the use of fluoxetine in children.
[c]For ages ≥ 8 yr, start with 25 mg h.s.
[d]Not approved by United States Food and Drug Administration for children; also available as an oral suspension of 10 mg/5 mL.
[e]For ages ≥ 6 yr, start with 25 mg h.s.; available as an oral concentrate of 20 mg/mL.
[f]Not currently approved for obsessive-compulsive disorder; however, literature exists to support its use in both children and adults.

for the OCD indication. Occasionally, patients respond well to other agents (e.g., **trazodone**, monamine oxidase inhibitors, **lithium, buspirone**). Combinations of this group of proserotonergic agents (e.g., **buspirone** added to **fluoxetine, lithium** added to **clomipramine, citalopram** added to **clomipramine**), when used for augmentation when a single agent has not proven effective, have also been beneficial to some refractory patients. Most clinicians start with an SSRI and then add in or switch to **clomipramine** when the response to the SSRI is not sufficient. **Clomipramine** typically has more adverse effects than the SSRIs.

The theoretical value of these proserotonergic agents is supported by the research finding of increased cerebrospinal fluid levels of 5-hydroxyindoleacetic acid, a product of the metabolism of serotonin, in OCD patients. Moreover, **metergoline**, a serotonin antagonist, can promote relapse in treated patients or worsening in untreated OCD patients. Imaging studies increase glucose utilization (hyperactivity) in orbitofrontal and frontostriatal pathways in some persons who have OCD.

When large groups of OCD patients are treated with SSRIs or **clomipramine**, from 40% to 80% generally show improvement, with an overall reduction from baseline symptomatology of 25% to 50%. Some do quite well; others do not. No predictors of success exist, and the duration for pharmacotherapy has not been set with OCD. Many patients receiving pharmacotherapy alone relapse fairly promptly when the medication is discontinued. One approach to the duration is to continue pharmacotherapy (in the absence of side effects) until a suitable behavior therapy program can be initiated and is found to be effective. The medication dose is then tapered very gradually. In some refractory patients, augmentation of proserotonergic agents with **lithium** or low doses of an atypical antipsychotic agent may be beneficial.

For some patients, combining cognitive-behavior therapy (CBT) with medication that modifies serotonergic tone may result in a better outcome than either treatment alone. Some patients fail to comply with behavioral regimens (see section III.B.2). When CBT is not available or when it is ineffective, pharmacotherapy may need to be continued indefinitely, with thoughtful monitoring and follow-up to avoid long-term toxicity from drug accumulation.

2. **Cognitive-Behavior Therapy**. Effective **CBT** for OCD requires the following two techniques: exposure and ritual or response prevention. Exposure decreases anxiety and other forms of distress associated with obsessions, whereas response prevention decreases the time involved in a need for rituals. Anxiety management training may provide additional benefit. For children with OCD, family interventions (e.g., psychoeducation, avoiding inadvertent reinforcement of any rituals, habit reversal, behavioral rewards) (see Chapter 21) are useful.

As an example of behavior therapy, consider a patient who fears that, if he raises the toilet seat before he urinates, he may contract a human immunodeficiency virus infection, even in his own home. Being a considerate person, he regularly raises the toilet seat before urinating. Having done so, he can only quell his anxiety by then washing his hands for 5 minutes—a ritual that he detests both because of the time that is consumed and the conspicuous nature of the ritual. Exposure therapy has him raise the toilet seat with his hand (instructing the patient to use his hand and to resist the temptation to use his shoe or a paper towel is important), thereby "running the risk" that he may get a human immunodeficiency virus infection (in reality, the probability of contracting it in this manner is virtually absent). His anxiety level predictably increases with this exposure task, and he is then asked to decrease his washing ritual to 4 minutes. Education and the support of the therapeutic relationship augment the patient's motivation to change and help him to bear the discomfort associated with this treatment approach. With repetition, both the anxiety about raising the toilet seat and the discomfort of reducing the ritual diminish, and the patient learns that he can control his anxiety without ritualizing.

About 25% of patients decline behavior therapy as too time consuming, too frightening, or too stressful. For the 75% who try to comply faithfully, about half will have at least a 70% reduction in the severity of their rituals and obsessions, and an additional 40% will have reductions of 30% to 69%. Sixty percent of patients treated with exposure and response prevention therapy maintain at least moderate gains for up to 6 years in follow-up, a striking contrast to the almost certain and relatively rapid relapse associated with pharmacotherapy alone (e.g., SSRIs or combinations of agents). To maintain the positive benefits from CBT over time, it is essential for patients to continue to practice the cognitive and behavioral strategies that have worked for them.

Relaxation, which is often taught as a technique for the reciprocal inhibition of anxiety, is actually an inert component of CBT. As a coping tactic that helps patients face the things they fear, it may be of indirect benefit. Some patients, by contrast, prefer rapid and complete exposure with no attempts to reduce or minimize anxiety, a technique known as **flooding**. The level of anxiety experienced, whether low or high, does not correlate with improvement.

Despite long traditions of the use of psychoanalysis, other nonbehavioral psychotherapies, and hypnosis to treat OCD, little nonanecdotal evidence exists to support the efficacy of these treatments when given alone (i.e., without medication or behavioral treatment). Their use should be reserved for those patients with OCD who have failed to respond to treatments that have been established as effective by controlled clinical trials. All patients deserve and benefit from supportive care in which they are provided with an explanation of their disorder, empathy for their emotional pain and suffering, and hope for improvement.

Finally, although scant and sometimes contradictory evidence for the effectiveness of **electroconvulsive therapy** (see Chapter 24) and anterior cingulate gyrus or limbic leucotomy exists, both have been used in severe cases of OCD. The effects of electroconvulsive therapy are at best modest and transitory. Leucotomy, which is reserved for severe or life-threatening self-injurious behaviors and which putatively acts through interruption of the thalamofrontal tracts, appears to produce full remission in a few instances. The use of leucotomy is consistent with the hypothesis that overactivity of the cingulate region (just dorsal to the corpus callosum) is associated with compulsive acts and behaviors. An obvious concern is whether these "psychosurgical" treatments cause significant decrements in overall mental functioning. Limited data suggest that, although certain frontal lobe functions may be compromised, global cognitive abilities remain comparable with those of nonsurgically treated patients with OCD.

IV. Clinical and Diagnostic Considerations

For a better understanding of this category of disorders, some additional comments are warranted. When obsessions and compulsions appear in their mildest forms, a defensive value may seem apparent. As in displacement, obsessions distract, preoccupy, and shift the focus from other, perhaps less bearable, sources of anxiety or distress. Most people can remember simple ritualistic games from childhood (e.g., avoiding stepping on cracks in the sidewalk, perhaps while reciting "step on a crack, break your mother's back"). Rituals may mitigate fears of loss of control or concerns about rage and anger. In addition, one cannot, given the current limitations in knowledge about the pathophysiology of obsessions and compulsions, exclude the possibility that rituals are protective behaviors that have gone awry. Perhaps the ego "perceived" some subtle deficit in functioning, whether neurologic or otherwise, and instituted actions that were meant to reduce harm (e.g., checking); however, now that behavior is not under appropriate control or internal monitoring (e.g., a perseverative action in the presence of altered frontal lobe functioning). In any case, true OCD patients are in agony. The repetitive nature of their irresistible thoughts and behaviors causes so much suffering that any defensive or protective value, if indeed any exists, is lost. The automatic involuntary nature of these thoughts and actions seems quite tic-like at times. As a clinician who has had considerable experience with patients with varying degrees of obsessions and compulsions, the author is convinced of the clinical and theoretical value of seeing minimal to mild forms (those previously called "neurotic") as separate (i.e., not on a continuum) from OCD. A lack of linearity or a continuum of severity is also supported by the previously mentioned low frequency of OCPD in the histories of patients with OCD.

Finally, a contrast to simple and social phobias (see Chapter 14) seems in order. Phobias, like obsessions and compulsions, curtail freedom. In both, the patient is aware that the disquieting ideas, thoughts, or actions are generated from within and that they are unrealistic. The obsessive, as has been noted earlier, cannot control them. The compulsive would like to stop checking or counting or eating or not eating, but he or she cannot (e.g., "Jack Sprat would eat no fat, his wife would eat no lean"). Simply willing oneself to stop, unless one is supported and enabled by a therapist as part of an exposure and response prevention program, typically produces incremental anxiety, at least initially. When an appropriate treatment plan is in place and when the symptoms are still at a level that can be helped by behavior therapy, the initial anxiety increment diminishes with practice, time, and the support of the therapist.

When a patient with simple phobia successfully avoids the feared object (i.e., if Miss Muffet could have avoided the spider all together), no overt anxiety or discomfort is present. Most simple phobias (i.e., phobias involving a specific feared object, situation, or location that can generally be avoided or encountered infrequently) produce little anxiety in everyday living. The patient with a simple phobia usually can be helped with progressive exposure to the fear-provoking stimulus, coupled with relaxation strategies. This is technically referred to as desensitization. The patient with a social phobia, however, cannot readily avoid his or her discomfort that surfaces in gatherings of people and that is linked to feelings of being observed, an expectation of being criticized, or worry about being embarrassed or doing something personally embarrassing. The socially phobic patient also has frequent anxiety and distress, but the suffering and disability are seldom as intense as what is felt by the patient with OCD.

Further information for patients and families may be obtained online at *http://www.ocfoundation.org/* and *http://www.adaa.org/*.

ADDITIONAL READING

Angst J. The epidemiology of obsessive compulsive disorder. In: Hollender E, Zohar J, Marazziti D, et al., eds. *Current insights in obsessive compulsive disorder.* New York: John Wiley & Sons, 1994:93–104.

Barr LC, Goodman WK, Price LH, et al. The serotonin hypothesis of obsessive compulsive disorder. Implications of pharmacologic challenge studies. *J Clin Psychiatry* 1992;53:17–28.

Bejerot S, Bodlund O. Response to high doses of citalopram in treatment-resistant obsessive-compulsive disorder. *Acta Psych Scand* 1998;98:423–424.

Clomipramine Collaborative Study Group. Clomipramine in the treatment of patients with obsessive-compulsive disorder. *Arch Gen Psychiatry* 1991;48:730–738.

Cumming S, Hay P, Lee T, et al. Neuropsychological outcome from psychosurgery for obsessive-compulsive disorder. *Austr N Z J Psychiatry* 1996;29:293–298.

Degonda M, Wyss M, Angst J. The Zurich study. XIII. Obsessive-compulsive disorders and syndromes in the general population. *Eur Arch Clin Neurosci* 1993;243:16–22.

Dominguez RA, Jacobson AF, de la Gandara J, et al. Drug response assessed by the modified Maudsley obsessive-compulsive inventory. *Psychopharmacol Bull* 1989;25: 215–218.

Flament MF, Rapoport JL, Berg CJ, et al. Clomipramine treatment of childhood obsessive compulsive disorder: a double-blind controlled study. *Arch Gen Psychiatry* 1985;42:977–983.

Goodman WK, Price LH, Rasmussen SA, et al. The Yale-Brown obsessive-compulsive scale. I. Development, use, and reliability. *Arch Gen Psychiatry* 1989;46:1006–1011.

Grados MA, Riddle MA. Pharmacological treatment of childhood obsessive-compulsive disorder: from theory to practice. *J Clin Child Psychology* 2001;30:67–79.

Greist JH. Treatment of obsessive compulsive disorder. Psychotherapies, drugs, and other somatic treatments. *J Clin Psychiatry* 1990;51:44–50.

Hewlett WA, Vinogradov S, Agras WS. Clomipramine, clonazepam, and clonidine treatment of obsessive-compulsive disorder. *J Clin Psychopharmacol* 1992;12:420–430.

Hewlett WA, Vinogradov S, Agras WS. Clonazepam treatment of obsessions and compulsions. *J Clin Psychiatry* 1990;51:158–161.

Jenike MA, Baer L, Summergrad P, et al. Sertraline in obsessive-compulsive disorder: a double-blind comparison with placebo. *Am J Psychiatry* 1990;147:923–928.

Jenike MA, Hyman S, Baer L, et al. A controlled trial of fluvoxamine in obsessive-compulsive disorder: implications for a serotonergic theory. *Am J Psychiatry* 1990; 147:1209–1215.

Karno M, Golding JM, Sorenson SB, Burnam MA. The epidemiology of obsessive-compulsive disorder in five US communities. *Arch Gen Psychiatry* 1988;45:1094–1099.

Kronig MH, Apter J, Asnsi G, et al. Placebo-controlled multicenter study of sertraline treatment for obsessive-compulsive disorder. *J Clin Psychopharmacol* 1999;19: 172–176.

Leonard HL, Swedo SE, Rapoport JL, et al. Treatment of obsessive-compulsive disorder with clomipramine and desipramine in children and adolescents. A double-blind crossover comparison. *Arch Gen Psychiatry* 1989;46:1088–1092.

Levine R, Hoffman JS, Knepple ED, Kenin M. Long-term fluoxetine treatment of a large number of obsessive-compulsive patients. *J Clin Psychopharmacol* 1989;9:281–283.

March JS, Biederman J, Wolkow R, et al. Sertraline in children and adolescents with obsessive-compulsive behavior: a multicenter randomized controlled trial. *JAMA* 1998;280:1752–1756.

McDougle CJ, Goodman WK, Price LH. Dopamine antagonists in tic-related and psychotic spectrum obsessive compulsive disorder. *J Clin Psychiatry* 1994;55:24–31.

Montgomery SA, Kasper S, Stein DJ, et al. Citalopram 20 mg, 40 mg, 60 mg are all effective and well tolerated compared with placebo in obsessive-compulsive disorder. *Int Clin Psychopharmacol* 2001;16:75–86.

Murphy DL, Pigott TA. Obsessive-compulsive disorder. Treatment with serotonin-selective uptake inhibitors, azapirones, and other agents. *J Clin Psychopharmacol* 1990;10:91S–100S.

Perse TL, Greist JH, Jefferson JW, et al. Fluvoxamine treatment of obsessive-compulsive disorder. *Am J Psychiatry* 1987;144:1543–1548.

Price BH, Baral I, Cosgrove GR, et al. Improvement in severe self-mutilation following limbic leucotomy: a series of 5 cases. *J Clin Psychiatry* 2001;62:925–932.

Price LH, Heninger GR. Lithium in the treatment of mood disorders. *N Engl J Med* 1994;331:591–598.

Rasmussen SA, Eisen JL. Epidemiology of obsessive compulsive disorder. *J Clin Psychiatry* 1990;51:10–13.

Skoog G, Skoog I. A 40-year follow-up of patients with obsessive-compulsive disorder. *Arch Gen Psychiatry* 1999;56:121–127.

Tippin J, Henn F. Modified leukotomy in the treatment of intractable obsessional neurosis. *Am J Psychiatry* 1982;139:1601–1603.

Trivedi MH. Functional neuroanatomy of obsessive-compulsive disorder. *J Clin Psychiatry* 1996;57:26–35.

Turner SM, Jacob RG, Beidel DC, Himmelhoch J. Fluoxetine treatment of obsessive-compulsive disorder. *J Clin Psychopharmacol* 1985;5:207–212.

Westphal C. Dwangforstellungen. *Arch Psych Nervenkr* 1878;8:734–750.

Zohar J, Insel TR, Zohar-Kadouch RC, et al. Serotonergic responsivity in obsessive-compulsive disorder: effects of chronic clomipramine treatment. *Arch Gen Psychiatry* 1988;45:167–172.

7. TICS, TOURETTE DISORDER, AND RELATED PROBLEMS

Barbara J. Coffey
Richard I. Shader

Tics are characterized by stereotyped, rapid, recurrent motor movements or vocalizations that are nonrhythmic, seemingly involuntary, and sudden in onset. Tic disorders, including transient tics, chronic motor or vocal (phonic) tic disorder, and Tourette disorder (TD), are childhood onset disorders that most often begin in the first decade of life. TD, the most complex of the tic disorders, is characterized by multiple motor and vocal tics and, in clinical settings, a variety of behavioral and emotional symptoms. Although tic disorders may be quite common, limited epidemiologic data suggest a highly variable prevalence rate of TD ranging from 0.4% in Israel to 3% in the United Kingdom. Prevalence rates decline with age from about 4 in 10,000 in childhood to about 0.5 in 10,000 in adulthood. A recent community-based survey reported that about 3% of school-aged children meet the criteria for TD. Although TD is commonly thought to be a lifelong disorder, limited and somewhat contradictory information exists on its longitudinal course. Several recent studies suggest that although tics may persist into adulthood, the tic severity often declines significantly during adolescence.

The past two decades have been marked by significant progress in the understanding of the clinical phenomenology, epidemiology, and comorbidity of TD. Treatment studies have expanded to include the atypical antipsychotic agents and, most recently, targeted combined pharmacotherapy. Nevertheless, TD and tic disorders continue to pose many challenges, especially in the areas of pathophysiology, genetics, developmental neuroscience, psychopathology, and treatment.

This chapter briefly reviews the classification, clinical phenomenology, epidemiology, genetics, etiology, differential diagnosis, clinical assessment, and treatment of TD and chronic tic disorders.

I. **Classification and Clinical Phenomenology**
Tics typically involve one muscle (simple tic) or a group of muscles (complex tics), and they can be characterized by anatomic location, number, frequency, intensity, and complexity. For tic frequency or intensity to vary during the day is not unusual; afternoon or evening worsening is common. Tics can occur in volleys; many patients report having fewer tics during summer months. Table 7.1 lists some common examples of simple and complex tics. Tic disorders can be classified as transient (i.e., lasting at least 4 weeks but less than 1 year) or chronic (i.e., lasting longer than 1 year). Current diagnostic criteria for TD, chronic motor or vocal tic disorder, and transient tic disorder are detailed in Tables 7.2, 7.3, and 7.4, respectively.

II. **Natural History**
Most youth with TD experience the onset of symptoms before adolescence, typically by about the age of 6 or 7 years. Most children will experience a progression of simple to complex and rostral to caudal tics over several years, with typical waxing and waning of tics over days to months. Many children with TD who are evaluated in clinical settings will also meet the criteria for attention deficit hyperactivity disorder (ADHD), obsessive-compulsive disorder (OCD), or other psychiatric disorders. Recent data suggest that the tics in TD may abate or may show reduced severity in many youths over time. Chronic motor tic disorder typically has a similar natural history, and it is often considered a variant of TD.

III. **Comorbid Disorders**
Most youth seen in clinical settings will meet full or subthreshold criteria for at least one psychiatric comorbid disorder. The most common comorbid diagnoses are ADHD and OCD. Excessive motoric hyperactivity, inattention, and impulsivity are also problematic for many clinically referred TD patients; some investigators report that from 50% to 75% of TD patients also meet criteria for

TABLE 7.1. SOME EXAMPLES OF TICS

	Motor	Vocal
Simple	Eye blinking Nose twitching Shoulder shrugging	Throat clearing Coughing Grunting Sniffing
Complex	Touching objects or self Squatting or jumping	Uttering syllables or words Uttering phrases Swearing

TABLE 7.2. DIAGNOSTIC FEATURES OF TOURETTE DISORDER

1. Both multiple motor and one or more vocal tics are present at some time during the illness, although they are not necessarily concurrent.
2. The tics occur many times a day (usually in bouts), nearly every day, or intermittently throughout a period of more than 1 yr; no tic-free intervals lasting longer than 3 consecutive mo should occur.
3. The anatomic location, number, frequency, complexity, and severity of the tics change over time.
4. The symptoms cause significant distress in terms of social, educational, or occupational functioning.
5. Age at onset is before 18 yr.
6. Symptoms are not the result of a medical condition, such as Huntington chorea or postviral encephalitis; substance intoxication; or a medication-induced movement disorder.

From the American Psychiatric Association. *Diagnostic and statistical manual of mental disorders,* 4th ed., Text revision. Washington, D.C.: American Psychiatric Association, 2000, with permission.

TABLE 7.3. DIAGNOSTIC FEATURES OF CHRONIC MOTOR OR VOCAL TIC DISORDER

1. Either motor or vocal tics, but not both, are present at some time during the illness.
2. The tics occur many times a day, nearly every day, or intermittently throughout a period that is longer than 1 yr; no tic-free intervals lasting longer than 3 consecutive mo should occur.
3. The symptoms cause significant distress in terms of social, educational, or occupational functioning.
4. Age at onset is before 18 yr.
5. Symptoms are not the result of a medical condition, such as Huntington chorea or postviral encephalitis; substance intoxication; or a medication-induced movement disorder.

From the American Psychiatric Association. *Diagnostic and statistical manual of mental disorders,* 4th ed., Text revision. Washington, D.C.: American Psychiatric Association, 2000, with permission.

TABLE 7.4. DIAGNOSTIC FEATURES OF TRANSIENT TIC DISORDER

1. Single or multiple motor and/or vocal tics that occur many times a day, nearly every day for at least 4 wk, but for no longer than 12 consecutive mo.
2. No history of signs or symptoms lasting 1 yr or more and meeting criteria for Tourette disorder or chronic motor or vocal tic disorder.
3. The symptoms cause significant distress in terms of social, educational, or occupational functioning.
4. Age at onset is before 18 yr.
5. Symptoms are not the result of a medical condition, such as Huntington chorea or post-viral encephalitis; substance intoxication; or a medication-induced movement disorder.

From the American Psychiatric Association. *Diagnostic and statistical manual of mental disorders,* 4th ed., Text revision. Washington, D.C.: American Psychiatric Association, 2000, with permission.

ADHD. Recognition of other comorbid emotional disorders in TD, such as mood and non-OCD anxiety disorders, has also been increasing. Although the nature of the relationship between TD and comorbid disorders is still not clear, tics and behavioral, cognitive, or emotional dysfunction may represent manifestations of an underlying disinhibition problem. Comorbid disorders are often the primary clinical concern when these youths are evaluated in clinical settings.

A bidirectional relationship between TD and OCD in which OCD is a risk factor for TD and TD is a risk factor for OCD has been described. As many as 90% of clinically referred TD patients meet either the full or subthreshold criteria; up to 40% may meet the full OCD criteria. In addition, family studies indicate that OCD is found at a higher rate in close relatives of patients with TD than it is in control patients. Clinically, making the distinction between complex motor tics and compulsions (e.g., walking forward and then backward through a doorway, four paces in each direction) with certainty can be difficult. The increasing recognition of the subjectively experienced component of tics (e.g., sensory tics or premonitory urges) can also confound these distinctions.

Recently, mood and anxiety disorders in clinically referred TD patients have been described, including major depression, bipolar disorder, panic attacks, panic disorder, and simple and social phobias. Furthermore, some youths with TD who are evaluated in clinical settings may meet criteria for explosive outbursts.

IV. **Epidemiology**

As was noted above, prevalence estimates for TD vary greatly. Most recent lifetime prevalence rate estimates are 4 to 10 in 1,000 for TD and 1 in 200 for the full spectrum, including chronic motor tics and TD. Across the developmental spectrum, males are at least three to four times more likely than females to manifest TD. Limited data suggest that adults reveal the syndrome approximately one-tenth as often as children and adolescents.

V. **Genetics**

Genetic data derive from family pedigree, twin studies, and studies of sibling pairs. That TD, chronic tic disorders, and OCD congregate in families is well established. Twin studies have shown a high concordance rate for tic disorders among monozygotic pairs (ranging from 50% to 90%), in contrast to a relatively low rate among dizygotic twins (approximately 10%). Other studies have shown that first-degree relatives of TD patients have a higher percentage of TD, chronic tics, and OCD than do those of normal control subjects. Historically, genetic analyses of family pedigrees have appeared to be consistent with an autosomal dominant mode with incomplete penetrance of inheritance of TD; other investigators have proposed a single major gene locus in combination with other genes or environmental factors. To date, no unique locus has been specifically identified for TD; however, early findings in a study of 110 sibling pairs suggest that the 4q and 8p regions might be involved, although the results of this study did not reach statistical significance.

VI. Etiology and Pathophysiology

The etiology and pathophysiology of TD and tic disorders remain unknown. Data from neuroimaging and neurochemical studies of TD accumulated during the past decade point to a diffuse process in the brain involving pathways in the basal ganglia, striatum, and frontal lobes. Several neurotransmitters and neuromodulators have been implicated, including dopamine, norepinephrine, serotonin, and endogenous opioids. Neuroimaging studies that use cerebral blood flow and energy (glucose) metabolism parameters (e.g., positron emission tomography and single photon emission tomography) suggest altered activity (increased or decreased, and at times unilaterally) in various areas of the brain, such as the frontal and orbital cortex, the striatum, and the basal ganglia (e.g., putamen), in TD patients compared with that of control subjects or across brain regions within TD patients. Magnetic resonance imaging studies have indicated volume or asymmetry abnormalities in caudate or lenticular nuclei in subjects with TD compared with results for control subjects. A recent functional magnetic resonance imaging study has indicated changes in signal intensity in the basal ganglia, thalamus, and connecting cortical regions during tics.

In 1998, Swedo et al. described a putative subgroup of children with TD and OCD with hypothetical antecedent group A β-hemolytic *Streptococcus* (GABHS) infection who experienced symptom onset or exacerbation that was precipitated by streptococcal infection (pediatric autoimmune neuropsychiatric disorders associated with *Streptococcus* [PANDAS]). The Swedo group provided specific diagnostic criteria for PANDAS, including prepubertal onset, sudden explosive onset, and/or exacerbations and remissions, as well as a temporal relationship between symptoms and GABHS. One double-blind, placebo-controlled, crossover study of prophylactic oral **penicillin** that attempted to reduce recurrences of PANDAS failed to show any differences between the drug and the placebo; low **penicillin** doses and the time of year have made some clinicians question the relevance of the findings from this study. Some investigators believe that the connection of GABHS infection to TD is not direct; instead, they view it as indirect and postulate that the linkage is through ADHD comorbidity.

VII. Differential Diagnosis

Differential diagnosis of TD and tic disorders can be challenging; no specific laboratory tests are confirmatory. Diagnosis is made on clinical grounds, including the characteristic historical features and the clinical examination. Table 7.5 lists other involuntary movement disorders that must be considered in the differential diagnosis.

TABLE 7.5. DIFFERENTIAL DIAGNOSIS OF TIC DISORDERS

Descriptive Terms	Observable Movement Patterns
Akathisia	Motor restlessness (an unpleasant need to move), usually in the lower extremities
Athetosis	Slow writhing movements, usually in the hands and fingers
Ballismus	Large amplitude, jerking, shaking, flinging
Chorea	Irregular, spasmodic, usually limbs or face
Dyskinesia	Choreiform or dystonic, stereotyped, and not suppressible
Dystonia	Sustained tonic contraction that progresses to abnormal postures
Myoclonus	Sudden, brief, clonic, shock-like jerks or spasms, that usually involve the limbs
Periodic movements of sleep	Periodic dorsiflexion of the foot and flexion of the knee that occur during sleep
Stereotypy	Repetitive, usually meaningless, gestures, habits, or automatisms

Other movement disorders that are sometimes confused with TD include the following:

1. Sydenham chorea, a neurologic complication of streptococcal infection in which choreiform, writhing, often truncal movements are observed;
2. Huntington disease, an autosomal dominant disorder presenting with chorea and dementia that typically has its onset in the fourth or fifth decade of life;
3. Parkinson disease, typically a disorder of late life, that is characterized by flat facies, gait disturbance, rigidity, cogwheeling, and "pill-rolling" resting tremor;
4. PANDAS.

In psychiatric settings, patients who have been exposed to conventional antipsychotic agents (i.e., those showing the extrapyramidal effects at typical therapeutic doses) are at risk for drug-induced dyskinesias, including tardive and withdrawal dyskinesias. These undesirable effects may be seen in TD patients who have been treated with conventional antipsychotic agents. Careful baseline evaluation for and documentation of abnormal movements before initiating any form of therapy (especially before the use of conventional antipsychotic agents) for patients with tic disorders are essential.

VIII. Evaluation and Assessment

A comprehensive detailed history with observations derived from multiple sources is the cornerstone of the clinical evaluation of patients with tic disorders. Because TD is a diagnosis made primarily on the basis of its unique history and since tics may be suppressed during physical examination, reliable sources of information are essential.

Historical inquiry should include detailed medical and developmental information, past experiences with medications (including substances of abuse or recreation), educational and occupational data, social and interpersonal history, and a thorough family pedigree covering at least three generations. A careful, descriptive, longitudinal assessment of the movement disorder is important. The physical examination should include height, weight, presence or absence of dysmorphic features, posture, gait, reflexes, and a systematic rating of current abnormal movements. The Abnormal Involuntary Movement Scale is a systematic assessment procedure and rating form that can be adapted for use with children's tics.

Psychiatric evaluation should include a formal assessment of the comorbid disorders that frequently occur with TD, including OCD, ADHD, and mood and non-OCD anxiety disorders (see Chapters 6, 14, 21, and 22). The use of structured or semistructured diagnostic interviews, such as the Schedule for Affective Disorders and Schizophrenia for Children, the Diagnostic Interview Schedule for Children, and the Diagnostic Interview for Children and Adolescents, can improve the classification and assessment of comorbidity, especially in a research context. Standardized global rating scales developed specifically for the TD population have improved diagnostic reliability in research studies, and they can be easily administered by the clinician. The Yale-Global Tic Severity Scale is a clinician-administered ordinal scale that rates tic number, frequency, intensity, complexity, and interference in the past week; it has an established reliability and validity. Specific rating scales for OCD (e.g., the Leyton Obsessional Inventory, the Yale-Brown Obsessive-Compulsive Scale, the OCD Inventory) and ADHD (e.g., the Conners) can also be used for assessing the severity of these comorbid disorders when they are present.

Auxiliary data from outside sources are extremely useful. Pediatric and medical records may document the developmental and medical history, the adequacy of medication trials and responses, hospitalizations, and laboratory findings. A review of school records is essential for children, because many TD patients manifest their difficulties in school settings. Report cards can document academic performance; direct phone contact with teachers may provide data about attentional, social, and emotional functioning. Neuropsychologic or speech and language testing may be indicated for patients with impairments in school or occupational functioning.

IX. Treatment
A. General Guidelines
Treatment goals should be to reduce symptoms, to support adaptive functioning and strengths, and to enhance developmental progress. Some clinicians do not advocate treatment unless they are confident that an improved outcome will occur. Treatment should not be forced on either the parents or the child.

1. **Self-esteem** must always be supported because most patients with tic disorders will have at least some sense of personal and emotional vulnerability.
2. **Education** focusing on the phenomenology, natural history, and treatment options for TD is essential.
3. **Clarification** that the patient's symptoms are not voluntary eases the psychologic burdens for both the patient and the family. This is especially important because families observe that tics can be suppressed at times. A practical goal involves personal management of and responsibility for symptoms and behavior, regardless of their origins.
4. **Containment** and management comprise another cornerstone of treatment. Even with the use of effective medication, complete remission of tics is rare. Use of a "tic room" or a "time out" area at home or school provides a way to contain problematic tics or compulsions. Because emotional conflicts and stress frequently increase symptom intensity, time-limited withdrawal from stressful situations can be beneficial.

B. Specific Medications
1. **General comments**. The decision to treat tic disorders should be based on a thorough and comprehensive assessment. Patients with symptoms that significantly interfere with adaptation to family, school, work, peer relationships, or developmental progress should be treated. Patients who suffer significant emotional distress may also be candidates for treatment, even when the symptoms are relatively mild. Most patients with very mild tics will need monitoring, education, guidance, and support. Moderate to severe tics are usually treated more aggressively.

   In general, patients should be started on the lowest possible dose of any medication and should be titrated upward gradually. Most maximum doses for TD patients will be low compared with the dosages needed for other indications for the same agent. Table 7.6 lists specific drugs and dosages. When possible, monotherapy should be attempted initially. However, given the complexity and frequent comorbidity in most TD patients seeking treatment, targeted combined pharmacotherapy with two or more medications more often is the rule rather than the exception.

   Determining an adequate duration for a medication trial for patients with tics can be quite challenging because the natural course of TD involves the waxing and waning of tics over time. As a general guideline, one should wait at least several weeks after dosage adjustment before drawing conclusions about a given dose efficacy. External stressors as potential determinants of increased tic symptomatology must be taken into account and addressed accordingly. In general, achieving complete remission of tics with pharmacotherapy is rare, but attempting to reduce tics substantially is reasonable.

2. **Recommended pharmacotherapies for TD and other tic disorders**
   a. **α-Adrenergic agonists**. **Clonidine**, a centrally acting α_2-adrenergic receptor (presynaptic) agonist, has been used for about two decades for the treatment of TD. **Clonidine** is the recommended first-line treatment for mild to moderate tics, with or without comorbid ADHD. Unfortunately, this is not a United States Food and Drug Administration-approved indication (i.e., in the approved wording for the product label) for **clonidine** or any other agents in its class. When given in low doses, the postulation is that the presynaptic noradrenergic effects mediate the regularly observed clinical improvement in tics. In addition, unlike the antipsychotic agents, **clonidine**

TABLE 7.6. RECOMMENDED PHARMACOTHERAPIES FOR TOURETTE DISORDER AND OTHER TIC DISORDERS

Class Agent	Typical Range (mg)	Starting Dose (mg)	Maximum Recommended Dose	Common Side Effects
Partial α_2-adrenergic agonists				
Clonidine	0.05–0.45	0.025–0.05	0.45 mg	Sedation, headaches, dysphoria
Guanfacine	0.5–4	0.25–0.5	4 mg	Like clonidine but less sedating
Atypical antipsychotic agents				
Risperidone	0.5–4	0.25–0.5	6 mg	Weight gain, sedation, prolactinemia
Olanzapine	2.5–5	1.25–2.5	10 mg	Similar to risperidone
Conventional antipsychotic agents				
Haloperidol	0.25–5	0.25–0.5	5 mg	Sedation, weight gain, dysphoria, extrapyramidal effects
Pimozide	1–10	0.5–1	10 mg	Sedation, weight gain, ECG changes
Antidepressants: selective serotonin reuptake inhibitors				
Fluoxetine	5–40	2.5–10	60–80 mg	Behavioral activation, insomnia, gastrointestinal distress
Sertraline	25–200	12.5–25	200–250 mg	Same as fluoxetine
Fluvoxamine	50–300	12.5–25	300 mg	Same as fluoxetine
Antidepressants: tricyclics				
Clomipramine	50–200	25–50	250–300 mg	Dry mouth, sedation, weight gain, ECG changes
Desipramine	50–300	10–25	5 mg/kg/d	Same as clomipramine
Nortriptyline	25–100	10–25	2.5/mg/kg/d	Same as clomipramine

(continued)

TABLE 7.6.   (*Continued*)

Class Agent	Typical Range (mg)	Starting Dose (mg)	Maximum Recommended Dose	Common Side Effects
Psychostimulants				
Methylphenidate	5–40	2.5–10	Individualized	Insomnia, anorexia, dysphoria
d-amphetamine	2.5–30	2.5–5	Individualized	Same as methylphenidate

Abbreviation: ECG; electrocardiogram.

also ameliorates the disinhibition, impulsivity, hyperarousal, and motoric overactivity often seen in TD patients.

Clonidine should be started at 0.025 mg once or twice a day for prepubertal children and should be increased by 0.025 mg every 1 to 2 weeks. **Clonidine** is typically administered to prepubertal children three or four times a day. **Clonidine's** half-life varies from 10 to 30 hours; in younger children, it tends to have shorter half-lives. In adolescents, it tends to have intermediate values (i.e., 13 to 14 hours). Adolescents or adults can be started on 0.05 mg once or twice a day, and the dosage may be increased by 0.05 mg increments. Older patients may require less frequent dosing. The total daily dose typically is 0.05 to 0.45 mg (up to 8.0 µg per kg per day). Sedation, headaches, or stomach discomfort are the common side effects. Sedation usually will diminish over several weeks; when it does not, dosage reduction may be helpful. Cardiovascular effects (i.e., hypotension) are minimal in this dosage range, but an electrocardiogram, the blood pressure, and pulse should be evaluated before the initiation of treatment and should be monitored periodically. A withdrawal syndrome can occur after abrupt discontinuation. This complication is usually seen in patients taking more than 0.3 mg per day over an extended time period. A transdermal form of **clonidine**, Catapres TTS, is available for children who cannot swallow pills or for those who require very frequent dosing or more even absorption.

Guanfacine, another α_2-adrenergic receptor (presynaptic) agonist, is an alternative when **clonidine** has not been effective or when the response has been limited by side effects. **Guanfacine** appears to have a longer half-life than **clonidine**, and thus it can be given on a twice a day schedule. Additionally, it appears to cause sedation about half as often as **clonidine**. **Guanfacine** is also less likely than **clonidine** to lead to a withdrawal syndrome after abrupt discontinuation. Nevertheless, tapering is advised. **Guanfacine** is preferred by some clinicians.

b. **Antipsychotic agents.** Since the late 1960s when orally administered **haloperidol** was first introduced as a treatment for motor and vocal tics in TD patients, conventional antipsychotic agents have been the only medications that are formally approved for labeling for TD. These agents, including **haloperidol** and **pimozide** (see Chapter 4), antagonize dopamine (D_2) receptors in the basal ganglia. From the risk-versus-benefit perspective, they are effective and they are relatively safe for children, adolescents, or adults with moderately severe to severe tics. However, conventional antipsychotic agents are not recommended for mild to moderate tics because of the possibility of long-term side effects, such as tardive dyskinesia. When an antipsychotic

TABLE 7.7. APPROXIMATE RATIOS OF 5-HYDROXYTRYPTAMINE 2^a TO DOPAMINERGIC RECEPTOR AFFINITIES^a FOR SELECTED ANTIPSYCHOTIC AGENTS

Agent	5-HT$_{2a}$	D$_2$	Approximate Ratio (5-HT$_{2a}$/D$_2$)
Haloperidol	36.0	4.0	9.0
Pimozide	13.0	2.5	5.2
Risperidone	0.2	3.3	0.06
Ziprasidone	0.4	4.8	0.09
Olanzapine	4.0	11.0	0.36

^{a}Affinities are based on published data from product literature and are expressed as approximate K$_i$ values in μM. Lower values of K$_i$ indicate higher receptor affinities.
Abbreviations: D$_2$, dopamine-2 receptor; 5-HT$_{2a}$, 5-hydroxytryptamine-2a.

agent is necessary for a given child, an atypical antipsychotic agent should be tried first.

(1) **Atypical antipsychotic agents**. A characteristic of atypical antipsychotic agents is their stronger affinity for 5-hydroxytryptamine-2 (5-HT$_2$) receptors compared with their affinity for D$_2$ receptors. Table 7.7 compares the ratios of these affinities for some of the antipsychotic agents used in tic disorders. Remembering that antipsychotic agents also differ from each other in many other ways is also important; another key difference among them is their degree of receptor occupancy at therapeutic concentrations. **Haloperidol's** usual occupancy rate is greater than 80%, the level above which extrapyramidal side effects are more likely.

Open studies of **risperidone** suggest that it can be beneficial for TD at low to moderate doses (1.5 mg per day). **Risperidone** can be initiated at 0.25 mg per day in children and can be titrated upward gradually. Older youth and adults can be started on 0.5 mg per day. Open-label studies and case reports also suggest that **olanzapine** can be beneficial in the treatment of TD, with doses in the 2.5-mg to 10-mg range. A placebo-controlled trial of **ziprasidone** showed that agent to be significantly more effective than the placebo, and some clinicians report favorable use of **quetiapine**.

The most common and potentially problematic side effect with the atypical antipsychotic agents is weight gain, which can be significant in young patients. Increased insulin resistance may develop as a secondary side effect. These effects should be anticipated with parents so that an active exercise program and dietary monitoring can be initiated with treatment.

(2) **Conventional agents**. Children can be started at doses of 0.25 mg per day of **haloperidol**, an amount that can be increased by 0.25 mg weekly or biweekly. Adolescents or adults can be started on 0.5 mg per day, with weekly or biweekly increases in 0.5 mg increments. Most patients will respond to a total daily dose of 5 mg or less, although a few adults may need a higher daily dose (i.e., up to 10 to 15 mg).

Pimozide (see Chapter 4) is an alternative agent that may cause fewer side effects than **haloperidol**. However, because **pimozide** also has T-type calcium channel blocking properties, normal cardiac function, which can be ascertained from cardiac assessment and an electrocardiogram, is a prerequisite to its use. **Pimozide**, which is approximately half as potent as **haloperidol**, should be started at 0.5 to 1 mg per day for children and at about 1 mg per day for adolescents or adults. Most patients will require less than 10 mg per day.

The common side effects of conventional antipsychotic agents include weight gain, sedation, and dysphoric syndromes. Dosage reduction or switching to an alternative drug is the best way to respond to these side effects. Fortunately, acute dystonic reactions and tardive dyskinesia do not appear to be common sequelae of conventional antipsychotic agent use at the typical dosages used for tic disorder patients; nevertheless, clinicians should be alert to the possibility of these reactions and should consider appropriate interventions (e.g., antiparkinsonian agents, dosage reduction) as needed.

   c. **Alternative treatments**. **Nicotine** has been reported to reduce tics through cholinergically mediated effects when administered in a transdermal form either alone or in combination with an antipsychotic agent. **Mecamylamine**, a nicotinic cholinergic receptor antagonist, has also been reported to reduce tics in recent studies. Additionally, **baclofen**, which has γ-aminobutyric acid (GABA)ergic effects, was found in a recent double-blind placebo-controlled trial to reduce some TD symptoms more effectively than the placebo.

   d. **Proserotonergic agents**. Some of these agents, such as **fluoxetine, fluvoxamine, sertraline**, and **clomipramine**, represent alternative treatments for some of the OCD symptoms in TD. Because many TD patients have obsessions or compulsions as their primary symptoms of clinical concern, they are candidates for treatment with a selective serotonin reuptake inhibitor (SSRI). **Fluvoxamine, sertraline**, and **fluoxetine** have been studied in pediatric OCD (see Chapter 21), and thus they are recommended as first-line agents if a therapeutic trial is indicated. The established efficacy and side effect profiles are quite similar; the choice of agent may rest on pharmacokinetic or drug interaction differences (see Chapter 29).

   Fluoxetine typically is started at 2.5 to 5 mg per day for children and at 5 to 10 mg per day for adolescents or adults. **Sertraline** is typically started at 12.5 to 25 mg per day in children and at 50 mg per day in adolescents or adults; **fluvoxamine** is started at similar doses. An SSRI used in combination with an antipsychotic agent can be useful for controlling both tics and obsessive-compulsive symptoms. Common side effects in youths include behavioral activation, agitation, insomnia, headaches, gastrointestinal effects, or sexual dysfunction. Because the behavioral activation may abate over time, reducing the dose temporarily for observation is helpful. Switching to another SSRI or to **clomipramine** may be necessary if the OCD symptoms do not abate.

   When several SSRI trials have not been helpful, a trial of **clomipramine** should be considered. Its efficacy in pediatric OCD has been established since the mid-1980s. **Clomipramine** should be started at 10 to 25 mg per day for children and 25 to 50 mg per day for adolescents or adults and should then be titrated gradually upward. Total dosage ranges are typically 100 to 300 mg per day; blood levels may be obtained, but, at present, no therapeutic range is established. Common side effects are those seen typically with other tricyclic antidepressants, including sedation, dry mouth, constipation, blurring of vision, and weight gain. Baseline and follow-up electrocardiograms should be monitored.

3. **Attention deficit hyperactivity disorder treatments** (see Chapter 22). Historically, controversy has existed about the role of stimulants in the treatment of tic disorders and TD; older reports indicated that stimulants may induce or increase tics in children. However, several investigators recently reported the significant beneficial effects of stimulants either alone or in combination with **clonidine** when the ADHD symptoms are the primary clinical concern. Results of a recently completed National Institutes of Health-sponsored randomized clinical trial comparing **methylphenidate, clonidine**, and their combination with a placebo indicated that the combination was more effective than the placebo in treatment of both tics and ADHD symptoms. Results also indicated that **methylphenidate** treatment did not increase tics when used either alone or in combination with **clonidine**. In addition, tricyclic antidepressants, such as **desipramine** and **nortriptyline**, have been reported in both open and double-blind trials to be effective in children with ADHD and comorbid tics.

C. **Behavioral Therapies**

Behavioral paradigms can be useful for some patients with tic disorders. Simple behavioral approaches can be used to reduce stress and to contain the tic symptoms. Specific paradigms are indicated for obsessions, compulsions, and possibly some complex motor tics. Relaxation techniques, such as deep breathing, guided imagery, and the use of relaxation tapes, can be useful for the anxious or stressed TD patient. Habit reversal therapy, which consists of isometric muscle tensing to oppose motor tics, may be useful in the treatment of tic disorder. Opposing muscles are contracted when the urge to have a tic develops (e.g., having a child chew gum [preferably sugarless] to reduce facial tics). This competing response theoretically prevents the emergence of the tic. Preliminary results of a study currently underway comparing habit reversal therapy with monitoring indicate that habit reversal may be an effective behavioral treatment for tics in older patients. Tic substitution (i.e., substituting a more socially tolerable tic for a less socially tolerable one) is another alternative that may be helpful.

Contingency management emphasizes positive reinforcement and avoids increased guilt or anxiety. Massed negative practice (i.e., self-imposed forceful repetition of the tic) for a period of time (with intervals for rest) is beneficial for some patients. The patient performs the tic deliberately for as many times as possible. The ensuing tiredness theoretically produces a decrease in tic frequency. Although behavioral approaches typically work best for older youth and adults, even younger children can be taught some of the basic techniques with their parents. Behavioral treatment may be more acceptable than pharmacotherapy to some families, especially when the tic symptoms are mild.

D. **Psychoeducational Approaches**

Education of patients and their families is always essential. Opportunities for discussion of patients' questions and concerns should be made available early in the diagnostic process and in ongoing treatment. Referral to the national Tourette Syndrome Association (TSA) or to local chapters of the TSA is an excellent way to maintain ongoing education and support. The national TSA is located at 40-42 Bell Boulevard; Bayside, New York, 11361 (718-224-2999). The TSA provides useful information through its website (*http://www.tsa-usa.org*).

E. **Psychotherapy**

Individual, group, and family therapies are supportive adjuncts to pharmacotherapy. Individual supportive therapy that incorporates the principles of cognitive-behavior therapy is indicated for patients having difficulty adjusting to their disorder with their peers or family or with school or occupational functioning. Supportive therapy is particularly useful when evidence of moderate stress or anxiety or another comorbid psychiatric disorder responsive to this form of psychotherapy (e.g., mild depression) is observed. It can help to restore or to maintain self-esteem or to promote mastery and coping.

Family work or therapy is extremely useful in TD. Both parents and any other involved family members should be seen at least once as part of the initial evaluation. Ongoing family therapy is indicated when family development (i.e., growth and maturation) has slowed or halted because of the focus on the patient with the tic disorder. It may also be helpful with maladaptive reactions from or to siblings or with specific symptoms that are affecting the entire family.

Group therapy is another important adjunct. Support and education for parents and family members of patients with TD can be found in support groups sponsored by the national TSA. Informal, unstructured activities can be arranged through local TSA chapters. Formal structured support is also possible through psychoeducationally oriented groups.

F. School and Occupational Interventions

Learning problems and classroom difficulties are seen frequently in patients with tic disorders. Specific developmental disorders and ADHD-related or OCD-related symptoms may interfere with academic performance. Clinicians should be available to provide consultation, guidance, and education to teachers or employers of patients with tic disorders. Useful special educational interventions include creating moderate task-oriented support and individualized work or lesson plans. Flexibility is a key element in educational and occupational intervention. To promote tic control, optional time-outs from class or work settings might be needed. Time limits may have to be extended or eliminated for exams. Adaptive (as opposed to regular) physical education can be particularly helpful for children with TD; this can be arranged through special education departments in local schools. Programs should be tailored to each child's needs, strengths, and weaknesses. Specific workplace interventions include structured tasks, organization of tasks into smaller units, flexible time limits, and ample physical space.

ADDITIONAL READING

Apter A, Pauls DL, Bleich A, et al. An epidemiologic study of Gilles de la Tourette's syndrome in Israel. *Arch Gen Psychiatry* 1993;50:734–738.

Bruun R, Budman C. The course and prognosis of Tourette syndrome. In: Jankovic J, ed. *Tourette syndrome.* Philadelphia: WB Saunders, 1997:291–298. Neurologic Clinics series. Vol. 15.

Burd L, Kerbeshian J, Wikenheiser M, et al. Prevalence of Gilles de la Tourette's syndrome in North Dakota adults. *Am J Psychiatry* 1986;143:787–788.

Coffey B, Biederman J, Geller D, et al. The course of Tourette's disorder: a literature review. *Harv Rev Psychiatry* 2000;8:192–198.

Coffey B, Miguel E, Savage C, et al. Tourette's disorder and related problems: a review and update. *Harv Rev Psychiatry* 1994;2:121–132.

Garvey M, Perlmutter S, Allen AJ, et al. A pilot study of penicillin prophylaxis for neuropsychiatric disorders triggered by streptococcal infections. *Biol Psychiatry* 1999;45:1564–1571.

Leckman J, Zhang H, Vitale A, et al. Course of tic severity in Tourette syndrome: the first two decades. *Pediatrics* 1998;102:14–19.

Robertson M. Tourette syndrome, associated conditions, and the complexities of treatment. *Brain* 2000;123:425–462.

Singer H. Current issues in Tourette syndrome. *Move Disord* 2000;6:1051–1063.

Spencer T, Biederman J, Coffey B, et al. The four-year course of tic disorders in boys with ADHD. *Arch Gen Psychiatry* 1999;56:842–847.

Swedo S, Leonard H., Garvey M, et al. Pediatric autoimmune neuropsychiatric disorders associated with streptococcal infections: a clinical description of the first 50 cases. *Am J Psychiatry* 1998;155:264–271.

Tourette Syndrome Association International Consortium for Genetics. A complete genome screen in sib pairs affected by Gilles de la Tourette syndrome. *Am J Hum Genet* 1999;65:1428–1436.

Tourette's Syndrome Study Group. Treatment of ADHD in children with tics: a randomized controlled trial. *Neurology* 2002;58:527–536.

The following brochures are available from the Tourette Syndrome Association and its local chapters:

Coping with Tourette Syndrome—a Parent's Viewpoint
Coping with Tourette Syndrome in the Classroom
Facts You Should Know About the Genetics of Tourette Syndrome
Know Your Rights: Financial Resources
Know Your Rights: Services Available
Tourette Syndrome: Questions and Answers

8. DISORDERS OF EATING: ANOREXIA NERVOSA, BULIMIA NERVOSA, AND BINGE-EATING DISORDER

W. Stewart Agras

Eating behavior is modulated by cultural, social, familial, and biologic factors. These influences guide taste preferences, dietary choices, and patterns of food intake. Social learning may lead to food choices that would be aversive to members of another culture and may overcome natural aversions (e.g., to bitter taste or to certain food smells, such as ripe cheeses). Thus, in any culture, a wide range of eating behavior is considered normal. Similarly, children may demonstrate marked variation in their food intake from meal to meal, sometimes consuming only a single food during a meal, but they demonstrate much less variation over successive 24-hour periods. Aversions to various foods may persist for several months during childhood, only to disappear eventually.

Some psychiatric disorders are accompanied by minor to more extreme pathologic eating patterns. In depression, for example, the most common pattern is diminished interest in food and poor appetite, accompanied by weight loss (see Chapter 18). A second pattern, which is seen less commonly in depression, consists of excessive eating that is often accompanied by sleepiness and lethargy. Anxiety disorder patients (see Chapter 14) may also have diminished appetite and weight loss, although a few may increase their food intake, often consuming "junk food." Avoidance of foods that is most commonly based on a fear of choking may be seen in phobic disorders. Phobic patients typically avoid solid foods that are difficult to swallow. In paranoid disorders, food avoidances based on delusional thinking, often concerning poisoning, may also be seen.

Many neurochemical systems are involved in the regulation of feeding behavior. Serotonin, for example, modulates satiety, and high levels lead to the cessation of eating. Adrenergic compounds may either decrease or increase feeding, depending on the state of the organism at the time of feeding. Neuropeptide Y stimulates eating behavior; leptin appears to be inhibitory; and opioids and dopaminergic mechanisms are involved in the reinforcing properties of feeding. Cholecystokinin also plays a role in satiety.

Given these various control mechanisms, the fact that medications commonly used in psychiatric practice may affect eating behavior is not surprising. For example, the use of many antipsychotic agents, such as **clozapine, olanzapine**, and **risperidone**, can lead to weight gain, a troublesome problem for schizophrenic patients, who may need to be maintained on medication for many years. Some patients treated with antidepressants, such as **amitriptyline** or **mirtazapine**, may experience weight gain, presumably due to appetite stimulation. Paradoxically, patients with eating disorders often experience appetite suppression when they receive antidepressants. The benzodiazepines sometimes alter eating behavior by increasing food intake; an occasional patient will notice weight gain as a consequence. **Amphetamines**, most frequently those used for the treatment of attention deficit hyperactivity disorder (see Chapter 22) and occasionally those used for treatment of resistant depressions, diminish the appetite, and their use may lead to weight loss. In some patients, **topiramate**, an anticonvulsant that is sometimes used as a mood stabilizer, is also associated with weight loss.

Cultural preferences for body shape, particularly for women, strongly affect eating behavior. In undeveloped countries, a plump body shape is preferred. On the other hand, in the developed countries, the current cultural preference is for a thin body shape for women. In Western countries, researchers have shown that most adolescent females develop a fear of becoming fat and that they experience dissatisfaction with their body shape and weight. These fears and dissatisfactions, which are seen less frequently in males, lead most high school girls to diet from time to time in attempts to control their body shape and weight. However, relatively few young women develop an eating disorder. Thus, although a continuum of concern about body weight and shape that influences dietary behavior undoubtedly exists, eating disorders probably should be regarded as distinctly separate psychopathologic entities with risk factors that can add to the effects of simple dietary restriction. Such risk factors, in addition to weight and shape concerns and restrictive dieting, include genetic factors; a family or personal history of being overweight or obese; family influences, such as maternal concerns about a daughter's weight and shape; and peer teasing about weight and shape. Less specific factors include low self-esteem, sexual or physical abuse, and stressors of various types.

The disorders of eating, which range in frequency from relatively rare to quite common, consist of **anorexia nervosa, bulimia nervosa,** and **binge-eating disorder**; the latter condition is frequently observed in the overweight. Although these three conditions are usually considered the core eating disorders, a further clinical problem, **ruminative vomiting,** that is seen in infancy and in the institutionalized mentally retarded, is also considered in this chapter.[1] The core eating disorders are seen far more commonly in females than in males, which mirrors the dietary concerns of the general population, and, with the exception of ruminative vomiting, they have increased in prevalence during the past 30 years. The behaviors involved in the core eating disorders include overvaluation of a thin body shape and low weight, restriction of food intake, binge eating, and purging. One should note that the treatment of the eating disorders is as costly as that for conditions such as obsessive-compulsive disorder. Hence, recognition of these disorders early in their development is important.

I. Disordered Eating Behaviors
A. Definitions and Concepts

1. **Overvaluation of body shape and weight**. The **overvaluation of body shape and weight** seen in the eating disorders is partly a response to the changes in the fashion cycle noted above; thinness has become desirable for women. The most recent cyclical change toward a thin body shape began in the late 1960s. Unlike a similar cycle in the 1920s in which the thin look was attained by changes in dress style that included binding the breasts to achieve a boyish silhouette, in the most recent cycle thinness is attained by dieting. This change in societal values has led most females to become dissatisfied with their body shape and weight and to diet. However, cultural and socioeconomic differences in response to these societal demands do exist, with upper-class and middle-class white women being the most responsive. The patient with an eating disorder appears to be more concerned with her body shape and weight than are "normal" women of the same race and socioeconomic class.

2. **Dietary restriction**. The dietary restriction seen in anorexia nervosa, bulimia nervosa, and binge eating is a response to overvaluing body shape and weight. The degree of restriction is most extreme in the anorexic and is least in the overweight binge eater. These patients elaborate various rigid food rules, many of which are unreasonable. For the most part, the foods that are avoided are those considered "fattening" by each individual, and hence they vary from patient to patient. Anorexics use various techniques to enhance their control over food intake. They tend to eat slowly, and they may make food less attractive by cutting it into small pieces or sometimes by garnishing it with pepper or salt. In the bulimic and binge eaters, episodes of dietary restriction alternate with binge eating.

3. **Binge eating**. This is defined as an eating episode that the patient perceives as being "out of control" as the individual is not able to resist the temptation to eat certain foods or to stop eating unless food is no longer available, unless he or she is interrupted by someone, or unless the patient is physically unable to eat more. Binge eating is a consequence of excessive caloric restriction or the attempt to attain such restriction, with the consequent disruption of normal feeding patterns. Thus, attempts at dieting precede binge eating in patients with bulimia nervosa.

---

[1] Another eating disorder, **pica** (the persistent ingestion of non-nutritive substances such as paint, plaster, or dirt), is sometimes considered important. Its frequency in adults and adolescents, however, is quite low, and the decision to omit it was made with this chapter's author.

Severe dietary restriction can usually be sustained only for a limited time, and then various factors lead to a breakdown of control and to binge eating. Factors leading to a loss of control include the sight and smell of particularly desired foods and emotional arousal secondary to stressful life events. A large amount of food is often eaten in a binge, although wide variation in size, from small (100 calories) to large (several thousand calories), is observed. Most binges occur in time-limited episodes, although some episodes may take up most of the day, with the patient typically eating small amounts of food almost continuously, a pattern sometimes referred to as **grazing**. The food chosen is usually easily swallowed, often consisting of breads, pastries, ice cream, or snack items. Binges are usually carried out in private for fear of discovery or interruption. Binge eating should be distinguished from overeating, which usually occurs in the context of a special social occasion, such as Thanksgiving, although overeating may be more frequent and habitual in some people. In the case of overeating, the individual has no sense of having lost control of eating. Because overeating usually is socially sanctioned, little anxiety or guilt is associated with it. In addition, the food consumed in episodes of overeating more closely resembles a normal meal than does the food eaten in a binge.

4. **Purging**. This may be defined as any activity aimed at ameliorating the perceived negative effects of a binge on body shape and weight. Purging may consist of self-induced vomiting, the use of laxatives, the use of diuretics, or enemas. A rarer form consists of spitting out food that has been chewed but not swallowed. Excessive exercise or fasting may also be used to compensate for binge eating. These latter behaviors are now termed **nonpurging compensatory behaviors**. Patients who induce vomiting often drink large amounts of fluids during and after the binge to facilitate purging. Although most bulimics become adept at inducing vomiting without emetics, a few use **ipecac**; this practice occasionally results in death from **ipecac** toxicity.

II. Anorexia Nervosa
A. Definitions and Concepts

The cardinal features of anorexia nervosa are a weight that is at least 15% below the ideal body weight, a strong fear of gaining weight, a perception of being fat even at a low weight, and, in the female, amenorrhea. The low body weight is achieved via a relentless pursuit of thinness through dieting, excessive exercise, and often purging. The degree of weight loss and the accompanying weakness and fatigue are often denied. The differential diagnosis includes weight loss accompanying severe depression, although no preoccupation regarding body shape or size is observed in this condition; in the weight loss accompanying schizophrenia, the food avoidance is based on delusional thinking.

The initial visit by a patient with this disorder usually stems from family concern about excessive weight loss, although a few patients present with physical complaints, such as orthopedic problems due to excessive exercise or cardiovascular problems secondary to starvation and potassium deficiency.

Anorexia nervosa is a relatively rare disorder with an incidence of about 15 new cases per 100,000 population per year in the United States. The disorder is seen far more frequently in females than in males, in whom it is quite rare. Because it is a chronic disorder, the lifetime prevalence is higher, ranging from 0.1% and 0.7%. The peak onset is during adolescence, although the first episode may occur in childhood or in early adult life.

Genetic factors may play a significant etiologic role. Twin studies reveal a concordance rate of approximately 70% for monozygotic twins. Family studies reveal that anorexia nervosa is about eight times more common in the relatives of anorexics than it is in the relatives of patients without anorexia. An excess of affective disorder is also observed in the families of bulimic anorexics, but the two disorders appear to be transmitted separately.

Comorbid obsessive-compulsive disorder with the usual range of obsessions and compulsions (e.g., dirt, infection, harming others, and associated rituals) occurs in 10% to 20% of anorexics. Because of the obsessional thinking and compulsive behavior regarding food that occur in all anorexics, some view the obsessional traits as a major contributor to the disorder (see Chapter 6). A concurrent episode of major depression is seen frequently, as is social phobia.

Many of the behavioral and physiologic changes seen in anorexia nervosa are a consequence of starvation; these are also seen in any starving population. They include intense preoccupation with food; slow eating; depression; a loss of energy; a loss of sexual interest; social withdrawal; and cognitive impairments resulting in diminished concentration, diminished performance on tests of intellectual function, and poor judgment. About half of all anorexics also binge eat and purge. This behavior is more likely to occur in the impulsive, less inhibited anorexic.

Physical examination reveals the evident cachexia, slow pulse rate, hypotension, cold and blue extremities, dry skin, and, at times, the appearance of fine body hair known as **lanugo**. Although many alterations in metabolic function occur, all are secondary to starvation. Thus, gonadotropin levels are decreased, the luteinizing hormone levels assume a prepubertal pattern, and the follicle-stimulating hormone and estrogen levels are also low. Growth hormone levels may be high in some patients, and the resting plasma cortisol levels are elevated. Triiodothyronine levels are below normal. All of these changes may be viewed as compensatory adaptations to starvation. Osteopenia and osteoporosis are common, and they may be accompanied by fractures in severe cases. Other changes that may be noted are elevated levels of cholesterol and carotene, leukopenia, and anemia. Potassium levels may also be low, particularly in the purging anorexic. These low levels (less than 3.0 mEq per L) may, in turn, give rise to cardiac arrhythmias that can lead to death when they are not corrected by supplemental potassium and the restoration of a normal fluid balance. In the low-weight anorexic, as opposed to the bulimic, this should be accomplished by intravenous infusion.

B. Treatment

The first step in the treatment of anorexia nervosa is to persuade both the patient and the family that treatment is necessary and to explain the nature of the treatment carefully. Most anorexics can be treated on an outpatient basis with short-term hospital admissions to remedy medical instability. Conceptualizing treatment as having the following two phases can be useful: an acute phase during adolescence and a more chronic phase for those who have not recovered within a few years of the initial episode. A specialized form of family therapy has been shown to be quite successful for the adolescent anorexic in controlled trials. The prime aim of this therapy is to help the parents regain control of their child's eating behavior so that he or she steadily regains weight. Once the child's weight has been stabilized, therapy enables the parents to loosen their control and to address ongoing family issues that may maintain the anorexic behaviors. In the chronic form of the disorder, therapy is aimed at increasing caloric intake and in dealing with the social isolation that characterizes the anorexic. Partial hospitalization may be useful for such patients.

Hospitalization in a specialized inpatient unit may be required in the very low weight anorexic (i.e., more than 25% below an ideal body weight). The first step is to correct metabolic abnormalities and to begin weight restoration. The usual program takes the form of systematic reinforcement of weight gain in which access to certain activities is contingent on a specified daily amount of weight gain (e.g., 0.2 kg per day). Reward activities (e.g., leaving the hospital room for a specified period of time) are limited at first. Later, they may include access to visitors other than family members, passes off the unit, and so on. A contract specifying the amount of weight gain and the contingent privileges must be worked out with the patient and should then be renegotiated at frequent intervals during hospitalization. Patients are encouraged to take an active role in such negotiations so that the reinforcements are personalized. Failure to gain weight usually signifies that the contingencies are not sufficiently rewarding, and it points to the need to discover more effective reinforcers.

Contingent reinforcement of this type has been shown to lead to increased caloric intake and weight gain in controlled studies. Such treatment has been shown to be more successful than the usual hospital care in a controlled study, although it may be more effective with patients who are less severely ill.

Fluid retention may occur during the initial stages of refeeding. For the first week or 10 days, the caloric intake should not exceed 2,000 calories per day and fluid intake should be carefully monitored. Once the individual's weight has begun to increase, family therapy and individual psychotherapy, if it is needed, is begun.

Medication *has relatively little place in the treatment of the anorexic.* One study has shown that nonbulimic anorexics respond better to **cyproheptadine**, a serotonin antagonist that stimulates the appetite, in doses up to 32 mg per day than to a placebo; but the response is often clinically insignificant. For the most part, the symptoms of depression usually remit with weight gain, and no pharmacologic treatment is necessary.

Tube feeding, which was once commonly used in the treatment of anorexia nervosa, is now rarely used because it may be complicated by inhalation pneumonia. The indications for parenteral feeding include dehydration and electrolyte imbalance, an intercurrent medical emergency necessitating weight gain, and failure to gain weight after an adequate trial of therapy. If parenteral feeding is indicated, it is best carried out on a medical ward so that, once the emergency has been treated, the patient can continue in a weight restoration program. Separation of medical and psychiatric treatments limits the opportunities for manipulation of the treatment system by these patients. Tube feeding may, on occasion, be used as negative reinforcement (i.e., by gaining weight at a certain rate or above a certain threshold, the patient can avoid tube feeding).

Long-term outpatient treatment should be provided after discharge from the hospital and should be continued until a satisfactory weight has been attained and has been stabilized for at least 6 months. Such treatment usually consists of **cognitive-behavior therapy** (CBT) aimed at providing support for the patient, modifying the distorted patterns of thinking about weight and shape, and dealing with the ongoing problems of living. Although most patients gain weight in such a treatment program, many will relapse within a few months and will require further hospitalization. Some evidence indicates that **fluoxetine** may be useful in enabling the maintenance of weight gains.

Less than half of the patients with this disorder recover fully, although vocational functioning is often preserved.

C. Caution

Anorexia nervosa has the highest mortality rate of any psychiatric disorder. In some long-term follow-up studies, the mortality rate from anorexia nervosa has been as high as 15%, although the usual figure that is given is 5%. In about half of the cases, death is due to suicide (see Chapter 17), a reminder that mood disorder is prevalent in this population and that suicidal risk should be carefully evaluated. Obesity is a rare complication of treatment, occurring in approximately 2% of patients.

III. Bulimia Nervosa

A. Definitions and Concepts

The following two types of bulimia nervosa are now recognized: **purging** and **nonpurging** syndromes. In the nonpurging syndrome, the compensatory behaviors are fasting and/or excessive exercise. Bulimia nervosa consists of severe dietary restriction, binge eating, and compensatory behaviors, whether purging or nonpurging, combined with dissatisfaction about body weight and shape and a fear of weight gain.

Binges are preceded in some 70% of episodes by a negative mood that is often induced by faulty interpersonal interactions. In the remaining cases, binge eating is preceded by acute dietary restriction. Binges are followed by feelings of guilt and depressed mood. The typical dietary pattern is to eat little or no breakfast, to have a very light lunch, and then to lose control and binge eat and purge in the late afternoon or evening.

The disorder usually begins in late adolescence with dieting and binge eating that precede the onset of purging by several months. Bulimia nervosa appears to run a chronic, sometimes episodic, course. Seeing patients who have suffered from the disorder for 30 years or more is not uncommon. Most bulimics are normal weight, and about 10% are overweight. About one-fourth of bulimics have a prior history of anorexia nervosa. A history of major depressive disorder, current major depressive disorder, and borderline personality disorder or impulsive traits are common in these patients. Other comorbid conditions are **alcohol** and drug abuse or dependence.

Like anorexia nervosa, bulimia nervosa is far more common in females than in males, with a prevalence of approximately 1% for patients meeting strict diagnostic criteria. Although the specific etiology of the disorder is unknown, the societal value of a thin body shape clearly appears to have influenced the increase in the number of cases of bulimia nervosa that have been seen in clinics since the late 1970s. Excessive dieting leads to a loss of control over eating, as has been demonstrated in laboratory experiments, and to binge eating. When faced with the threat of weight gain, some binge eaters then begin to purge. Dysregulation of serotonin metabolism may possibly be associated with bulimia nervosa, as bulimics appear to have low serotonin levels. Binge eating leads to the intake of tryptophan (a precursor of serotonin)-containing foods, thus raising the serotonin levels. In turn, this leads to satiety and to correction of the bulimic's low mood. However, whether the serotonin abnormalities are a result of the dietary dysregulation or a cause of it is not known.

One of the most frequent complications of bulimia nervosa is dental caries and periodontal disease as a consequence of the consumption of sweet foods. Serum amylase levels are increased in about two-thirds of patients, and swollen parotid glands are a distinguishing feature in a few. About one-fourth of all bulimics suffer from menstrual irregularity or amenorrhea. About 5% of patients will have a low serum potassium level that requires oral potassium supplementation. Other rarer complications associated with self-induced vomiting are chronic hoarseness, gastrointestinal reflux, and esophageal tears and bleeding. The use of laxatives as a method of purging leads to physiologic adaptation with slowed intestinal mobility and constipation. Many bulimic patients deny their laxative use. When covert laxative use is suspected, urine testing for phenolphthalein, a common ingredient in many over-the-counter and prescription laxatives (e.g., Ex-Lax, Medilax, Modase), is useful. However, the fact that another common laxative, **bisacodyl** (e.g., Dulcolax), is not detected by this method should be noted.

B. Treatment

The following three treatment approaches to bulimia nervosa have been demonstrated to be successful in controlled trials: antidepressant medications, CBT, and interpersonal therapy. CBT appears to be more successful than antidepressant medication, and its onset of action is faster than interpersonal therapy. Hence, CBT is generally recognized as the first-line treatment for bulimia nervosa.

1. **Antidepressants** were first used on the assumption that bulimia nervosa was a disorder closely related to depression. However, bulimics who are not overtly depressed and who have no history of major depressive disorder respond as well to antidepressant treatment as do depressed bulimics. Thus, the belief that the success of antidepressants in bulimia nervosa is not secondary to their efficacy in ameliorating symptoms of depression is now generally accepted. Antidepressants, including the tricyclic antidepressants (e.g., **imipramine, desipramine**), the monoamine oxidase inhibitors (e.g., **phenelzine**), and the serotonin reuptake

inhibitors (e.g., **citalopram, fluoxetine, fluvoxamine, paroxetine, sertraline**), have all been found to be effective in the treatment of bulimia nervosa. The tricyclic antidepressants and the monamine oxidase inhibitors are used at usual antidepressant doses. **Fluoxetine**, on the other hand, is used at higher doses than is usual in the treatment of depression (e.g., 60 rather than 20 mg per day). On average, binge eating and purging decline by about 80%, and some 30% of patients become symptom free for some period of time.

Unfortunately, relapse often occurs when medication is withdrawn and, in about one-fourth of cases, even when the medication is maintained. Thus, bulimics should be maintained on an adequate dosage of an antidepressant for at least 1 year to prevent relapse.

2. **The main aims of CBT** are to enhance food intake; to decrease avoidance of specific foods; and to deal with distorted thinking about foods, body image, and weight. Binge eating and purging are expected to decline once dietary restriction is eased. These aims are facilitated by detailed self-monitoring of food intake and the precipitants and consequences of binge eating. In the later stages of treatment, relapse-prevention techniques are used (e.g., learning how to cope with high-risk situations). Patients are usually seen weekly for about 20 sessions over a 6-month period. Overall, half of the patients will become symptom free after treatment, and another one-fourth will demonstrate significant improvement. The treatment of laxative abuse is best accomplished by acute withdrawal. Patients should be alerted to potential side effects of such withdrawal, including constipation, bloating and bowel discomfort, and edema. These symptoms usually persist for between 7 and 10 days. A recent study found that patients who did not reduce their purging behavior by 70% after six sessions of treatment were likely to fail treatment. For such patients, the clinician might consider adding an antidepressant to CBT.

IV. Binge-Eating Disorder

A. Definitions and Concepts

As was noted above, some adolescents who binge eat do not purge. Instead, many of them go on to struggle with weight gain for much of their lives. This syndrome is now considered a disorder that requires further research in the *Diagnostic and Statistical Manual of Mental Disorders,* 4th edition; it is similar to that of bulimia nervosa, except the individual does not engage in compensatory behaviors and hence has no medical complications attributable to purging. Like bulimics, these patients alternate between episodes of binge eating and dietary restriction, although the degree of such restriction is less than that seen in the bulimic patient. In other respects, the psychopathology of binge-eating disorder appears similar to that of bulimia nervosa. However, these patients tend to present for treatment later in life (often in the context of weight-reduction attempts), and they are more likely to be seen in medical clinics than in psychiatry clinics. The prime medical comorbidities of this disorder are those associated with obesity, such as essential hypertension, type II diabetes mellitus, hypercholesterolemia, and cardiovascular disease.

The **night eating syndrome**, a relatively uncommon disorder, should be considered in the differential diagnosis of binge-eating disorder. In this syndrome, patients present with morning anorexia, evening overeating, and insomnia. Compared with obese control subjects, those with night eating syndrome consume more calories, and over 50% of their daily caloric intake is eaten after 10 p.m., compared with control subjects whose post-10 p.m. caloric intake is 15%. Recent studies have found that those with night eating syndrome lack the usual nocturnal rise in leptin levels. They also have lower than usual nocturnal melatonin levels, which perhaps explains their nighttime eating (in the absence of leptin inhibition of eating) and their sleep disturbance. No treatments for this condition have been described.

Although the prevalence of binge-eating disorder in the general population is approximately 2%, between one-fourth and one-third of all obese people binge eat, and the frequency of binge eating increases with increasing levels of adiposity. This suggests that binge eating may be a risk factor for the development of obesity and that a significant minority of the obese has an eating disorder.

B. Treatment

Antidepressant medication, CBT, and interpersonal psychotherapy all appear effective in the treatment of the overweight binge eater. Unlike the findings for bulimia nervosa, CBT and interpersonal therapy appear to be equally effective in binge-eating disorder. Antidepressant therapy appears to promote greater weight losses when it is added to CBT. Moreover, if the cessation of binge eating is maintained, it is associated with larger weight losses than for those patients who do not stop binge eating.

V. Ruminative Vomiting

A. Definitions and Concepts

As was noted earlier, this is a relatively rare disorder that usually affects infants, in whom it is life threatening. The usual presentation is early failure to thrive, accompanied by regurgitation of milk. The infant appears to have "learned" to provoke regurgitation so that he or she is able to enjoy the taste of milk doubly. Unfortunately, the milk then flows out of the infant's mouth, depriving him or her of needed nutrition. The etiology of this disorder is unknown, although clinical observation suggests that the maternal relationship is often unsatisfactory, sometimes bordering on outright rejection by the mother.

B. Treatment

One treatment approach, which is based on the preceding observation, is to give the infant extra attention in a hospital environment. Although successes have been reported with this treatment, no controlled studies of its effectiveness exist. An alternative approach is to follow the regurgitative behaviors with an aversive event. Regurgitative behaviors include curling the tongue into the back of the mouth, a behavior that is often accompanied by movements of the throat and facial muscles. Various aversive stimuli have been used, including sour or bitter tastes (e.g., lemon juice). These procedures have been shown to be effective in single-case controlled studies as they rapidly eliminate regurgitation and are followed by weight gain. Clearly, the maternal relationship should be carefully investigated, and educational, social, or psychotherapeutic interventions should be offered if needed.

VI. Comment

The website of the Academy for Eating Disorders provides useful information about the Academy, as well as links to sites providing information about eating disorders (*http://www.aedweb.org/*).

ADDITIONAL READING

Agras WS, Apple RF. *Overcoming eating disorders: a cognitive-behavioral treatment for bulimia nervosa and binge eating disorder. Therapist guide*. San Antonio, TX: The Psychological Corporation, 1997.

Attia E, Haiman C, Walsh BT, et al. Does fluoxetine augment the inpatient treatment of anorexia nervosa? *Am J Psychiatry* 1998;155:548–551.

Dare C, Eisler E, Russell GM, et al. Family therapy for anorexia nervosa: implications from the results of a controlled trial of family and individual therapy. *J Marital Fam Ther* 1990;16:39–57.

Fairburn CG. *Overcoming binge eating*. New York: The Guilford Press, 1995.

Fairburn CG, Welch SL, Doll HA, et al. Risk factors for bulimia nervosa. A community-based case-control study. *Arch Gen Psychiatry* 1997;54:509–517.

Fluoxetine Bulimia Nervosa Study Group. Fluoxetine in the treatment of bulimia nervosa. *Arch Gen Psychiatry* 1992;49:139–147.

Herzog DB, Greenwood DN, Dorer DJ, et al. Mortality in eating disorders: a descriptive study. *Int J Eating Disord* 2000;28:20–26.

Keel PK, Mitchell JE, Miller KB, et al. Long-term outcome of bulimia nervosa. *Arch Gen Psychiatry* 1999;56:63–69.

Spitzer RL, Yanovski S, Wadden T, et al. Binge eating disorder: its further validation in a multisite study. *Int J Eating Disord* 1993;13:137–153.

Striegel-Moore R, Leslie D, Petrill SA, et al. One-year use and cost of inpatient and outpatient services among female and male patients with an eating disorder: evidence from a national database of health insurance claims. *Int J Eating Disord* 2000;27:381–389.

Walsh BT, Wilson GT, Loeb KL, et al. Medication and psychotherapy in the treatment of bulimia nervosa. *Am J Psychiatry* 1997;154:523–531.

Zipfel S, Lowe B, Deter HC, et al. Long-term prognosis in anorexia nervosa: lessons from a 21-year follow-up study. *Lancet* 2000;355:721–722.

9. TREATMENT OF PHYSICAL DEPENDENCE ON BARBITURATES, BENZODIAZEPINES, AND OTHER SEDATIVE-HYPNOTICS

Richard I. Shader
Domenic A. Ciraulo
David J. Greenblatt

I. General Information

The number of persons who abuse prescription drugs in the United States is estimated to be about 2% to 4%. Although the stereotypic drug abuser is portrayed as an inner city male, data suggest that whites, particularly those with psychiatric disorders and those between the ages of 18 and 25 years, are more likely to abuse prescribed agents intentionally. Unintentional misuse is more common among the elderly than it is among the young. Nevertheless, concern about physical dependence on sedative-hypnotic agents among both older persons and those of middle age, the age cohorts in which indefinite use of "sleeping pills" is most common, is widespread.

However, as the overall data on prescription drug abuse might lead one to expect, the population that most often seeks or is required to obtain treatment for a drug "habit" of "downs" or "downers" is adolescents and young adults. Short-acting and intermediate-acting barbiturates; benzodiazepines, including **flunitrazepam** or Rohypnol; other sedative-hypnotics, including γ-**hydroxybutyrate**; and **alcohol** are used by this younger cohort as mood modifiers, either alone or in combination with **cocaine**, amphetamines, or opioids. Usage alone rarely applies to the benzodiazepines. In the jargon of this cohort, such illicit drugs are commonly referred to according to the colors of their capsules as follows: "yellow jackets," "red birds," "red devils," "rainbows," and "blue heavens" (Table 9.1). Such street names go in and out of fashion. Some names refer to any agent with central nervous system depressant properties.

Although United States pharmaceutical companies have discontinued the manufacture and sale of some sedative-hypnotics (e.g., **methaqualone, glutethimide, halazepam, prazepam**) or some dosage strengths or they have temporarily withdrawn some from the market (e.g., some oral barbiturates), many licit forms remain. Others in the illicit market either appear as imports from other countries or as illegally manufactured street drugs.

Dependence is a general term used to describe the subjective sensation of a perceived need for regular doses of a drug. Dependence on a substance is usually present when the following characteristics exist: (a) a strong desire or need to continue with the drug or its substitutes, which is sometimes called "craving"; (b) a tendency to increase the dose that is usually related to tolerance; (c) psychic dependence, which is sometimes associated with "drug-seeking" behavior or the need to have the drug available at all times; and (d) physical dependence. Emphasizing that the presence of craving does not predict physical dependence (strong craving may exist without tolerance or dependence) is important, nor does the presence of the first three characteristics necessarily imply the fourth. Physical dependence refers to abstinence or withdrawal symptoms that appear when a drug is abruptly stopped. This is a physiologic phenomenon that does not imply abuse or "addiction." Therefore, discussions of the general concept of drug dependence need to include more descriptive specificities of the characteristics of the particular syndrome and of the patients. Table 9.2 compares these properties among classes of central nervous system depressants (see also Chapters 3, 10, and 14).

When patients reporting or suspected of physical dependence are initially seen by a clinician, they must be medically evaluated for symptoms and signs of overdose, intoxication, or abstinence. An accurate history, which is often difficult to obtain, is invaluable; questioning the patient or other informants about

TABLE 9.1. SEDATIVE-HYPNOTICS: STREET NAMES OF SOME COMMONLY ABUSED FORMS

Generic Name	Trade Name	Street Name
Amobarbital[a]	Amytal	Blue angels, blue birds, blue devils, blue dolls, blue clouds, blue heavens, blue tips, blue velvet
Amobarbital and secobarbital[b]	Tuinal	Double trouble, rainbows, reds and blues, tooies, tuie
Chloral hydrate	Noctec	Chorals, coral, green frog, mickey finn
Ethchlorvynol	Placidyl	Pickles, Mr. Green Jeans
Methaqualone[c]	—	Q, quads, ludes, 714s, sopers
Pentobarbital	Nembutal	Nembies[d], nemmies, nimbies, yellows, yellow bullets, yellow jackets
Secobarbital	Seconal	Marshmallow reds[e], Mexican reds, reds, red bullets, red devils, redbirds, seggy, seccy
Flunitrazepam	Rohypnol	Circles, forget-me drug, forget pill, forget-me pill, La Rocha, pingus, reynolds, rib, roach-2, robutal, rochas dos, roche, roofies, rope, rophies, rophy, ropies, roples, row-shay, ruffies, ruffles,
γ-Hydroxybutyrate	Xyrem[f]	Cherry meth, easy lab, everclear, G.B., gamma oh, Georgia homeboy, great hormones at bedtime, grievous bodily harm, jib, liquid E, liquid ecstasy, liquid X, max, salt water, scoop, sleep-500, soap, somatomax
Nonspecific (class) terms	Depressants, especially barbiturates	Bambs, bank bandit pills, barbs, barbies, block busters, busters, downers, downie, drowsy high, gangster pills, goofers, gorilla pills, green dragons, idiot pills, lay back, mother's little helper, Mighty Joe Young, peanut, peter, phennies, phenos, stoppers, stumbler, tranq, ups and downs

[a]The formulation of amobarbital that is legally available in the United States in 2001 is for i.v. use.
[b]Temporarily withdrawn, but reintroduced in late 1991 in 100 and 200 mg oral forms.
[c]No longer legally manufactured in the United States.
[d]An orange-and-white 50 mg capsule is also manufactured.
[e]Currently manufactured as an orange pulvule.
[f]Proposed name; not currently marketed in the United States.

the amount of drug taken, the time of ingestion of the last dose, and the chronicity of use is important. In addition, knowledge of the events leading to the referral or admission; of what environmental supports are available; of any history of prior or current psychiatric or drug-related problems; and of whether **alcohol** or stimulants, such as **cocaine** or amphetamines, were also recently ingested is helpful. The patient's motivation should be assessed; examining carefully the realistic quality of his or her plans is also useful.

Among sedative-hypnotic drugs, **pentobarbital, secobarbital**, and **methaqualone** are disproportionately abused; **meprobamate** and the benzodiazepines are abused less often, even though they are widely available. As was noted above, **methaqualone** is no longer available as a licit drug in the United States. However, it remains available as a "street" drug in some areas of the

TABLE 9.2. COMPARATIVE UNWANTED PROPERTIES[a] OF VARIOUS CENTRAL NERVOUS SYSTEM DEPRESSANTS

Drug	Abstinence or Withdrawal Syndrome (after 3 mo)	Therapeutic Dose Tolerance	Psychologic Dependence (at Therapeutic Doses)	Physical Dependence (at Supra-Therapeutic Doses)
Barbiturates and barbiturate-like drugs	+++	++	+	+++
Benzodiazepines	+	+	++	++
Alcohol (ethanol)	+++	++	++	+++
Opioids	++++	+++	++++	++++

[a]Variation exists within each class.
Increased number of + represents an increased degree.

country, and overdose victims are seen in emergency departments (see Chapter 3). The barbiturates provide a paradigm for discussing the difficulties that clinicians encounter when treating persons dependent on any of these agents.

II. Medical Evaluation
  A. Abstinence (the Withdrawal Syndrome)
    The character of a person's physical dependence results in part from the type of drug ingested, its dose, the length of time it was used, and whether that use was continuous or intermittent. Physical dependence does not usually develop with short-term usage at therapeutic dosages; it may develop when therapeutic dosages are ingested over months or years. Physical dependence may develop sooner if large doses are consumed at a steady or escalating rate. Thus, persons taking nightly doses of 200 mg of a short-acting barbiturate rarely become physically dependent. Routine ingestion of 400 mg per day of **pentobarbital** or **secobarbital** can lead to tolerance development and mild withdrawal symptoms after a period of 90 days. Persons consuming 600 to 800 mg per day of either drug for 35 to 120 days may have grand mal seizures upon withdrawal, even though they usually do not show symptoms of delirium. Table 9.3 illustrates the relationship between the barbiturate dosage level and the intensity of physical dependence.

TABLE 9.3. RELATIONSHIP OF DOSAGE OF SECOBARBITAL OR PENTOBARBITAL TO ABSTINENCE MANIFESTATIONS[a]

Daily Dose (mg)	Duration of Ingestion (d)	Percentage of Patients Showing		
		Convulsions	Delirium	Minor Symptoms
200	365	0	0	0
400	90	0	0	5.5
600	35–57	11	0	50
800	42–57	20	0	100
900–2,200	32–144	78	75	100

[a]Data derived from 61 patients.
From Wikler A. Diagnosis and treatment of drug dependence of the barbiturate type. *Am J Psychiatry* 1968;125:758–765, with permission.

Table 9.4 summarizes the doses of sedative-hypnotic drugs that reportedly can lead to physical dependence. Remembering that documented experience with nonbarbiturate sedative-hypnotics is limited and is largely anecdotal is important.

The syndrome of barbiturate abstinence is similar to that which is seen after **alcohol** withdrawal (see Chapter 12); it is characterized by tremulousness; anxiety; insomnia; anorexia; nausea; vomiting; sweating; postural hypotension; tendon hyperreflexia; excessive sensitivity to light and sound; and, in some cases, convulsions and delirium (Table 9.5). Some authors also include progression to hyperpyrexia, electrolyte abnormalities, cardiovascular collapse, and death in this list. The character and intensity of the withdrawal state should differentiate this state from that of a return of anxiety symptoms or from a temporary rebound state after drug discontinuation.

The examining clinician must carefully separate subjective symptoms from those that have been verified by the physical examination. The abstinence syndrome, if it occurs, usually begins 16 to 72 hours after the cessation of drug intake. Typically, the onset of abstinence symptoms is related to the elimination half-life of the particular drug. Grand mal convulsions, when they occur, generally are noted 3 to 7 days after drug cessation, usually as single episodes but occasionally in multiple bursts. (*Note:* Convulsions after longer-acting benzodiazepine use tend to come later in the abstinence syndrome.) Convulsions may be accompanied by a loss of consciousness and cyanosis and occasionally by progression to delirium. When delirium is present, it most often begins between the fourth and sixth days with fluctuating consciousness, visual and auditory hallucinations, unsystematized delusions, mood fluctuations, restlessness, insomnia, fever, and hyperreflexia with marked blepharospasm. Delirious patients often have no understanding of their situation. They may be combative and difficult to manage. Physical restraints may be required to protect both the patient and staff (see Chapter 26). The intensity of the withdrawal syndrome lessens gradually, and almost all of the symptoms are gone by 2 weeks after the cessation of drug intake.

Electroencephalographic examination of patients with increased barbiturate blood levels sometimes reveals a "spiky" pattern with abnormal fast activity. Photic stimulation can produce occasional paroxysmal bursts of activity. During abstinence, the electroencephalogram can become distinctly abnormal. One early report found that 12% of abstinent patients had paroxysmal activity without photic stimulation; two-thirds showed paroxysmal activity with photic stimulation.

TABLE 9.4. EXAMPLES OF DOSAGE AND DURATION ASSOCIATED WITH WITHDRAWAL SYMPTOMS FROM SEDATIVE-HYPNOTICS[a]

Generic Name	Dose (g)	Duration (mo)
Ethchlorvynol[b]	2–4	7–8
Glutethimide[c]	2.5	3
	5	0.5
Methaqualone[c]	0.6–0.9	≥ 1
Meprobamate	2.4	9
	3.2–6.4	1.3
Chlordiazepoxide	0.3–0.6	5–6
Diazepam	0.1–1.5	Several

[a]Data derived from case reports.
[b]Usually over four times the therapeutic dose.
[c]Not legally available in the United States.

TABLE 9.5. BARBITURATE ABSTINENCE (WITHDRAWAL) SYNDROME[a]

Clinical Phenomenon	Frequency (%)	Time of Onset	Duration (d)	Remarks
Apprehension	100	1st day	3–14	Vague uneasiness or fear of impending catastrophe
Muscle weakness	100	1st day	3–14	Evident on mildest exertion
Tremors	100	1st day	3–14	Coarse, rhythmic, non-patterned; evident during voluntary movement and subsiding at rest
Postural faintness	100	1st day	3–14	Evident on sitting or standing suddenly; associated with marked fall in systolic and diastolic blood pressure and with pronounced tachycardia
Anorexia	100	1st day	3–14	Usually associated with repeated vomiting
Twitches	100	1st day	3–14	Myoclonic muscle contractions or spasmodic jerking of one or more extremities; sometimes bizarre patterned movements
Seizures[b]	80	2nd–3rd day	8	Up to a total of four grand mal episodes, with loss of consciousness and postconvulsive stupor
Psychoses or delirium[b]	60	3rd–8th day	3–14	Usually resemble "delirium tremens"; occasionally resemble schizophrenia or Korsakoff syndrome; acute panic states may occur

[a]Seen after abrupt withdrawal in 19 persons exposed to experimental addiction to secobarbital or pentobarbital using chronic intoxication at dose levels of 0.8–2.2 g/d p.o. for 6 wk or more.
[b]Four persons developed seizures without subsequent psychosis—one exhibited delirium without antecedent seizures, and three escaped both seizures and delirium.
From Wikler A. Diagnosis and treatment of drug dependence of the barbiturate type. *Am J Psychiatry* 1968;125:758–765, with permission.

B. Intoxication

Intoxicated patients range in appearance from those who are sleeping but are easily aroused to those who are alert, with fine lateral nystagmus as the only sign of recent use. Drowsiness, slurred speech, coarse nystagmus, hyporeflexia, and ataxia characterize moderate intoxication. Intoxicated patients may be aggressive, uncooperative, or even violent.

C. Overdose

The treatment of an overdose of sedative-hypnotics is reviewed in Chapter 3.

III. Detoxification: Assessment and Management

When assessing a patient for   ie clinician must carefully examine (a) the context of the patient's admission, (b) the events leading to admission, (c) the availability of social supports, (d) the purpose for which the patient used the drug, (e) the patient's past history of drug detoxification, (f) the patient's expectation of difficulties without the drug, and (g) the realistic quality of the patient's plans and motivations. Objective validation of the recency and quantity of drug exposure based on a plasma barbiturate measurement may be highly desirable or even essential. Urine drug screening may also be helpful. From this assessment, an attentive clinician may foresee some of the problems that may arise after the detoxification regimen is begun. Similarly, careful assessment may allow the clinician to recognize patients who may be taking multiple drugs. Because multiple-drug users may be taking drugs with different elimination rates (half-lives), knowing what the patient has taken facilitates making decisions about which detoxification to undertake first.

Detoxification of a person as either an inpatient or an outpatient is possible. Although hospitalization offers more safety and control, particularly when the reliability of the patient is uncertain, outpatient care may be the only means of engaging the patient in treatment. A stable environment and strong motivation may permit withdrawal to take place without excessively disturbing the patient's daily life routines. Detoxification must not be carried out perfunctorily. Information about the actual amounts and types of drugs taken is frequently unavailable to the treating clinician, or the information that is available may be unreliable; close observation of the patient's responses and conducting a thorough physical examination are essential. Individuals respond differently to medication. What may be an adequate withdrawal schedule for one person can heavily sedate another.

With any form of drug detoxification, the patient should be informed at the outset that this is an uncomfortable procedure that is often accompanied by malaise, anxiety, increased heart rate, "shakiness," insomnia, and nightmares. Nightmares may at times be so distressing that the patients will interrupt the drug withdrawal to suppress their nightmares by taking more drugs. Some complain of anorexia, nausea, and mild abdominal cramps. The clinician must separate these from the symptoms of other physical ailments. The insomnia from sedative-hypnotic detoxification or withdrawal may last for weeks, and it is associated with a "dream rebound" ("REM rebound"), in which the patient has many anxious nightmarish dreams.

A. Initiation of a Planned Withdrawal

Three methods for withdrawing patients from barbiturates are available. The first two rely on an estimation of the patient's level of drug requirement, based either on estimated equivalencies to **phenobarbital** or on the results of a **pentobarbital** challenge test. The third method uses a loading dose of **phenobarbital** to achieve sedation and mild toxicity.

1. Test dose (pentobarbital challenge test). The patient is given 200 mg of **pentobarbital** orally, and changes in the neurologic examination are assessed after 1 hour. Table 9.6 presents possible findings on the physical examination, the associated degree of tolerance, and the estimates of 24-hour pentobarbital requirements. If no physical changes are observed after 1 hour, the level of the habit is probably above 1,200 mg per day of **pentobarbital**. The test is then repeated 3 to 4 hours later, using 300 mg of pentobarbital. No response to the 300 mg dose suggests a "habit" above 1,600 mg per day.

TABLE 9.6. CLINICAL RESPONSE PATTERNS TO TEST DOSE OF 200 mg OF PENTOBARBITAL GIVEN ORALLY: RELATIONSHIP TO TOLERANCE

Patient's Condition 1 h After Test Dose	Degree of Tolerance	Estimated 24-h Pentobarbital Requirement (mg)
Asleep but arousable	None or minimal	None
Drowsy, slurred speech; coarse nystagmus; ataxia; marked intoxication	Definite	400–600
Comfortable; fine lateral nystagmus is only sign of intoxication	Marked	800
No signs of drug effects; perhaps persisting signs of abstinence; no intoxication	Extreme	1,000–1,200 or more

After 2 to 3 days of stabilization, either **phenobarbital** or **pentobarbital** can be used for withdrawal, but the course of withdrawal is often smoother with **phenobarbital**, because it causes fewer variations of the blood barbiturate level. The estimated daily requirement of **pentobarbital** is divided into four equal doses and is administered orally every 4 to 6 hours. Smaller total doses of **phenobarbital**, usually one-third of the amount of **pentobarbital**, are required due to its longer duration of action. **Phenobarbital** is given orally in equally divided amounts every 8 hours. Both the **pentobarbital** and the **phenobarbital** can be reduced at a rate of one-tenth the starting dose per day (e.g., an initial daily dose of 600 mg of **pentobarbital** would be decreased by 60 mg per day; the equivalent 200 mg of **phenobarbital** would be lowered by 20 mg per day). Reducing the dosage at this slow rate typically results in a minimal and tolerable withdrawal syndrome.

Stabilization doses of 500 to 600 mg per day of either **phenobarbital** or **pentobarbital** should rarely be exceeded. The risk-to-benefit ratio above this range is not favorable.

2. **Phenobarbital equivalents**. Another technique for determining the baseline level of drug that is required daily was developed for outpatients who have refused admission but who nonetheless seek detoxification. Table 9.7 gives the empirically established amounts of **phenobarbital** that correspond to some of the abused drugs. With this method, knowing the names and quantities of the drugs that are frequently abused (Table 9.1) becomes important. By totaling the number of daily hypnotic doses that are reported and calculating their equivalent, the clinician can estimate the patient's initial requirement for **phenobarbital**. After 2 to 3 days of stabilization, the dose is divided on an every-8-hour schedule and is tapered, with a total daily decrement of about 10%. Many clinicians are reluctant to use this procedure because of the possibility that a patient may misuse the prescribed amounts. Another problem with this approach is that drug histories are frequently unreliable; moreover, some drug-seeking patients may exaggerate the amounts they have been using. In instances of mixed sedative abuse or when **alcohol** is also used, thus complicating the clinical presentation, the calculation of equivalencies is also likely to be inexact. In these patients, the challenge test or a loading-dose strategy is more appropriate. Furthermore, some argue that, when the **phenobarbital**-equivalents procedure is used in outpatients, the risks to the patient and the medicolegal risks from seizures, automobile accidents, or cardiac arrhythmias are too high.

TABLE 9.7. ESTIMATED OR APPROXIMATE "PHENOBARBITAL SUBSTITUTION" WITHDRAWAL DOSAGE EQUIVALENCIES FOR SOME SEDATIVE-HYPNOTIC AGENTS

Generic Name	Dosage (mg)
Phenobarbital	30
Pentobarbital	100
Secobarbital	100
Chloral hydrate	500
Meprobamate	200
Alprazolam	1
Chlordiazepoxide	25
Clonazepam	0.5
Clorazepate	15
Diazepam	5
Estazolam	2
Flurazepam	15–30
Lorazepam	1
Oxazepam	15–30
Quazepam	15
Temazepam	15–30
Triazolam	0.25
Zaleplon	10
Zolpidem	10

When withdrawal is impending, the patient may be given a single intramuscular loading dose of 100 to 200 mg of **phenobarbital**. The first oral dose is then begun after the patient has gone several hours without significant physical signs of intoxication.

3. **Loading dose**. A third approach to detoxification involves an oral loading dose of **phenobarbital**; the clinician then tries to reach the level of early sedation and toxicity by adding further increments of **phenobarbital** (i.e., titrating up to this level). Usually a dose of 120 mg (smaller amounts [e.g., 40 mg] are advocated by some clinicians) is given every hour until the patient becomes dysarthric, ataxic, sedated, or labile or until the individual shows nystagmus. Typically, three of these findings are considered sufficient for determining that the intoxication threshold has been reached. Reaching this level may take 15 to 20 hours; thus, this method is best reserved for hospital situations or for those in which the patient can be confined and can be continuously supervised by trained personnel. Some clinicians have found that an accumulated initial dose with this method ranges from 1,300 to 1,500 mg. The **phenobarbital** is then slowly eliminated, and the resulting withdrawal is quite mild. Patients requiring 500 mg per day or less of **phenobarbital** usually do not require intervention other than support and observation.

B. **Mixed Physical Dependence ("Addiction")**

When a patient is dependent on both an opioid and a barbiturate or a barbiturate-like sedative-hypnotic, the best approach is to withdraw the hypnotic gradually while maintaining the opioid at a constant level (e.g., **methadone**, usually 20 mg per day, if the patient has verifiable opioid dependence). Decreasing both drugs at once is possible, but this simultaneous weaning occasionally complicates the clinical picture. Some barbiturates (or **meprobamate**) may induce the metabolism of **methadone** (see Chapter 29), as may other drugs, such as **carbamazepine** and **phenytoin**. Restabilizing the **methadone** concentrations in the blood and tissues after the discontinuation of the barbiturate or barbiturate-like drug may take time.

A person withdrawing from opioids (see Chapter 10) usually has dilated reactive pupils; an elevated pulse rate, blood pressure, and respirations; muscle aches and twitches; and tremulousness, nausea, vomiting, diarrhea, tearing, runny nose, yawning, restlessness, chills, and gooseflesh ("cold turkey"). By carefully examining the patient's eyes; pulse; blood pressure, both while lying and standing; reflexes, including the blink reflex; and mental status, separating one withdrawal syndrome from the other should be possible. Nonetheless, an accurate clinical distinction is often difficult. Although opioid withdrawal is uncomfortable, it rarely leads to convulsions, and it is not lethal. Abstinence from a sedative-hypnotic clearly is more dangerous.

C. Psychologic Adjuncts

Psychologic interventions may be helpful in both acute withdrawal and in the longer term treatment of underlying or withdrawal-related anxiety. Several general principles can be derived from studies of benzodiazepine-dependent patients, even though the number of such studies is small. Most clinicians recommend frequent contact with the patient during the withdrawal phase. For inpatients, daily contact is recommended; once-weekly or twice-weekly appointments and telephone availability are appropriate for most outpatients. The clinician, both through discussion and written materials, should provide the patient with information about the nature of the withdrawal syndrome and the distinctions between withdrawal symptoms and a return of underlying anxieties. Success rates are usually highest in patients who are able to develop alternative coping skills that help them to achieve a sense of control over their worries, stresses, and drug cravings. With this in mind, offering patients at least one trial for determining their own rate of withdrawal through setting their own "targets" may be helpful. The goals should be flexible, and they should be reviewed with the clinician. One strategy is suggesting that the first dosage reduction may be set by omitting the dose the patient feels that he or she least needs. In some instances, the omission of a full dose is not tolerated, and a partial reduction may be chosen instead.

Many clinicians recommend the use of a diary to help patients distinguish between withdrawal symptoms and anxiety and to help them see what situational stresses or precipitants trigger or augment their anxiety or promote an urge to return to drug taking. This approach can increase a patient's sense of mastery over his or her anxiety. Discussing the diary entries with the patient may alert the clinician to maladaptive coping strategies or to compensatory increases in **alcohol** consumption. Other cognitive-behavioral approaches (e.g., relaxation training, systematic desensitization, graded *in vivo* exposure, and cognitive restructuring) have been proposed as additional adjuncts.

IV. Benzodiazepine Dependence

In recent years, considerable media and regulatory attention has been paid to benzodiazepine dependence (see Chapters 3 and 14). Contrary to what would be expected from popular reports, actual physical dependence on benzodiazepines is not a common problem when benzodiazepines are taken at their therapeutic doses. Dependence at therapeutic doses is infrequent, and it is rarely seen in patients who have taken benzodiazepines for less than 3 months. When dependence does develop on therapeutic dosing regimens, it is most likely idiosyncratic, although a personal or family history of sedative-hypnotic or alcohol abuse or misuse may be more common in those who develop it. Based on clinical experience, some clinicians argue that **diazepam**, **alprazolam**, and **lorazepam** have a higher abuse potential than **clonazepam**, **chlordiazepoxide**, **clorazepate**, and **oxazepam**. (*Note:* No credible scientific evidence supports this impression.) In general, patients who gradually taper the dosage of any benzodiazepine at the time of drug discontinuation will reveal minimal withdrawal symptoms. When symptoms do appear, they most likely reflect a return of the original anxiety disorder for which the benzodiazepines were prescribed. In general, if dependence and withdrawal do occur, the patient has likely exceeded the therapeutic dose by at least a factor of 2 or 3 for 1 month or more.

The clinical presentation of benzodiazepine withdrawal is basically identical to that which is seen with barbiturates and other sedative-hypnotics. Some clinicians believe, however, that hyperacusis (sensitivity to sound), photophobia (sensitivity to light), myoclonic jerks, and urinary incontinence in an apparently alert patient are seen more frequently in benzodiazepine withdrawal than in barbiturate withdrawal. Withdrawal can be treated with barbiturate substitution as reviewed above; by reinstituting the prediscontinuation dose of benzodiazepine and beginning a gradual tapering of the dosage (usually a 10% to 20% reduction every second or third day); or by substituting a longer-acting benzodiazepine, such as **clonazepam**, and then beginning the tapering strategy.

What is sometimes improperly called "interdose dependence" (i.e., withdrawal symptoms, such as anxiety symptoms and tachycardia) is sometimes reported by patients taking shorter-acting benzodiazepines at widely spaced dosing intervals. Decreasing the dosage interval while maintaining the same total daily dose is an appropriate corrective strategy. An alternative is increasing the 24-hour dosage to ensure that the patient remains above the minimum therapeutic concentration at all times—a strategy that may unfortunately result in a greater likelihood of dependence over time. A sustained-release form of **alprazolam** might obviate the occurrence of interdose withdrawal symptomatology.

For patients who do not adequately respond to tapering or substitution, "covering" the final stages of the withdrawal with oral **carbamazepine** (100 to 300 mg per day for the last 5 to 10 days) may prove beneficial. The latter strategy is supported by anecdotal case reports, small-sample uncontrolled studies, and at least one animal model study.

The oral administration of other anticonvulsants is another option that may be used to ease patient discomfort during a planned withdrawal from benzodiazepines. Some clinicians believe that **gabapentin** use reduces somatic complaints and improves sleep, although the specific withdrawal symptoms (e.g., hyperacusis) may not be alleviated. A common regimen reflects the typical anticonvulsant range for **gabapentin** (900 to 3,600 mg per day). A more aggressive regimen involves a higher maximum dose (e.g., 5,400 mg per day). **Gabapentin** is then tapered after the benzodiazepine has been discontinued. **Divalproex sodium** (500 to 2,500 mg per day) has been used in a similar manner. Antidepressants (e.g., **trazodone** [100 to 500 mg per day], **nefazodone** [200 to 600 mg per day]) have also been used successfully by some clinicians. Unfortunately, the limited number of published observations for these anticonvulsants and antidepressants is insufficient for providing the evidence that is needed for strongly recommending their use.

Because some patients "forget" to tell their clinicians that they are taking benzodiazepines, **alcohol**, or other sedative-hypnotics, specific inquiry before surgery or hospitalization is essential to avoid the complications of withdrawal during recovery or the possible confusion of withdrawal symptoms with the underlying disorder or some other untoward reaction.

V. Flunitrazepam

Flunitrazepam is a benzodiazepine hypnotic that is not marketed in the United States. However, it is imported illegally into this country, especially from Central and South America. It has received wide publicity as a "date rape" drug, because of reported cases of individuals who have unknowingly ingested the drug with alcohol, which renders the victim sedated, unable to resist sexual activity, and often amnestic for the assault. That **flunitrazepam** is unique among benzodiazepines in producing this effect is unlikely; **clonazepam**, for example, is sometimes sold as "roofies" (so-called because of the trade name for **flunitrazepam**, Rohypnol; see Table 9.1 for some other common street names). Withdrawal syndromes, including seizures, have been reported in individuals abusing **flunitrazepam**.

A related drug, γ-**hydroxybutyrate** (GHB), is abused for its sedative effects; liquid GHB combined with alcohol has also been linked to sexual assaults. Some street names for GHB are given in Table 9.1. GHB is now available in the United States under the trade name Xyrem for the treatment of narcolepsy. GHB is easily synthesized from γ-butyrolactone or 1,4-butanediol, which has increased the illegal access to GHB. GHB can produce the abstinence syndrome characteristic of sedative-hypnotics, although some authorities believe that it is milder than that which is induced by barbiturates, **alcohol**, or benzodiazepines. The abstinence syndrome most commonly presents with anxiety and insomnia, although more severe symptoms may also occur. The recommended treatment is stabilization on benzodiazepines, followed by gradual tapering. Complicating the assessment is the difficulty that one may have in distinguishing acute intoxication from withdrawal. At low doses, GHB appears to be a central nervous system depressant; at higher doses, it is excitatory and it may even induce seizures. This reflects the complexity of the pharmacologic actions of GHB, which are different than those of drugs that act on the γ-aminobutyric acid A receptor. GHB naturally occurs in the body, where it acts as a neuromodulator or neurotransmitter. A GHB receptor has been identified, but the drug's actions affect many neurotransmitter systems, including the **dopamine, serotonin**, opioid, and γ-aminobutyric acid B receptors.

VI. **Zolpidem**

This is an imidazopyridine hypnotic that has a rapid onset of action. Although some studies suggest that its abuse potential may be lower than that of the benzodiazepine hypnotics, instances of abuse and physiologic dependence have been reported. At the present time, it is the most commonly prescribed hypnotic in the United States. **Zaleplon** is a pyrazolopyrimidine hypnotic that has a short duration of action, thus allowing patients to take the medication in the middle of the night as long as they are able to avoid activities for at least 4 hours. Little or no psychomotor impairment appears to be present the following day, and some studies have found no evidence of rebound insomnia or withdrawal when the drug is taken in prescribed doses. When dependence with **zolpidem** or **zaleplon** develops, treatment of the abstinence syndrome should follow the guidelines for benzodiazepine withdrawal.

VII. **Longer Term Treatment**

Treatment of patients with sedative-hypnotic dependency must be individualized. In general, most patients develop their dependence either as part of a problem with polysubstance abuse or in the context of their treatment for a medical condition, such as chronic pain or a psychiatric condition.

The authors' impression is that many of the latter group of patients do not fare well in standard drug or **alcohol** abuse treatment programs. Treatment must be directed not only at their problem of dependence but also at their underlying medical or psychiatric problem. In some cases, this is easily accomplished; for example, **Fiorinal** could be replaced by a nonsteroidal antiinflammatory agent in some patients with chronic headache or by an antidepressant (e.g., **venlafaxine XR**). A β-adrenergic receptor antagonist could be substituted for a benzodiazepine in a chronically anxious patient. Often, however, the situation is sufficiently complex that individual psychotherapy or cognitive-behavioral therapy is also needed.

Unfortunately, many polysubstance-abusing patients who begin detoxification from sedative-hypnotic agents do not complete their course of treatment, and some of those who do quickly return to a drug-dependent state. Discussions with barbiturate and other sedative-hypnotic abusers often reveal that their use of drugs substitutes or compensates for unsatisfying or unpredictable relationships. A common theme is the avoidance of interpersonal frustration. Some constrict their relationships, avoiding strong ties; others evolve tortuous associations. Their treatment, if it is successful, often requires involvement in some form of a 12-step program modeled after Alcoholics Anonymous; individually tailored combinations of individual, group, and cognitive-behavioral therapies (e.g., social skills training); and, when appropriate, psychotropic medications other than sedative-hypnotics (see Chapter 11).

For some patients, especially licensed health care practitioners, contingency contracting is an effective therapeutic adjunct. Upon entering a treatment program, a "contract" is generated and signed that outlines the program the patient must follow; it includes monitoring by an appropriate agency (e.g., a state medical society in the case of a physician). If the patient does not comply with the contract or shows evidence of relapse (e.g., a verified positive urine screen), the appropriate licensing board is notified and the practitioner's license is suspended or revoked.

Inpatient detoxification and rehabilitation programs may be necessary when complicated detoxification strategies are anticipated (e.g., in patients with significant medical or psychiatric impairment). Inpatient care may also be important for patients who would have to return to environments that could not support abstinence. However, one must remember that substance abuse disorders are often chronic disorders and that inpatient care *per se* is rarely sufficient. Inpatient treatment should be followed by one of the longer-term outpatient treatment plans noted above.

ADDITIONAL READING

Addolorato G, Caputo F, Capristo E, et al. A case of gamma-hydroxybutyric acid withdrawal syndrome during alcohol addiction treatment: utility of diazepam administration. *Clin Neuropharmacol* 1999;22:60–62.

Bonnet U, Banger M, Leweke FM, et al. Treatment of alcohol withdrawal syndrome with gabapentin. *Pharmacopsychiatry* 1999;32:107–109.

Ciraulo DA, Nace EP. Benzodiazepine treatment of anxiety or insomnia in substance abuse patients. *Am J Addictions* 2000;9:276–284.

Ciraulo DA, Sarid-Segal O. Sedative-, hypnotic-, or anxiolytic-related abuse. In: Sadock BJ, Sadock VA, eds. *Comprehensive textbook of psychiatry,* 7th ed. Philadelphia: Lippincott Williams & Wilkins, 2000:1071–1085.

Crockford D, White WD, Campbell B. Gabapentin use in benzodiazepine dependence and detoxification. *Can J Psychiatry* 2001;46:287.

Dodes LM, Khantzian EJ. Psychotherapy and chemical dependence. In: Ciraulo DC, Shader RI, eds. *Clinical manual of chemical dependence.* Washington, D.C.: American Psychiatric Press, 1991:345–358.

Dooley M, Plosker GL. Zaleplon: a review of its use in the treatment of insomnia. *Drugs* 2000;60:413–445.

Dyer JE, Roth B, Hyma BA. Gamma-hydroxybutyrate withdrawal syndrome. *Ann Emerg Med* 2001;37:147–153.

Harris JT, Roache JD, Thornton JE. A role for valproate in the treatment of sedative-hypnotic withdrawal and for relapse prevention. *Alcohol Alcoholism* 2000;35:319–323.

Marlatt GA, George WH. Relapse prevention: introduction and overview of the model. *Br J Addict* 1984;79:261–273.

McElroy SL, Keck PE Jr, Lawrence JM. Treatment of panic disorder and benzodiazepine withdrawal with valproate. *J Neuropsychiatry Clin Neurosci* 1991;3:232–233.

Moroz G, Rosenbaum JF. Efficacy, safety, and gradual discontinuation of clonazepam in panic disorder: a placebo-controlled, multicenter study using optimized dosages. *J Clin Psychiatry* 1999;60:604–612.

Myrick H, Brady KT, Malcolm R. Divalproex in the treatment of alcohol withdrawal. *Am J Drug Alcohol Abuse* 2000;26:155–160.

Nelson J, Chouinard G. Guidelines for the clinical use of benzodiazepines: pharmacokinetics, dependency, rebound and withdrawal. Canadian Society for Clinical Pharmacology. *Can J Clin Pharmacol* 1999;6:69–83.

Nicholson KL, Balster RL. GHB: a new and novel drug of abuse. *Drug Alcohol Depend* 2001;63:1–22.

Pages KP, Ries RK. Use of anticonvulsants in benzodiazepine withdrawal. *Am J Addict* 1998;7:198–204.

Pollack MH, Mathews J, Scott EL. Gabapentin as a potential treatment for anxiety disorders. *Am J Psychiatry* 1998;155:992–993.

Rickels K, Schweizer E, Garcia Espana F, et al. Trazodone and valproate in patients discontinuing long-term benzodiazepine therapy: effects on withdrawal symptoms and taper outcome. *Psychopharmacology* 1999;141:1–5.

Spiegel DA. Psychological strategies for discontinuing benzodiazepine treatment. *J Clin Psychopharmacol* 1999;19:17S–22S.

Volpicelli JR, Pettinati HM, McLellan AT, O'Brien CP. *Combining medication and pyschosocial treatment for addiction: the BRENDA approach.* New York: Guilford Press, 2001.

10. OPIOID ABUSE AND DEPENDENCE: ACUTE AND CHRONIC TREATMENT

Richard I. Shader
John A. Renner, Jr.

Papaver somniferum, the **opium**-yielding poppy, is native to many parts of the world. Documentation of the use of **opium** for pain relief in Asia Minor can be found in writings from as early as 1500 B.C. The specific cultivation of **opium** began more than 2,000 years ago when settlers bordering the Mediterranean began to understand its sedative, pain-relieving, and antidiarrheal properties. Recognition of the antitussive properties of **codeine** and the positive role for **morphine** in cardiac-related pulmonary edema came later.

The opium poppy contains a number of active alkaloids, including **morphine**, **codeine**, and **thebaine**. **Thebaine**, which is usually derived from *Papaver bracteatum*, can be converted into **codeine** or a number of semisynthetic **opioids**, including **hydrocodone** (e.g., Hycodan), **oxycodone** (e.g., Percodan), and **oxymorphone** (e.g., Numorphan). **Codeine** is metabolized to **morphine**; one should note, however, that a small proportion of the overall population in the United States—perhaps 10%—lacks a functional hepatic microsomal enzyme (cytochrome P-450 [CYP] 2D6) necessary to carry out this catabolic step. Two highly abusable semisynthetics derived from the opium poppy are **heroin**, which is metabolized to **morphine**, and **hydromorphone** (Dilaudid).

Numerous synthetic opioids, such as **meperidine** (Demerol), **methadone** (Dolophine), **pentazocine** (Talwin), and **propoxyphene** (e.g., Darvon), are currently manufactured. **Alfentanil** (Alfenta, Rapifen) and **sufentanil** (Sufenta) are examples of rapidly acting synthetic opioids that are given intravenously (i.v.). **Alfentanil** is also available in a lollypop formulation that is designed to facilitate pain relief for small children. In this chapter, the inclusive term **opioids** is generally used to describe the naturally occurring **opiates**, the semisynthetic and synthetic compounds, and the **endogenous opioids**. Because of low frequency or site-specific usage, not all of the available opioids are considered in this chapter.

Knowledge about the wanted and unwanted actions of the opioid compounds and the endogenous opioids (e.g., enkephalins, endorphins, endomorphins 1 and 2) at clinical and molecular levels has expanded dramatically over the last two decades. A comprehensive review of these issues is beyond the scope of this chapter. In brief, a variety of receptors throughout both the central and peripheral nervous systems that appear to be important to the actions of endogenous, natural, and synthetic opioids has been identified. For example, β-endorphin and **morphine** are agonists at μ receptors, which are named after the affinity of **morphine** for this receptor. They also have some agonist activity at the δ receptors, which are named after their presence in the *vas deferens,* but the met-enkephalins and leu-enkephalins are the major endogenous agonists at the latter receptors. Two μ receptor subtypes, μ_1 and μ_2, appear to exist. The μ_1 subtype likely mediates the analgesic effects. The marketed antagonists, **naloxone** and **naltrexone**, are synthetic congeners of **oxymorphone**, and they act primarily at the μ receptor sites. They also have some antagonist activity at the κ receptors. Antagonism at the μ_2 subtype is likely the basis for the reversal of the respiratory depression and for most other changes seen in opioid overdosage and withdrawal.

At least two subtypes of the δ receptors also exist; the δ receptors appear to be involved in opioid-induced sedation. κ Receptors, of which at least three subtypes exist, are fundamental to the agonist actions of other endogenous opioids (e.g., dynorphin), but no pure κ agonists are currently available for use in humans. κ Receptors derive their name from the agonist ligand **ketazocine**; they appear to mediate analgesia at the level of the spinal cord. Other opioid receptor subtypes whose functions are not fully established also have been found. Among these are the τ receptors, which play some role in mydriasis and possibly in delirium.

Some mixed agonist–antagonists (e.g., **pentazocine**) act at both the μ and κ receptors, such as κ agonists with weak μ antagonism. κ Agonism likely plays some part in the dysphoric and psychotomimetic properties, including hallucinations, nightmares, and anxiety, that are seen with some κ-active synthetics (e.g., **pentazocine**) in abuse and overdosage. Some opioids are mixed agonists (κ and μ) with weak antagonist properties (e.g., **butorphanol**). Finally, some opioids are partial agonists[1] (e.g., **buprenorphine** [Buprenex], a partial agonist at the μ receptors). The highest concentrations of opioid receptors are found in the periaqueductal gray matter and in the thalamus, limbic cortex, locus coeruleus, caudate nucleus, and medulla.

The focus of this chapter is the accidental misuse or deliberate abuse of opioids. The dangerous complications of opioids are most commonly associated with **heroin**, but they apply equally to other opioids under circumstances in which they are misused or abused. In the United States, the current estimate is that 0.4% to 0.7% of adults will become dependent on **heroin** at some point in time. Although about one-fourth of those exposed to **heroin** will become dependent on it, very few patients who have been prescribed **morphine** or other opioids as a needed analgesia or during anesthesia will become dependent. Initial illicit or nonmedical use of any opioid is a much more significant risk factor for the development of opioid dependence than is exposure *per se*.

I. Acute Overdosage

A. Diagnosis

Overdosage with opioids (usually **heroin** or **methadone**) can be deliberate or accidental. The patient typically is young, and he or she generally is brought to the emergency department by police or friends. The following clinical picture of overdose is similar for most opioids: depressed respiration, depressed consciousness, pinpoint (miotic) pupils (*note: **the pupils may not be miotic after meperidine overdose or they may be dilated [mydriatic] if severe hypoxia is present or if the opioid was taken with other drugs***), possibly hypotension, and possibly pulmonary edema (or pulmonary congestion). Venous sclerosis or track marks (old or new) are supplementary evidence of opiate use, but their absence does not refute the diagnosis, because heroin may be smoked or taken intranasally and **methadone** and other opioids, such as **hydromorphone**, may be taken orally. The presence of ice packs near the testicles or milk in the mouth may also suggest opioid use; these methods are sometimes used as "street" remedies for overdose. This combination of findings, together with other history that is available, usually is sufficient to establish the diagnosis; nevertheless, other causes of coma, including the intake of more than one drug, must be considered. (See Chapter 3 for a further discussion of the diagnosis and medical treatment of the comatose patient.)

B. Treatment

Emergency treatment consists of supporting or restoring vital functions and of promptly administering an **opioid antagonist**.

1. **Adequacy of airway, breathing, and circulation (ABCs)** should be assessed immediately. If these functions are inadequate, resuscitation should begin at once. Intubation should be performed if it is clinically indicated (see Chapter 3). If intubation is not performed, care should be taken to prevent aspiration. Support of vital functions should continue while further diagnostic and therapeutic procedures are undertaken.

2. **A reliable i.v. route should be established**. Blood should be taken for appropriate laboratory studies, including blood **glucose**. The serum should be screened for common drugs of abuse, including **acetaminophen** and **aspirin**. As a conservative procedure, a 50% dextrose–water solution

---

[1]Although more than one definition of the term partial agonist may exist, here it refers to a receptor ligand that binds to a receptor and elicits a response that is submaximal when compared with a full agonist for the same receptor. By occupying the receptor in this manner, a coadministered full agonist cannot bind as well to its receptor; the net result is that the partial agonist functions as an antagonist to the full agonist.

may be injected rapidly, even when hypoglycemia is not thought to be the primary cause of the coma.

3. Depending on the particular clinical situation, **gastric lavage** may occasionally be helpful when evidence of recent ingestion of drugs is observed. This procedure should not be undertaken in a patient who has evidence of respiratory depression unless the airway has been protected by previous intubation.

4. **Naloxone** is the current short-acting antagonist of choice for the immediate reversal of the respiratory depression accompanying opioid overdosage. The usual adult dose is 0.4 to 2 mg i.v. A good response to **naloxone** is indicated by the reversal of the respiratory depression within one minute, followed by a lighter consciousness or level of sedation, decreased hypotension, and a widening of the pupils. Repeat doses may be given every 2 to 3 minutes, but these should be administered only if the previous dose appears ineffective. If no clinical improvement is observed after administering **naloxone** (up to a total of 10 mg), the clinical condition is usually not due solely to an opioid, and other causes of coma, such as trauma and other drugs, should be considered.[2] Because the withdrawing patient can become agitated, combative, and violent when emerging from the coma, the emergency use of **physical restraints** (see Chapter 26) may be required. A nonintubated patient should only be restrained in a position that minimizes the likelihood of aspiration. *Naloxone does not appear to be effective, however, in relieving respiratory depression after overdosage with the partial agonist buprenorphine.*

5. **Naloxone** *should be administered cautiously* to an opioid-dependent person, because an excess may precipitate withdrawal symptoms. When withdrawal symptoms do appear, they may be severe, but they should last only as long as the effect of the **naloxone** (about 30 to 90 minutes). **Clonidine**, a centrally acting α_2-adrenergic receptor agonist, can be administered to minimize any discomfort (see section II.C.7). Because **naloxone** is a "pure" antagonist, it should have no intrinsic pharmacologic activity in patients not taking opioids.

6. **A syndrome of interstitial or alveolar pulmonary congestion** can accompany acute overdosage. Manifestations range from asymptomatic congestion that is seen only by x-ray to severe life-threatening pulmonary edema. The heart is of normal size, and cardiac function is unimpaired. **Digitalis** and **diuretics** are of no value, and their use should not be attempted. Treatment consists of **oxygen**, assisted ventilation, and intubation, if necessary.

7. **Patients should be hospitalized**, preferably with continuous observation in an intensive care unit, for at least 24 hours after acute overdosage to minimize the dangers of relapse into coma and to provide for full medical evaluation, particularly when multiple-drug use is suspected.

8. **Because most opiates have a longer duration of action than naloxone**, respiratory depression and coma can recur after the initial doses of **naloxone**. This is particularly true with an oral **methadone** or **propoxyphene** overdose. The depressant effects may last for 24 to 48 hours after the overdose. The patient should be carefully observed, and **naloxone** should be readministered as required after the initial positive response.

9. **Even after a positive response to naloxone**, the physician should remember that the patient may have taken more than one drug, and monitoring should continue accordingly.

---

[2] Although the authors have not found documentation in the literature, the authors have received an anecdotal report of rare cases of apparently massive **methadone** overdoses that seemed to require further doses of **naloxone** to produce an initial response (W. Leigh Thompson, M.D., *personal communication*).

10. **Before discharge** from the intensive care unit or its equivalent, the advisability and availability of specialized follow-up medical and psychiatric care, including evaluation by a physician competent in substance abuse treatment and hospitalization in a dedicated substance abuse treatment unit, should be made clear to the patient. This is especially important, and it may enhance the chances for recovery for the patient whose overuse has been life threatening. Unless adequate attention is paid to the process of referral for aftercare and comprehensive aftercare programs are available, many opioid-addicted patients will not return for follow-up care.

II. Withdrawal

A. Diagnosis of Opioid Dependence

The diagnosis of opioid dependence is based on a history of or evidence of opioid use, followed by the abrupt cessation of use and the development of the characteristic symptoms of withdrawal (the abstinence syndrome). See Chapter 9 for a discussion of key elements in the diagnosis of physical dependence.

1. **Heroin or morphine abstinence syndrome.** The typical heroin or morphine abstinence syndrome begins approximately 8 to 12 hours after the last dose. Relatively early signs and symptoms include drug-seeking behavior, an increased respiratory rate, sweating, fever, yawning, lacrimation, rhinorrhea, "gooseflesh," piloerection, tremor, anorexia, irritability, and dilated (mydriatic) pupils. More advanced signs and symptoms that occur 48 to 72 hours after the last dose include insomnia; nausea; diarrhea; weakness; abdominal cramps; vomiting; tachycardia (typically higher than 90 beats per min); hypertension (typically greater than or equal to 160/95 mm Hg in the absence of a known history of hypertension); and involuntary muscle spasms and limb movements, which were the basis for the expression "kicking the habit." The syndrome subsides gradually over a period of 7 to 10 days. Some patients may have protracted withdrawal that lasts 6 to 9 months, and they may be quite troubled by mood dysregulation and greater sensitivity to life's stresses during this time.

2. **Methadone or propoxyphene abstinence syndrome.** The **methadone** or **propoxyphene** abstinence syndrome is qualitatively similar to that of **morphine** or **heroin**, but it follows a different time course. The first signs and symptoms of abstinence after regular use are seen later, generally 22 to 48 hours after the last dose. Although measuring blood concentrations of **methadone** typically is not part of the routine clinical assessment, data suggest that withdrawal symptoms typically appear when the blood concentrations of **methadone** fall below 100 ng per mL. The peak intensity appears on the third day or later. The syndrome gradually subsides, but it may continue for 3 weeks or more. Deep bone pain has been reported in the **methadone** abstinence syndrome. **Clonidine** (see section II.C.7) may relieve some of the bone pain, as may **ibuprofen** (600 mg every 6 hours). These patients may also experience a protracted withdrawal syndrome.

3. **Pentazocine abstinence.** This is clinically similar to abstinence from other **opioids.** However, it is not well antagonized by **methadone** substitution. **Pentazocine's** affinity for the κ receptors may explain this. Some clinicians recommend reinstituting **pentazocine** and then tapering the dose as the best treatment for a **pentazocine** abstinence syndrome.

B. Diagnosis of Opioid Dependence in the Neonate

An infant born to a **heroin**-dependent or a **methadone**-dependent mother may develop a withdrawal syndrome of hypertonicity, tremor, irritability, vomiting, fever, respiratory distress, high-pitched cry, hyperbilirubinemia, and convulsions. This typically occurs within the first 48 to 72 hours after birth (for treatment recommendations, see section II.C.12).

C. Treatment of Withdrawal (Detoxification)

Opioids should be withdrawn from a dependent person gradually, and oral **methadone** or **buprenorphine** should be given to attenuate the abstinence syndrome. When the use of opioids is precluded, **clonidine** may be used instead (see section II.C.7). Optimally, detoxification should be performed in conjunction with a comprehensive treatment program to reduce the likelihood of recidivism.

1. **The initial evaluation** of a patient should include at least a complete medical and drug abuse history, a physical examination, and careful urine screening for drugs of abuse.

2. **Attempts to establish the magnitude of a patient's habit** are rarely helpful. In addition to the fact that the patient's reporting may be misleading, any formula for the conversion of "bags" of street **heroin** to a **methadone** dose will vary as a function of the quality of the street drug, which is usually unknown. In the last few years, the **heroin** available in most parts of the United States has become much more potent. More accurate estimates of the level of physical dependence can be made in the case of **methadone** maintenance patients who are taking a known amount of **methadone**. **Before beginning a patient's detoxification at a given methadone level, attempting to confirm the date and amount of the last dose is important**. Because patients do not always take their prescribed amounts, dividing the first day's dose to avoid accidental overdosage may be prudent. If the dose cannot be confirmed, the safest course is to follow the regimen described in section II.C.4.

3. **Detoxification** may be done on either an inpatient or outpatient basis. Some facilities reserve inpatient detoxification for patients who are dependent on more than one drug, for those who plan to enter a halfway house or a drug-free residential treatment community, for individuals who are being withdrawn from high-dose methadone maintenance, or for those who are psychotic or seriously depressed. Because of the high rate of relapse after outpatient detoxification, many facilities favor inpatient detoxification for most opioid-addicted patients. Detoxification is usually performed with long-acting opioids, such as **methadone** or **buprenorphine**. The addition of an α_2-adrenergic receptor agonist (e.g., **clonidine**) may help to attenuate the autonomic withdrawal symptoms and may permit a more rapid detoxification using lower doses of opiates. Patients generally prefer **methadone** or **buprenorphine** for detoxification because **clonidine**, when used alone, does *not* reduce the subjective opiate craving.

4. **When methadone is used**, an initial dose of 10 to 20 mg of oral **methadone** is administered after the appearance of withdrawal symptoms, such as (a) an increase in heart rate of at least 15 beats per min above baseline or a rate above 100 beats per min; (b) a diastolic blood pressure greater than 100 mm Hg, a systolic level above 160 mm Hg, or an increase in either of 15 mm Hg or more; or (c) an obvious pupillary dilatation. These determinations should be made after the patient has been observed at rest for at least 5 minutes, because some patients may use exercise to increase their heart rate and blood pressure. A single dose of **methadone** typically reaches peak levels in 30 to 60 minutes, and its effects on opioid withdrawal symptoms may last for 24 to 36 hours. Signs of intoxication, such as drowsiness, after the initial dose may indicate the use of too much **methadone**. Incremental doses of 10 mg are given over the next 24 hours when further signs of abstinence occur, but no more than 20 mg should be required in any 12-hour period, unless the patient has a documented history of tolerance to more than 40 mg of methadone per day. This first 24-hour amount is then administered as a single daily dose or in divided doses as the initial dosage strategy. Within the first few days of detoxification, the **methadone** dose is adjusted to reach stabilization.

   Methadone is sometimes administered to outpatients in a more routine fashion that varies somewhat from program to program. Some clinicians supplement **methadone** with **dicyclomine** to relieve abdominal cramps, at a dose of 40 mg orally (p.o.) every 6 hours as needed for

48 hours and then of 20 mg every 6 hours for the next 48 hours, as needed. Other useful symptomatic medications include **ibuprofen**, 600 to 800 mg every 6 to 8 hours, for headache, muscle or joint pain; **methocarbamol**, 750 mg, for muscle spasm; **lorazepam**, 1 to 2 mg p.o., for anxiety; and **trazodone**, 50 mg p.o., for insomnia.

5. **Once stabilization is achieved**, detoxification can begin. Many schedules call for a reduction of 5 mg per day or a maximum of 20% reduction per day and complete withdrawal within 7 to 10 days; other protocols involve more gradual detoxification schedules for some patients. One well-tolerated protocol uses 5 mg per day decrements until a daily dose of 10 mg is reached; at that point, the reduction is shifted to 2.5 to 5 mg per day. Patients should be told that they may experience some mild withdrawal symptoms, which are similar to a mild case of the "flu," during detoxification. During detoxification, the patients' urine should be monitored for drugs of abuse. Detoxification without a comprehensive care plan is seldom useful.

6. The clinician should remember that **methadone** metabolism can be induced by the coadministration of **carbamazepine, phenobarbital, rifampin**, or **phenytoin**, even though such drug combinations are not frequently encountered. The acute or chronic use of these medications may precipitate withdrawal or may lead to a need for higher dosages of **methadone**.

7. **Clonidine** can be helpful in reducing many of the distressing hyperadrenergic (autonomic) symptoms associated with withdrawal. As it has some intrinsic analgesic effects, it may also lessen bone and muscle pain. However, **clonidine** does not reduce subjective withdrawal symptoms or relieve opiate craving. Most patients strongly prefer detoxification protocols that use opioids. Because of the potential for hypotension and excessive sedation, **clonidine** administration is sometimes initiated with the patient in bed in a clinical setting for the first 24 to 36 hours, but **clonidine** has also been successfully used in outpatient settings. Initial amounts of 0.1 to 0.3 mg every 6 to 8 hours (not exceeding 2.5 mg per day) are given p.o., depending on the severity of the patient's symptoms. Once the symptoms are reasonably controlled, the clonidine dosage is tapered by 0.1 to 0.2 mg per day. In some clinical settings, detoxification is conducted with **clonidine** alone. An alternative protocol begins with oral **clonidine** and then adds the **clonidine** patch, which is continued over 3 weeks, using the 2 transdermal therapeutic system, 0.2 mg dose, (TTS-2) patches for 2 weeks and then 1 TTS-2 patch for the final week. When time and resources allow a longer detoxification strategy, the patient can first be stabilized on **methadone**, and **clonidine** can be added to alleviate any withdrawal symptoms that appear during the **methadone** detoxification (see section II.C.4.).

   Rapid opioid detoxification, using crossover dosing of **clonidine** and **naltrexone**, has been proposed. On day 1, patients are given 0.1 to 0.2 mg of **clonidine** p.o. every 4 hours (up to 1.2 mg), plus **naltrexone**, 12.5 mg p.o.; on day 2, the **clonidine** dose is 0.1 to 0.2 mg p.o. every 4 hours (up to 1.2 mg), and 25 mg of **naltrexone** is administered p.o. The **clonidine** dose is tapered on day 3 (0.1 to 0.2 mg p.o. every 4 hours), with the addition of **naltrexone**, 50 mg p.o.

   Ultrarapid detoxification protocols have been described; these involve (a) inducing and maintaining sleep with a **benzodiazepine** (e.g., i.v. **midazolam**), (b) precipitating withdrawal with **naloxone** while the patient is sleeping, and (c) reversing the sleep with the benzodiazepine receptor antagonist **flumazenil**. Little data have been published on this approach, and it should be considered highly experimental.

8. **After detoxification**, patients should be offered continued outpatient or residential rehabilitative care to prevent relapse. Many clinicians believe that patients in outpatient treatment should have daily visits for counseling and urine screens for at least 3 months.

9. **Patients being withdrawn from methadone maintenance**, especially those on doses greater than 50 mg per day, are often detoxified over a more prolonged period. These patients can be detoxified with a reduction of 5 mg per day until the level of 20 mg per day is reached. At this level, they are often detoxified more gradually. A slower **methadone** taper over 3 to 6 months is favored by most clinics. An alternative approach consists of adding a **clonidine** patch for the final 2 weeks of a gradual **methadone** taper and then continuing the patch for the first **methadone**-free week. Some facilities favor inpatient detoxification once the 20 mg level is reached. Some clinicians have advocated the combined use of **clonidine** and **naltrexone** (see sections II.C.7 and III.D.1) on an inpatient basis to ease the distress of withdrawal in patients taking modest doses of **methadone**.

10. **The detoxification of patients** who are dependent on both **opioids** and **sedative-hypnotics** is discussed in Chapter 9.

11. Some **pregnant women** on opioids (see also section III.B) are at high risk for hepatitis B, hepatitis C, and human immunodeficiency virus (HIV) infection. Staff involved in their care must be aware of these risks, and they should follow the appropriate procedures. Some data suggest that pregnant women in **methadone** maintenance programs, compared with addicted women who are not in such programs, have, on average, fewer birth complications, larger newborns, and longer pregnancies (i.e., closer to full term).

12. **The infant born to an opioid-dependent mother** should be observed for signs of withdrawal. Such signs typically occur within 72 hours after birth. Treatments include **paregoric** where available and **phenobarbital**. Breast-feeding can be carried out by women in **methadone** maintenance programs for the first 6 months after delivery. No data beyond 6 months are available.

III. Longer Term Treatment

Follow-up treatment for opioid use is particularly important because of the public health threat of hepatitis and HIV infection through needle sharing. It should involve efforts at rehabilitation and the prevention of recidivism. Such care should be given by experienced programs that include at least the following services:

- Group and individual psychotherapy, family counseling, supplementary education, job training and placement, legal aid, and welfare assistance, as necessary;
- Psychiatric treatment for comorbid psychiatric disorders because up to 70% of all opioid-dependent patients may have a mood disorder at some point in their lives;
- Medical treatment for the complications of addiction;
- Attempts at helping the patient to overcome the drug craving that has been described in addicts after withdrawal;
- Involvement in a 12-step program, such as Narcotics Anonymous.

Drug abuse treatment programs can be categorized according to their overall approach to treatment.

A. Drug-Free Programs

These programs do not use pharmacotherapy in their treatment regimen. Instead, they try to stimulate a "change" in opioid-dependent patients that will allow them to remain drug free. Treatment usually begins after detoxification, and it often includes a phase of full-time residence in the program. A variety of programs exists, including "therapeutic communities" using peer counseling and confrontational and cognitive-behavior therapy approaches to change attitudes and behaviors and to promote drug-free living. These programs are arduous, and they require a high level of motivation and commitment to change.

Many **opioid-addicted** patients are treated with a staged approach. The inpatient stay includes detoxification, educational experiences, participation in Narcotics Anonymous, psychotherapy, and relapse-prevention training. The next step frequently is placement in a halfway house for 3 to 12 months. This phase may be followed by "three-quarter-way" house placement. Finally, "drug-free apartments" are used. Patients are usually moved along as cohorts of peers, and 12-step principles and relapse-prevention training continue in all stages. Patients are told that the road to recovery is known to be difficult, and this is also reflected in staff attitudes. As the patient progresses, the level of the "holding environment" is gradually decreased, and the patient assumes increasing degrees of responsibility. Long-term success depends on the development of an effective support system in the community that will help the addicted person sustain a drug-free life-style after the completion of the residential phase of treatment.

Rehabilitation and a return to independent living frequently take 6 to 24 months. These programs are expensive, and they are extremely demanding on the patients and treatment staff; experience suggests that only the most highly motivated patients stay in treatment. For those who do stay in treatment, however, the outcome may include a significant enhancement of social and psychologic functioning. Many graduates of these programs later become effective workers in drug abuse programs.

B. **Opiate Substitution Therapy Programs**

Initially developed using methadone maintenance, opiate substitution therapy (OST) programs now provide a variety of pharmacologic options for facilitating the addiction recovery process. Oral medication—**methadone, levacetylmethadol (*l*-acetyl-α-methadol [LAAM]), or buprenorphine**—normalizes the addicted person's altered physiologic processes and provides a foundation for other rehabilitative activities. Extensive research has demonstrated that OST reduces mortality and illicit drug use, reduces the transmission of HIV and hepatitis, and reduces both unemployment and crime. At appropriate dosage levels, these medications prevent opioid withdrawal, block the euphoric effects of illicitly used opioids, and prevent opioid craving. Patients in OST show a significant improvement in psychologic and physical health. OST has been proven most effective for those patients who have chronic histories of addiction, who have demonstrated repeated relapses after detoxication, and who have failed in drug-free treatment modalities. OST is usually provided to outpatients and is augmented by the various rehabilitative services listed earlier. Many successful programs require daily attendance for at least 3 months in which random checks of urine are conducted to detect lapses and a well-defined continuing program of group and individual counseling.

1. **Methadone** is an orally effective synthetic μ-opioid receptor agonist that was originally developed for the treatment of severe pain. Because of its long elimination half-life, it prevents opioid withdrawal for 22 to 36 hours and it can be administered for OST in a single daily dose. **Methadone** is an effective substitute for short-acting opioids. Patients maintained on **methadone** become tolerant to most of its effects at the maintenance dosage, and they can carry out their usual functions without any evidence of intoxication or functional impairment.

Methadone is begun without prior detoxification. Research has demonstrated that maintenance doses in the range of 60 to 80 mg per day or higher are required to block the effect of injected illicit opiates, to eliminate opiate craving, and to curtail the use of illicit opiates. Common side effects include constipation, a decreased sexual drive (libido), and excessive sweating. Most patients adapt to these side effects. Fertility is often improved in successfully maintained patients. Many patients can be successfully maintained on daily doses below 40 mg per day once they have achieved several years of stability at higher doses. Gradual detoxification from maintenance is recommended for younger addicts with briefer histories of addiction. Unfortunately, an 80% relapse rate within 12 months after detoxification is observed for even the most successful maintenance patients. Clinicians should use great caution in recommending detoxification for chronic addicts. Opioid-addicted persons who have not achieved drug-free status by the age of 35 years rarely remain abstinent after detoxification. Indefinite OST should be recommended for such chronic and vulnerable patients.

Methadone maintenance remains the most widely applicable medical treatment available today. In the United States, federal regulations define admission standards for OST programs; describe appropriate doses; delineate the take-home supply; and specify the need for urine testing, record keeping, and supportive services. Each program must be approved before it can provide OST. In some countries (e.g., Germany), specific qualifications are needed to prescribe **methadone**, and all prescriptions are monitored centrally by an agency comparable with the United States Food and Drug Administration.

Some programs maintain **heroin-dependent pregnant women** on low doses of **methadone** (20 to 40 mg per day) to reduce the likelihood both of continued i.v. opioid use by the mother and of a severe withdrawal reaction in the infant. Maintaining a steady dose of **methadone** also protects the fetus from the changing concentrations of any opioid that the mother might abuse if she was not taking **methadone**. With such patients, however, ensuring that the low dose chosen is effective is important; otherwise, their "craving" for opioids may be increased. A concern that detoxification could terminate the pregnancy often exists. Some programs believe that very gradual detoxification and referral to a halfway house specializing in treating pregnant patients is beneficial. With the latter approach, the fetus is detoxified *in utero* and is born to a drug-free mother. Further studies are still needed to give more information on the optimal treatment of these patients.

2. **Levacetylmethadol** (**LAAM**) is a synthetic μ-opioid receptor agonist that is a longer-acting derivative of **methadone**. It is similar to **methadone** in its clinical efficacy, side effects, and drug interactions; but it has a slower onset of action. **LAAM** has two active metabolites, **nor-LAAM** and **dinor-LAAM**. Because these metabolites are eliminated more slowly than the parent drug, they produce a longer duration of action. In adequate doses, **LAAM** prevents opiate withdrawal for 48 to 72 hours. It is used clinically on an every other day (q.o.d.) or three times per week dosing schedule. Treatment begins with a 20 to 40 mg q.o.d regimen, with increases of 5 to 10 mg until a dose in the range of 80 to 100 mg or higher is achieved. Some clinics prefer to stabilize patients on **methadone** initially and then to convert them to a **LAAM** dose that is 1.2 to 1.3 times the **methadone** maintenance dose. A 30% to 40% higher dose is administered for the first 72-hour interval. Many patients prefer **LAAM** to **methadone**, reporting that they feel more "normal" (probably because of the longer duration of action) and that three times a week dosing is less disruptive to work and family responsibilities than is the daily dosing that is required for **methadone** treatment.

LAAM availability has ended in European Union countries. This action was taken because these countries concluded that **LAAM** had an unacceptable benefit-to-risk ratio, with the risk coming from increases in QTc intervals and, in some cases, of the ventricular tachyarrhythmia *torsade de pointes*. In the United States product, labeling for **LAAM** has been revised to include a "black box" warning, and it has been downgraded to non–first-line therapy status. **LAAM** should not be prescribed for patients with preexisting QTc interval prolongation or for those taking medications that inhibit CYP 3A4. Patients should be given a 12-lead electrocardiogram before starting **LAAM**. Initial biweekly electrocardiographic monitoring with subsequent periodic monitoring is prudent. **LAAM** is not approved for use in pregnant women; those on **LAAM** who become pregnant must be switched to **methadone**.

3. **Buprenorphine**. The most recent addition to the group of medications proposed for OST is **buprenorphine**. This semisynthetic partial agonist has an extremely high affinity for μ-opioid receptors, and it is also a potent antagonist at the κ receptors. It dissociates slowly from these receptors, giving it a long duration of action (24 to 48 hours) and a unique safety profile that includes a reduced likelihood of withdrawal reactions.

Buprenorphine is a hybrid of the agonist **etorphine** and the antagonist **diprenorphine**. It produces subjective opioid effects after acute use, but it causes only limited dependence and mild withdrawal reactions in humans. In overdoses, an apparent ceiling effect at the μ receptor appears to prevent fatal respiratory depression despite the escalated intake. Like **LAAM**, doses can be administered three times a week. Its clinical efficacy is comparable with **methadone**. Addicted persons can be administered an initial dose of **buprenorphine** at 12 to 24 hours after their last heroin dose. Sublingual doses of 2 to 4 mg can be administered every 2 to 4 hours up to a maximum dose of 8 mg for the first day. An additional 2 to 4 mg can be added daily until the initial target maintenance dose of 12 to 16 mg per day is reached.

In addition to its use for OST, **buprenorphine** appears to be an effective medication for opioid withdrawal. Although a gradual 10-day to 14-day detoxification protocol is preferred, 3-day protocols have been well accepted by patients. Using the parenteral analgesic form of buprenorphine, patients have been dosed according to the following regimen: 0.3 to 0.6 mg intramuscularly three times a day on day 1, 0.15 to 0.3 mg intramuscularly three times a day on day 2, and 0.15 mg intramuscularly once or twice a day on day 3. Using the sublingual (SL) tablets, patients can be dosed with 12 mg SL (days 1 and 2) and then 6 mg SL on day 3.

In a major departure from the **methadone** maintenance clinic model, sublingual **buprenorphine** distributed as a combination tablet with **naloxone** has been proposed as a take-home medication for use by stable OST patients in office-based clinical practices. However, until the United States Food and Drug Administration grants final regulatory approval, this use of **buprenorphine** for the treatment of opioid addiction is precluded in the United States.

C. **Multimodality Programs**

Many drug abuse treatment programs use more than one treatment track or option. Such options might include drug-free residential treatment, OST treatment, **methadone** detoxification with continued outpatient treatment, or various combinations of these. All patients in these different settings have access to common social and rehabilitation services as described earlier. The growing recognition in drug-free residential programs has been that attention must be paid to the concomitant psychiatric and medical disorders, such as depression and chronic pain. Special consideration must be given to selecting nonaddicting medications for treating accompanying disorders in these so-called dual diagnosis patients.

D. **Other Chemotherapy Maintenance Treatments**

1. **Naltrexone** is a long-acting competitive opioid antagonist. It has little intrinsic activity, although it may produce miosis in some patients. It has minimal effects on craving and no reinforcing properties. **Naltrexone** acts for more than 24 hours after a single oral dose, usually of 50 mg. Some have suggested that **naltrexone**, which antagonizes the effects of an administered opioid, can be taken by the detoxified patient until the likelihood of a relapse to opioid use is diminished.

Naltrexone is generally administered only after a patient remains opioid free and without clinical signs of withdrawal for 5 to 10 days and then shows no signs of precipitated withdrawal after a **naloxone** challenge. The usual waiting period is 10 to 14 days after **methadone** discontinuation. The challenge procedure often involves an initial injection of 0.2 mg of **naloxone** i.v., followed by a second dose of 0.6 mg. Treatment is then begun at 10 mg per day, with increases to 150 mg per day over the initial 10 days. Maintenance dosing schedules, such as 50 mg of **naltrexone** every 24 hours, with additional dosing (i.e., an additional 50 to 100 mg) on "vulnerable" days, such as weekends, are typical. Spaced dosing with larger doses (i.e., 100 to 150 mg every 2 or 3 days) sometimes helps with adherence.

Many experienced clinicians believe that **naltrexone** maintenance is the approach of choice when treating opioid-dependent physicians and other health care professionals. Clearly, the use of **naltrexone** is most successful in highly motivated patients who believe that they have a great deal to lose if treatment does not work. Less-motivated patients rarely participate in naltrexone programs. At times, legal or penal system involvement is beneficial. Considerable care must be given to educating patients about the benefits and risks of naltrexone use. They must understand that it is different from **methadone**; **naltrexone** can precipitate withdrawal in an addicted person, and this withdrawal cannot be easily overridden. The use of **naltrexone** in patients abusing more than one substance poses special risks.

2. **Nalmefene** is a new opioid antagonist that has shown some promise in reducing relapse in alcoholics, and it has the potential for usefulness in the treatment of opioid addiction. It appears to produce no hepatotoxicity or other serious side effects; it is also a longer-acting agent than is **naltrexone**.

E. **Needle Exchange Programs**

Needle exchange programs are one example of a "harm reduction" approach to the problem of opioid abuse. Many health care providers believe that, in the absence of more effective strategies and treatments to reduce recidivism rates, harm reduction is a more workable goal than is complete abstinence for some opioid abusers. Needle exchange programs have demonstrated their effectiveness in reducing the transmission of HIV and hepatitis; they may also be helpful in recruiting addicted persons into treatment programs. Currently no evidence indicates that such needle exchange initiatives encourage or spread i.v. drug use.

ADDITIONAL READING

Ball J, Ross A. *The effectiveness of methadone maintenance treatment.* New York: Springer-Verlag, 1991.

Barthwell A, Senay E, Marks R, et al. Patients successfully maintained with methadone escaped human immunodeficiency virus infection. *Arch Gen Psychiatry* 1989;46: 957–958.

Bell J, Seres V, Bowron P, et al. The use of serum methadone levels in patients receiving methadone maintenance. *Clin Pharmacol Ther* 1988;43:623–629.

Camacho LM, Bartholomew NG, Joe GW, et al. Maintenance of HIV risk reduction among injection opioid users: a 12 month post-treatment follow-up. *Drug Alcohol Depend* 1997;25:11–18.

Caplhorn JRM, Ross M. Methadone maintenance and the likelihood of risky needle sharing. *Int J Addict* 1995;28:983–998.

Charney DS, Heninger GR, Kleber HD. The combined use of clonidine and naltrexone as a rapid, safe, and effective treatment of abrupt withdrawal from methadone. *Am J Psychiatry* 1986;143:831–837.

Church SH, Rothenberg JL, Sullivan MA, et al. Concurrent substance use and outcome in combined behavioral and naltrexone therapy for opiate dependence. *Am J Drug Alcohol Abuse* 2001;27:441–452.

Comer SD, Collins ED, Fischman MW. Buprenorphine sublingual tablets: effects on IV heroin self-administration in humans. *Psychopharmacology* 2001;154:28–37.

Cooper J, Altman F, Brown B, et al. *Research on the treatment of narcotic addiction: state of the art.* Rockville, MD: National Institute on Drug Abuse, 1983.

D'Aunno T, Folz-Murphy N, Lin X. Changes in methadone treatment practices: results from a panel study, 1988–1995. *Am J Drug Alcohol Abuse* 1999;25:681–699.

National Institutes of Health Consensus Development Conference. Effective medical treatment of opiate addiction. *NIH consensus statement.* November 17–19, 1997. 1997;15:1–38.

Geraghty B, Graham EA, Logan B, et al. Methadone levels in human breast milk. *J Hum Lactation* 1997;13:227–230.

Gowing L, Ali R, White J. Buprenorphine for the management of opioid withdrawal (Cochrane review). *Cochrane Database Syst Rev* 2000;3:CD002025.

Harding-Pink D. Methadone: one person's maintenance dose is another's poison. *Lancet* 1993;341:665–666.

Jasinski DR, Johnson RE, Kocher TR. Clonidine in morphine withdrawal: differential effects on signs and symptoms. *Arch Gen Psychiatry* 1985;42:1063–1066.

Johnson RE, Jaffe JH, Fudala PJ. A controlled trial of buprenorphine for the treatment of opioid dependence. *JAMA* 1992;267:2750–2755.

Joranson DF, Ryan KM, Gilson AM, et al. Trends in medical use and abuse of opioid analgesics. *JAMA* 2000;283:1710–1714.

Kosten TR, Kleber HD. Buprenorphine detoxification from opioid dependence: a pilot study. *Life Sci* 1988;42:635–641.

Ling W, Charuvastra C, Collins JF, et al. Buprenorphine maintenance treatment of opiate dependence: a multicenter, randomized clinical trial. *Addiction* 1998;93:475–486.

Ling W, Wesson DR, Charuvastra C, et al. A controlled trial comparing maintenance in opioid dependence. *Arch Gen Psychiatry* 1996;53:401–407.

Maddux JF, Desmond DP. Methadone maintenance and recovery from opioid dependence. *Am J Drug Alcohol Abuse* 1992;18:63–74.

Mason BJ, Salvato FR, Williams LD, et al. A double-blind, placebo-controlled study of oral nalmefene for alcohol dependence. *Arch Gen Psychiatry* 1999;56:719–724.

Mello NK, Mendelson JH, Kuehnle JC. Buprenorphine effects on human heroin self-administration: an operant analysis. *J Pharmacol Exp Ther* 1982;223:30–39.

Metzger D, Woody G, McLellan A, et al. Human immunodeficiency virus seroconversion among intravenous drug users in- and out-of-treatment: an 18 month prospective follow-up. *J Acquir Immune Defic Syndr* 1993;6:1049–1056.

O'Connor PG, Carroll KM, Shi JM, et al. Three methods of opioid detoxification in a primary care setting. *Ann Intern Med* 1997;127:526–530.

O'Connor PG, Kosten TR. Rapid and ultra rapid opioid detoxification techniques. *JAMA* 1998;278:229–234.

O'Connor PG, Oliveto AH, Shi JM, et al. A randomized trial of buprenorphine maintenance for heroin dependence in a primary care clinic for substance users versus a methadone clinic. *Am J Med* 1998;105:100–105.

Pasternak GW. Opioid receptors. In: Meltzer H, ed. *Psychopharmacology: the third generation of progress.* New York: Raven, 1987:281–288.

Peachy JE. The role of drugs in the treatment of opioid addicts. *Med J Australia* 1986; 145:395–399.

Rosen MI, Kosten TR. Buprenorphine: beyond methadone? *Hosp Comm Psychiatry* 1991; 42:347–349.

Rounsaville BJ, Kleber HD. Untreated opiate addicts. *Arch Gen Psychiatry* 1985;42: 1072–1077.

Sees KL, Delucchi KL, Masson C, et al. Methadone maintenance vs 180-day psychosocially enriched detoxification treatment of opioid dependence. *JAMA* 2000;283: 1303–1310.

Senay EC. Methadone maintenance treatment. *Int J Addict* 1985;20:803–821.

Umbricht A, Montoya ID, Hoover DR, et al. Naltrexone shortened opioid detoxification with buprenorphine. *Drug Alcohol Depend* 1999;56:181–190.

Ward J, Hall W, Mattick RP. Role of maintenance treatment in opioid dependence. *Lancet* 1999;353:221–226.

Woods JH, Winger G. Opioids, receptors, and abuse liability. In: Meltzer H, ed. *Psychopharmacology: the third generation of progress.* New York: Raven, 1987: 1555–1564.

Zweben JE. Counseling issues in methadone maintenance treatment. *J Psychoactive Drugs* 1991;23:177–190.

11. ALCOHOLISM AND ITS TREATMENT

Domenic A. Ciraulo
Richard I. Shader
Ann Marie Ciraulo

Alcoholism remains a major public health problem in the United States. An estimated 14 million Americans meet the diagnostic criteria for **alcohol** abuse or alcoholism, resulting in economic costs of over 184 billion dollars annually according to the *Tenth Special Report to the United States Congress on Alcohol and Health* (2000). Using a sampling of adults from five metropolitan areas, the Epidemiologic Catchment Area survey estimated that the lifetime prevalence of **alcohol**-related disorders is 13.5%, with consistently higher rates for men than for women (for lifetime, 1-year, and 1-month prevalence). Somewhat higher rates were found in the National Comorbidity Survey, which sampled a relatively younger population and found a lifetime prevalence of **alcohol** dependence of 20.1% for men and 8.2% for women. The Joint Committee of the National Council on Alcoholism and Drug Dependence and the American Society of Addiction Medicine defines **alcoholism** as a primary, chronic, often progressive and fatal disease having genetic, psychosocial, and environmental factors that influence its development and manifestations. Impaired control over drinking; preoccupation with **alcohol**; use of **alcohol** despite adverse consequences; or cognitive distortions, such as denial, may be continuous or periodic. Although per capita **alcohol** consumption in the United States has declined somewhat since 1981, **alcohol** is the most abused substance in this country, and the lifetime risk for **alcohol** abuse is between 13% and 20%, with men at greater risk than women. For perspective, one should remember that **alcohol**, at the brain concentrations experienced during intoxication, has both specific and nonspecific effects on many cellular processes, including both excitatory and inhibitory transmission. The **alcohol** withdrawal (or abstinence) syndrome (see Chapter 12) is a state of overactivity of the central nervous system that is marked by increased firing of sympathetic neurons; enhanced production of norepinephrine and cortisol; and increased activity of excitatory amino acids, such as glutamate.

This chapter presents an overall treatment approach to the patient who misuses or abuses or who is dependent on **alcohol**. In Chapter 12, the recognition and treatment of the **alcohol** withdrawal syndrome and its complications are reviewed. The approach taken throughout this chapter is based on the view that alcoholism is a multidetermined social and medical phenomenon requiring careful diagnosis and evaluation, as well as individualized treatment. The primary clinician must be familiar with, and open to, a variety of applicable techniques, ranging from individual and group psychotherapy to Alcoholics Anonymous (AA), family therapy, pharmacotherapy, or behavioral treatments, and he or she must be prepared to use consultants in these fields when this becomes necessary. Although the first goal is to have the patient stop drinking, understanding a patient's feelings, conflicts, relationships, experiences, relevant family interactions, expectations, and history is essential in planning a treatment program. Secondary diagnosis (e.g., anxiety, familial tremor, depression, schizophrenia) is necessary to determine whether and when pharmacologic intervention is appropriate.

I. Diagnosis
Table 11.1 lists the *Diagnostic and Statistical Manual of Mental Disorders,* 4th edition (DSM-IV), criteria for the diagnosis of **alcohol** dependence. From a clinical standpoint, an affirmative answer to the question, "*Did you ever think or did anyone ever tell you that you had a problem with alcohol?*" is usually enough to make a presumptive diagnosis of **alcohol** abuse or dependence. Finding out how many drinks a person must have to feel "high" and whether this amount has changed can also be helpful as an indication of tolerance development, in which increasing amounts of **alcohol** are needed to produce the desired effect. More detailed questioning should focus on social disruptions (e.g., problems

TABLE 11.1. DIAGNOSTIC FEATURES OF ALCOHOL (ETHANOL) DEPENDENCE

A maladaptive pattern of alcohol use lasting at least a year and leading to clinically significant impairment or distress as manifested by at least 3 of the following features:

1. Tolerance to the effects of alcohol as reflected by
   a. A need for markedly increased amounts of alcohol over time to achieve a desired effect or level of intoxication.
   b. Markedly diminished effects from continued use of the same amount.
   c. **Functioning adequately at amounts of alcohol or blood concentrations that would produce significant impairment in a casual or naive drinker**.
2. Withdrawal as reflected by either of the following:
   a. A characteristic alcohol withdrawal syndrome as manifested by at least 2 of the following:

Tremor	Insomnia
Autonomic hyperactivity	Nausea or vomiting
Psychomotor agitation	Anxiety
Transient illusions or hallucinations	Tonic-clonic seizures

   This syndrome should appear shortly (usually within a few hours) after the cessation of or a clear cut reduction in the amount of alcohol consumed.
   b. Alcohol has been used to avoid or relieve the symptoms of the withdrawal syndrome.
3. Alcohol is taken in larger amounts or over a longer period than intended (i.e., reflecting loss of control or tolerance).
4. A history of unsuccessful efforts to contain or reduce alcohol use or to be a "controlled" drinker.
5. A great deal of time is spent in the following:
   a. Drinking.
   b. Recovering from the effects of drinking.
   c. **Activities necessary to obtain alcohol**.
6. Important activities (i.e., social, occupational, recreational) are given up or reduced because of alcohol use.
7. Continued use of alcohol despite knowledge of persistent or recurrent physical or emotional problems caused or aggravated by alcohol use.
8. **A pattern of recurrent use of alcohol in hazardous situations (e.g., driving an automobile, using equipment that requires coordination or prompt reactions)**.
9. **Recurrent alcohol-related legal or interpersonal problems**.

From the American Psychiatric Association. *DSM-IV options book: work in progress.* Washington, D.C.: American Psychiatric Press, 1993, with permission. The authors of this chapter feel that this criteria set has more clinical utility than the more generic criteria seen in *Diagnostic and statistical manual of mental disorders,* 4th ed., Text revision (2000) (DSM-IV-TR). **Items 1c, 3c, 8, and 9 do not appear in the final version of the DSM-IV-TR.**

in employment, family relationships, and social functioning) and signs and symptoms of physical dependence (e.g., tremulousness, abstinence symptoms).

Another useful screening tool is the **CAGE** system (see Additional Reading). CAGE is a mnemonic for the following four questions that are easily included in a clinical interview:

C: "Have you ever felt you should **cut down** on your drinking?"
A: "Have people **annoyed** you by criticizing your drinking?"
G: "Have you ever felt bad or **guilty** about your drinking?"
E: "Have you ever had a drink first thing in the morning to steady your nerves or to get rid of a hangover (an '**eye opener**')?"

If a patient answers yes to two or three of these questions, a presumptive diagnosis of alcoholism can be made in about 90% of patients.

Another commonly used assessment scale is the Michigan Alcohol Screening Test, a 25-item questionnaire that covers the psychosocial complications of alcoholism. (*Note:* Briefer 13-item and 10-item forms are also available.) The MacAndrew Alcoholism Scale, a 49-item scale derived from the Minnesota Multiphasic Personality Inventory, is another commonly used self-report screening instrument.

A. Alcoholism as a Disease

Alcoholism is a complex disease with biologic, psychologic, and social components. The concept of alcoholism as a disease is useful from a variety of perspectives. Having the patient focus on this concrete issue facilitates engagement in psychotherapy and helps to reduce the overwhelming and sometimes obsessive feelings of guilt. This approach also allows the clinician to address the problem drinking directly. The disease concept, however, should not connote that alcoholism is a unitary phenomenon with a single etiology or treatment, any more than the term **psychosis** connotes a single disease with one specific treatment. Also consistent with the disease concept are data suggesting a genetic vulnerability to alcoholism in some individuals, particularly in males who show an earlier onset of **alcohol** use, develop tolerance and physical dependence, and exhibit marked antisocial behavior in childhood and adolescence.

The disease concept should not imply that a person has no control of his or her drinking and behavior. As with most medical illnesses, a person's behavior influences the course of the illness (e.g., diabetes mellitus and hypertension). Even when excessive drinking is a symptom of an underlying psychiatric illness, if the problem drinking persists long enough, it takes on a life of its own; and, almost invariably, ending the drinking must become the focus of any initial therapy.

B. Genetics and Alcoholism

Early twin studies had suggested that the heritability of alcoholism was approximately 50% in men, although a genetic link in women was not established. More recently, a study of adult Australian twins suggested that about two-thirds of the risk is genetically mediated in both men and women, with the remainder being determined by environmental factors.

The mechanism of genetic risk is unknown. The strongest evidence linking genes to alcoholism is the finding of specific polymorphisms of the **alcohol** dehydrogenase genes, *ADH2* and *ADH3*. **Alcohol** is first metabolized to acetaldehyde by the hepatic enzyme **alcohol** dehydrogenase (Fig. 11.1). Acetaldehyde in turn is metabolized to acetic acid by aldehyde dehydrogenase. Alleles of *ADH2* and *ADH3* encode forms of alcohol dehydrogenase that metabolize the **alcohol** to acetaldehyde more rapidly than do other forms of the enzyme. As a consequence, acetaldehyde accumulates and produces toxicity. The alleles are common in Asian populations, in which they provide a partial protective effect against the development of alcoholism. Other genes may also be involved in the development of alcoholism. Although early studies suggested that dopamine receptor gene *DRD2* polymorphisms were associated with the risk for alcoholism, later studies have not confirmed this relationship. Other studies have linked genes coding for serotonin 5-hydroxtryptamine 1B [5-HT$_{1B}$] receptors (and the serotonin transporter) to certain subtypes of alcoholism. Additional studies have found an association between alcoholism and the allele of the tyrosine hydroxylase gene. Further studies are required to validate these findings.

C. Associated Psychiatric Illnesses

A careful differential diagnosis must always include consideration of concomitant or underlying psychiatric illnesses. Depressive symptoms (see Chapters 18 and 19) are found in many alcoholic patients, either as a consequence of chronic drinking or, less commonly, as a predisposing factor to **alcohol** abuse. Transient symptoms of depression frequently occur after the cessation of drinking. Some epidemiologic evidence suggests a connection between depression and alcoholism. However, other studies note that the

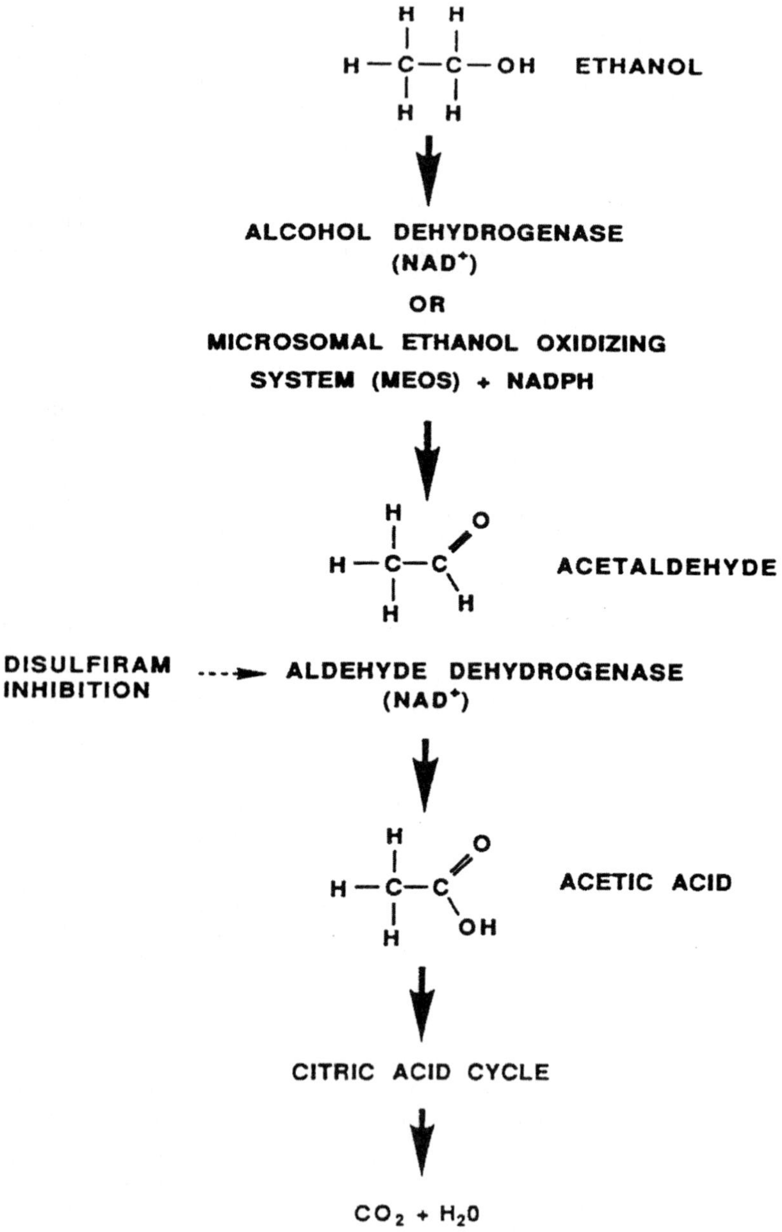

FIG. 11.1. Disulfiram and the metabolic pathway of alcohol (ethanol).

prevalence of mood disorders in alcoholic patients does not differ from their rates in the general adult population. Several studies have shown an increased prevalence of affective disorders in the families of alcoholic patients. Suicide, especially after any significant loss (e.g., a loved one, a job), is frequent in alcoholic patients (see Chapter 17). Depression is often the reason that an alcoholic patient seeks treatment. Schizophrenia and other major psychoses, such as involutional melancholia, psychotic organic brain syndrome, and bipolar disorder, also commonly occur in alcoholic patients. Binge drinking frequently accompanies the manic phase of a bipolar affective disorder; it can also be linked to the luteal phase of the menstrual cycle in some women. On psychiatric units that treat alcoholic patients (i.e., Dual Disorder or Psychiatrically Impaired Substance Abuse units), bipolar disorder, major depressive disorder, and schizophrenia are the most common concomitant major diagnoses (i.e., DSM-IV axis I). On dedicated substance abuse units (i.e., those that typically screen out patients with psychiatric disorders), the most common additional axis I diagnoses are major depressive disorder and anxiety disorders. Careful evaluation of any accompanying psychiatric disorder is central to the proper treatment of the alcoholic patient.

D. Multidisciplinary Approach

Ideally, diagnosis and treatment of the alcoholic patient are pursued in a multidisciplinary setting. A physician and nurse familiar with the medical problems associated with acute withdrawal and chronic **alcohol** consumption should be part of the diagnostic and treatment team. Often the alcoholic patient's presenting complaint is medical, and the diagnosis of alcoholism is made only by an alert clinician with a high index of suspicion. Commonly associated conditions are hypertension, pneumonia, gastrointestinal problems, impotence, insomnia, and neuropathies. Among patients on general medical wards (depending on the type of institution and the population served), between 12% and 60% will have an **alcohol** problem. Thus, the importance of an alert medical practitioner can hardly be overemphasized.

Serum γ-glutamyl transferase (SGGT) or transpeptidase is a sensitive indicator of the effects of **alcohol** on the liver. In a person who has been drinking heavily, this enzyme typically remains elevated (i.e., over 30 U per L) for 4 to 5 weeks after the cessation of drinking. If no confounding explanation for an elevation in SGGT is present, this test can be used to aid in the diagnosis of alcoholism or in monitoring abstinence. SGGT may also be elevated in liver disease from other causes, as well as in obesity, inflammatory bowel or thyroid disease, diabetes, pancreatitis, acute renal insufficiency, trauma, or other illnesses. (*Note:* SGGT levels may also be increased from the use of high doses of benzodiazepines or **phenytoin**.) Elevated SGGT, especially in the presence of macrocytic anemia, should alert the clinician to the potential of **alcohol** abuse. Although several other biologic markers or combinations of markers have been used to identify alcoholic patients in general hospitals, none are commonly used in clinical practice. Carbohydrate deficient transferrin, a widely used marker for heavy drinking in research studies, may also have clinical utility. This test is not widely available at present, and it does not have adequate sensitivity in women unless it is used in conjunction with SGGT.

To ensure a comprehensive diagnostic and treatment evaluation, a psychiatrist should be a member of the treatment team. In addition, social workers should be available for family evaluations and therapy and to aid in community and aftercare placement. Finally, an **alcohol** counselor (often a recovering alcoholic) who is familiar with AA is an invaluable asset to the treatment team. He or she also provides concrete evidence that recovery is possible. The counselor can also be a valuable link to community and aftercare resources.

Most office-based psychiatric physicians find the team approach impractical. In such instances, the psychiatrist must be prepared to fill several roles, including inquiry about medical problems and referral to appropriate treatment alternatives when necessary. Evaluating available family members and, on occasion, engaging in family therapy may also be valuable. Most importantly, the psychiatrist must be cognizant of the importance of the support and group involvement provided by programs such as AA to many alcoholic patients, and he or she should encourage such patients to attend meetings regularly and to participate actively. Although the comments in this paragraph target the office-based psychiatrist, they apply to many other physicians and mental health clinicians as well.

II. Therapeutic Modalities for Alcoholism

A. Psychosocial and Behavioral Treatments

These are the primary forms of therapy for alcoholism. Although the efficacy of many types of behavioral treatments is well established, no specific type is superior. In a large sample study, the following three treatments were compared: 12-step facilitation therapy, which was modeled on the principles of AA; cognitive-behavior therapy (CBT); and motivational enhancement therapy (National Institute on Alcohol Abuse and Alcoholism [NIAAA], Project MATCH, 1998). All the treatments were effective; however, 12-step facilitation therapy was slightly more effective than the other therapies in one particular subgroup in which the subjects were recruited from outpatient settings as opposed to those recruited from aftercare programs. A follow-up study of the Project MATCH sample found that all of the therapies were also associated with lower medical costs (comparison of pretreatment and posttreatment), although the motivational enhancement therapy did not fare as well in certain subgroups (e.g., patients with a diagnosis of **alcohol** dependence, high psychiatric severity, or low social support). In clinical practice, psychotherapy for **alcohol** dependence is usually based on one of two conceptual models, social learning theory or psychodynamic theory. Both approaches often include aspects of motivational enhancement therapy, community reinforcement, contingency contracting, pharmacotherapy, and network therapy (i.e., involvement of the patient's social network).

B. Individual Psychotherapy

CBT is based on social learning theory (see Bandura, 1977; Marlatt and Gordon, 1985), but it may also incorporate aspects of motivational (see Miller and Rollnick, 1991) and change theories (see DiClemente and Prochaska, 1982). An example of this approach is the COMBINE Behavioral Intervention, which was designed by an expert panel participating in the NIAAA study *Combining Medications and Behavioral Interventions*. It incorporates many of the therapeutic interventions used in Project MATCH. COMBINE Behavioral Intervention is based on the principles that people pass through a series of stages in the course of modifying behavior and that different therapeutic interventions should be used depending on the stage of change. These stages are as follows:

1. **Precontemplation**, in which the person is not considering a change;
2. **Contemplation**, in which the individual realizes that a problem exists but has ambivalence about change;
3. **Action**, in which the person engages in efforts to change the behavior;
4. **Maintenance**, in which strategies are used to support the change and to prevent relapse.

COMBINE Behavioral Intervention consists of four phases that correspond to the stages of change. In the first phase, techniques of motivational interviewing are used to enhance a person's readiness for change. In the second phase, a shift from building motivation for change to development of a plan for change occurs. Early in the second phase, the therapist examines the common antecedents and consequences of drinking and assesses psychosocial functioning. Later in the second phase, a treatment plan is negotiated with the individual. In the third phase, the plan is implemented using various coping skills modules (e.g., assertiveness training, mood and craving management, relationship skills training, social or recreational counseling, job finding training). After the modules are completed, the fourth phase, which focuses on the maintenance of abstinence and the psychosocial gains achieved in prior phases, begins. When relapse occurs, the treatment is modified by repeating or adding the appropriate modules from the earlier treatment phases.

Although many clinicians treating alcoholism have embraced CBT as a first-line psychotherapy, others favor a psychodynamically oriented approach. An inherent disadvantage of the psychodynamic approach is the extensive training that is needed to acquire adequate skills. This approach cannot be "manualized" for use in treatment centers—this and other factors make evaluation of psychodynamically oriented treatment in controlled studies impossible. Nevertheless, the authors have observed many patients who did not respond to CBT but who later responded to individual or group therapy using modified psychodynamic approaches. Recent psychodynamic theories of substance abuse have emphasized deficits in the ego (see Chapter 1). Under one such formulation, deficits in ego defenses result in overwhelmingly painful affects, such as anxiety, depression, rage, and shame, that are being muted by drug and **alcohol** use. The use of **alcohol** and other chemical substances may allow such vulnerable persons to believe that they have more control over their suffering. Narcissistic deficits are also viewed as important by some clinicians. In this formulation, feelings of rage or shame are triggered by disappointment by or "in the eyes of" important persons ("idealized objects") or by challenges to a grandiose sense of oneself; these lead to **alcohol** or drug use as a means of containing the resulting distress. Other psychodynamic formulations address deficiencies in self-care functions and difficulty in experiencing and tolerating affects.

Individual psychodynamic psychotherapy may be helpful to many alcoholic patients; however, some modifications of technique are necessary. The initial phases of psychotherapy need a "here and now" focus to help the patient deal with the problems that have arisen from **alcohol** abuse and to suggest practical techniques for avoiding relapse. This first phase is crucial in establishing rapport; general agreement is found on the principle that an active, nurturing therapist is more likely to be effective than one who is not. Therapist empathy, a positive therapeutic alliance, and a nonconfrontational style, which are sometimes referred to as a "client-centered approach," correlate with positive outcomes.

Often, one of the earliest issues in therapy is establishing whether total abstinence is the only acceptable treatment goal. The authors' recommendation is that total abstinence is the goal of treatment. Although the ability of some alcoholic patients to return to controlled drinking has been documented, predicting who can return to moderate drinking and who will lose control is impossible. Some research suggests that the patients with more severe alcohol problems are less likely to achieve controlled drinking.

With regard to drinking episodes that occur during the course of treatment, the authors' approach is flexible. Even though the first goal of treatment is to stop drinking, expecting an alcoholic patient to stop drinking as soon as he or she enters treatment is unrealistic. Occasional drinking episodes are not, in and of themselves, sufficient reason for hospitalization. If the patient "slips" during the course of treatment, psychotherapy should explore the circumstances surrounding the episode; this can result in the patient's greater awareness of high-risk situations and mood states that lead to drinking. The clinician must accept that alcoholism is a chronic disease and that relapses are common.

In general, when the patient is intoxicated at a treatment session, an evaluation of safety and of the need for hospitalization should be made, along with reasonable efforts to ensure safe transportation home when inpatient treatment is not indicated. Although, on occasion, the intoxicated state may provide useful information about the alcoholic patient's behavior while drunk, typically very little can be accomplished and these sessions are canceled.

An initial task in treatment involves confronting the patient's denial of a problem with **alcohol**. Admitting one is an alcoholic can be a narcissistic injury, implying loss of control and powerlessness. Empathic confrontations, family meetings, and participation in AA are often helpful in confronting denial. The authors discourage large group interventions to coerce patients into treatment; however, carefully selected family members or friends, working in collaboration with clinicians, can help motivate patients for treatment. The authors find that two clinicians and one person with close personal ties to the patient provide a workable, and perhaps optimal, group composition. The selected friend or family member should meet with the clinicians before the intervention to understand the process and the principles of motivational interviewing.

AA should also be discussed in the early stages of treatment. The clinician should introduce AA in a general way and should explore the patient's feelings about it. The more first-hand knowledge of AA the clinician has, the more effective he or she will be in confronting the patient's rationalizations and negative impressions about AA. AA Facilitation, a therapeutic intervention that encourages AA participation and reinforces AA principles, was established as an effective psychosocial intervention in Project MATCH.

At an early stage in treatment, addressing the issue of a balanced life-style is also important. Although a balance between work and recreational activities has never been directly linked to substance abuse problems, many authorities believe that achieving this balance is important to avoid chronic resentments about overworking. Brooding resentment is one of the negative emotional states that often leads to drinking.

Many clinicians believe that spirituality has a key place in the treatment of some patients and that it should be addressed early on. That conversion experiences facilitate abstinence has long been recognized, and religious reform groups have been successful in helping some alcoholic patients achieve and maintain abstinence.

In later stages of treatment, the focus shifts from an emphasis on supportive and directive techniques to the development of self-understanding, insight, and mastery. In practice, these progress concurrently, although as the length of time in recovery increases, the proportion of the effort focused on self-understanding, insight, and mastery increases.

Readers interested in a detailed discussion of psychosocial treatment approaches should refer to the Additional Reading section.

C. Group Psychotherapy

Groups are a useful treatment modality for alcoholic patients; however, no specific type of group therapy is consistently superior to others. Group work is especially useful in this population because of the difficulties that some alcoholic patients have in tolerating the intense feelings toward the treating clinician that they develop in individual therapy. Some clinicians also believe that confrontation of the alcoholic patient's denial and rationalization by the group is a more powerful and less-threatening intervention than when this is done by an individual clinician.

Other benefits may result from the positive effects that a group experience can have on the alcoholic patient's self-esteem and self-image. In the group setting, the patient helps others by listening and sharing and by offering advice and insights. By being with people who have recovered and maintained abstinence and with those who relapse but recover, the group experience can also instill hope. In addition, it provides an opportunity to discuss fears of intimacy and to acquire useful interpersonal skills. Finally, many groups fulfill an important educational function—the patient can learn about alcoholism, its treatment, and the availability of other resources.

D. Family Therapy

Whenever an evaluation of the alcoholic patient's family is possible, this should be conducted. Experienced clinicians may also use family therapy as a primary or adjunctive treatment. Family therapy may take many forms, including meeting with the entire family in therapy sessions, seeing only the marital dyad, or encouraging group therapy for couples or spouses. For the clinician practicing outside of an alcoholism treatment center, making an initial family evaluation and, on that basis, coming to a decision about the value and extent of family involvement seems reasonable.

Al-Anon, Ala-Teen, and Adult Children of Alcoholics are specialized self-help groups that address family issues. They arose as parallel, but separate, groups from AA, and they bear much similarity to AA. They stress a caring detachment from the alcoholic patient, emphasizing that the family member is powerless over both **alcohol** and the patient; and they work to establish

TABLE 11.2. THE TWELVE STEPS OF ALCOHOLICS ANONYMOUS

Step 1	Admitted we were powerless over alcohol—that our lives had become unmanageable.
Step 2	Came to believe that a Power greater than ourselves could restore us to sanity.
Step 3	Made a decision to turn our will and our lives over to the care of God **as we understood Him**.
Step 4	Made a searching and fearless moral inventory of ourselves.
Step 5	Admitted to God, to ourselves, and to another human being the exact nature of our wrongs.
Step 6	Were entirely ready to have God remove all these defects of character.
Step 7	Humbly asked Him to remove our shortcomings.
Step 8	Made a list of all the persons we had harmed and became willing to make amends to them all.
Step 9	Made direct amends to such people wherever possible, except when to do so would injure them or others.
Step 10	Continued to take a personal inventory and, when we were wrong, promptly admitted it.
Step 11	Sought through prayer and meditation to improve our conscious contact with God **as we understood Him**, praying only for knowledge of His will for us and the power to carry that out.
Step 12	Having had a spiritual awakening as the result of these steps, we tried to carry this message to alcoholics and to practice these principles in all our affairs.

From Alcoholics Anonymous (AA) World Services. *Twelve steps and twelve traditions.* New York: AA World Services, 1952. The Twelve Steps are reprinted with permission of Alcoholics Anonymous World Services, Inc. (AAWS). Permission to reprint this material does not mean that AAWS has reviewed or approved the contents of this publication or that AAWS agrees with the views expressed herein. AA is a program of recovery from alcoholism only—use of the Twelve Steps in connection with programs and activities that are patterned after AA but that address other problems, or in any other non-AA context, does not imply otherwise.

independence from the patient and reliance on a "higher power." They are usually supportive and nonconfrontational, and some resemble traditional therapy groups more than they do AA meetings.

E. Alcoholics Anonymous

AA is a worldwide fellowship of an estimated 1.6 million recovering alcoholics who are dedicated to helping others recover from alcoholism. The foundation of the program is the Twelve Steps (Table 11.2). The steps help the recovering alcoholic to accept the diagnosis of alcoholism, to make abstinence his or her goal, to develop humility, and to learn reliance on others. The Twelve Steps encourage self-examination, absolve guilt, and promote altruism by helping other persons struggling with their use of **alcohol**.

AA has speaker meetings, discussion meetings, and step meetings. Speaker meetings are often "open" (i.e., nonalcoholics may attend). Small group discussions are "closed," and these provide a forum for a more intimate exchange among recovering people. Special meetings address the needs of the newcomer. Step meetings are also usually closed and structured; each meeting focuses on one of the Twelve Steps. In these sessions, sometimes a chapter is read from the *Twelve Steps and Twelve Traditions* and then the members discuss it; other step meetings may be less structured. In addition to these types of meetings, informal networks develop for socialization, outreach, and spiritual renewal.

New members are encouraged to choose a sponsor, an AA member with long-term abstinence. The roles of the sponsor include staying in close contact with the new member, clarifying the tenets of the AA program, offering practical advice on maintaining abstinence, sharing his or her experiences in early recovery, and being a role model for the newcomer. Sponsorship is also an important therapeutic factor for the sponsor; it keeps the suffering associated with active drinking in view and at the same time affirms the effectiveness of the AA program.

The AA program is one of the most powerful treatment programs for alcoholism, although AA does not view itself as treatment. The steps provide a guide for recovery, and they bear much similarity to the stages of psychotherapy that are often recommended for alcoholic patients. The early steps encourage the confrontation of denial and the admission of loss of control, whereas the later steps encourage self-examination. The goal is to replace dysfunctional defense mechanisms with more mature coping styles.

AA offers much practical advice that the clinician can and should reinforce. Alcoholic patients in early recovery are told to avoid major life changes and new intimate relationships. The plan for recovery is simple—**do not drink, go to meetings**, and **get a sponsor**. AA stresses the role of negative emotional states in provoking relapse. The acronym **HALT** warns members that they should not get **h**ungry, **a**ngry, **l**onely, or **t**ired, because these states are triggers or cues to drinking. As the length of sobriety increases, the focus of the program shifts to character change.

AA is an invaluable resource for both alcoholic patients and treatment programs. Clinicians who treat alcoholic patients should be familiar with AA and the types and locations of meetings in their area. They differ in membership (e.g., educational background, socioeconomic status), dogmatism, and the acceptance of various forms of therapies and in their inclusion of patients with dual diagnoses, especially those who may require treatment with psychotropic medications. Knowledge of the availability of focused AA meetings (e.g., for physicians, women, youth, gays, or lesbians) is also important.

Some clinicians provide their alcoholic patients with a directory of available meetings. These can be obtained by contacting the local AA chapter listed in the telephone directory. The referring clinician should be aware of the difficulty that many patients have with going to their first meeting. In some cases, arranging telephone or personal contact between an active AA member and the patient may be necessary. Recovering physicians are often helpful in arranging such meetings.

F. Alternative Support Groups

Several alternative mutual support groups that reject some of the basic tenets of AA or that integrate other therapies, such as cognitive-behavioral techniques or medication, have developed. The major areas of divergence from AA philosophy are rejection of several key AA beliefs, including the disease concept of alcoholism, the spiritual component of AA, the labeling of participants as "alcoholics," the need to identify with the culture of recovery, and the concept of a person's powerlessness over **alcohol**. Alternative groups may provide opportunities for treatment for individuals who refuse to attend AA because they do not accept the AA philosophy. The clinician must explore with the patient whether the reluctance to attend AA is related to philosophic differences or whether it is instead a reflection of ambivalence about entering treatment. Access to alternative groups may be limited in some areas of the country, and clinicians should become familiar with the more common programs, such as Rational Recovery and Self Management and Recovery Training (SMART), to determine their availability and their compatibility with other therapeutic interventions.

G. Community Reinforcement Approach

The community reinforcement approach (CRA) is a therapeutic approach to alcoholism and drug abuse that uses a variety of techniques to make abstinence more rewarding than drinking. The initial phases of treatment attempt to remove barriers to treatment, such as legal, financial, or other social problems. Treatment may include individual and group psychotherapy, family therapy, social clubs, vocational rehabilitation, housing assistance, or medication. CRA is often linked with contingency contracting to enhance treatment adherence and to decrease drinking directly. Although

CRA programs differ, the basic principle remains the same—environmental reinforcers (e.g., treatment and social services) are available when a person is abstinent but not when he or she is drinking. CRA is often provided by clinical teams that use community outreach, especially for patients with **alcohol** dependence and severe persistent mental illness. Evidence for the efficacy of CRA in alcoholism and drug dependence is well established.

H. Pharmacotherapy for Alcoholism

Pharmacotherapy for abstinent alcoholic patients falls into the following two broad categories: relapse prevention and treatment of psychiatric comorbidity. Drugs for relapse prevention may decrease **alcohol** craving, treat persistent withdrawal symptoms or **alcohol**-induced toxicity, or block alcohol's reinforcing effects. Psychopharmacologic agents are valuable in the treatment of coexisting psychiatric disorders. In the presence of alcoholism, however, psychotropic drugs must be carefully selected. Attention must be paid to abuse liability, overdose risk, toxicity, and any potential for interaction with **alcohol**. In alcoholic patients, monitoring plasma levels may be crucial for evaluating the effectiveness and safety of some drugs, such as tricyclic antidepressants or other oxidatively metabolized drugs. Chronic exposure to **alcohol** may induce some metabolic pathways. The following subsections are guidelines that are intended to enhance the effective and safe use of specific drug classes that may be prescribed to alcoholic patients.

1. **Naltrexone. Naltrexone** is a nonspecific opioid antagonist that has efficacy in the treatment of alcoholism. Agonist effects are minimal, but they may include miosis and dysphoria. In clinical practice, this does not pose limitations to its use. Some patients experience nausea and headaches, especially during the initiation of therapy, but this can be minimized by beginning with a 25 mg per day dose or by delaying drug therapy until the most severe symptoms of **alcohol** withdrawal have passed.

The usual therapeutic dose is 50 mg per day, but some clinicians prescribe higher doses of 150 to 200 mg per day. These higher doses (i.e., those greater than 50 mg) are usually reserved for treatment-resistant cases, and they are mainly used by clinicians with extensive experience in the treatment of alcoholism. Although these higher doses are approved by the United States Food and Drug Administration for the treatment of opioid dependence, the rationale for higher doses in alcoholism derives from animal models that suggest a dose–response relationship to **alcohol** consumption. Craving for **alcohol**, although this has not been studied rigorously, may predict drug response.

Variability in the metabolism of **naltrexone** is observed, with levels of **6-β-naltrexol**, the major metabolite, being approximately 10 times higher than those of **naltrexone** (with great intersubject variability). Oral bioavailability ranges from 5% to 40%. Peak concentrations of **naltrexone** and its major metabolite occur within 1 hour of oral administration. The potency of **6-β-naltrexol** is less than that of **naltrexone** (in animal models, potency ratios of from 1 to 12 to 1 to 53 have been reported), but some preliminary studies in humans suggest that both the efficacy and adverse effects correlate with higher levels of 6-β-naltrexol. Elimination half-lives range from 1 to 10 hours for **naltrexone**, with no accumulation after customary multiple dosing regimens.

Clinical trials in alcoholic patients have produced a consistent profile of adverse effects, with nausea and headache being the most commonly reported. The most serious adverse effect is hepatotoxicity; hepatotoxicity was reported in studies of obesity at doses of 300 mg per day. In fact, a long-term tolerability study indicated that the liver enzymes decline with time in alcoholics who are treated with **naltrexone**. Nevertheless, monitoring of liver function tests is recommended, especially because most alcoholics achieve a reduction in the amount consumed rather than total abstinence. Furthermore, cases of hepatotoxicity in patients taking **naltrexone** do occur, and these require immediate discontinuation of the drug. Other adverse effects include neuroendocrine changes, including increased serum cortisol, luteinizing hormone, and β-endorphin with no change in corticotropin or follicle-stimulating hormone. Some studies have reported an increase in prolactin and testosterone. The clinical significance of these changes is unknown.

Precipitated **opioid withdrawal** is a potential effect of **naltrexone** administration to alcoholic patients who are also using opioids. This can be avoided by obtaining a urine screen, although certain assays may not be sensitive to low opioid levels. The authors recommend that clinicians know the limits of sensitivity of the drug assay screens that they are ordering so that adverse interactions can be avoided. Alternatively, some treatment programs use a **naloxone challenge** when opioid dependence is suspected. This is done before administration of **naltrexone**. For the challenge procedure, **naloxone** is administered either intravenously or subcutaneously. For the intravenous challenge, 0.8 mg of **naloxone** is drawn into the syringe. After the injection of one-fourth of the syringe contents (0.2 mg), the patient is observed for 30 seconds for evidence of precipitated withdrawal. If no symptoms are noted, the remainder is injected and the observation period is extended for another 20 minutes. When symptoms do occur after either step, the patient is considered ineligible for **naltrexone** until he or she is opioid free. The subcutaneous challenge is conducted with the whole 0.8 mg and an observation period of 20 minutes. Usually, when either test method has been "positive" for opioids, a 24-hour interval is imposed before the challenge is repeated.

Patients taking **naltrexone** may not achieve analgesia from typical doses of opioids for as long as 72 hours after the last dose. The duration of opioid antagonism is related to dosage, with the general guideline that 50, 100, and 150 mg produce antagonism for 24, 48, and 72 hours, respectively. Therefore, emergency situations require the use of opioid analgesias with respirator monitoring.

Naltrexone is currently being tested in depot formulations, as is **nalmefene**, another opioid antagonist that may have efficacy in the treatment of **alcohol** dependence. **Nalmefene** (a μ-opioid and κ-opioid antagonist), when administered at 40 mg per day in one clinical study, was more effective in inducing abstinence than was the 10 mg per day dose or the placebo (see Chapter 10).

2. **Acamprosate (calcium acetylhomotaurinate).** This synthetic drug shows structural similarity to γ-aminobutyric acid and taurine. Many clinical trials in Europe and the United States have established its efficacy in the treatment of **alcohol** dependence. It is typically administered in three divided doses totaling 2 to 3 g per day. Titrating the dosage is not necessary. The formulations that have been tested to date are poorly absorbed, with oral bioavailability of approximately 11% and peak concentrations after oral dose occurring at 1 to 2.5 hours. Mean elimination half-life after oral dosing has been reported to be about 33 hours. One should note, however, that the pharmacokinetic properties of the preparation available in the United States are proprietary at the present time. Despite its limited clinical use in the United States, some general clinical principles can be derived from its use abroad. Because the drug is not metabolized and because it is cleared entirely by renal elimination, disturbed hepatic function, with the exception of hepatic failure, should not affect the dosing. Steady-state levels are reached within 5 days. Neither gender nor age appears to affect the elimination unless the renal function is impaired. Data regarding drug interactions are inadequate; however, bioavailability may be decreased when the drug is taken with food. No evidence of an interaction with **alcohol, diazepam, imipramine,** or **disulfiram** has been observed. Common adverse effects include diarrhea and headache. Some patients also report pruritus

and a rash. **Acamprosate** by itself does not affect the electroencephalogram, although it may affect the sleep architecture changes induced by **alcohol**. No sedative effects, abuse, or impairments of psychomotor performance have been reported. The mechanism of action of **acamprosate** is uncertain; however, current research suggests that the drug may normalize glutamate hyperexcitability during withdrawal. A similar mechanism may be responsible for its putative effect in reducing cue-induced craving.

3. **Disulfiram (Antabuse).** This drug may be a useful adjunct in the treatment of chronic alcoholism. When combined with **alcohol**, **disulfiram** causes a reaction that ranges from mild discomfort to a severe reaction consisting of flushing, throbbing in the head, respiratory difficulty, nausea and vomiting, sweating, chest pain, palpitations, dyspnea, hypotension, syncope, vertigo, confusion, and blurred vision. In severe cases, unconsciousness, respiratory arrest, cardiovascular collapse, convulsions, and death can occur.

Either **disulfiram** or its metabolites interferes with the normal metabolism of **alcohol** (Fig. 11.1). Aldehyde dehydrogenase is inhibited, and, as a result, acetaldehyde accumulates and causes many of the symptoms of the **alcohol-disulfiram** reaction. Inhibition of dopamine β-hydroxylase, xanthine oxidase, succinic dehydrogenase, and catalase activity may also account for parts of the syndrome.

Disulfiram is given to the alcoholic patient as a deterrent to further drinking. Once the individual is aware that even small amounts of **alcohol** may precipitate an unpleasant reaction, he or she is less likely to drink impulsively. The decision not to drink is made **once** a day when the pill is taken, instead of each time a craving is experienced. Because the patient is aware that the duration of action of **disulfiram** is as long as 5 to 14 days, he or she must wait before resuming drinking, which further decreases the likelihood of an impulsive drinking binge. **Disulfiram**, when it is ingested as part of a total treatment plan, can be extremely effective in decreasing drinking relapses in some chronic alcoholic patients. Placebo-controlled studies are difficult to conduct with a drug whose effectiveness depends on **anticipated** actions. Even after so many years of use and study, no placebo-controlled studies of **disulfiram** have unequivocally established its efficacy. Nevertheless, for some patients, disulfiram use is worthwhile, especially early in treatment. Studies using the monitored administration of **disulfiram** have generally produced superior results to those that have not used monitors. Thus, many programs suggest that patients who are prescribed **disulfiram** should take their daily doses under the supervision of a monitor, preferably a person who has a strong investment in the patient's abstinence and who is willing to attend some therapy sessions.

Disulfiram use is contraindicated in the presence of severe myocardial disease and certain psychoses. It has the ability to exacerbate schizophrenia, mania, or depressions, possibly as a result of its action on the enzymes involved with catecholamine synthesis and degradation. **Disulfiram** inhibits dopamine β-hydroxylase, the enzyme that converts dopamine to norepinephrine, and low pretreatment levels of this enzyme may be associated with psychotic reactions to the drug. Preexisting differences in the biogenic amine enzyme systems may predispose certain patients to behavioral toxicity.

Before starting any patient on **disulfiram**, the rationale for its use should be fully explained. The patient must be reliable enough for the physician to be assured that **alcohol** has not been consumed during the previous 12 hours. The patient should be warned to avoid **alcohol** in disguised forms, such as sauces, vinegars, cough and cold mixtures, mouthwashes, aftershave lotions, sunscreens, back rubs, or fumes.

Patients should also be told that certain medications, when taken with **alcohol**, may cause a **disulfiram**-like reaction. These include the genitourinary tract antiinfective agent **metronidazole** (Flagyl), some additional antifungal and antibiotic agents (e.g., **chloramphenicol** [Chloromycetin]), and some oral hypoglycemic agents (e.g., **chlorpropamide** [Diabinase], **tolbutamide** [Orinase]).

When patients are well selected and well motivated, socially stable, "obsessively" careful, and not depressed or suicidal and low doses of disulfiram (e.g., 250 mg) are used, severe **alcohol-disulfiram** reactions will be minimized. If they occur, supportive measures to restore blood pressure and treatment of any signs or symptoms of shock should be initiated. One gram of **vitamin C** (as ascorbic acid) administered intravenously may act as an antioxidant and may reduce acetaldehyde production, thereby promoting the excretion of unmetabolized **alcohol**. Intravenous **ephedrine sulfate** and antihistamines (e.g., **diphenhydramine**, 25 to 50 mg) may also be administered, although the rationale for this is not well-established. The potassium levels should be monitored because hypokalemia sometimes occurs.

Side effects from **disulfiram** are usually minor; they include a garlic or metallic aftertaste during the first few weeks of therapy, dermatitis, headache, drowsiness, and impotence. More serious adverse reactions include hepatotoxicity, optic neuritis, peripheral neuropathy, and polyneuritis. Liver function tests should be monitored for several weeks after **disulfiram** is started. **Disulfiram** may inhibit the metabolism of concomitantly administered oxidatively metabolized medications.

4. **Ondansetron.** This drug, which is a 5-HT$_3$ receptor antagonist, may reduce drinking in early-onset alcoholic patients; however, additional studies are required.

5. **Antianxiety (sedative-hypnotic) agents.** Benzodiazepines are clearly useful and effective for treating the **alcohol** abstinence syndrome (see Chapter 12). Less clear, however, is their role in chronic alcoholism. A growing body of evidence seems to suggest that many types of anxiety antedate the onset of alcoholism. From these observations, one can infer that symptomatic anxiety may have etiologic significance in **alcohol** abuse and dependence. Once **alcohol**-induced withdrawal anxiety has been ruled out, anxiolytics may be prescribed. In general, agents with a lower abuse potential should be used first. β-Adrenergic receptor antagonists or **buspirone** can be good first choices. However, their efficacy in panic disorder and some forms of social phobia may be limited or inconsistent.

The benzodiazepines have considerable abuse liability for alcoholics, but some patients may nevertheless benefit from them. Among the benzodiazepines, a spectrum of abuse potential exists. Those agents with a rapid onset of euphoric effect and a short duration of action may present the greatest risk. **Diazepam** and **alprazolam**, for example, may produce a rapid initial euphoric effect and may increase the craving for **alcohol** in abstinent alcoholics. **Chlordiazepoxide** and **oxazepam**, as benzodiazepines that have a slower onset of action and less intense initial subjective effects, may present a lower risk for abuse. No matter which benzodiazepine is chosen, only single-source dispensing of limited supplies should be permitted, and frequent patient contact is essential.

Antidepressants may also be of value in some forms of anxiety. However, the clinician must remember that, in the alcoholic patient, an overdose with a tricyclic antidepressant or even with other antidepressants, such as **bupropion**, which may lower seizure threshold, may lead to serious morbidity or death. Monoamine oxidase inhibitors, selective serotonin reuptake inhibitors (e.g., **fluoxetine**, **sertraline**, **paroxetine**, **citalopram**), and mixed-action agents (e.g., **venlafaxine**) may be helpful when anxiety, phobic symptoms (e.g., social phobia), and panic attacks accompany a depressed or dysphoric mood. Monoamine oxidase inhibitors should be used cautiously and only by physicians who are experienced in their use. Sedating antidepressants, such as **mirtazapine, nefazodone,** or **doxepin,** are also commonly prescribed for these patients.

6. **Antidepressants.** Depression in alcoholic patients is a serious problem requiring vigorous treatment. Although many alcoholic patients undergo a time-limited withdrawal depression lasting 2 to 3 weeks, some depression may persist. In a small proportion of patients, depression that lasts may represent persistent withdrawal-related depression. More likely, however, enduring depressive symptoms indicate the presence of a major depression, they are the consequence of chronic residual effects of **alcohol** on the brain, or they are a reflection of the psychologic and social disruptions caused by alcoholism (e.g., loss of relationships, jobs, or self-esteem; demoralization). Suicide is a serious problem, with 6% to 21% of alcoholic patients committing suicide, compared with an estimated 1% of the general population (see Chapter 17).

The authors' practice is to observe a depressed alcoholic patient without an established diagnosis of major depression for 3 weeks after the discontinuation of **alcohol.** When the patient's depressive symptoms persist, an antidepressant is started. In patients showing a clinical picture consistent with major depressive disorder that antedates the onset of alcoholism or that was present in periods of prolonged abstinence, an antidepressant may be started sooner than 3 weeks. No specific antidepressant has been shown to be superior in the treatment of depression in alcoholics, although serotonergic agents, such as selective serotonin reuptake inhibitors, are often tried first because some studies suggest that they may decrease **alcohol** consumption in problem drinkers and that they may increase the days of abstinence.

7. **Lithium.** Although some evidence has suggested that **lithium** use may reduce relapse in alcoholics and may block the euphoric effects of **alcohol,** this use of **lithium** has not gained wide clinical acceptance for this population. **Lithium** is most often prescribed for alcoholic patients with bipolar disorder, major depression, or a family history of mood disorder and for highly impulsive episodic drinkers. It is also occasionally used to treat patients with impulsive angry outbursts. **Carbamazepine, oxcarbazine, or valproate** may also be useful in certain impulsive alcoholic patients (see also Chapter 13).

8. **Antipsychotic agents.** These agents offer an advantage over benzodiazepines for the relief of agitation and anxiety in some patients because they have little intrinsic abuse potential. This potential benefit must be weighed against the risk of tardive dyskinesia from conventional antipsychotic agents (e.g., **chlorpromazine**) and the discomfort from other side effects. Studies that compared the two classes of drugs and that found several of the conventional antipsychotic agents to be superior have used low doses of benzodiazepines, thus obscuring findings due to problems of cross-tolerance (i.e., benzodiazepines are cross-tolerant with **alcohol**; antipsychotic agents are not).

The authors do not recommend the use of conventional antipsychotic agents for alcoholic patients unless the patient has an accompanying psychiatric illness for which this class is more clearly indicated (e.g., in a patient with schizophrenia who has a concomitant **alcohol** problem). Even in these cases, atypical antipsychotic agents are preferred over conventional agents. **Clozapine,** for example, may reduce **alcohol** consumption in patients with schizophrenia and schizoaffective disorder. Similarly, **tiapride,** a dopamine-2 (D_2) receptor antagonist, is used in the treatment of **alcohol** withdrawal and relapse prevention in Europe.

III. Comment

Outcome results are influenced by a variety of factors, including motivation to stop drinking, amount and duration of **alcohol** use, and availability of treatment resources and personal supports. The highest recovery rates (approximating 75%) are found in those who acknowledge their drinking problem and have adequate financial and emotional (e.g., family) support.

ADDITIONAL READING

Agarwal DP, Goedde HW. *Alcohol metabolism, alcohol intolerance, and alcoholism.* Berlin: Springer-Verlag, 1990.

Bandura A. *Social learning theory.* Englewood Cliffs, NJ: Prentice Hall, 1977.

Brewer C, Meyers RJ, Johnsen J. Does disulfiram help to prevent relapse in alcohol abuse? *CNS Drugs* 2000;14:329–341.

Ciraulo DA, Nace EP. Benzodiazepine treatment of anxiety or insomnia in substance abuse patients. *Am J Addict* 2000;9:276–284.

Ciraulo DA, Shader RI, eds. *Clinical manual of chemical dependence.* Washington, D.C.: American Psychiatric Press, 1991.

DiClemente CC, Prochaska JO. Self-change and therapy changes of smoking behavior: a comparison of processes of change in cessation and maintenance. *Addictive Behaviors* 1982;7:133–142.

Enomoto N, Takase S, Yasuhara M, et al. Acetaldehyde metabolism in different aldehyde dehydrogenase-2 genotypes. *Alcohol Clin Exp Res* 1991;15:141–144.

Heath AC, Bucholz KK, Madden PA, et al. Genetic and environmental contributions to alcohol dependence risk in a national twin sample: consistency of findings in women and men. *Psychol Med* 1997;27:1381–1396.

Heinälä P, Alho H, Kiianmaa K, et al. Targeted use of naltrexone without prior detoxification in the treatment of alcohol dependence: a factorial double-blind, placebo-controlled trial. *J Clin Psychopharmacol* 2001;21:287–292.

Kranzler HR. Pharmacotherapy of alcoholism: gaps in knowledge and opportunities for research. *Alcohol Alcoholism* 2000;35:537–547.

Kranzler HR, Tennen H, Penta C, Bohn MJ. Targeted naltrexone treatment of early problem drinkers. *Addictive Behaviors* 1997;22:431–436.

Kranzler HR, Van Kirk J. Efficacy of naltrexone and acomprosate for alcoholism treatment: a meta-analysis. *Alcohol Clin Exp Res* 2001;25:1335–1341.

Larimer ME, Palmer RS, Marlatt GA. Relapse prevention. An overview of Marlatt's cognitive-behavioral model. *Alcohol Res Health* 1999;23:151–160.

Marlatt GA, Gordon JR, eds. *Relapse prevention.* New York: Guilford Press, 1985.

Mason BJ, Ownby RL. Acamprosate for the treatment of alcohol dependence: a review of double-blind, placebo-controlled trials. *CNS Spectrums* 2000;5:58–69.

Mendelson JH, Mello NK, eds. *The diagnosis and treatment of alcoholism,* 3rd ed. New York: McGraw-Hill, 1992.

Miller WR. COMBINE Behavioral Intervention (NIAAA, unpublished).

Miller WR, ed. *Combined behavioral intervention; therapist manual.* Bethseda, MD: National Institute on Alcohol Abuse and Alcoholism (*in press*).

Miller WR, Meyers RJ, Hiller-Sturmhofel S. The community-reinforcement approach. *Alcohol Res Health* 1999;23:116–121.

Miller WR, Rollnick S, eds. *Motivational interviewing: preparing people to change addictive behavior.* New York: Guilford Press, 1992.

Morse RM, Flavin DK. The definition of alcoholism. *JAMA* 1992;268:1012–1014.

Nutt D. Alcohol and the brain. Pharmacological insights for psychiatrists. *Br J Psychiatry* 1999;175:114–119.

Project MATCH Series. *Twelve step facilitation therapy manual.* Vol. 1. NIH Publ. No. 94-3722, 1995; *Motivational enhancement therapy manual.* Vol. 2. NIH Publ. No. 94-3723, 1994; *Cognitive-behavioral coping skills therapy manual.* Vol. 3. NIH Publ. No. 94–3724, 1995. Washington, D.C.: National Institutes of Health.

Slutske WS, Heath AC, Madden PA, et al. Personality and the genetic risk for alcohol dependence. *J Abnorm Psychol* 2002;111:124–133.

Spanagel R, Zieglgansberger W. Anti-craving compounds for ethanol: new pharmacological tools to study addictive processes. *Trends Pharmacol Sci* 1997;18:54–58.

Swift RM. Drug therapy for alcohol dependence. *N Engl J Med* 1999;340:1482–1490.

Thome J, Gerwitz JC, Weijers HG. Genome polymorphism and alcoholism. *Pharmacogenomics* 2000;1:63–71.

Tiffany ST, Conkin CA. A cognitive processing model of alcohol craving and compulsive alcohol use. *Addiction* 2000;95:S145–S153.

Vaillant GE. *The natural history of alcoholism.* Cambridge, MA: Harvard University Press, 1983.

12. TREATMENT OF ALCOHOL WITHDRAWAL

Richard Saitz
Domenic A. Ciraulo
Richard I. Shader
Ann Marie Ciraulo

Most withdrawal syndromes develop in chronic alcoholic patients who stop drinking or who reduce their intake for whatever reason. However, the development of withdrawal symptoms is possible in any person with any pattern of regular **alcohol** consumption who ceases drinking or who reduces the level of intake. Clinicians must remember that some patients conceal their use of **alcohol**. Unanticipated **alcohol** withdrawal is a not infrequent complication in the care of patients admitted to the hospital for various urgent or elective reasons.

I. **Signs and Symptoms of Alcohol Withdrawal**

Manifestations of **alcohol** withdrawal typically are divided into the following two varieties: the mild symptoms and signs that tend to occur early in the course of withdrawal and the more severe symptoms, or complications. Some clinicians think that mild manifestations, if untreated, progress to severe ones and that severe manifestations are invariably preceded by milder ones. However, evidence suggests that these relationships are by no means invariable. Physicians who approach all patients expecting this progression of symptoms may make unnecessary errors. Although delirium (see Chapter 5) is often preceded by progressive adrenergic symptoms, most cases of **alcohol** withdrawal, even those that manifest with mild symptoms, do not progress to **alcohol** withdrawal delirium, even without treatment. Treatment can, however, ameliorate the symptoms and can prevent complications of **alcohol** withdrawal.

A. **Mild or Early Symptoms**

These can begin any time between a few hours and 10 days after the last drink. Typically, they appear 6 to 48 hours after the cessation of **alcohol** ingestion. They can be suppressed by continued drinking. Possible manifestations are listed in Table 12.1. Many are not specific to withdrawal, and they should raise concern for coexisting **alcohol**-related illnesses (e.g., gastritis when abdominal discomfort is prominent; hypophosphatemia, hypocalcemia, or hypokalemia with muscle weakness or cramping). The severity of these symptoms can be quantified with simple-to-use standardized scale, the Clinical Institute Withdrawal Assessment for Alcohol, revised (CIWA-Ar). Scores are useful when communicating with nurses and other physicians caring for the patient, for assessing worsening and improvement, and for helping with decisions regarding medication (Table 12.2). Scores of 8 to 10 or greater usually require treatment with medication, and higher scores represent a risk for severe withdrawal. Although most of the early symptoms are mild, noting that some of the most troubling and significant symptoms, convulsions and hallucinations, can occur in the first 24 to 48 hours is important. *Both seizure and hallucinosis can occur without being preceded by mild withdrawal symptoms.*

B. **Severe Manifestations or Complications**

As was previously mentioned, although some withdrawing alcoholic patients have mild or early symptoms before progressing to more advanced or more severe manifestations, others may start with severe symptoms (Table 12.3). Advanced or severe symptoms typically begin 48 to 96 hours after the cessation of drinking. **Delirium tremens (DTs)** is the classic term that is used to describe the most advanced or severe toxic state. Unfortunately, this term is exceedingly vague, and it conveys numerous nondiagnostic implications, as does the term **rum fits**. Because of the limitations of the currently popular

TABLE 12.1. MILD OR EARLY SYMPTOMS OF ALCOHOL WITHDRAWAL

Gastrointestinal symptoms
  Anorexia
  Nausea
  Vomiting
  Abdominal discomfort
  Diarrhea

Sleep disturbances
  Insomnia
  Nightmares

Autonomic nervous system hyperactivity
  Tachycardia
  Systolic hypertension
  Diaphoresis
  Tremor

Behavioral changes
  Anxiety
  Irritability
  Agitation

Neurologic consequences
  Difficulty concentrating
  Easy distractibility
  Memory impairment
  Impaired judgment
  Seizures
  Hallucinosis

terminology, the diagnosis must be approached with caution and an open mind. **Alcohol** withdrawal delirium is characterized by confusion and disorientation, as well as by hyperautonomia. It is often preceded by mild symptoms of withdrawal and progressive tachycardia, diaphoresis, and tremor. Alcoholic hallucinosis occurs with an otherwise clear sensorium. Prodromal manifestations can be subtle; slight irritability or intransigence in the patient's demeanor may be the only clues. In some patients, severe tremulousness and auditory hallucinosis can develop without progression to delirium or panic. In others, a grand mal seizure may be the very first manifestation of withdrawal. The differential diagnosis of withdrawal seizures includes head trauma, metabolic disturbances, infection (e.g., meningitis), and other causes of seizures. Untreated or inadequately treated withdrawal can be fatal. The current mortality rate attributed to DTs is about 1%.

C. **Predictors of Alcohol Withdrawal Delirium**

The **alcohol** withdrawal (abstinence) syndrome must be understood as a heterogeneous clinical concept with numerous possible combinations of signs, symptoms, and time courses; terms such as impending DTs should be used only when the aspects of the disease process to which they refer are clearly understood. Given the individual variability in timing and duration of **alcohol** consumption, the varied amounts and concentrations of **alcohol** in the beverages consumed, and the amount of food eaten with or between drinks, predicting those at high risk for withdrawal seems chancy. Nevertheless, one recent study noted that withdrawal delirium occurred, despite benzodiazepine treatment, only in patients who had the following five risk factors: evidence of a current infection, heart rate above 120 beats per min, the presence of signs of withdrawal when **alcohol** blood levels were above 100 mg per dL, previous seizures by history, and previous episodes of delirium. Other

TABLE 12.2. THE CLINICAL INSTITUTE WITHDRAWAL ASSESSMENT SCALE FOR ALCOHOL, REVISED[a]

Nausea and vomiting—Ask "Do you feel sick to your stomach? Have you vomited?"
Observation:

0 = no nausea with no vomiting
1
2
3
4 = intermittent nausea with dry heaves
5
6
7 = constant nausea, frequent dry heaves and vomiting

Tremor—Arms extended and fingers spread apart.
Observation:

0 = no tremor
1 = not visible, but can be felt fingertip to fingertip
2
3
4 = moderate, with patient's arms extended
5
6
7 = severe, even with arms not extended

Paroxysmal sweats
Observation:

0 = no sweats visible
1 = barely perceptible sweating, moist palms
2
3
4 = beads of sweat obvious on forehead
5
6
7 = drenching sweats

Visual disturbances—Ask "Does the light appear to be too bright? Is its color different? Does it hurt your eyes? Are you seeing anything that is disturbing to you? Are you seeing things you know are not there?"
Observation:

0 = not present
1 = very mild sensitivity
2 = mild sensitivity
3 = moderate sensitivity
4 = moderately severe hallucinations
5 = severe hallucinations
6 = extremely severe hallucinations
7 = continuous hallucinations

Agitation
Observation:

0 = normal activity
1 = somewhat more than normal activity
2
3

(continued)

TABLE 12.2. (*Continued*)

	4 = moderately fidgety and restless 5 6 7 = paces back and forth during most of the interview or constantly thrashes about
Tactile disturbances—Ask "Have you any itching, pins and needles sensations, any burning, or any numbness, or do you feel bugs crawling on or under your skin?" Observation:	0 = none 1 = very mild itching, pins and needles, burning or numbness 2 = mild itching, pins and needles, burning or numbness 3 = moderate itching, pins and needles, burning or numbness 4 = moderately severe hallucinations 5 = severe hallucinations 6 = extremely severe hallucinations 7 = continuous hallucinations
Headache, fullness in head—Ask "Does your head feel different? Does it feel like there is a band around your head?" Do not rate for dizziness or lightheadedness. Otherwise rate severity:	0 = not present 1 = very mild 2 = mild 3 = mildly severe 4 = moderately severe 5 = severe 6 = very severe 7 = extremely severe
Auditory disturbances—Ask "Are you more aware of sounds around you? Are they harsh? Do they frighten you? Are you hearing anything that is disturbing to you? Are you hearing things you know are not there?" Observation:	0 = not present 1 = very mild harshness or ability to frighten 2 = mild harshness or ability to frighten 3 = moderate harshness or ability to frighten 4 = moderately severe hallucinations 5 = severe hallucinations 6 = extremely severe hallucinations 7 = continuous hallucinations
Anxiety—Ask "Do you feel nervous?" Observation:	0 = no anxiety, at ease 1 = mildly anxious 2 3

TABLE 12.2. (*Continued*)

	4 = moderately anxious or guarded, so anxiety is inferred
	5
	6
	7 = equivalent to acute panic states, such as those seen in severe delirium or acute schizophrenic reactions
Orientation and clouding of sensorium—Ask "What day is this? Where are you? Who am I?"	0 = oriented and can do serial additions
	1 = cannot do serial additions
	2 = disoriented for date by no more than 2 calendar days
	3 = disoriented for date by more than 2 calendar days
	4 = disoriented for place and/or person

aAlso known as CIWA-Ar.
Total score is a simple sum of each item score (maximum score = 67).
From Sullivan JT, Sykora K, Schneiderman J, et al. Assessment of alcohol withdrawal: the revised Clinical Institute Withdrawal Assessment for Alcohol scale (CIWA-Ar). *Br J Addict* 1989;84:1353, with permission. The scale is not copyrighted and may be used freely.

studies have shown that the number of prior episodes of withdrawal delirium correlates positively with the intensity of symptoms in subsequent episodes of withdrawal delirium.

II. Criteria for Hospitalization

Abstinent alcoholic patients usually present at acute treatment facilities (emergency departments) of general or psychiatric hospitals with some symptoms already apparent. Admitting physicians must recognize which patients require hospitalization and must treat the least ill patients on an outpatient basis. Because of the unpredictable natural history of the withdrawal syndrome, this is not always an easy choice; errors in judgment are made in both directions. Outpatient detoxification has gained wider acceptance in recent years, as it offers substantial cost savings. For patients with mild to moderate withdrawal and no concurrent active medical or psychiatric conditions, outpatient withdrawal may be as effective as inpatient treatment as long as a significant other is available to assess the patient and daily contact with the health care provider is feasible. Table 12.4 lists criteria for hospitalizing the withdrawing alcoholic patient. Guidelines for treatment of those who are not hospitalized are given in Table 12.5.

III. Hospital Treatment of Alcohol Withdrawal

All newly hospitalized abstinent alcoholic patients should receive the following minimum evaluation: (a) history (from patient, available family and friends, and any previous hospital records); (b) physical examination; and (c) venous blood samples for determinations of the complete blood count with differential; international normalized ratio (INR); blood urea nitrogen; glucose, sodium, potassium, chloride, and bicarbonate levels; serum calcium, magnesium, phosphate, and liver enzymes; bilirubin; and albumin. Measurement of amylase is often indicated when abdominal pain is present. A urine or serum toxic screen for other drugs of abuse is essential because intoxication with some drugs may mimic **alcohol** intoxication or may alter the signs, symptoms, or course of **alcohol** withdrawal. Concurrent abuse of long-acting benzodiazepines, for example, may delay the onset of withdrawal symptoms or DTs. Further workup is dictated by the clinical situation. For example, a chest x-ray is indicated when pulmonary symptoms are present or after a seizure; because withdrawal can

TABLE 12.3. LATER OR MORE SEVERE COMPLICATIONS OF ALCOHOL WITHDRAWAL

Worsening of mild symptoms
  Tremor
  Diaphoresis
  Tachycardia
  Hypertension
  Agitation

Delirium
  Usually preceded and accompanied by progressive autonomic symptoms
    (e.g., those above) and fever
  Occurs 48 to 72 h after onset of withdrawal
  Usually lasts 2 to 3 d
  Disorientation, clouded sensorium
  Frequent fluctuation of symptoms, signs, and severity
  Impaired cognition

Hallucinations
  Can occur with a clear sensorium
  Visual, tactile, or auditory
  Can be threatening

Delusions
  Usually paranoid
  Merge with or are reinforced by hallucinations
  Can cause agitation and terror

Seizures
  Often occur without warning and without prior autonomic symptoms, hallucinations,
    or delirium
  Usually generalized, not focal
  May have focal or lateralizing start, though this should raise suspicion for intracranial
    lesion
  No prior seizure disorder necessary
  Usually single and self-limited; additional seizures rarely occur 6 h after the first
  Occur within 48 h
  Status epilepticus can occur

precipitate angina or arrhythmia, an electrocardiogram (ECG) should be conducted for those at the age of 40 years and over or when symptoms or risk factors for heart disease are present. Urinalysis is indicated when electrolytes reveal an acid-base disturbance or renal insufficiency; computed tomography of the brain is indicated when the focal neurologic signs of brain injury are present, particularly with signs of head trauma. Examination of the cerebrospinal fluid is warranted when meningeal signs or fever and confusion are present. The following sections detail the fundamental elements of the medical treatment plan.

A. Vitamin Use

Vitamin deficiencies, either clinical or subclinical, exist in many, if not all, chronic alcoholic patients. Because administration of appropriate amounts of water-soluble vitamin supplements carries no hazard, all patients should receive them whether or not clinical manifestations are present.

1. **Assessment and testing**
   a. **Neurologic examination** will reveal signs of Wernicke encephalopathy when it is present; these include nystagmus, internuclear ophthalmoplegia, cerebellar ataxia, and a characteristic pattern of intellectual deterioration. Immediate administration of **thiamine**

TABLE 12.4. CRITERIA FOR HOSPITALIZATION OF THE WITHDRAWING ALCOHOLIC

Severe tremulousness, other autonomic symptoms, or hallucinosis
Significant volume depletion, acid-base or electrolyte disturbance
Fever and delirium or seizure
Fever above 38.1°C (100.5°F)
First seizure ever or seizure without prior evaluation
Delirium
Prior alcohol withdrawal delirium
Wernicke encephalopathy (e.g., ataxia, nystagmus, internuclear ophthalmoplegia)
Head trauma with loss of consciousness
Failure to respond to initial outpatient treatment
Presence of significant comorbidity requiring hospitalization
    Decompensated liver disease
    Respiratory compromise or failure
    Pneumonia
    Gastrointestinal bleeding
    Pancreatitis
    Severe malnutrition
    Angina
    Multiple seizures, particularly with incomplete recovery
    Unstable psychiatric illness, such as severe depression, suicide risk, active
      schizophrenia or bipolar disorder
Need for pharmacologic management with inability to take appropriately as an outpatient
    No responsible other person available to help with medication
    No health care services available to manage as outpatient

Pharmacologic management is indicated for significant symptoms (i.e., Clinical Institute Withdrawal Assessment Scale for Alcohol, revised [CIWA-Ar] score > 8–10), prior or current seizure during withdrawal, prior or current delirium or hallucinosis, coexisting acute medical or psychiatric disorder, or preoperative prophylaxis. Significant symptoms of withdrawal (and therefore need of medication) are unlikely when symptoms have not developed after 36 h of abstinence or when dependence duration is 6 or fewer yr. **While not absolutely required, hospitalization should be strongly considered for the elderly and for those withdrawing with a blood alcohol level of 150 mg/dL or greater.**

TABLE 12.5. OUTPATIENT MANAGEMENT OF MILD ALCOHOL WITHDRAWAL

History, physical, and laboratory evaluation to look for indications for hospitalization and
    cooccurring disorders
Intramuscular thiamine, 100 mg, followed by daily multivitamin; folate, 1 mg, and
    thiamine p.o.
Initial dose of benzodiazepine (chlordiazepoxide [50–100 mg p.o.] or lorazepam
    [1–2 mg, any route])
Observation for 1–2 h for signs of symptom relief
Provide a 1-d supply of benzodiazepine to be used for symptoms or on a regular basis
    (e.g., 4–8 doses)
Explanation of instructions to reliable, responsible, caring adult family member or friend
Daily contact with health care provider
Linkage to outpatient alcoholism treatment, primary medical care, and psychiatric care
    as needed

mononitrate (vitamin B_1) can prevent irreversible brain damage. All patients should receive **thiamine** (see section III.A.2.a), even when Wernicke encephalopathy is not detected.

b. The **megaloblastic anemia** characteristic of folic acid deficiency is revealed by complete blood count, determination of serum or red blood cell folate levels, study of the peripheral blood smear, and bone marrow aspiration when indicated.

c. Elevated INR, in the absence of cirrhosis or other causes of hepatic insufficiency, suggests **vitamin K** deficiency.

d. **Signs and symptoms of other deficiency states**, such as hypovitaminosis C or scurvy (corkscrew hairs, perifollicular hemorrhages, gingival hemorrhage), are not infrequently encountered. Fractures and osteopenia can be seen in vitamin D deficiency, which is not uncommon in alcoholic patients. The diagnosis is made with a serum 25-hydroxy-vitamin D level.

2. Treatment

a. **All patients should receive thiamine**. An initial dose of 100 to 200 mg intramuscularly (i.m.) or intravenously (i.v.) should be given immediately, before the administration of any glucose-containing solutions. This amount is repeated, parenterally or orally, for at least the next 3 consecutive days. (*Note:* Oral multivitamin preparations usually contain only 5 mg of **thiamine**.)

b. **All patients should receive folic acid**, 1 mg per day i.m. or orally, until normal indexes are obtained.

c. **All patients should receive a daily multivitamin supplement**. Tablets containing thiamine or an equivalent may be given once oral intake is tolerated. Typical oral multivitamin preparations contain minimum amounts of B vitamins (e.g., **cyanocobalamin** [B_{12}], **niacinamide, pyridoxine** [B_6], and **riboflavin** [B_2]) and **vitamin C** as ascorbic acid (75 to 100 mg). The latter amount should be adequate to treat scurvy. Various parenteral multivitamins are also available. If pellagra is suspected, ensure that the patient has an adequate intake of **niacin** (100 to 200 mg per day).

d. **If the INR is elevated, vitamin K**, 5 to 10 mg, is given subcutaneously; this is repeated at least once because this route may be less effective than oral or i.v. dosing. Intravenous vitamin K, 1 mg, may be given slowly in the case of an urgent need (e.g., bleeding) to correct the INR. Intravenous dosing is rarely associated with anaphylaxis. Oral vitamin K, 5 mg, may be used; this is effective if malabsorption does not occur. Larger doses are of no additional benefit, although, if the INR decreases, repeat dosing is advisable. Failure of this dose to normalize or shorten the prothrombin time over the course of the next 8 hours to 3 days suggests that significant hepatic disease may be present.

e. **When serum 25-hydroxy-vitamin D is low**, replenish this with the administration of 50,000 IU of vitamin D weekly for 1 month, followed by a daily multivitamin containing a standard 400 IU of vitamin D.

3. Hazards from short-term vitamin treatment are essentially nonexistent.

B. Sedation

More than ample evidence suggests that the administration of sedative-hypnotics to abstinent alcoholic patients during withdrawal makes the subjective experience less unpleasant and decreases the morbidity of the withdrawal syndrome. However, in nonmedical settings, alcoholic patients in mild withdrawal are often cared for without sedative-hypnotics. These programs are safe and effective, as long as patients do not have medical or psychiatric illnesses or a history of DTs or seizures (complicated withdrawals). Generally, treatment with sedative-hypnotics is most beneficial when it is begun as early as possible. Alcoholic patients with moderate to severe withdrawal symptoms should receive sedative-hypnotics, as should patients at high risk of complicated withdrawal or those who would tolerate complications poorly (e.g., past seizure, concurrent acute medical or psychiatric illness, heart disease). These drugs, however, must be used with caution when cirrhosis and its complications or significant hepatic synthetic dysfunction (e.g., elevated INR, depressed serum albumin) are present. (*Note:* γ-Aminobutyric acid A agonists [e.g., benzodiazepines] have been known to aggravate hepatic encephalopathy.)

1. **Assessment**. Therapy must be carefully titrated and individualized; fixed regimens alone cannot be considered rational. Larger doses of sedative-hypnotics and more frequent monitoring are needed when the symptoms are severe than when they are mild. The dosage and frequency of administration should be adjusted and titrated so that symptoms are suppressed; a state of light sleepiness is usually desirable. When therapy is inadequate, the symptoms continue, whereas excessive treatment may produce respiratory depression, obtundation, or coma. Achieving the desired therapeutic effect, which is between the two extremes, is not always easy. One way to individualize the treatment is by using a standardized scale, the CIWA-Ar (Table 12.2; see section I.A), to monitor withdrawal.

2. **Treatment**. A number of sedative-hypnotics has been successfully used in treating **alcohol** withdrawal. Each has its benefits and hazards. With whatever drug is chosen, the suggested dosage (Table 12.6) should be given every 1 to 2 hours until adequate sedation is achieved. An alternative strategy is to dose the patient every 6 hours, while providing additional medication when needed between the doses and tapering the regular dose over several days. Initial parenteral therapy is sometimes necessary. Once the symptoms are suppressed, the doses may be reduced in size and the time between them may be lengthened; any further sedative-hypnotic use should occur on an as-needed basis, taking into account the pharmacokinetic properties of the chosen drug.

   Although, in general, only symptomatic patients (i.e., CIWA-Ar score of 8 to 10 or greater, seizures or delirium) should receive sedative-hypnotic treatment, those at a high risk for complications as noted above (Tables 12.4 and 12.6) should be treated with at least one dose, even in the absence of symptoms, to prevent the progression of the withdrawal syndrome.

   Some clinicians recommend the use of a loading procedure. For example, a long half-life benzodiazepine (e.g., **diazepam** [20 mg] or **chlordiazepoxide** [100 mg]) is administered every 1 to 2 hours until mild sedation occurs. Typically, at least three doses (cumulative loading dose of 60 mg of **diazepam** or 300 mg of **chlordiazepoxide**) are given under close medical supervision. Proponents of this approach assert that once sedation is achieved, additional doses are rarely necessary. Shorter-acting drugs may be used as long as they are carefully tapered once symptom control is achieved. Rapid or no tapering has been associated with the occurrence of seizures during withdrawal.

   a. **Benzodiazepines**. Benzodiazepines remain the drugs of choice for the treatment of **alcohol** withdrawal (Table 12.6). They are safe and effective, and they produce minimal or infrequent cardiovascular or respiratory depression. They are the only drugs that have been proven to prevent seizures and delirium in clinical trials.

   The pharmacokinetic characteristics of different benzodiazepines influence drug therapy. The longer-acting agents most frequently used to treat withdrawal are **diazepam** and **chlordiazepoxide**, although any longer-acting benzodiazepine would be effective. The longer-acting agents have the advantage of being somewhat self-tapering because of their own long-acting active metabolites. This can be a disadvantage, however, when drug metabolism is slowed (e.g., in the elderly or in patients with cirrhosis). The shorter-acting agents, which in-

TABLE 12.6. RECOMMENDED REGIMENS FOR THE MANAGEMENT OF ALCOHOL WITHDRAWAL

Dosing

Fixed (or regular) schedule dosing: administer drug q.i.d., taper by 50% each d for 2–3 d, and then stop. Reassess frequently and give additional medication as needed (i.e., when Clinical Institute Withdrawal Assessment Scale for Alcohol, revised [CIWA-Ar] score ≥ 8–10).

Symptom-triggered (front-loading) dosing: administer medication every 1–2 h as needed (i.e., when CIWA-Ar ≥ 8–10). When no symptoms are present, provide one dose of sedative (see text).

Available agents

Drug	Dosage	Comments
Benzodiazepines		
Long acting		
Chlordiazepoxide	50–100 mg p.o.	Many active metabolites provide smooth taper; metabolism prolonged in elderly or those with hepatic synthetic dysfunction; avoid i.m. route due to erratic absorption
Diazepam	10–20 mg p.o., 5 mg i.v.	Less desirable for outpatients because of initial euphoria. i.v. dose should be used every 5 min for delirium; metabolic issues same as for chlordiazepoxide
Short acting		Initial dosing same as for other sedatives listed, but important to taper administration of a regularly scheduled dose (e.g., q.i.d.) over 2–3 d to avoid late withdrawal; choose when significant hepatic synthetic dysfunction or tenuous respiratory function is present
Lorazepam	1–2 mg p.o., i.v., i.m., s.l.	
Oxazepam	30–60 mg p.o.	No parenteral forms available
Barbiturates		
Phenobarbital	100–200 mg p.o.	No randomized trial evidence for efficacy; long acting; induces hepatic microsomal enzymes; narrow toxic-therapeutic index (respiratory depression), which makes this option less desirable

Abbreviations: i.m., intramuscular; i.v., intravascular; p.o., orally; q.i.d., four times a day; s.l., sublingual.

clude **lorazepam** and **oxazepam**, are metabolized directly to their glucuronide conjugates, which are water soluble and which are eliminated by the kidney. The metabolism of **lorazepam** and **oxazepam** is not influenced by cirrhosis or aging. However, they usually require multiple doses over a 24-hour period, and they must be tapered more carefully than **diazepam** or **chlordiazepoxide**. Other shorter-acting benzodiazepines may also be used, and recent experience suggests that the use of **midazolam**, given i.v., may be effective in severe **alcohol** withdrawal, though it offers no advantage over **diazepam** or **lorazepam**. For **alcohol** withdrawal seizures, one dose of a benzodiazepine, preferably **lorazepam**, should be administered regardless of symptoms. For agitated **alcohol** withdrawal delirium, i.v. **lorazepam** or **diazepam** should be given every 5 minutes until a calm, but awake, state is achieved. Continuous monitoring of vital signs, oxygen saturation, and the ECG are essential. Restraints (on the patient's side or prone with the head of the bed elevated to avoid aspiration) may be necessary for patient safety (see Chapter 26).

Benzodiazepine receptor antagonists have also been used to reverse the effects of **alcohol** in overdose, both with and without concomitant benzodiazepine ingestion. **Flumazenil** is commonly used for this purpose. Although results with **flumazenil** (0.1 to 0.2 mg per kg i.v.) in normal volunteers who are intoxicated solely with **alcohol** have not been promising, positive outcomes have been observed in actual emergency department use, especially when sedative-hypnotics have also been ingested. The use of **flumazenil** may transiently increase the risk of seizures, especially in the withdrawing patient or in the patient receiving concomitant antidepressant therapy with **imipramine** or **bupropion**, for example.

b. **β-Adrenergic receptor antagonists (beta-blockers)**. Both **propranolol**, 10 to 40 mg four times daily, and **atenolol**, 50 to 100 mg per day, have been used to treat **alcohol** withdrawal, but they are rarely used as sole therapy except in the mildest cases. Many centers use β-adrenergic receptor antagonists, in addition to benzodiazepines, because of their antiarrhythmic effects. β-Adrenergic receptor antagonists may also reduce the required dose of a given benzodiazepine. Caution is advised, however, because β-adrenergic receptor antagonists do not prevent seizures or delirium. Furthermore, **propranolol** is contraindicated in patients with asthma, insulin-dependent diabetes, or congestive heart failure. Toxic confusional states have also been reported with **propranolol** use in **alcohol** withdrawal.

Because **atenolol** is a relatively cardioselective β_1-adrenergic receptor antagonist, alcoholic patients with mild asthma may tolerate lower doses of this drug, but a β_2-adrenergic receptor agonist (i.e., a bronchodilator, such as **albuterol**) should be readily available. (*Note:* Receptor selectivity diminishes with increasing amounts of **atenolol**.) The main utility of β-adrenergic receptor antagonists in **alcohol** withdrawal is in patients with ischemic heart disease, severe tachycardia, or hypertension unresponsive to benzodiazepine treatment.

c. **Barbiturates**. Before the introduction of the benzodiazepines, barbiturates were a first-line treatment for **alcohol** withdrawal. Some clinicians still use phenobarbital as their primary agent for detoxification. Dosage guidelines for the use of **phenobarbital** are given in Table 12.6. Because barbiturates are more likely than benzodiazepines to cause respiratory depression, because they also interact with many other drugs via their enzyme-inducing properties (see Chapter 29), and because controlled trials do not exist to support their efficacy for preventing withdrawal complications, most clinicians view barbiturates as second-line treatments.

An additional problem in the United States has been inconsistent availability of the oral formulations of the short-acting and intermediate-acting barbiturates, such as amobarbital. In the rare patients who are unresponsive to benzodiazepines, some clinicians choose **amobarbital**, preferring this agent over **phenobarbital** because of its shorter duration of action that gives the clinician greater control of the level of sedation. However, as with the short-acting benzodiazepines, careful tapering is required.

d. α_2-**Adrenergic agonists**. **Clonidine** (0.1 mg twice a day to 0.2 to 0.3 mg three times a day) and other α_2-adrenergic agonists can be given to reduce the hyperadrenergic symptoms of **alcohol** withdrawal. Although these drugs may reduce anxiety, tension, blood pressure, heart rate, tremor, or sweating, they do not prevent seizures, delirium, or hallucinations. That clonidine may cause hypotension and drowsiness should be noted, however. α_2-Adrenergic agonists may be useful adjuncts for treating severe hypertension in **alcohol** withdrawal or for coexisting opiate withdrawal, but they are not recommended as first-line therapy.

e. **Carbamazepine.** This drug is an anticonvulsant (see Chapter 19) that is structurally related to the tricyclic antidepressants. Although it is approved by the United States Food and Drug Administration for use in partial complex seizures, generalized tonic-clonic seizures, mixed seizures, or trigeminal neuralgia, several studies have noted efficacy in the **alcohol** withdrawal syndrome. A typical approach is to administer **carbamazepine** in doses of 600 to 800 mg per day during the first 48 hours of abstinence and then to reduce the dose by 200 mg per day. The most common early adverse reactions encountered are dizziness, sedation, unsteadiness, nausea, and vomiting. Fewer rebound withdrawal symptoms and less sedation may occur than are seen with lorazepam, but experience with **carbamazepine** use in alcoholic patients is limited. When taken for other disorders, its most serious adverse reaction is suppression of the hematopoietic system; furthermore, the risk of developing aplastic anemia and agranulocytosis is estimated to be five to eight times greater in patients taking **carbamazepine** than in the general population. In the general population, the risk of agranulocytosis is approximately 6 per 1 million population per year; the risk of aplastic anemia is 2 per 1 million population per year. The actual frequency of these reactions during **carbamazepine** treatment of **alcohol** withdrawal is unknown.

Cardiovascular, dermatologic, and hepatic toxicities have also been reported with **carbamazepine** use. Given its potential for toxicity, **carbamazepine** is not recommended as a first-line agent for treatment of the **alcohol** withdrawal syndrome.

f. **Chloral hydrate.** This agent is also effective in **alcohol** withdrawal, but its associated adverse effects make it unacceptable for routine use. Gastric irritation leads to nausea and vomiting; gastric necrosis may occur with toxic doses. **Chloral hydrate** interacts with **alcohol** and displaces drugs like warfarin from their protein-binding sites. The typical initial oral doses in **alcohol** withdrawal are 1 to 2 g. No parenteral form is currently available.

g. **Paraldehyde.** Once a mainstay of treatment in the **alcohol** withdrawal syndrome, **paraldehyde** is no longer used in the United States. It is a noxious, malodorous liquid that may cause gastric irritation, hepatotoxicity, and respiratory depression. Large volumes were necessary when it was given parenterally, and injection site complications sometimes developed.

h. **Chlormethiazole.** This sedative-hypnotic agent is used in some countries for the treatment of **alcohol** withdrawal; it is not approved for use in the United States, and it has been withdrawn from use in some other countries. The usual doses are three capsules or tablets, each containing 192 mg of **chlormethiazole** base, every 6 hours for 2 days, followed by two capsules or tablets every 6 hours for the next 4 days. Treatment usually lasts no longer than 9 days. It may cause oversedation in some cases; fatalities have also been reported. It has a high potential for abuse and dependence.

i. **Antipsychotic agents.** When delirium occurs in the course of **alcohol** withdrawal, antipsychotic agents may be indicated (see Chapters 5 and 20). With some of these agents (e.g., **chlorpromazine, thioridazine**), clinicians must be concerned about avoiding hypotension or lowering the seizure threshold. The risk of hypotension can be reduced by avoiding certain conventional antipsychotic agents, such as the aliphatic phenothiazines (e.g., **chlorpromazine, promazine**) and the aliphatic thioxanthenes (e.g., **chlorprothixene**).

Loxapine may also cause hypotension and may lower the seizure threshold. Of these two adverse effects, hypotension is the more serious, and some fatalities have been reported following i.m. or i.v. use of **chlorpromazine** in DTs.

Although delirium during **alcohol** withdrawal should primarily be treated with benzodiazepines, **haloperidol** is often added in doses of 0.5 to 5 mg i.m. or i.v. every 2 hours to treat psychotic symptoms and hallucinations. A reasonable strategy is to begin with lower **haloperidol** doses and to increase them as necessary. Augmenting the effects of **haloperidol** by the judicious use of i.v. benzodiazepines (e.g., **lorazepam**, 1 to 2 mg i.v. every 5 minutes) may also be helpful. (*Note:* Any benzodiazepine use may cause greater than usual sedation or respiratory depression when evidence of compromised hepatic function [e.g., elevated serum ammonia or INR or depressed serum albumin] is seen.)

   j. **Miscellaneous agents**. Other agents have been used to treat **alcohol** withdrawal, but none has proved superior to the benzodiazepines. **Valproate**, **bromocriptine**, antihistamines, and calcium channel blocking agents have been employed, but none of these are recommended for routine clinical use. **Gabapentin** has shown some promise because it does not affect mental status as often as the benzodiazepines, but its efficacy remains to be established. **Ethanol** should not be used for **alcohol** withdrawal except in the setting of **methanol** or **ethylene glycol** ingestion. **Ethanol** is toxic and difficult to administer appropriately, and it may interfere with engagement with the overall treatment plan.

C. **Volume Repletion**

   Although many concomitant conditions, such as rhabdomyolysis, alcoholic ketoacidosis, starvation, vomiting, and diarrhea, in alcoholic patients in **alcohol** withdrawal require i.v. fluid administration, one cannot assume all patients are volume depleted. Administration of volume (i.e., saline solution) could be dangerous if the patient is not volume depleted and when unrecognized alcoholic cardiomyopathy coexists. In young, healthy adults who are volume depleted, little danger exists in administering fluids. Treatment should clearly be individualized.

   1. **Assessment**. Appraisal of the withdrawing alcoholic's state of fluid balance is notably difficult. Usually reliable indicators can be misleading.
      a. **Skin turgor** assessment must be approached with caution. Poorly nourished alcoholic patients may have reduced subcutaneous connective tissue, and they may thus appear to be volume depleted when they in fact are not. The inner aspect of the thigh is the most reliable location for this assessment.
      b. **Body weight** is useful, if a recent weight from a previous admission is available. However, weight loss may be due to poor nutrition as much as to volume depletion. Once a baseline weight has been obtained on admission, daily changes in weight are a valuable indicator of volume status. For this reason, all withdrawing alcoholic patients should be weighed daily. Unless the initial volume depletion was severe, weight gain should be no greater than 0.5 to 1 kg per day.
      c. **Blood urea nitrogen** levels also can be deceiving. They may be inappropriately high if renal disease is present or if blood is present in the gastrointestinal tract. Misleadingly low values can occur because of poor protein intake or from failures in urea synthesis secondary to liver disease.
      d. **Thirst or dry mucous membranes** also are not reliable markers. Hyperventilation is common in **alcohol** withdrawal, and this can produce drying of mucous membranes in the absence of volume depletion.
      e. **Postural vital signs** (a seated or standing and supine blood pressure and pulse) with a significant drop in blood pressure or a rise in pulse indicate a significant volume deficit.

    f. Hematocrit values appear normal in many alcoholic patients who are anemic when in a normal state of hydration. Because of hemoconcentration, their hematocrit values then appear normal when they are dehydrated.

    g. Urinalysis is valuable if renal function is normal. A urine specific gravity greater than 1.025 or a sodium concentration of less than 10 mEq per L in a spot urine sample strongly suggests volume depletion. Ketonuria can occur with decreased oral intake or persistent vomiting.

2. Treatment. When the patient is not seriously ill and he or she can tolerate oral intake, the individual will correct fluid deficits and will maintain normal hydration when given *ad libitum* access to water and a diet containing normal amounts of sodium chloride. Patients who cannot eat or drink or who are significantly volume depleted must be given parenteral fluids. If the history, physical examination, body weight, and laboratory studies suggest that a fluid deficit is present, the deficit must be corrected in addition to the administration of maintenance fluids.

    a. Approximate daily maintenance requirements are **water** (30 to 40 mL per kg), **sodium** (40 to 80 mEq), and **potassium** (30 to 60 mEq). These should be given by continuous infusion with 5% **dextrose** in a normal saline solution so that calories are provided and hypoglycemia is avoided (see section IV.B.2). **Potassium chloride** (20 to 40 mEq) and **magnesium sulfate** (1 to 2 g) can be added to each liter of fluid provided renal function is normal.

    b. Fluid and electrolyte deficits should be corrected as indicated. Deficits developing during hospitalization from vomiting, fever, diaphoresis, or marked hyperactivity can be avoided by increasing the maintenance therapy.

3. Hazards. The approach to parenteral fluid and electrolyte administration must be modified when cirrhosis is present or when **sodium** metabolism is abnormal (see section IV.B.1 and V.B.5).

D. Potassium Balance

Even when parenchymal liver disease is not present, most chronic alcoholic patients have a total body potassium deficit. This can contribute to symptoms such as depression, fatigue, and muscle weakness. When the deficit is severe and when it is superimposed on sympathetic nervous system hyperactivity during **alcohol** withdrawal, fatal cardiac arrhythmias may ensue. Most patients, therefore, should receive **potassium** supplementation.

1. Assessment. Serum **potassium** is the only measurement readily available to most clinicians. **Potassium** is primarily an intracellular cation. Of a normal total body **potassium** content of 3,000 to 3,500 mEq, less than 1% is found in serum. Consequently, serum **potassium** can appear to be normal despite a total body deficit. In addition, when the serum **potassium** is less than 3.0 to 3.2, the total body deficit may be several hundred milliequivalents or more. Patients who have received long-term diuretic therapy without potassium supplementation invariably have a potassium deficit. This is especially likely with thiazide diuretics and **furosemide**. Furthermore, alcoholic patients are often **magnesium** deficient, and **magnesium** is required for renal reabsorption of **potassium**. The influence of pH on serum **potassium** must also be remembered. Respiratory alkalosis due to hyperventilation is frequently found in **alcohol** withdrawal. This results in an influx of **potassium** into cells, thus lowering the serum concentration without changing the total body store. Systemic acidosis does the reverse, and serum **potassium** rises.

2. Treatment. Potassium chloride is the supplement of choice.

    a. When serum potassium is normal (above 4.0 in a patient with heart disease), the danger of cardiac arrhythmias due to hypokalemia is slight. Replacement can proceed slowly at a rate of 60 to 100 mEq per day. A normal diet usually contains ample **potassium**, and supplements should not be necessary once oral intake resumes.

b. **A low serum potassium** in the absence of alkalosis almost always indicates a total body deficit. **Potassium** chloride concentrations of more than 60 to 80 mEq per L are extremely irritating when given i.v. The maximum replacement rate is 30 to 40 mEq per h. This should be continued until the serum **potassium** is 3.5 mEq or more. The usual replacement dose is 100 to 140 mEq per day. Oral therapy is preferable whenever possible.

c. **Potassium replacement** is futile when **magnesium** deficiency coexists and is left untreated.

3. **Hazards.** The risks are those of hyperkalemia. **Potassium** should not be given unless urine output is adequate. Renal insufficiency necessitates caution and a reduced dosage. Serum **potassium** concentrations should be determined at least daily during replacement therapy, but more frequent determination is preferred until a safe range (e.g., greater than 3.3 mEq but less than 6.0 mEq) is achieved. Intravenous **potassium chloride** should be given by continuous infusion, **never** by bolus injection. The ECG should be monitored if large amounts of **potassium** are given i.v. Administration of **potassium chloride** with **potassium**-sparing diuretics, such as **spironolactone**, **amiloride**, and **triamterene**, or other medications such as angiotensin-converting enzyme inhibitors that promote **potassium** retention may be hazardous, even when thiazide diuretics are coadministered, and patients should be closely monitored.

E. **Magnesium Balance**

The metabolism of **potassium** and **magnesium** is similar. Most alcoholic patients are **magnesium** depleted regardless of serum concentrations. **Magnesium** deficiency can contribute to symptoms of lethargy and weakness and to hypokalemia. Hypomagnesemia has also been suggested to lower the seizure threshold and to lead to cardiac arrhythmias. **Magnesium** sulfate (1 to 2 g i.v., added to i.v. fluids) is preferable when i.v. fluids are being given. Several oral preparations (e.g., **magnesium** gluconate, **magnesium** oxide, and **magnesium** hydroxide as commonly found in antacids) are available. Their use is limited by their main side effect, diarrhea. The **aluminum** that is often combined with antacids counteracts this effect, but it should be avoided because it can exacerbate hypophosphatemia. Combination antacids containing **calcium** carbonate rather than **aluminum** are preferable for minimizing diarrhea. Treatment is continued until the **magnesium** levels normalize and clinical improvement occurs. If **magnesium** deficiency or hypokalemia is present, one can assume that the total body deficit is approximately 1 to 2 g of elemental **magnesium**. Ideally, this should be replaced over 4 or 5 days, keeping in mind that half of the replaced **magnesium** is excreted in the urine.

F. **Phosphate**

Hypophosphatemia is common in persons withdrawing from **alcohol**. Serum levels can be misleading when rhabdomyolysis or starvation coexist, as these result in a false elevation that rapidly drops with the administration of **glucose** and fluids or refeeding. Oral supplementation is preferable; milk contains about 1 g per L of **phosphorus** and **calcium**. For patients who cannot tolerate oral fluid intake (skim milk, **potassium** phosphate tablets, or oral **carbonated phosphates** as found in cathartics), several parenteral phosphorous preparations are commercially available. These should be used only with close monitoring of serum **calcium** and **phosphorus** when the patient cannot take anything orally and when the serum **phosphorus** is less than 1 mg per dL due to the risk of hypocalcemia and cardiac effects. A total daily oral dose of 2 to 3 g of **elemental phosphorus** is given in two to four divided doses. Mild diarrhea is a frequent adverse effect. Supplemental treatment is continued until the phosphate levels return to normal.

G. Calcium

Hypocalcemia is commonly seen in alcoholic patients. Hypomagnesemia causes reversible hypoparathyroidism, which can cause a depressed serum **calcium**. The serum **calcium** may appear to be even lower because of a low serum albumin. When the corrected serum **calcium** is low, treatment with **magnesium** will usually correct the abnormality. Treatment with oral or i.v. **calcium** is futile because the problem is not the body stores of calcium, even though osteopenia is not uncommon, but rather the regulation of the serum level. **Calcium** supplementation will not raise the serum levels.

H. Prophylactic anticonvulsants

The indications for prophylactic anticonvulsant therapy in **alcohol** withdrawal are extremely limited.

1. **Assessment depends largely on history**.

    a. **Most patients** either have no history of seizures, or they have had convulsions only during prior episodes of **alcohol** withdrawal.

    b. **A smaller subgroup** of patients is known to have grand mal seizures that occur apart from the **alcohol** abstinence syndrome. Almost all of these individuals are or should be receiving maintenance anticonvulsant therapy. However, many have stopped taking their medication. Categorizing these patients into the following two groups may be useful: those who have continued taking anticonvulsants up to the present and those who have stopped taking them 5 or more days earlier.

2. **Treatment** depends on the category into which the patient falls.

    a. **With no seizure history or with seizures during alcohol withdrawal only**, no evidence exists to suggest that prophylactic **phenytoin** or other anticonvulsants will prevent withdrawal seizures. Sedative-hypnotics have anticonvulsant activity in themselves. Adequate treatment of the abstinence syndrome with sedative-hypnotics minimizes the likelihood of seizures.

    b. **Patients known to have an underlying seizure disorder** are at risk of developing convulsions during **alcohol** withdrawal.

       (1) **When patients have been taking phenytoin** or another anticonvulsant **reliably**, their daily maintenance doses should be continued. Most patients require 300 to 400 mg per day of **phenytoin**. The dose can be given as a single dose. When oral intake is precluded, the maintenance dose of **phenytoin** should be given i.v. at a rate not exceeding 50 mg per minute. **Phenytoin** should not be given by i.m. injection because it is incompletely absorbed. However, an ester preparation, **fosphenytoin** (75 mg = 50 mg of **phenytoin**), can be given i.m. As soon after admission as possible, the serum **phenytoin** concentration should be determined and should be used to guide therapy. The effective serum concentration range is 10 to 20 µg per mL or whatever level has previously been associated with seizure control for that individual. The dosage should be adjusted to keep serum concentrations in this range, rather than keeping them fixed according to an arbitrary dosing regimen.

       (2) **If phenytoin or another anticonvulsant maintenance was stopped 5 or more days before admission**, then the total body anticonvulsant stores are usually depleted. In this circumstance, a **loading dose of phenytoin** should be given (**phenytoin**, 10 to 15 mg per kg i.v., should be administered slowly—not faster than 50 mg per min). This procedure requires about 20 minutes in a 70-kg patient. Each injection of **phenytoin** into a vein or catheter should be followed by an injection of sterile **saline** through the same needle or catheter to avoid local venous irritation. After the loading dose, an oral maintenance dose of 100 mg is given every 6 to 8 hours. In the absence of status epilepticus, a slower rate of administration of the loading dose

may be preferable (e.g., 10 to 15 mg per kg over 4 to 6 hours). Intravenous **phenytoin** can cause mild atrioventricular block or hypotension; the blood pressure and ECG should be monitored continuously. Although **fosphenytoin** avoids these effects, it is also considerably more expensive. **Phenytoin** is the drug of choice, even when the patient has required another anticonvulsant, because adequate serum levels can be achieved rapidly. **Phenobarbital** is a reasonable alternative for this purpose.

(3) **The hazards** of parenteral **phenytoin** are that it is given in a propylene glycol solvent vehicle that can cause bradycardia or hypotension when given in a rapid bolus. For this reason **i.v. phenytoin** should be given at **no faster than 50 mg per min**. Addition of **phenytoin** to i.v. fluids should be avoided because solubility problems may lead to precipitation. Long-term administration of **phenytoin** can produce malabsorption of **folic acid** and **vitamin D**. These possibilities should be considered in newly admitted alcoholic patients who have already received **phenytoin** as outpatients.

I. Aftercare

Withdrawal from **alcohol** or acute detoxification is only the first step in management for the alcoholic patient. Detoxification does not reduce the rate of relapse. All patients treated for withdrawal should be offered treatment for **alcohol** dependence, including counseling or pharmacotherapy, such as supervised **disulfiram** or **naltrexone** (see Chapter 11). Active psychiatric disorders, most commonly mood disorders, coexist in half of all patients with addictions; these should be treated without delay. Finally, alcoholic patients should avoid **acetaminophen** because of the risk of hepatic necrosis and fulminant liver failure due to toxic metabolites that accumulate as a result of fasting and underlying liver disease leading to depleted **glutathione** stores. No dose of **acetaminophen** is known to be safe in the setting of **alcohol** use.

IV. Recognition and Therapy of Complications

Complications of the **alcohol** withdrawal syndrome must be assessed and dealt with promptly. Sequelae such as infection and metabolic derangements can be rapidly fatal when they are unrecognized, but they are readily reversible with sound medical treatment. Multiple complications often coexist, and they may go unrecognized because they are mistakenly attributed to the withdrawal syndrome.

A. Fever

Fever during **alcohol** withdrawal becomes more common with the increasing severity of the withdrawal syndrome. Hyperpyrexia *per se* is a symptom, not a disease. Epidemiologic studies suggest that fever in this setting is commonly due to volume depletion or pulmonary infection. Alcoholic hepatitis is another common cause of low-grade fever; acute pancreatitis can also be associated with fever. However, statistics do not apply to individual patients. In any abstinent alcoholic patient, a fever greater than 38.1°C (100.5°F) should suggest infection until this has been proved otherwise. A systematic search for a source of infection must be undertaken. Common sites of infection are the lungs (e.g., *Streptococcus pneumoniae, Haemophilus influenzae, Klebsiella pneumoniae,* mixed bacterial, *Mycobacterium tuberculosis*); the meninges; the peritoneum; and the urinary tract, especially with Foley catheters or obstruction. Infection can also be catheter related. Aspiration pneumonias are not uncommon. *M. tuberculosis* is becoming more prevalent, and it should be suspected in patients who have been homeless or have lived in shelters. Fever during an acute confusional state necessitates examination of the cerebrospinal fluid. Fever and ascites indicate examination of the peritoneal fluid to identify spontaneous bacterial peritonitis.

B. Metabolic disturbances

Recognition and therapy of abnormalities in fluid, **potassium** balance, and **magnesium** balance were discussed earlier in sections III.D.2 and III.E. Common metabolic disturbances include the following.

1. **Hyponatremia** can be iatrogenic, due to excessive parenteral administration of **sodium**-free solutions, but it may also be seen in beer drinkers. It is often observed when patients have been vomiting and have been replacing losses with water or other hypotonic fluids. Treatment consists of the restriction of free water if its nature is iatrogenic; however, in the case of volume depletion with hyponatremia, treatment consists of i.v. isotonic **saline**. When hyponatremia is severe (less than 110 mEq per L) or when it is accompanied by objective neuropsychiatric symptoms, hypertonic **sodium chloride** solution can be given i.v. with caution. Rapid administration of hypertonic **sodium chloride** solution has been associated with central pontine myelinolysis. The serum **sodium** should increase by no more than 0.5 mEq per h.

2. **Hypoglycemia** is a significant danger in abstinent alcoholic patients. Glycogen depletion, hepatic disease, and poor caloric intake can contribute to the hypoglycemia. All parenteral solutions should contain 5% **dextrose** in addition to other needed solutes. Whenever unexplained obtundation occurs, a blood sample should be drawn to determine the **glucose** level, and a 50 mL bolus of 50% **glucose** solution should immediately be given i.v. while awaiting the results of the test.

3. **Alkalosis** is usually due to hyperventilation (i.e., respiratory alkalosis). Alkalosis is important because it lowers extracellular **potassium** and **magnesium** concentrations, causing weakness and possibly a lowered seizure threshold. Therapy consists of sedation and supplements of **potassium** and **magnesium**, as described in sections III.D.2 and III.E.

4. **Acidosis** is important to recognize because it may be the only clue of a toxic ingestion of **ethylene glycol**, antifreeze (glycolic acidosis), or methanol (formic acidosis). These toxic acids are osmotically active. When an anion gap is present, measured serum osmolality should be compared to calculated osmolality to determine whether a significant gap exists to detect these ingestions. Anion gap acidosis may also occur after a seizure, as a sign of sepsis (lactic acidosis), or as a result of diabetic or alcoholic ketoacidosis. Alcoholic ketoacidosis can present with hypoglycemia or hyperglycemia and a mild or severe acidosis, and this should be treated with i.v. **dextrose** (5%) in isotonic **saline**, with in**sulin** as needed according to the blood sugar, accompanied by monitoring of the serum pH or serum **bicarbonate**. Urine ketones are often undetectable initially because β-hydroxybutyrate predominates at the outset and this is not detected by urine dipstick tests. The most common nonanion gap acidosis in alcoholic patients is due to diarrhea.

C. Alcoholic Hepatitis

Alcoholic hepatitis is a complication not of **alcohol** withdrawal *per se* but of the drinking episode before abstinence. Clinical characteristics include an enlarged and tender liver, low-grade fever, leukocytosis, mild hepatic function abnormalities, and fatty infiltration of the liver on histologic study. Elevated serum γ-glutamyl transferase and an elevated ratio (i.e., greater than 1.0) of aspartate aminotransferase to alanine aminotransferase are indicators of liver inflammation or necrosis. The syndrome can occur in all individuals after an **alcohol** binge, and, in theory, it is completely reversible once drinking stops. Repeated episodes of alcoholic hepatitis in chronic alcoholic patients can lead to irreversible damage (cirrhosis) eventually. Most patients presenting with clinical episodes of alcoholic hepatitis have some degree of cirrhosis. Fatality rates in hospitalized patients are quite high. At the present time, the only specific therapy for all cases is cessation of drinking. Corticosteroids (**prednisolone**) have been shown to reduce mortality in severe cases of alcoholic hepatitis, when INR and bilirubin are significantly elevated and hepatic encephalopathy is present without gastrointestinal bleeding. **Pentoxifylline** also shows promise for this indication. Malnutrition is strongly related to mortality in patients with alcoholic hepatitis. Caloric intake should be ensured, and, when significant malnutrition is present,

oxandrolone, an anabolic steroid, can be added to decrease mortality. **Propylthiouracil** and **colchicine** may help once cirrhosis is present, although this has not yet been reliably established. Liver transplantation is an option for end-stage liver disease once the patient has achieved a stable abstinence.

D. Hematologic disorders

Several hematologic abnormalities occur in alcoholic patients, and these can complicate **alcohol** withdrawal.

1. **Coagulopathy**. This can occur on the basis of liver disease or **vitamin K** deficiency. Coagulopathy associated with intractable bleeding requires the administration of plasma.

2. **Thrombocytopenia**. **Alcohol** ingestion can transiently reduce the platelet count to extremely low levels. This effect is rapidly reversible, and it probably is of little consequence. A rebound thrombocytosis is often noted after several days of abstinence.

3. **Impaired granulocyte function**. **Alcohol** depresses granulocyte function. This may explain the increased susceptibility of alcoholics to bacterial infection or the occasional finding of a slightly low or normal white blood cell count during serious systemic infection.

4. **Anemia**

   a. **Anemia in alcoholic patients** is assessed by the following methods.

      (1) **Examination of a peripheral blood smear**.

      (2) **Reticulocyte count, mean corpuscular volume, and red cell distribution width**.

      (3) **More expensive less essential measures**, including serum concentration determinations of **iron, iron-binding capacity, ferritin, vitamin B$_{12}$**, and folate.

   b. **Common etiologies of anemia** are as follows:

      (1) **Iron deficiency** secondary to chronic gastrointestinal blood loss.

      (2) **Megaloblastic processes** that are usually due to **folic acid** deficiency or poor utilization. **Vitamin B$_{12}$** deficiency is rarely the cause.

      (3) **Idiopathic anemia** that apparently is secondary to bone marrow depression by **alcohol**.

   In most alcoholic patients, anemia is due to a combination of all three.

   c. **Treatment depends on the etiology**, and ultimately it involves treatment of the underlying causes.

      (1) **If bone marrow aspirate or a combination of serum indicators, history, and physical examination (e.g., blood loss) reveal iron deficiency**, then **iron** therapy is given. Oral therapy is preferable.

      (2) **All alcoholics should be assumed to be folate deficient**, whether they are anemic or not. **Folic acid** (1 mg per day) is given.

      (3) **Cessation of alcohol ingestion** is the only therapy for acute alcoholic thrombocytopenia and idiopathic alcoholic anemia.

V. Modifications of Therapy when Major Associated Diseases Coexist

Several disease states are notoriously common in alcoholic patients. Some, such as cirrhosis and gastrointestinal bleeding, are a direct consequence of alcoholism; others, like chronic obstructive pulmonary disease, are not causally related, but they are frequently associated with alcoholism. Treatment of **alcohol** withdrawal may have to be modified when one or more of these problems is present. Not infrequently, hospital admission occurs because of an associated disease, and a withdrawal syndrome develops only after the patient is hospitalized.

A. Neurologic Problems

1. **Head trauma**, even when it is seemingly minor, should always raise the question of intracranial bleeding. Patients with any evidence of head trauma should be observed carefully for the appearance of focal neuro-

logic signs, such as focal weakness, unilateral mydriasis, lateralizing seizures, increased intracranial pressure, papilledema, vomiting, hypertension, bradycardia, or depression of consciousness. Findings consistent with any of these conditions necessitate urgent neurologic or neurosurgical consultation and brain imaging.

2. **Wernicke encephalopathy** is an acute neurologic illness characterized by ophthalmoplegia, ataxia, and confusion. Eye signs include nystagmus, lateral rectus palsies, conjugate gaze palsies, anisocoria, and slowly reactive pupils. Treatment is with parenteral **thiamine**, 50 to 100 mg per day. Maximum improvement may take several weeks. Unfortunately, some symptoms, such as ataxia and nystagmus, may persist. During the acute phase, the mortality rate may be 15% to 20%.

3. **Most patients who survive Wernicke encephalopathy go on to develop Korsakoff syndrome (alcohol amnestic disorder).** Korsakoff syndrome is characterized by amnesia; recent memory is affected to a greater extent than is the remote memory. Patients may appear indifferent to their memory loss, filling in memory gaps with fabrications (confabulation). Even after thiamine treatment and the cessation of drinking, the amnestic syndrome may not improve in about half of patients with the disorder.

4. **Alcoholic dementia** is an impairment of both short-term and long-term memory that is accompanied by impaired judgment, a personality change, or other disturbances in abstract thinking. It should be differentiated from Korsakoff syndrome, which affects the memory but spares the other intellectual functions.

5. **Hepatic encephalopathy** is not usually confused with **alcohol** withdrawal, but agitation and tremor may be the only signs in the early stages. The characteristic tremor is asterixis. The later stages involve obtundation, and these could be confused with an atypical presentation of **alcohol** withdrawal delirium. When cirrhosis is present in a patient with suspected **alcohol** withdrawal, precipitants of encephalopathy, such as gastrointestinal bleeding, infection, and recent sedative use, should be sought.

6. **Other neurologic consequences of alcoholism include cerebellar degeneration, corpus callosum degeneration (Marchiafava-Bignami disease), and central pontine myelinolysis.**

B. **Gastrointestinal Effects**

1. **Alcoholic patients commonly develop esophagitis, gastritis, duodenitis, or peptic ulcerations,** all of which can lead to serious blood loss. Superficial gastritis due to **alcohol** or aspirin or both is the usual cause of gastrointestinal bleeding in alcoholic patients, but the etiology must be determined by carefully conducted endoscopy. Superficial gastritis usually ceases rapidly after antacid administration and abstinence from **alcohol**. Nasogastric suction may be used for comfort. Peptic ulcer disease is the next most common cause of bleeding. Treatment with a proton pump inhibitor and antibiotics when *Helicobacter pylori* infection (an important etiology factor in most duodenal and many gastric ulcers) is present is usually successful. Conservative therapy (e.g., H_2-receptor blocking agents) is usually successful.

Bleeding from esophageal varices is catastrophic, intractable, and often fatal. Initial emergent management after i.v. access is obtained and blood products are transfused is endoscopic ligation, banding, or sclerosis. **Somatostatin** or **octreotide** (50 μg per h) should be started and continued for 1 to 3 days. **Vasopressin** is no longer used for this indication because of its unclear efficacy in the acute setting and its association with vasospasm and cardiac ischemia. Balloon tamponade is the next step, but this is fraught with complications. Transjugular intrahepatic portosystemic shunts can decrease the bleeding when endoscopy fails, although these shunts do increase the risk of encephalopathy and their long-term safety and efficacy are not known. β-Adrenergic receptor antagonists (e.g., **propranolol, nadolol**) and **isosorbide mononitrate** can decrease recurrent variceal bleeding. Surgical portosystemic shunts can also decrease recurrence, but they increase the risk for encephalopathy and do not decrease mortality.

2. **Alcoholic steatosis (fatty liver)** presents as an enlarged, nontender, smooth liver. This is a direct consequence of **alcohol**, and it is reversible with abstinence. Dietary restriction of fat may be beneficial.

3. **Alcoholic hepatitis**, as discussed earlier, usually presents as fever, anorexia, nausea, vomiting, weight loss, right upper quadrant pain, jaundice, or leukocytosis (see section IV.C). Most patients have concurrent cirrhosis. The presence of ascites, encephalopathy, elevated INR (prolonged prothrombin time), hyperbilirubinemia, and rising serum creatinine are poor prognostic signs. Although mild cases usually show clinical recovery, repeated episodes may lead to irreversible liver injury.

4. **Hepatitis C** is more prevalent in alcoholic patients than it is in the general population. Risk factors include injection drug use and blood transfusion. Although sexual transmission in monogamous relationships is rare, multiple sex partners confers a greater risk of hepatitis C. The clinical course of hepatitis is indolent over 15 to 20 years, but **alcohol** use and human immunodeficiency virus infection both independently and synergistically increase the rapidity of progression to cirrhosis, end-stage liver disease, and hepatocellular carcinoma. Current treatment for alcoholic patients in remission is polyethylene glycolated (pegylated) **interferons** with **ribavirin** for 1 year. Side effects include hemolysis, depression, and flu-like symptoms.

5. **Alcoholic cirrhosis** usually causes a slow development of symptoms in patients over the course of many years of drinking **alcohol**. The symptoms may begin as weakness, fatigue, anorexia, or a loss of muscle mass. As the disease progresses, bruising, jaundice, ascites, gastroesophageal varices, or encephalopathy may develop. Renal dysfunction may occur in the later stages of the illness. On physical examination, the liver is nodular; it may be enlarged, of normal size, or even smaller than normal. Secondary signs include spider angiomas, palmar erythema, splenomegaly, or clubbing fingers. In men, hormonal changes may result in testicular atrophy, gynecomastia, or decreased body hair.

Coexistence of the **alcohol** withdrawal syndrome with cirrhosis is prognostically grave. This indicates continued **alcohol** consumption, despite irreversible **alcohol**-induced liver damage. The following modifications in therapy are necessary.

a. **Medications**

(1) **Sedative-hypnotics** must be administered with the utmost caution. Even small doses can precipitate hepatic coma. Careful titration is the only rational approach, with underdosage preferred to oversedation. When cirrhosis is present, benzodiazepines are the safest choice of drugs, particularly **lorazepam and oxazepam**. The belief that **paraldehyde** is safe in liver disease is unfounded—only a small proportion of **paraldehyde** excretion is via the lungs; hepatic metabolism is its major route of elimination.

(2) **Antidepressants, such as fluoxetine and sertraline**, should be used with caution, even at lower-than-usual doses. Some clinicians suggest that they not be used at all. Cirrhotic liver impairment typically reduces biotransformation. **Fluoxetine's** elimination half-life, for example, may be increased from its usual range of 2 to 3 days to 7 to 8 days.

(3) **Acetaminophen** use should be avoided because of the risk of hepatic necrosis even with usually recommended doses. **Aspirin** and nonsteroidal antiinflammatory agents should also be

avoided, not only because of the antiplatelet effects and the risk of bleeding but also because of **sodium** retention.

b. **Fluid and electrolyte therapy**. In cirrhosis, these therapies must take into account any abnormalities in sodium metabolism. In cirrhotic patients, **sodium** retention occurs despite total body sodium overload. **Sodium** intake should be restricted. Total body **sodium** and water excess may occur when the intravascular volume is depleted. In general, **sodium**, either orally or parenterally, should be avoided. However, when significant volume depletion (e.g., hypotension, poor organ perfusion) occurs, isotonic **saline** should not be withheld, even though it will expand the extracellular space and worsen the peripheral edema and ascites. **Blood** is the volume-expanding agent of choice when anemia coexists because it remains in the intravascular space. **Albumin**, although it has a role in large volume paracentesis and in helping to replace intravascular volume, has very short-lived effects; it is not used for diuresis or routine volume replacement. All i.v. solutions should contain 5% **dextrose** to provide calories and to avoid hypoglycemia. **Potassium** depletion can be very severe in cirrhosis, and supplements are invariably required. Hyponatremia is common, and, although it is generally well tolerated, **sodium** and free water restriction are often necessary. Diuresis of ascitic fluid should be undertaken gently with a weight loss of no more than 1 kg per day. **Spironolactone**, 100 to 400 mg per day, is the diuretic of choice. The addition of **furosemide** helps the diuresis and assists in avoiding hyperkalemia. Large-volume paracentesis (4 to 6 L), followed by i.v. **albumin** to avoid renal insufficiency and hyponatremia, is associated with fewer complications than is treatment with diuretics. The hazards of coadministration of **potassium chloride** with **spironolactone** must be remembered.

c. **Infection.** Infection can precipitate a hepatic coma, so it must be treated aggressively. Ascitic fluid is an ideal culture medium, and it should always be examined in the evaluation of fever. Spontaneous bacterial peritonitis may be present even if leukocytosis, abdominal pain, and tenderness are not present. High-risk patients with ascites, particularly those who have had spontaneous bacterial peritonitis, should take prophylactic **norfloxacin or ciprofloxacin**.

6. **Hepatorenal syndrome** is acute renal insufficiency secondary to severe liver disease. Signs include mild hypotension, oliguria, low urinary sodium (i.e., less than 10 mEq per L), and hypertonic urine. Signs of advanced hepatic disease are also present. The kidneys themselves are normal, and no characteristic histopathologic changes have occurred. Renal hypoperfusion due to vasoconstriction is thought to be the primary etiologic factor. No effective treatment exists for the hepatorenal syndrome at this time. Surgical procedures, such as placement of a peritoneovenous shunt or liver transplantation, are the only approaches that have had any degree of success. Neither dialysis nor medical approaches, such as volume expansion, steroids, antibiotics, pressor agents, prostaglandins, or transfusions, seem to benefit these patients. However, every patient should receive a trial of volume expansion with isotonic fluids or blood products, as if volume depletion was the cause of the renal insufficiency, because prerenal azotemia is often indistinguishable from the hepatorenal syndrome initially.

7. **Pancreatitis**, especially the acute form, should be suggested by the presence of severe abdominal pain, fever, and leukocytosis. Serum amylase and lipase levels should be determined when pancreatitis is suspected. Chronic pancreatitis can present with pain and normal amylase and lipase levels.

a. **As with gastrointestinal bleeding**, sedative-hypnotics must be given in doses that are sufficient to prevent the patient from pulling out the nasogastric tube or i.v. catheters. Because many patients may require opioid analgesics as well (i.e., **meperidine** is usually preferred to avoid sphincter of Oddi problems from **morphine**), the possibility of additive central nervous system depression should be considered.

   b. Fluid and electrolyte therapy must be vigorous. Patients with acute pancreatitis can lose large amounts of fluid volume into the retroperitoneal space. The hematocrit should be taken frequently. **Hypocalcemia** can occur in pancreatitis and can lower the seizure threshold. Serum calcium should be measured in all patients with pancreatitis. Calcium supplements (1 g **calcium chloride** or **gluconate**) are given i.v. when the level of calcium is critically low.

   c. Malabsorption syndromes are common in chronic pancreatitis, and they can produce deficiencies of **vitamins A, D, and K**. Hypocalcemia can result from hypovitaminosis D; this emphasizes the importance of measuring serum calcium. **Vitamin K** deficiency increases the possibility of coagulopathy and bleeding. The INR should be measured, and parenteral **vitamin K**, 5 mg, should be given when indicated.

   d. Hyperglycemia can be associated with acute or chronic pancreatitis due to inadequate insulin secretion. Fingerstick blood **glucose** levels should be measured in all patients with pancreatitis, and insulin should be given when indicated.

   e. Although exocrine deficiency in chronic pancreatitis can be diagnosed by the N-benzoyl-L-tyrosyl-p-aminobenzoic acid test to detect chymotrypsin deficiency or the reference standard secretin test to detect impaired duodenal bicarbonate secretion, these tests are not often conducted. Exocrine deficiency is usually diagnosed clinically by the symptoms of greasy stools and chronic pain in the setting of recurrent pancreatitis and by calcifications on abdominal radiograph. In addition to vitamin supplementation, particularly of the fat-soluble vitamins, patients should be placed on a low-fat diet (less than 50 g of fat per day) and should be given oral pancreatic enzyme supplements. The pain is quite difficult to manage, and it often requires opioids, medications used for neuropathic pain, or nerve blocks.

   f. Fever may result from pancreatic abscess or necrosis, an infected pseudocyst, or aspiration pneumonia.

   g. Surgical therapy may be indicated in some cases of severe necrotizing or hemorrhagic pancreatitis or when abscesses or pseudocysts develop.

   h. Adult respiratory distress syndrome may develop. This is characterized by high-permeability pulmonary edema, and it is typically treated with mechanical ventilation.

 8. Other gastrointestinal effects of **alcohol** include an increased risk of many types of cancer, including those of the upper digestive tract.

C. Cardiovascular Effects

 1. Patients with alcoholic cardiomyopathy present with fatigue, dyspnea on exertion, orthopnea, or palpitations. On an ECG, they may show atrial fibrillation, conduction defects, abnormal P waves, or decreased QRS voltage. Chest x-ray reveals cardiomegaly. Echocardiography is often conducted. The heart tissue shows muscle fiber hypertrophy and degeneration, fibrosis, and endocardial fibroelastosis. Some systolic function may return with abstinence from **alcohol**.

 2. Atrial fibrillation, which is sometimes called the **holiday heart syndrome**, may develop in patients without heart disease during periods of excessive **alcohol** consumption or withdrawal.

 3. Hypertension is commonly seen in **alcohol** dependence and in alcoholic patients during withdrawal, but this typically resolves without specific drug treatment. Chronic medication treatment may be necessary if hypertension persists after the resolution of **alcohol** withdrawal.

D. Endocrine Effects

Plasma cortisol is increased in alcoholic patients, and a cushingoid syndrome may develop. Other endocrine effects may be influenced by liver disease. In male alcoholic patients, **testosterone** clearance is enhanced, and its synthesis is depressed, while **estrogen** levels rise. One clinical presentation includes testicular atrophy, breast enlargement, loss of facial hair, impotence, or decreased libido. Women with alcoholism may have amenorrhea, luteal phase dysfunction, anovulation, early menopause, or hyperprolactinemia.

E. Chronic Obstructive Pulmonary Disease

The nonsmoking alcoholic patient is a rarity, particularly at urban hospitals. Chronic obstructive pulmonary disease, therefore, usually coexists with alcoholism. When significant pulmonary disease is present, arterial blood gas determinations should be a routine aspect of assessment.

1. **Sedative-hypnotics** again require careful titration. Oversedation can precipitate **carbon dioxide** retention, narcosis, or coma. Benzodiazepines are the safest of the currently available drugs. When **carbon dioxide** retention is present, shorter-acting benzodiazepines are preferred. Barbiturates are hazardous. Hypoxia or **carbon dioxide** narcosis or both should be considered whenever an alteration in mental status occurs. Hypoxia can cause agitation, both of which are made worse by treatment with sedative-hypnotic drugs rather than oxygen.

2. **Fluid and electrolyte therapy** must account for the possibility of *cor pulmonale*. Physical examination, chest x-ray, and ECG can diagnose this entity. **Sodium** must be administered cautiously when *cor pulmonale* is present.

3. **Infection** is a significant threat to the patient with chronic obstructive pulmonary disease. Pulmonary infection should be carefully considered as the etiology of fever when fever occurs. **Superinfection** with hospital-acquired antibiotic-resistant organisms is prognostically grave. This usually occurs during ongoing antibiotic therapy in patients receiving assisted ventilation through tracheostomies or endotracheal tubes.

F. Alcohol-Related Birth Defects (Fetal Alcohol Syndrome)

Maternal **alcohol** ingestion is associated with central nervous system effects, growth deficiency, and facial abnormalities in the fetus. Children show a characteristic facial appearance; they have short palpebral fissures (eye openings), thin hypoplastic upper lips, and an absent or diminished philtrum (the depression in the center above the upper lip). Their ears are often posteriorly rotated and they have an altered shape, and the midface is flattened. Central nervous system effects include impaired intellectual functions that persist throughout development.

The amount of maternal **alcohol** ingestion that leads to the fetal **alcohol** syndrome is unknown, but most clinicians conservatively advise women to avoid **alcohol** during pregnancy. A continuum of dysmorphic and dysfunctional effects likely occurs, ranging from subtle deficits to the full syndrome. The rate of fetal **alcohol** syndrome seems to be particularly high in African Americans and Southwest Plains Indians. The effects of paternal alcoholism on conception and fetal development are unknown.

G. Trauma

Trauma and related orthopedic complications, such as ankle fracture, and multiple trauma from motor vehicle crashes and interpersonal violence are not uncommon. Interventions for alcoholism are known to decrease these consequences. The management of withdrawal is often complicated by the need for anesthesia and brain injury, making the assessment and dosing of prophylaxis and treatment with sedation difficult.

H. Pneumonia

A common reason for hospitalization in alcoholic patients is pneumonia. As with other acute medical, surgical, and psychiatric illnesses, prophylactic sedation should be administered to prevent complicated withdrawal in these high-risk patients. Common causes of community-acquired pneumonia in patients with alcoholism are aspiration of anaerobic and micro-aerophilic oral flora; the so-called atypical bacteria, such as mycoplasma, chlamydia, and legionella; tuberculosis; and pneumocystis.

I. **Human immunodeficiency virus**

Human immunodeficiency virus is more prevalent in persons with alcoholism than it is in the general population. **Alcohol** consumption has been associated with high-risk sexual practices. Consideration should be given to human immunodeficiency virus testing when risk factors are present and when the patient is ready to hear the results.

J. **Pellagra**

This condition is difficult to diagnose, and it can occur in alcoholic patients with nutritional deficiencies. Symptoms can include a rash in sun-exposed areas, diarrhea, abdominal discomfort, nausea and vomiting, glossitis, cognitive impairment, insomnia, anxiety, depression, psychosis, seizure, ataxia, and paraparesis. The diagnosis is clinical, and treatment is with niacin. Because of the difficulty with diagnosis, the difficulty in distinguishing symptoms caused by withdrawal from **alcohol** from other coexisting illnesses, and the simplicity of treatment, a multivitamin is routinely recommended, although additional niacin may be required if symptoms persist (see section III.A.2).

ADDITIONAL READING

Ciraulo DA, Shader RI, eds. *Clinical manual of chemical dependence.* Washington, D.C.: American Psychiatric Press, 1991.

Goldstein DB. *Pharmacology of alcohol.* New York: Oxford University Press, 1983.

Imperiale TF, McCullough AJ. Do corticosteroids reduce mortality from alcoholic hepatitis? A meta-analysis of the randomized trials. *Ann Intern Med* 1990;113: 299–307.

Krystal JH, Tabakoff B. Ethanol abuse, dependence, and withdrawal: neurobiology and clinical implications. In: Davis KL, Charney D, Coyle JT, et al., eds. *Neuropsychopharmacology: the fifth generation of progress.* Philadelphia: Lippincott Williams & Wilkins, 2002:1423–1443.

Lieber CS. Medical disorders of alcoholism. *N Engl J Med* 1995;333:1058–1065.

Malcolm R, Roberts JS, Wang W, et al. Multiple previous detoxifications are associated with less responsive treatment and heavier drinking during an index outpatient detoxification. *Alcohol* 2000;22:159–163.

Mayo-Smith MF. Pharmacological management of alcohol withdrawal: a meta-analysis and evidence-based practice guideline. American Society of Addiction Medicine Working Group on Pharmacological Management of Alcohol Withdrawal. *JAMA* 1997;278;144–151.

Mendelson JH, Mello NK, eds. *The diagnosis and treatment of alcoholism,* 3rd ed. New York: McGraw-Hill, 1992.

Mendenhall CL, Moritz TE, Roselle GA, et al. A study of oral nutritional support with oxandrolone in malnourished patients with alcoholic hepatitis: results of a Department of Veterans Affairs Cooperative study. *Hepatology* 1993;17:564–576.

Myrick H, Malcolm R, Brady KT. Gabapentin treatment of alcohol withdrawal. *Am J Psychiatry* 1998;155:1632.

National Institute of Alcohol Abuse and Alcoholism. Fetal alcohol syndrome. *Alcohol Alert* 1991;13:1–4.

National Institute on Alcohol Abuse and Alcoholism. Alcohol withdrawal. *Alcohol Health & Research World* 1998;22:5–12.

Palmstierna T. A model for predicting alcohol withdrawal delirium. *Psych Serv* 2001; 52:820–823.

Saitz R, O'Malley SS. Pharmacotherapies for alcoholism: withdrawal and treatment. *Med Clin North Am* 1997;81:881–907.

Sereny G, Sharma V, Holt J, Gordis E. Mandatory supervised Antabuse therapy in an outpatient alcoholism program: a pilot study. *Alcoholism* 1986;10:290–292.

Sullivan JT, Sykora K, Schneiderman J, et al. Assessment of alcohol withdrawal: the revised Clinical Institute Withdrawal Assessment for Alcohol scale (CIWA-Ar). *Br J Addict* 1989;84:1353–1357.

Spohr HL, Willms J, Steinhausen HC. Prenatal alcohol exposure and long-term developmental consequences. *Lancet* 1993;341:907–910.

United States Department of Health and Human Services. *Tenth special report to the US Congress on alcohol and health.* Bethseda, MD: United States Department of Health and Human Services, 2000.

Vaillant GE. *The natural history of alcoholism.* Cambridge, MA: Harvard University Press, 1983.

Vaillant GE. *The natural history of alcoholism revisited.* Cambridge, MA: Harvard University Press, 1995.

Annual special report to the U.S. Congress on alcohol as well as other relevant resources. National Institute on Alcohol Abuse and Alcoholism website. Available at: *http://www.niaaa.nih.gov/.* Accessed October, 2002.

13. PHARMACOLOGIC TREATMENT OF PERSONALITY DISORDERS: A DIMENSIONAL APPROACH

James M. Ellison
Richard I. Shader

Personality disorders affect between 5% and 10% of the general adult population in the United States. Most such persons are unaware of their disorder, and thus they seek no treatment; nonetheless, they sustain a chronic impairment of social and occupational functioning, an increased propensity to substance abuse, and frequent legal complications. Patients with personality disorders often present treatment requests that are not well addressed by the established uses of pharmacotherapy. Some of the most challenging dilemmas encountered in clinical practice are balancing patients' goals with the potential risks and benefits of available pharmacotherapeutic agents. In the absence of any comprehensive and definitive explanatory model, portions of this chapter focus on a review of selected issues and hypotheses concerning personality disorders.

Many efforts have been made to capture the essence of personality and its disorders; in this process, the theoretic pendulum has swung to and fro between the domains of biology and psychology. The psychodynamic approach to personality disorders that was widely accepted during the preceding century attributes the origins of personality disorders to conflicts, ego deficits, or impaired object relations. From the time of Hippocrates, another view of personality disorders has suggested that they originate from biologic factors, either inherited or acquired, within the central nervous system.

The Hippocratic concept of temperaments (i.e., inherited physiologic predispositions to observable behavioral traits or patterns) resembles the more modern concept of personality dimensions. In the 1940s, Eysenck used factor-analytic mathematic techniques to demonstrate the validity of a model that accounted for much of the variance of personality on the basis of three dimensions: **introversion-extraversion**; **neuroticism**, an index of emotional instability; and **psychoticism**, a measure of antisocial tendencies. Other researchers have considered these dimensions useful and valid.

A somewhat different approach focuses on clinical observation and description to explain and codify personality and its disorders. One such system of classification pioneered by Schneider subsequently evolved into the system still present in the *International Statistical Classification of Diseases and Related Health Problems,* tenth revision. This system categorizes personality types and disorders descriptively on the basis of recurrent behaviors or traits. Grounded more solidly in clinical assessment methods than in the techniques of experimental psychology, it differs from dimensional approaches by building a syndromal description from a list of many behaviors, some of which may lack independence or perhaps even validity. Although the *Diagnostic and Statistical Manual of Mental Disorders,* 4th edition, (DSM-IV) classification uses some different categories, it does resemble the *International Statistical Classification of Diseases and Related Health Problems,* tenth revision, approach in that it is based on objective description rather than on etiologic inference.

In the multiaxial perspective of DSM, 3rd edition, revised (III-R), personality disorders were placed on an independent axis to differentiate what were considered more stable and persistent disorders from the axis I disorders, which were believed to be more florid and often more episodic. Another prominent goal of placing personality disorders on axis II was to ensure they would not be overlooked. However, this approach seems to ignore certain lines of evidence (e.g., genetic data associating schizophrenia with schizotypal personality disorder) that suggest that some axis II disorders may be milder forms of axis I disorders, not wholly distinct syndromes. DSM-IV tries to mitigate these issues by acknowledging this inherent weakness. As with DSM-III-R, DSM-IV delineates personality disorders according to the predominance of pervasive observable behavioral patterns (e.g., dramatic, odd, impulsive).

The categoric descriptive approach has stimulated clinical awareness and has contributed to a greater understanding of personality disorders. It has also fostered questioning about the nature of personality and the appropriateness of an etiology-free classification system. Embedded in the DSM-IV approach are a variety of unproved assumptions about the nature of personality that have implications for treatment and research. The very conceptualization of a specific personality configuration as a disorder implicitly assumes that these behavioral syndromes are illnesses rather than informed or voluntary lifestyle choices. The descriptive approach assumes also that these conditions can be identified on the basis of overt behaviors rather than be inferred through dynamic exploration and formulation. Furthermore, the assumption is that these disorders are sufficiently discrete so as to be distinguishable and stable enough that one does not transmute into another. Viewing them as enduring or chronic rather than episodic implies that personality disorders remain present even when they are clinically dormant during less symptomatic or asymptomatic intervals. As has been noted above, their placement on axis II and their separation from axis I disorders imply a discontinuity between the latter disorders (i.e., the more obvious and frequently episodic syndromes) and the chronic maladaptive behavior patterns of personality disorders. To some extent, this separation mirrors treatment approaches that have emphasized somatic therapies for axis I disorders while discouraging them for personality disorders.

In addition to these theoretic concerns, multiple practical difficulties accompany the use of a descriptive categoric model. Personality disorders, as research now clearly shows, often co-occur (i.e., they are comorbid), complicating both diagnosis and treatment. They are also found in the presence of axis I disorders, including depression and substance abuse, with unexpectedly high frequency. As was noted, the relationships between some of the axis I and axis II disorders (e.g., the aggregation within families of patients with schizotypal or paranoid personality disorders and schizophrenia) appear to be integral to the nature of a number of disorders, and this suggests continuity along a pathologic spectrum. When studying treatment interventions, a "pure culture" or homogeneous cohort of any personality disorder type is usually difficult to obtain. In the typical clinical settings, patients rarely fit neatly into the descriptive categories. Moreover, from a practical standpoint, these categories have been of limited value in pointing toward diagnosis-specific therapeutic approaches. When planning psychotherapeutic interventions, for example, diagnosis is viewed by some as having less value than the clinician's psychodynamic formulation.

Research into the pharmacotherapy of personality disorders has been facilitated by their acceptance and definition as diagnostic entities and by the subsequent availability of research interview protocols and symptom rating scales. Any advance in this knowledge base, however, may also have been impeded by the tendency of some of these disorders' definitions to follow psychologic and theoretic divisions, rather than biologically meaningful ones. Successful pharmacotherapy frequently focuses more on target symptoms than on syndromal diagnoses, treating similar symptoms with the same agent in varying diagnostic contexts. Aggressive or impulsive behavior may respond, for example, to **risperidone** or **carbamazepine** in a broad range of patients (e.g., personality disorders, mental retardation, brain damage, posttraumatic stress disorder, schizophrenia). Historically, much of the pharmacotherapeutic research on personality disorders has been carried out in patients diagnosed as borderline personality disorder (BPD) or schizotypal personality disorder (see Tables 13.1 and 13.2). This research approach may be less illuminating than a symptom-based approach to ameliorating target symptoms that are not unique to any specific personality disorder (e.g., impulsivity, lability of affect).

I. "Normal" Personality and Its Relationship to Personality Disorders

In general, personality refers to a stable configuration of patterns and modes of relating to oneself and others (i.e., behaviors central to one's life adaptation). From the many behaviors that typify any individual, clusters of related traits can be grouped together and can be used to define that individual's position along a behavioral dimension. Experimental psychologists have used factor analysis to develop models that explain much of the variance of personality on

TABLE 13.1. DIAGNOSTIC FEATURES OF BORDERLINE PERSONALITY DISORDER (BPD)

BPD is characterized by a pervasive and enduring pattern of unstable and impaired interpersonal relationships, self-image, affects, and impulse control that usually begins during adolescence or by early adulthood. Patients with BPD typically present with at least five of the following features:

1. Frantic and chaotic efforts to avoid real or imagined abandonment. (*Note:* It does not include the suicidal, self-mutilating, or other self-injurious behaviors in item 5.)
2. Unstable and intense interpersonal relationships characterized by alternations between the extremes of idealization and devaluation of these relationships.
3. Persistent and markedly disturbed, distorted, or unstable self-image or sense of self (e.g., feeling as if one does not exist or as if one embodies evil).
4. Potentially self-damaging impulsivity manifested in at least two activity areas (e.g., spending money, sexual activity, substance abuse, shoplifting, reckless driving, binge-eating). (*Note:* This does not include the suicidal, self-mutilating, or other self-injurious behaviors in item 5.)
5. Recurrent suicidal threats, gestures, or behavior or self-mutilating or other self-injurious behaviors.
6. Marked affective instability or reactivity of mood (e.g., intense, episodic dysphoria, irritability, or anxiety usually lasting a few hours and only rarely more than a few days).
7. Chronic feelings of emptiness that the patient frequently localizes to the abdomen or chest.
8. Inappropriate or intense anger or lack of control of anger (e.g., frequent displays of temper, constant anger, recurrent physical fights).
9. Severe dissociative symptoms or paranoid thoughts that are transient and typically stress related. (*Note:* Feeling abandoned is a common stress.)

From the American Psychiatric Association. *Diagnostic and statistical manual of mental disorders,* 4th ed. Text revision. Washington, D.C.: American Psychiatric Association, 2000, with permission.

the basis of a small number of fundamental dimensions. Implicit in this approach is the belief that a dimensional model of personality disorders can be expanded to illustrate a theoretic continuum that extends into axis I and axis II disorders.

Much has been learned about the biology of normal personality from longitudinal, observational, and family studies. One group, for example, identified nine dimensions of temperament and periodically assessed a selected cohort of toddlers until they reached early adulthood. Behavior at age 3 (i.e., behaviors so early in development as to suggest possible constitutional factors) was a stronger predictor of adult behavior than were parental child-rearing attitudes. An interaction between temperament and environmental factors was hypothesized to explain the contribution of each to a developing personality.

Other preliminary work to try to understand the biologic determinants of personality has been conducted by focusing on traits that could be assessed longitudinally. Studies of *shyness,* for example, have noted persistence of this trait from the toddler stage to later in childhood. In these studies, shy behavior was also correlated with a psychophysiologic profile of autonomic nervous system arousal in response to a novel situation.

Among genetic studies, investigations of personality traits measured in monozygotic and dizygotic twins separated at birth suggest that as much as 50% of the variance in these traits may be attributed to genotype. This indicates that a substantial component of personality is heritable.

An attractive explanation for the dimensionality of personality and the continuity of normal personalities with axis I and axis II disorders is the hypothesis that biologic factors produce a temperament that interacts with environmental factors. This interaction molds behavioral traits and coping styles. Personality,

TABLE 13.2. DIAGNOSTIC FEATURES OF SCHIZOTYPAL PERSONALITY DISORDER

Schizotypal personality disorder (SPD) is characterized by a pervasive and enduring pattern of social deficits and impaired interpersonal relationships that is manifested as acute discomfort with and reduced capacity for closeness and of cognitive or perceptual distortions and eccentricities of behavior; it usually begins in adolescence or by early adulthood. Patients with SPD typically present with at least five of the following features (*note:* these must not be present only during discrete periods in which mood is clinically altered [e.g., depression, anxiety, anger])[a]:

1. Ideas of reference, excluding delusions of reference;
2. Odd or unusual beliefs that are not consistent with cultural or subcultural norms or magical thinking that influences behavior (e.g., superstitiousness, belief in clairvoyance, telepathy, or "a sixth sense," belief that "others can feel my feelings"; in children and adolescents, bizarre fantasies or preoccupations may be present);
3. Unusual perceptual experiences, including somatosensory (bodily) illusions or distortions;
4. Odd or unusual thinking or speech that is not associated with loosening of associations or incoherence (e.g., vague, circumstantial, metaphoric, overelaborated, or stereotyped);
5. Suspiciousness or paranoid thoughts;
6. Inappropriate or constricted affect (e.g., appears distant, cold, aloof);
7. Behavior or appearance that is odd, eccentric, or peculiar;
8. An absence of close friends or confidants (or only one) other than first-degree relatives that results primarily from a lack of desire, pervasive discomfort with others, or eccentricities;
9. Excessive social anxiety (e.g., extreme discomfort in social situations that does not diminish with familiarity and that tends to be associated with paranoid fears rather than with negative judgments about self).

[a]These features must not occur exclusively during the course of schizophrenia or another psychotic disorder, a mood disorder with psychotic features, or a pervasive developmental disorder.
From the American Psychiatric Association. *Diagnostic and statistical manual of mental disorders,* 4th ed. Text revision. Washington, D.C.: American Psychiatric Association, 2000, with permission.

then, is the result of environmental shaping of temperamental possibilities. A greater or lesser expression of inherited tendencies through the overlay of environmentally shaped behavior could then account for a spectrum of personality configurations ranging from normative to pathologic.

II. Dysfunctional Personality Traits and Personality Disorders

The nature of maladaptive or dysfunctional personalities is still incompletely understood. Family studies of antisocial, paranoid, and schizotypal personality disorders suggest strong components of heritability. Some efforts have been made to trace traits such as impulsivity and affective instability among the relatives of patients with BPD. Still, many important aspects of these disorders (e.g., sensation-seeking, suspiciousness, cognitive slippage) require further study.

Although most work on the treatment of personality disorders has made categoric distinctions, some authors have sought to identify and to target for treatment the hypothetic dimensions of psychopathology that span multiple DSM-III-R axis II categories. These dimensions, unlike those used to define normal personality, have arisen from clinical observation rather than from factor analysis. The resulting dimensions appear to be heterogeneous and they may lack independence, yet they serve as a useful beginning in the development of a functional and potentially unifying perspective.

A. Cognitive and Perceptual Style and Organization

These may be defined as a person's capacity to receive, process, and respond selectively to important external stimuli and to use these inputs, along with previous experiences, to plan and implement subsequent actions. Impairment in this function could reveal itself, for example, as suspiciousness, paranoia, or distortion of others' intentions (see Chapter 4). Such dysfunction might lead to social isolation and further decrements in reality testing. Impairment along this dimension is particularly characteristic of schizotypal and paranoid personality disorders, but it may be seen in patients with other personality disorders (e.g., the "all or nothing" thinking of patients with BPD). Evidence suggesting a biologic basis of some alterations in this dimension in patients with schizotypal personality disorder continues to accumulate.

Abnormalities of smooth pursuit eye movements and impaired performance on tests of visual and auditory attention, similar to that which may be found in some patients with schizophrenia, have been associated with social withdrawal and other "deficit symptoms" in schizotypal patients. Psychotic exacerbations among some such patients have been associated with elevated levels of plasma and cerebrospinal fluid homovanillic acid, a finding consistent with the hypothesis of an underlying abnormality of dopaminergic activity.

B. Impulsivity and Aggression

These traits may be viewed as the consequences of a lowered threshold to respond with action in the face of external or internal stimuli. Some action-oriented persons seem to be stimulus seekers; their craving for and, at times, impulsive pursuit of excitement appear to be directed at achieving an altered internal state. Action-oriented stimulus-hungry persons seem to have a high need for novelty. Impulsive persons often have difficulty delaying action, they tend to externalize the sources of their difficulties, they express aggression or frustration easily, and they may be less likely to experience guilt or anxiety. Excessive impulsivity is frequently found in overdramatizing patients and is manifested variably as self-injurious behavior, suicidality, aggressive behavior directed at others, or substance abuse. Some studies suggest that antisocial personality disorder, which prominently features impulsivity and aggression, has a heritable component. Impulsivity has been found to be unusually frequent among the relatives of patients with BPD.

Impulsive or aggressive behaviors may represent a common pathway of expression for several different dysfunctional states. Among possible etiologies, the following appear to be of particular importance in treatment planning.

1. **Cerebral cortical dysfunction**. Some impulsive persons may suffer from cerebral cortical dysfunction. Early studies using electroencephalographic techniques and provocative testing with procaine injections attempted to correlate impaired control of impulsivity with temporolimbic seizures. Although subsequent investigations have not confirmed this hypothesis, positron emission tomography results have suggested a link between impulsive aggression and orbitofrontal hypometabolism.

2. **Serotonergic pathway alterations**. A number of studies suggest that a dysfunction of serotonergic neurotransmission underlies aspects of impulsive behavior. Some patients with personality disorder who have committed suicide by violent methods or who have displayed violent or aggressive behavior have been found to have decreased cerebrospinal fluid 5-hydroxyindoleacetic acid levels and a diminished prolactin response to the serotonin releaser **fenfluramine** (see Chapter 17).

3. **Adrenergic pathway alterations**. Some impulsive persons who exhibit a high degree of self-stimulating or sensation-seeking behavior may have dysfunctional noradrenergic neurotransmission. Evidence consistent with this hypothesis includes studies in which growth hormone responses to **clonidine** administration were correlated with the presence of aggressive behavior. The noradrenergic system may not be the primary site of dysfunction, however, because serotonergic, noradrenergic, and dopaminergic systems are interactive.

4. **Adult attention deficit hyperactivity disorder (ADHD)** (see Chapter 22). Some persons with impulsive or distractible behavior may be demonstrating elements of an adult form of ADHD. In such persons, a

childhood history of ADHD is typically present. This presentation may be misdiagnosed as antisocial personality disorder, or it may serve as an antecedent to personality changes consistent with that disorder.

C. **Affective Instability**

This disorder can be defined as a vulnerability to rapidly shifting mood states that are reversible and reactive to environmental events (e.g., separation, loss, frustration, rejection, criticism). Some affectively unstable persons appear highly "reward dependent"; they feel good when they are receiving praise or applause, even in symbolic forms. Their moods may rapidly plummet, however, when they feel neglected, unwanted, or unappreciated. At times, affective instability may form the basis for dysfunctional interpersonal sensitivity. Impairment of affective stability may result in fluctuating self-esteem, inhibited or avoidant behavior, or difficulties in modulating emotional responses. Disturbances of this dimension are particularly common among patients with histrionic, borderline, narcissistic, and antisocial personality disorders. Among the family members of some patients with BPD, the trait of affective instability has been shown to be relatively frequent. Some have hypothesized that this lability represents a variant form of mood disorder, because disordered mood is also frequent among the relatives of patients with BPD. This is consistent with the observation from sleep studies of shortened rapid eye movement latency, a putative marker of major depression, in some patients with BPD.

D. **Anxiety**

Anxiety (see Chapter 14), which may at times appear as high "harm avoidance," is most likely a dimension of personality with heterogeneous origins, involving physiologic and subjective responses to novelty or threat. Patients with avoidant, borderline, compulsive, dependent, or histrionic personality disorders may experience excessive anxiety. As noted earlier, one hypothesis is that heightened autonomic reactivity in the face of novel stimuli characterizes some individuals who are excessively shy. No unifying biologic basis, however, has been convincingly identified for this personality dimension. Panic attacks are frequent among overdramatizing patients with personality disorders; they can also occur in people of all ages who have no obvious underlying psychopathology. The free-floating anxiety seen in many anxious patients most likely has a different basis.

III. **A Dimensional Approach to the Use of Pharmacotherapy; Empiric Pharmacotherapy Findings from the Literature**

For many years in the United States, individual insight-oriented psychotherapy has remained the mainstay of treatment of personality disorders; this pattern has persisted even though studies confirming its efficacy are limited. Self-psychology, supportive therapy, cognitive-behavioral approaches, dialectic behavior therapy, and group therapy are also advocated and practiced. In recent years, some attempts have been made to elucidate shared or differentiating features of these disorders relevant to psychotherapeutic interventions.

Medications are still regarded by some patients and clinicians as superfluous or harmful to the treatment of personality disorders. Others regard pharmacotherapy as acceptable, but primarily in a symbolic sense—as a tangible manifestation of the therapist's effort to relieve the patient's suffering. This view is reflected in the following paraphrased statement of one such authority: "*Just as you cannot teach a foreign language by giving a medication, you cannot expect medication to change character.*" Results, however, from a growing body of empiric medication trials undertaken in patients with personality disorders suggest that pharmacotherapy can diminish the intensity or frequency of certain symptom patterns. These studies have been conducted in patient groups selected for their diagnostic homogeneity. Because of the unavoidable and inevitable comorbidity for additional personality disorders in these cohorts, however, considering them also to be studies of the treatment of symptom dimensions across these comorbid disorder categories seems plausible.

A. For Cognitive and Perceptual Abnormalities

The usefulness of low-dose treatment with antipsychotic agents was initially reported before DSM-III in a small cohort of patients termed "borderline," each of whom also had at least one persistent psychotic symptom. None had responded completely to any of a variety of prior medications. With conventional antipsychotic agents, however, improvement was observed across a range of symptoms, including tangentiality, distractibility, social withdrawal, thought slippage, cognitive dysfunction, and overt psychotic symptoms. In an uncontrolled trial in 80 outpatients with BPD, reductions of hostility and suspiciousness were observed after treatment with either **loxapine** (mean daily dose, 14 mg) or **chlorpromazine** (mean daily dose, 110 mg). In another uncontrolled study, **thiothixene** (mean daily dose, 9.4 mg) or **haloperidol** (mean daily dose, 3 mg) diminished psychoticism, illusions, ideas of reference, paranoid ideation, and derealization in 52 outpatients with BPD or schizotypal personality disorder. A subsequent uncontrolled trial suggested that **thioridazine** (mean daily dose, 92 mg) reduced paranoid ideation in a small group of outpatients with BPD. Among the atypical antipsychotic agents, **clozapine** (25 to 100 mg per day) has been reported to be helpful in a group of treatment-resistant BPD inpatients with psychotic symptoms, and **olanzapine** (2.5 to 10 mg per day) has been reported to be helpful in a group of outpatients with BPD and comorbid dysthymic disorder.

Several controlled studies have addressed the effects of antipsychotic agents on cognitive and perceptual dysfunction among patients with BPD or schizotypal personality disorder. Using **thiothixene** (mean daily dose, 8.67 mg) in 50 such outpatients, one group observed a significant reduction of illusions and ideas of reference. The composition of this cohort of patients was skewed toward schizotypal by a requirement that each patient must have at least one psychotic symptom. Another group compared **haloperidol** (mean daily dose, 7.24 mg) with **amitriptyline** (mean daily dose, 148 mg) and noted the superiority of **haloperidol** for treating paranoid ideation or psychoticism in 64 patients with BPD or schizotypal personality disorder.

In all of these studies, the clinical improvement has been significant but modest. Furthermore, a 16-week continuation-phase study in a cohort of patients with BPD who had initially improved on **haloperidol** revealed that the improvement was circumscribed and that the treatment discontinuation was disappointingly frequent.

B. Impulsivity and Aggressiveness

These traits, possibly reflecting a more heterogeneous group of behaviors than cognitive or perceptual impairments, have been treated with some success in various clinical populations with a variety of medications. The pathophysiology of aggressivity almost certainly cuts a swath across current personality disorder distinctions. Antipsychotic agents, psychostimulants, anticonvulsants, **lithium**, monoamine oxidase inhibitors (MAOIs), and selected proserotonergic agents may all have useful, but limited, roles in the treatment of this dimension.

On rare occasions, impulsivity and aggression are the consequences of emerging psychosis in some patients with personality disorders. More often, impaired integration of environmental cues by an individual with a limited repertoire of behavioral responses may lead to impulsive or aggressive reactions in overly frustrating situations. In some instances, antipsychotic agents reduce these symptoms through their antipsychotic actions. More frequently, however, they appear to modulate aggressive behavior in nonpsychotic patients via a nonspecific and inadequately understood quieting effect. Their use, although it has long been established, is increasingly recognized as less focal with respect to this target dimension. Reductions in anger attacks or other aspects of dyscontrol have been noted after the use of antipsychotic agents in patients with BPD or schizotypal personality disorder. In one study, patients with BPD viewed themselves as unchanged in impulsivity or suicidality when treated with **trifluoper-azine**, yet they were assessed to be less suicidal by their physicians. Although antipsychotic agents, both conventional and atypical, are not the first-line agents for impulsivity, at low doses they may still have a treatment role as an alternative or complementary intervention.

The use of proserotonergic medications arises from findings linking altered or deficient serotonergic functioning with aggression in patients with personality disorders. **Fenfluramine**, a serotonin agonist that is no longer available in the United States, was found to reduce suicidal behavior in a small series of patients with various psychotic diagnoses. **Fluoxetine**, a serotonin reuptake inhibitor, reduced impulsivity and self-injurious behavior in several studies of patients with BPD. Similarly, **sertraline**, **venlafaxine**, and **citalopram** have reportedly reduced aggressiveness, irritability, or self-injurious behavior in reports on small cohorts of patients.

Some aggressive patients may have a neurodevelopmental or neurologic impairment that hampers their capacity to cope with complex and potentially overwhelming external and internal stimuli. For those who suffer from an adult form of ADHD, treatment with stimulants may stabilize functioning and reduce impulsivity, hyperactivity, or hostility (see Chapter 22). When impulsivity is linked with an electroencephalographic abnormality or a history of seizures, a carefully monitored anticonvulsant trial may be of value. **Phenytoin**, although it is at present rarely used for this purpose, was previously assessed as a treatment for impulsivity. **Carbamazepine** (average dose of 820 mg per day) was found to improve behavioral dyscontrol, impulsivity, anger, and suicidality in one group of patients with mixed personality disorders. **Divalproex sodium** (daily dose range of 1,000 to 2,000 mg), **gabapentin** (mean daily dose, 900 mg), and **lamotrigine** (daily dose range, 75 to 300 mg) have each been reported as helpful in small series of patients with BPD. Interestingly, some patients without detectable electroencephalographic abnormalities may also respond to an anticonvulsant, thus suggesting that the mood-stabilizing effects of an anticonvulsant may be more relevant to its beneficial effects in these patients than are its antiseizure effects.

Lithium, another mood-stabilizing agent, was studied in a group of patients with emotionally unstable character disorder, a forerunner to the diagnosis of BPD. Its use reduced both impulsivity and mood lability. Another study that investigated the effects of **lithium** among a group of prison inmates found a reduction in aggressive behaviors with blood levels averaging about 0.9 mEq per L.

Although tricyclic antidepressants have not been shown to reduce aggression (*note:* **amitriptyline** was noted to increase suicidality and hostility in one study of patients with BPD), MAOIs have shown some efficacy in at least two relevant studies. One explored the use of **phenelzine** in patients considered to be suffering from hysteroid dysphoria and found a reduction in behavioral impulsivity at doses of 15 to 75 mg per day. Another noted lower levels of impulsivity among patients treated with **tranylcypromine** (mean daily dose, 40 mg).

C. Dysphoria and Affective Instability

Although they are often lumped together, these are distinctly different from each other. **Dysphoria**, an undifferentiated feeling of emotional discomfort, is a disturbance of mood content, and it may reflect underlying major depressive disorder, atypical depressive states, anxiety, rage, boredom, or emptiness. Dysphoria is found in many patients with personality disorders. **Tranylcypromine, phenelzine**, or **isocarboxazid** may be effective in alleviating some patients' dysphoria. Others may respond, possibly with less specificity, to benzodiazepines or antipsychotic agents.

The pharmacotherapy of **affective instability**, which can be considered a disturbance of mood maintenance, is becoming increasingly understood.

This dimension of personality has responded to several classes of medications. In several studies, antipsychotic agents have been shown to have mood-stabilizing effects. Some investigators have even claimed that the low-dose use of antipsychotic agents can result in a reduction of excessive rejection sensitivity. As early as the 1960s, **chlorpromazine** use was noted to have a stabilizing effect on affective functioning, and, in a comparison with **amitriptyline**, **haloperidol** has been shown to be more helpful in stabilizing mood. **Haloperidol** (mean daily dose, 3 mg) and **thiothixene** (mean daily dose, 9.4 mg) were both observed to improve interpersonal functioning in one uncontrolled comparison. In a placebo-controlled trial, **trifluoperazine** (mean daily dose, 7.8 mg) improved patient-rated depression and rejection sensitivity. More recently, **thioridazine** (mean daily dose, 92 mg) and **olanzapine** (mean daily dose, 7.7 mg) were separately reported in small cohorts to reduce dysfunctional interpersonal sensitivity.

Antidepressants of all categories have also been used to treat dysphoria or affective instability. Tricyclic antidepressant use has yielded mixed results. Both **amitriptyline** and **imipramine** have helped in some patients, but they may have worsened mood lability in others. Unfortunately, when increases in anger, hostility, or suicidality occur, determining whether such worsening reflects the underlying disorder or if it has arisen secondary to treatment is not possible. The presence or history of hypomanic symptoms in a patient probably should discourage the use of cyclic antidepressants for treating affective instability. **Mianserin**, an antidepressant that is not marketed in the United States and that is structurally related to **mirtazapine**, failed to reduce suicidality in a group of patients with personality disorders. (*Note:* One small-sample study in fact suggested that **mianserin** may be associated with an increased risk of suicide.)

The MAOIs, on the other hand, seem to be effective at stabilizing affective functioning in some patients with BPD. Interestingly, the presence of "borderline" traits in patients with atypical depression, which is defined operationally as the combination of mood reactivity with reversed (atypical) neurovegetative symptoms, leaden fatigue, or rejection sensitivity, predicts that **phenelzine** may outperform **imipramine**. In patients labeled as hysteroid dysphorics, many of whom have traits consistent with personality disorders, **phenelzine** was shown to improve mood reactivity, problems with being alone, and rejection sensitivity. In another study, both patients and physicians considered **tranylcypromine** to be helpful for depression or rejection sensitivity.

Lithium, as noted in section III.B, has been shown to be useful in reducing emotional lability among a group of young women diagnosed with emotionally unstable character disorder. Surprisingly, in view of its effectiveness in bipolar disorder, no study has yet demonstrated a strong effect of **carbamazepine** on affective instability, although, in one study, a few trial noncompleters did rate themselves as experiencing less rejection sensitivity while taking **carbamazepine**.

D. Anxiety
This very nonspecific symptom, has been treated with many classes of medications. Benzodiazepines, antipsychotic agents, antidepressants, and carbamazepine all appear to have had beneficial effects in some patients. Although many patients with generalized anxiety disorder respond well to benzodiazepines, a situation of greater complexity exists with anxious patients who have personality disorders and who also manifest aggressive or impulsive behaviors. In one study, **alprazolam** (mean daily dose, 4.7 mg) was associated with marked increases in self-destructive behavior in an outpatient group of women diagnosed with BPD and having a history of such behavior; however, in that study, a small number of patients rated **alprazolam** as beneficial. Another report noted an improvement of anxiety in three patients with BPD treated with moderate doses of **alprazolam** (0.5 to 1 mg, four times a day).

Avoidant personality disorder, in which anxiety is invariably prominent, has been compared with social phobia, a phenomenologically overlapping axis I disorder. Avoidant traits in patients with social phobia may respond to **alprazolam,** and anxiety in social phobia has also been successfully treated with MAOIs, **clonazepam,** or **buspirone.** By analogy, any of these medications merits consideration for the treatment of anxiety in patients with personality disorders. The potential for behavioral disinhibition from benzodiazepine use suggests caution, particularly when a history of self-injurious behavior is present.

An anecdotal report of patients with avoidant personality disorder made note of a reduction of social anxiety and an increased sense of well-being with **tranylcypromine, phenelzine,** or **fluoxetine.** Anxiety has also responded well to MAOIs in atypical depressive and hysteroid dysphoric patients, many of whom have personality disorder features. In a treatment study using **tranylcypromine,** patients with BPD rated their anxiety as improved. One authority hypothesized that the somatic components of anxiety are particularly responsive to MAOIs, whereas psychic anxiety may respond preferentially to benzodiazepines.

Antipsychotic agents are known to have a nonspecific anxiety-reducing or calming effect, yet they are not frequently prescribed for this purpose, perhaps because of concerns about acute and long-term side effects. Nevertheless, a reduction of anxiety has been repeatedly demonstrated in patients with BPD and schizotypal personality disorder who are receiving low doses of neuroleptics, including **loxapine, chlorpromazine, haloperidol, thiothixene, trifluoperazine,** and **thioridazine.** When the anxiety is accompanied by a thought disorder, the use of a low dose of an antipsychotic agent may be especially appropriate.

Lithium has not been shown to reduce anxiety in personality disorder patients. **Carbamazepine** and **gabapentin** were each rated as beneficial in separate small-sample studies. Table 13.3 summarizes some potentially useful pharmacotherapeutic interventions for treating symptom dimensions in patients with personality disorders.

IV. Caveats

The use of medications always carries with it a risk of untoward outcomes. Recognition of this is particularly important in patients with personality disorders for a number of reasons. In contrast to the treatment of mood disorders, psychosis, or anxiety disorders, the empiric basis of pharmacotherapeutic recommendations regarding personality disorders is more limited. The diagnostic specificity of these disorders is low, and treatment recommendations are only beginning to address the dimensions of behavior rather than the diagnostic categorization. Their chronicity entails the possibility of a need for extended pharmacotherapy. Because of their ego-syntonic nature, the personality disorders are construed by some to be lifestyle choices rather than as diseases requiring treatment; this complicates the clinician's attempts to differentiate the normal from the abnormal. Some clinicians view the effects of medications as potentially "cosmetic." In this view, medications can have positive effects that enhance already adequate functioning and that move the patient toward a more desirable state. The act of prescribing a medication to enhance a desirable quality rather than to alleviate a disturbing one is a dramatic alteration of the current role of pharmacotherapy (i.e., treating dysfunction, distress, or disease). Such a reframing of pharmacotherapy, which has already taken place among those who advocate so-called smart drugs (i.e., those reputed to enhance intelligence) or prosexual drugs (i.e., those reputed to enhance sexual performance), has far-reaching implications.

No medication currently carries a United States Food and Drug Administration-approved indication for the treatment of personality disorders or their common traits. As Appendix I discusses, the clinician must follow several important steps when he or she makes a decision to prescribe a medication for a nonapproved

TABLE 13.3. SOME POSSIBLE PHARMACOTHERAPIES FOR DIMENSIONS OF PERSONALITY PATHOLOGY[a]

Symptom Cluster	Suggested First-Line Medications	Suggested Second-Line Medications	Use with Caution or Not at All
Cognitive and perceptual impairment (e.g., transient psychotic symptoms, distractibility, thought slippage, suspiciousness)	**Antipsychotic agents** Olanzapine, 2.5–10 mg/d Haloperidol, 2–6 mg/d Clozapine, 25–100 mg/d	None are known	**Psychostimulants** (may exacerbate symptoms)
Impulsive symptoms (self-injurious behavior, suicidal behaviors)	**Mood-stabilizing anticonvulsants** Divalproex sodium, 50–100 μg/d[b] Lamotrigine, 75–300 mg/d Carbamazepine, 4–12 μg/d **Serotonergic agents** Fluoxetine, 5–80 mg/d Sertraline, 25–200 mg/d Citalopram, 5–80 mg/d Venlafaxine, 25–300 mg/d[c]	**Antipsychotic agents** Haloperidol, 2–6 mg/d **Psychostimulants** Dexedrine, 5–10 mg t.i.d. Methylphenidate, 5–15 mg t.i.d.	**Benzodiazepines** (may exacerbate impulsivity or self-injurious behavior)
Mood symptoms (instability, rejection sensitivity, dysphoria, related sleep disturbances)	**Mood-stabilizing anticonvulsants** Divalproex sodium, 50–100 μg/d Lamotrigine, 75–300 mg/d	**Serotonergic agents** Fluoxetine, 5–80 mg/d Sertraline, 25–200 mg/d Citalopram, 5–80 mg/d **Antipsychotic agents** Olanzapine, 2.5–10 mg/d Haloperidol, 2–6 mg/d	**Tricyclic antidepressants** (may exacerbate mood instability)
Anxious symptoms (free-floating, panic, or obsessive anxiety)	**Serotonergic agents** Fluoxetine, 5–80 mg/d Sertraline, 25–200 mg/d Citalopram, 5–80 mg/d Venlafaxine, 25–300 mg/d[c] **Mood-stabilizing anticonvulsants** Divalproex sodium, 50–100 μg/d Lamotrigine, 75–300 mg/d	**Antipsychotic agents** Haloperidol, 2–6 mg/d Olanzapine, 2.5–10 mg/d **Nonbenzodiazepine anxiolytics** Buspirone, 5–20 mg t.i.d.	**MAOIs** (may be associated with unacceptable risks) **Benzodiazepines** (may be associated with risk of misuse)

Abbreviations: MAOIs, monoamine oxidase inhibitors; t.i.d., three times a day.

[a]These recommendations are based on research with patients primarily diagnosed with borderline personality disorder and on the authors' clinical experiences.

[b]Note that, for some agents, concentration ranges are given.

[c]Experience is insufficient to provide dosage ranges for the venlafaxine XR formulation, but use of the XR formulation may be indicated once a dosage has been established for the patient.

indication, including complying with the requirement that the patient understands that the medication use in this role is "off label" and "innovative."

The actual effects of medications on personality disorders are often modest. The degree of benefit may be enough to allow improved functioning, better tolerance of affects, or fuller engagement in psychosocial treatment. Medication in this context is rarely, if ever, "curative." One should note, however, that patients may perceive subjective effects that they consider quite significant, even when effects only of a lesser magnitude are observed by "blind" evaluators. Clinical experience suggests that, in some instances, the medication effects on personality traits may dissipate over a period of months. Whether this decremental change, when it occurs, results from tolerance or adaptation to medication, nonadherence, use of concomitant medications, alcohol or substance abuse, or other factors is not known.

Some medications advocated for treating personality disorder traits are abusable. For example, psychostimulants that may provide significant benefit to an individual affected by ADHD may also provide a greater sense of well-being to patients with BPD without ADHD. Some patients who have heard or read about ADHD may have self-diagnosed a learning disability, which may more truly reflect a wish to function at a level higher than he or she has currently attained. Such a patient might be at risk for psychostimulant abuse.

Benzodiazepines also carry an abuse risk in some patients (see Chapters 9 and 14), in addition to their previously mentioned potential for infrequently causing behavioral disinhibition. When taken in overdose amounts in conjunction with other central nervous system depressants, they may contribute to untoward outcomes. Many other medications are even more dangerous in overdosage (e.g., MAOIs; see Chapter 3).

Adverse physical effects can occur with all agents discussed here. Antipsychotic agents are particularly prone to causing intolerable side effects, including weight gain, sedation, erectile dysfunction, or akathisia. Tardive dyskinesia is a potential long-term hazard. Other medications, such as **carbamazepine** and **lithium**, require careful periodic monitoring to reduce the risk of toxic effects. **Lamotrigine** must be prescribed and monitored with awareness of the potential for serious adverse dermatologic and systemic reactions.[1]

Adverse psychologic effects can also be seen, such as the unpleasantly over-tranquilized or oversedated effect that some patients experience even with very low doses of antipsychotic agents; the anxious, agitated, or paradoxically apathetic states sometimes seen with proserotonergic antidepressants; the increased self-injurious or disinhibited behavior occasionally seen during benzodiazepine use; the confusion, agitation, or hostility that has occasionally been seen in patients receiving **amitriptyline**; and the melancholia-like depressive states that have been observed in some patients taking **carbamazepine** or **thioridazine**.

In planning treatment and discussing objectives with a patient, emphasizing the fact that, as yet, no adequate long-term studies of medication effects on personality have been conducted is valuable. The stability of any beneficial effects, the relapse rates upon discontinuation, and the incidence of long-term adverse effects remain unknown.

V. Assessment of Patients for Treatment

Evaluating the patient with a personality disorder for pharmacotherapy differs in several respects from assessing a patient with an axis I disorder. The symptoms of personality disorders are chronic and ego syntonic, blurring the distinction between "normal" and "pathologic." Many of the personality disorder traits of greatest interest to the clinician wax and wane over time in relationship to such variables as the season, the menstrual cycle, contemporaneous stressors, and the availability of supportive relationships, thus necessitating the

---

[1] **Topiramate** is another anticonvulsant receiving anecdotal use for some behavioral symptoms, including mood lability and promotion of weight loss in patients with antipsychotic agent-induced or antidepressant-induced weight gain. Confusion and memory impairment not infrequently accompany any beneficial effects.

devotion of careful attention to longitudinal functioning. Comorbid axis I syndromes also may be present. Posttraumatic stress disorder, a particularly complex condition for multimodal treatment, is especially important to identify (see Chapters 14 and 27). Mood disorders, anxiety disorders, and psychotic disorders are among other commonly comorbid axis I conditions. The assessment process needs to unfold slowly enough to facilitate information gathering from the patient, a significant other, friends, relatives, and previous caregivers.

The identification of treatment-responsive target symptoms or dimensions requires careful inquiry and tactful negotiation as part of a working alliance. Many patients seeking pharmacotherapy have had prior medication trials. These must be reviewed with attention to their appropriateness for the target symptoms under consideration, the adequacy of dosage and duration, and issues of adherence. To enhance the likelihood of adherence and efficacy, the clinician must thoughtfully inform the patient about potential side effects, the expected duration of treatment, any interactions of the medication with foods or other drugs, the procedure for dealing with missed doses, and the safety or lack thereof from abrupt discontinuation of the medication. Helping the patient conceptualize the way in which pharmacotherapy will complement any other ongoing treatments is also useful.

VI. Treatment Integration: The Psychodynamics of Pharmacotherapy

The pharmacotherapy of personality disturbances offers a modest but significant opportunity to alleviate a spectrum of targeted behavioral disturbances and to promote greater stability. Medications, however, must be a component of a more comprehensive treatment plan that includes other psychosocial interventions, such as individual or group psychotherapy and inpatient care as needed.

The psychodynamic features of the pharmacotherapy relationship should not be overlooked. Even a treatment relationship that is primarily medication oriented has psychotherapeutic elements and exists within a psychodynamic framework. Without attention to elements such as transference (see Chapter 1), pharmacotherapy may have reduced value. As in all therapeutic relationships, a working alliance must be established to allow the treatment to proceed with greatest effectiveness. This "pharmacotherapeutic" alliance may be tested or strengthened when defining the goals for treatment and discussing side effects, the potential for abuse by the particular patient, or the clinician's availability for the resolution of medication-related and non–medication-related difficulties. In delineating the behavior chosen for modification, the clinician can frame the targeted symptom tactfully by identifying it as an alternative that is pursued with some ambivalence within a stressful context (e.g., "When you are overly stressed, you sometimes have trouble containing an urge to react with anger, even when you know that other ways of behaving would more likely help your situation"). This approach can be viewed as a form of "self-psychopharmacology" analogous to the "self-psychology" used by patients to protect themselves from unbearably disruptive injuries to their self image or sense of self that occur in treatment, as well as in other life situations. Attention to the therapeutic alliance also involves a number of practical matters (e.g., consistency, availability, willingness to discuss and to explain alternatives). The last is particularly important because the use of medications for treatment of personality disorders *per se* is not among the indications approved by the United States Food and Drug Administration.

The clinician must also be aware that any alliance may fluctuate and may reflect vacillations in the patient's internal state and relationships. At one time, the clinician may be idealized and at another time devalued and hated. Attempting to maintain consistency and stability throughout these fluctuations and to convey a secure presence and a willingness to remain available while continuing to set appropriate limits is important. Sustaining the alliance over time is often a critical factor in outcome, because multiple medication trials may be necessary and these may be accompanied by unexpected side effects, disappointing therapeutic effects, and frequent dosage adjustments.

Any relationship carries transference elements. Providing medication to a patient may intensify aspects of transference, particularly when patients have expectations and fantasies about the medication(s). Patients' responses vary greatly, however, and a variety of transference reactions may be seen, sometimes in sequence. A common response is for the patient to adopt an idealizing, positive transference toward the prescribing clinician, especially early in treatment when hope abounds. The prescribing clinician may, in fact, be an authoritative and knowledgeable figure, who presents a coherent and nonjudgmental explanation of the patient's difficulties and who seems not to confront the patient with a need to look inward or to face painful past and current experiences. Medication, which some may view with awe and suspicion, may initially be welcomed as a powerful ally. Unfortunately, the inconsistent and sometimes limited results from medication use within the context of longstanding and maladaptive personality traits may be disappointing to some patients, who, after an initial period of significant symptom reduction, may then feel even worse, possibly leading to increased despair and anger. An additional hazard of the initially positive transference toward the prescribing clinician is a concurrent devaluation of any other ongoing treatments, including psychotherapy. The psychotherapist, whose values may stress self-knowledge and long-term dynamic exploration and understanding rather than what he or she views as a "quick fix" from medication, may be toppled from a primary role in the patient's treatment life and may be relegated to a devalued or resented role. This "splitting," if it is unrecognized, may undermine the overall treatment plan.

Some patients seek pharmacotherapy out of a sense of pessimism about their psychotherapy. Others may see medications as agents of control or repression. Still others may experience the taking of pills as a form of identification with an ill relative. Pill taking also can become a way of acting out feelings about a prescribing clinician (e.g., they can be discarded or ingested in excess quantity). Alternatively, medication can be viewed as a comforting "transitional object" that symbolically represents the committed involvement of the concerned clinician.

Motivations for prescribing medications also deserve attention. Countertransference feelings need to be recognized and understood. Both the psychotherapist and the prescribing clinician must remain alert to countertransferential discouragement, particularly when they are the same person, and to wishes to help treatment progress more quickly or less painfully, to control the patient, or to give something tangible to the patient during a hopeless or helpless impasse. Lack of awareness of such factors may complicate and confound treatment.

ADDITIONAL READING

Ayd FJ Jr. Risperidone (Risperdal) treatment for aggressive behavior across the lifespan. *Int Drug Therapy Newslett* 2001;36:33–40.

Book HE. Some psychodynamics of non-compliance. *Can J Psychiatry* 1987;32:115–117.

Brinkley JR, Beitman BD, Friedel RO. Low dose neuroleptic regimens in the treatment of borderline patients. *Arch Gen Psychiatry* 1979;36:319–326.

Cloninger CR. A systematic method for clinical description and classification of personality variants. *Arch Gen Psychiatry* 1984;44:573–588.

Cowdry RW. Psychopharmacology of borderline personality disorder: a review. *J Clin Psychiatry* 1987;48:15–25.

Cowdry RW, Gardner DL. Pharmacotherapy of borderline personality disorder: alprazolam, carbamazepine, trifluoperazine, and tranylcypromine. *Arch Gen Psychiatry* 1988;45:111–119.

Deltito JA, Stam M. Psychopharmacological treatment of avoidant personality disorder. *Compr Psychiatry* 1989;30:498–504.

Faltus FJ. The positive effect of alprazolam in the treatment of three patients with borderline personality disorder. *Am J Psychiatry* 1984;141:802–803.

Frances AJ, Widiger T. The classification of personality disorders: an overview of problems and solutions. In: Frances AJ, Hales RE, eds. *Psychiatry update*. Vol. 5. Washington, D.C.: American Psychiatric Press, 1986:240–257.

Fuller RW. The influence of fluoxetine on aggressive behavior. *Neuropsychopharmacology* 1996;14:77–81.

Goodman M, New A. Impulsive aggression in borderline personality disorder. *Curr Psychiatry Rep* 2000;2:56–61.

Hermann N, Lanctôt K, Myszak M. Effectiveness of gabapentin for the treatment of behavioral disorders in dementia. *J Clin Psychopharmacol* 2000;20:90–93.

Hollander E. Managing aggressive behavior in patients with obsessive-compulsive disorder and borderline personality disorder. *J Clin Psychiatry* 1999;60:38–44.

Kagan J, Reznick JS, Snidman N. Biological bases of childhood shyness. *Science* 1988;240:167–171.

Lahmeyer HW, Reynolds CF III, Kupfer DJ, et al. Biologic markers in borderline personality disorder: a review. *J Clin Psychiatry* 1989;50:217–225.

Liebowitz MR, Fyer AJ, Gorman JM, et al. Phenelzine in social phobia. *J Clin Psychopharmacol* 1986;6:93–98.

Liebowitz MR, Quitkin FM, Stewart JW, et al. Antidepressant specificity in atypical depression. *Arch Gen Psychiatry* 1988;45:129–137.

Oquendo MA, Mann JJ. The biology of impulsivity and suicidality. *Psychiatric Clin North Am* 2000;23:11–25.

Pinto OC, Akiskal HS. Lamotrigine as a promising approach to borderline personality: an open case series without concurrent DSM-IV major mood disorder. *J Affect Disord* 1998;51:333–343.

Reich J, Noyes R, Yates W. Alprazolam treatment of avoidant personality traits in social phobic patients. *J Clin Psychiatry* 1989;50:91–95.

Rifkin A, Quitkin F, Carrillo C, et al. Lithium carbonate in emotionally unstable character disorder. *Arch Gen Psychiatry* 1972;27:519–523.

Schulz SC, Camlin KL, Berry SA, et al. Olanzapine safety and efficacy in patients with borderline personality disorder and comorbid dysthymia. *Biol Psychiatry* 1999;46:1429–1435.

Schulz SC, Cornelius J, Jarrett DB, et al. Pharmacodynamic probes in personality disorders. *Psychopharmacol Bull* 1987;23:337–341.

Shader RI, Scharfman EL, Dreyfuss DA. A biological model for selected personality disorders. In: Cooper AM, Frances AJ, Sacks MH, eds. *Psychiatry*. Vol. 1. New York: Basic Books, 1986:41–51.

Sheard MH, Marini JL, Bridges CI, et al. The effect of lithium on impulsive aggressive behavior in man. *Am J Psychiatry* 1976;133:1409–1413.

Siever LJ, Davis KL. A psychobiological perspective on the personality disorders. *Am J Psychiatry* 1991;148:1647–1658.

Silk KR, ed. *Biology of personality disorders*. Washington, D.C.: American Psychiatric Press, 1998.

Silverman JM, Pinkham L, Horvath TB, et al. Affective and impulsive personality disorder traits in the relatives of patients with borderline personality disorder. *Am J Psychiatry* 1991;148:1378–1385.

Soloff PH. Psychopharmacology of borderline personality disorder. *Psychiatric Clin North Am* 2000;23:169–192.

Tellegen A, Lykken DT, Bouchard TJ Jr, et al. Personality similarity in twins reared apart and together. *J Pers Soc Psychol* 1988;54:1031–1039.

Thomas A, Chess S. Genesis and evolution of behavioral disorders: from infancy to early adult life. *Am J Psychiatry* 1984;141:1–9.

Vaillant G, Perry JC. *Personality disorders*. In: Kaplan HI, Sadock BJ, eds. *Comprehensive textbook of psychiatry IV*. Baltimore: Williams and Wilkins, 1985:959–986.

Waldinger RJ, Frank A. Transference and the vicissitudes of medication use by borderline patients. *Psychiatry* 1989;52:416–427.

Zuckerman M. *Psychobiology of personality*. Cambridge: Cambridge University Press, 1991.

14. APPROACHES TO THE TREATMENT OF ANXIETY STATES[1]

Richard I. Shader
David J. Greenblatt

Anxiety is a ubiquitous experience. Many people function against a backdrop of anxiety generated by life's stresses, upheavals, stages, and phases every day. Anxiety is part of the internal signal system that alerts individuals to changes in their bodies and in the world around them. It can be adaptive or maladaptive, and it can generate concern or overconcern. Some degree of anxiety is experienced not only when things go wrong, but also when things are changed, unexpected, or just novel. Anxiety is an essential, but at times unpleasant, sense of tension, apprehension, or uneasiness that is experienced subjectively as apprehension or dread or that is observed in predictable, if idiosyncratic, physiologic changes, such as difficulty breathing, muscle tension, and shakiness. Most familiar is a pattern including clammy palms, "butterflies" in the stomach, racing pulse, and pounding in the chest that may occur when an imminent threat is sensed and the individual is alerted to cope with it. Another common presentation is the chronic worrier who looks tense and pale and whose brow is furrowed from the constant strain. Other typical complaints include intrusive thoughts (e.g., images, ruminations, frightening dreams), vigilance or trouble concentrating, or altered awareness of one's self or one's environment (e.g., depersonalization, derealization).

Coping with a serious threat or danger is usually accomplished through some form of **fight** or **flight**. The latter can take many forms, including escape and avoidance. Other responses, such as **freezing** and **fragmentation**, are less common, and thus they do not receive a comparable amount of attention. The still, crouched fawn "hiding" from danger is a familiar image. People seem to hide more to protect their sense of self (ego) than their bodies (see Chapter 1). Freezing and fragmentation are ego-protective responses, and these include distortion; displacement; and various forms of disconnection, including dissociation (see Chapter 4). Some anxious people may seem as if they pull the covers over their heads in much the same way that the ostrich buries its head in the sand. Dissociation is likely to occur when the threat feels overwhelming or when it comes from a trusted person.

Considerable overlap between anxiety and fear is observed when the threat or danger is external and real. In this context, anxiety has come to mean an exaggerated or excessive response that is disproportionate to the threat or the objective reality. The term anxiety is also used when the source of the threat is largely unrecognized, obscure, or unknown. This may occur when the anxiety reflects a conditioned response in which the connections to the original threatening stimulus are now suppressed, repressed, forgotten, or lost. Anxiety can also occur when one's sense of being able to take protective steps or effective action is blocked. Anxiety can be situational, intermittent or attack-like, or persistent; most often it is short-lived. When it reaches distressing levels and interferes with functioning, a clinical diagnosis of an anxiety disorder is made.

Clinical experience, controlled trials of pharmacologic treatment, and epidemiologic studies have led to a recognition of the need to separate anxiety as a symptom or momentary state from the more chronic or trait-like presentations. This has resulted in the development of a series of diagnostic criteria for various anxiety disorders and has increased recognition of their prevalence, natural history, and costs to society.

I. General Considerations

Widely accepted criteria for the diagnosis of anxiety disorders and their subtypes appear in currently used diagnostic manuals, such as the *Diagnostic and Statistical Manual of Mental Disorders,* 4th edition, (DSM-IV) and the *Inter-*

---

[1]This chapter is partly based on other publications by both authors that appear among the works listed under Additional Reading.

national Statistical Classification of Diseases and Related Health Problems, tenth revision (ICD-10). Such diagnostic criteria generally include qualitative or descriptive features, with quantitative requirements for how many specific symptoms must be present, how often they must occur, and how long they should be present (*note:* by themselves, descriptive criteria convey no information about etiology).

Some of the following distinctions about anxiety states may seem arbitrary, but they are consistent with and are derived from clinical observation and patients' reports. The clinician should also note that anxiety rarely occurs in isolation; other accompanying symptoms, such as depression, anger, and somatic complaints, are common. Table 14.1 lists some of the many descriptors and complaints that are mentioned by anxious people or that are observed by their clinicians. Table 14.2 provides a simplified approach to differentiating, at a clinical level, among categories of anxiety delineated in the DSM-IV. Some of these are also discussed below and in section III in more detail.

The following subsections consider presentations of anxiety that are descriptively useful but that do not always constitute or conform to recognized diagnostic categories. Because many of the presentations of anxiety respond to the same medications, the idea that they represent phenotypic variations of the same underlying pathologic processes is quite possible. Some intervention strategies are also noted for each broad category.

A. Situational Anxiety

Situational anxiety, which is also known as context-specific anxiety, describes reactions to a variety of stressful stimuli, such as interviews, tests, public speaking, planned presentations, auditions, and surgery. Such anxiety

TABLE 14.1. COMMON OBJECTIVE AND SUBJECTIVE DESCRIPTORS AND SYMPTOMS ASSOCIATED WITH ANXIETY STATES

Abdominal cramps	Nauseated
Anorexia	Overconcerned
Anxious	Pallor
Apprehensive	Palpitations
Breathless	Panicky
Butterflies in the stomach	Phobic
Chest pains	Preoccupied
Choking sensations	Pupils dilated
Churning inside	Rapid respirations or respiratory
Clutched up	distress (hyperpnea)
Diarrhea	Restless
Dizzy	Scared for no reason
Dread	Shaky
Dry mouth	Sweating
Easily startled	Syncope
Faint	Tense
Fearful	Terrified
Flushing	Threatened
Frightened	Tightness in the chest
Giddy	Tremulous
Headache	Troubled
Heart racing (tachycardia)	Uneasy
Impending doom feelings	Urge to urinate (and frequent urination)
Jittery	Vertigo
Jumpy	Vomiting
Keyed up	Weakness
Lightheaded	Worried
Muscle tension	Wound up

TABLE 14.2. A SIMPLIFIED APPROACH TO DIFFERENTIATING AMONG FORMS OF ANXIETY

Description	Diagnosis	Usual Age at Onset
Innate or conditioned or learned fears	Simple (specific) phobias	Childhood or later
Social discomfort, shyness, a sense of not fitting in	Social phobia (social anxiety disorder)	Peaks in mid-adolescence or later
Excessive worry about the consequences of what you have done or not done or excessive worry about what lies ahead or about things that have not yet happened	Generalized anxiety disorder	Late adolescence or later
Worry and discomfort or distress when away from familiar places (e.g., home) or out of contact with people to whom one is especially attached, even for brief periods of time; avoidance of anxiety-provoking contexts	Separation anxiety; likely also seen in borderline personality disorder; likely present in agoraphobia[a]	Childhood or later
Traumatic anxiety from experiences that overwhelm coping capacities	Posttraumatic stress disorder	Childhood or later
Rituals, acts, or repetitive thoughts (sometimes intended to ward off danger)	Obsessive-compulsive disorder	Childhood or later
Panic attacks that sometimes occur spontaneously or without apparent triggers or contexts	Panic disorder	Late adolescence or later
Panic attacks that culminate after incremental anxiety	Any of the above	Uncommon in childhood

[a]The authors consider agoraphobia to be a coping strategy rather than a diagnosis.

is usually short-lived, and it ends once the experience is started or completed. Situational anxiety can reflect worry about, or fear of, the unknown; it can also be colored by a patient's low self-esteem. In these instances, irrational fears of rejection, failure, criticism, and social or interpersonal catastrophe may be prominent. Clinical and research experiences suggest that preparing and informing the patient may quiet situational anxiety. Examples include preparation for surgery by preoperative discussions with anesthesiologists, role playing or rehearsal in preparation for job interviews, and assertiveness training. However, this approach is less likely to be adequate when sensitive self-esteem issues or a high degree of irrationality are involved. For many patients, their own use of denial and minimization is sufficient. Some patients may benefit from pharmacotherapy (e.g., the short-term use of β-adrenergic receptor antagonists for performance or public speaking anxiety). Some degree of situational anxiety is usually seen in all forms of formal anxiety disorders, including **generalized anxiety disorder** (GAD), **panic disorder** (PD), **specific phobia**, **social phobia**, **posttraumatic stress disorder** (PTSD), and **obsessive-compulsive disorder** (see Chapter 6).

So-called illness or cancer phobias are sometimes considered situational because they can occur after hearing of an illness in someone else. They are not true phobias (see section I.B) because nothing that can be avoided to bring relief is present. Similarly, a reassuring physical examination rarely brings relief. Cancer and other illness phobias sometimes have an obsessional or delusional component (see Chapters 4 and 6); they usually occur along with other evidence of obsessional thinking or depression. Such illness phobias may also result from the somatic delusions that may occur in psychotic depressions (see Chapter 18).

B. Phobic Anxiety

This condition is a form of situational or context-dependent anxiety in which the primary method of coping is avoidance. In some instances, the etiology of the phobia is clearly discernible, and how to help is straightforward. For example, if a child is bitten by a dog and thereafter she fears being in the presence of dogs, one suitable approach would be systematic desensitization as follows: a planned progressive exposure to the fear-inducing stimulus using a friendly dog or its facsimile (e.g., photographs of a dog). Carefully planned increments of exposure are augmented by teaching the patient how to relax before confronting the threat and sometimes by coadministration of the appropriate pharmacotherapy. In patients who fear open spaces, heights, or elevators, the etiology and treatment may be more complex. Exposure and desensitization techniques combined with pharmacotherapy can be beneficial, particularly when these situations trigger panic attacks.

The intensity of and impairment from phobic feelings vary greatly from person to person. For example, among people who actually fly in airplanes, about 75% have no fears of flying. About 15% are anxious when they fly. The remaining 10% are quite afraid when they fly, yet they manage to fly. What differentiates this last group from those whose fear of flying keeps them grounded or that even stops them from boarding an airplane that remains on the ground is not at all clear.

Even more complex are those phobias in which the feared object has a private, symbolic, or unconscious meaning. These types of phobias are most likely to develop in the context of interpersonal conflict; they involve coping mechanisms such as projection, displacement, and regression. When these are present, supplementing pharmacotherapeutic approaches with other psychotherapeutic techniques designed to help the patient understand the evolution of the phobic anxiety in terms of his or her particular life experiences may be important.

C. Anticipatory Anxiety

Anticipatory anxiety (worry, anxious apprehension) is frequently associated with phobic anxiety, situational anxiety, or panic attacks. This, at times, is an arbitrary distinction, but many patients can describe anxiety that precedes the actual contact with dreaded objects or situations or can relate fears of having attacks of anxiety or panic. The intensity of anticipatory anxiety is highly variable, ranging from a mild sense of anticipation to extreme vigilance. When an acute intervention is needed, benzodiazepine anxiolytics are often beneficial.

D. Free-Floating Anxiety

This anxiety bears no close temporal relationship to the precipitating events or fear-inducing stimuli. It can sometimes be intense enough to feel like an unfocused sense of dread. It can present as a pattern of indiscriminate worry or anxious apprehension, and it is a major component of GAD. Careful inquiry sometimes reveals precipitants for the anxiety; for example, something triggered the emergence of forbidden feelings or painful memories, which were quickly suppressed, but the anxiety remained. Free-floating anxiety may vary in duration from hours to days; most patients describe it as chronic and as persisting over weeks to months. Pharmacotherapy is often effective for free-floating anxiety.

E. Traumatic Anxiety

Traumatic anxiety is a distinctive type of anxiety that occurs in survivors of tragic and usually unanticipated experiences, such as natural disasters (e.g., sudden floods, tornadoes, and fires) and shipwrecks. It can also appear in those who are involved in wars or other overwhelming events, such as rape (see Chapter 27) or kidnapping. It is usually associated with sleep disturbances or nightmares that involve the overwhelming event and with a daytime syndrome of anxiety, restlessness, irritability, headache, overactive startle reflex, feelings of isolation and distrust, a sense of inadequacy, and the restriction of social contacts and activities that may include reliving parts of the experience. When its appearance is delayed and sufficient impairment of functioning occurs, a diagnosis of PTSD is made.

Traumatic anxiety is less common in those who are able to participate in a helpful or effective manner during or after the traumatic event. Group discussion and grief work (see Chapter 16) can be valuable. Pharmacotherapy should be delayed until a careful workup can be carried out to identify the presence of a postconcussion syndrome or occult intracranial or extracranial bleeding. When such complications can be ruled out, relief from the stressor and rest—sometimes assisted by the judicious use of antianxiety agents— are the cornerstones of initial care. In DSM-IV, traumatic anxiety can be classified as acute stress disorder or as PTSD.

F. Psychotic Terror

This can be quite dramatic in the acutely disorganized, frightened, and easily startled patient. Paranoia and hallucinations may be prominent. Visual hallucinations in such patients may indicate a toxic psychosis due to amphetamines, **cocaine**, or anticholinergic substances. Some schizophrenic patients describe an earlier stage in their decompensations during which they feel anxious and fear they are "going crazy." Treatment with antipsychotic agents is usually indicated (see Chapter 20), except in some toxic psychoses. When possible, the treatment of psychotic terror should include avoidance of overstimulation by providing a calm environment and familiar persons to stay with the patient. In rare instances, the use of seclusion may be beneficial (see Chapter 25).

G. Anxious Depression

In **anxious depression**, anxiety, tension, or agitation accompanies overt depressive affect. Over 60% of anxious patients eventually have symptoms of depression. Other patients are chronically depressed, with intermittent exacerbations of anxiety symptoms; they frequently complain of difficulty in falling asleep in addition to their early morning awakening (see Chapter 18). When the depressive picture is of minimal to mild intensity, psychotherapy aimed at altering negative styles of thinking and low self-esteem or at uncovering and articulating any underlying issues of disappointment, defeat, demoralization, or unresolved loss can be beneficial. Getting patients in touch with their anger and resentment may also be helpful because anxiety-bound hostility and guilt are sometimes prominent. Patients with concomitant anxiety and depression respond to a variety of pharmacotherapies, including benzodiazepines; selective serotonin reuptake inhibitors (SSRIs); more mixed inhibitors of monoamine reuptake (e.g., **venlafaxine**); tricyclic antidepressants (TCAs), such as **doxepin** and **amitriptyline**; and monamine oxidase inhibitors (MAOIs).

Caution is essential when treating elderly patients with anxiety and depression. Excessive sedation and resulting motor incoordination can have unwanted consequences, as can the anticholinergic, hypotensive, and arrhythmia-inducing properties of the TCAs. Combinations of low doses of antipsychotic agents and TCAs (e.g., **perphenazine** and **amitriptyline**) are still used in some countries and in some primary care settings, but few advantages appear to result from this approach unless psychotic elements are part of the presenting clinical picture.

H. Anxiety Secondary to Medical Conditions

These considerations must also include anxiety secondary to medical conditions. Table 14.3 lists medical conditions that may present with overt anxiety symptoms. Treatment should always be directed at the underlying medical condition. The anxiety associated with angina, for example, is best treated with **nitroglycerin**. Symptomatic treatment may be helpful in some

TABLE 14.3. SOME CONDITIONS THAT MAY PRESENT WITH PROMINENT ANXIETY SYMPTOMS

Akathisia secondary to dopamine receptor antagonists or selective serotonin reuptake inhibitors
Angina pectoris
Aspirin intolerance
Bad trips and drug intoxications
Behavioral toxicity from drugs
Caffeinism
Carcinoid
Cerebral arteriosclerosis
Congestive heart failure
Epilepsy, particularly psychomotor or temporal lobe epilepsy
Hyperdynamic β-adrenergic circulatory state (hyperventilation)
Hypoglycemia, hyperinsulinism
Hypoxic states (obstructive pulmonary disease, asthma)
Ménière disease
Mitral valve prolapse
Pain
Paroxysmal tachyarrhythmias and other cardiac arrhythmias
Pheochromocytoma
Premenstrual tension
Pulmonary embolism
Thyrotoxicosis (hyperthyroidism) or use of thyroid hormones
Use of monosodium glutamate
Use of stimulants or sympathomimetic agents (e.g., anorexigenics, decongestants)
Withdrawal from central nervous system depressant drugs

conditions. Low doses of antipsychotic agents (e.g., **risperidone, haloperidol**) may be beneficial in some patients who show anxiety and agitation associated with delirium or dementia (see Chapter 5). Hypoxic states that produce anxiety or agitation are best treated with **oxygen**, rather than with sedative-hypnotics, anxiolytics, or antipsychotic agents, some of which could actually produce a further degree of respiratory depression. Stress also may be a factor in the medical conditions not listed in Table 14.3. For example, some patients with chronic dermatologic conditions, hypertension, or peptic ulcer may benefit from antianxiety agents even in the absence of overt anxiety.

II. Stress

Stress is not an anxiety disorder, nor is it a normative concept (i.e., everyone experiences stress); a person typically is stressed when positive or negative (e.g., threatening) experiences temporarily strain or overwhelm adaptive capacities. Stress is highly individualized, and it depends on variables such as the novelty, rate, intensity, duration, or personal interpretation of the input and genetic or experiential factors. From the stress perspective, even too much of a good thing can quite possibly be a source of stress—one person's fun may be another person's stressor.

Both acute and chronic stress can intensify morbidity from anxiety disorders. Panic attacks, for example, are more frequent when the predisposed person is exposed to stressors. Stress-reduction strategies can be helpful to many anxious patients. Unfortunately, many anxious persons cannot concentrate enough to use such strategies for acute relief effectively. Most stress-reduction techniques have their greatest utility as elements of a prevention plan that attempts to raise one's threshold to anxiety-provoking experiences. Table 14.4 lists the **5Rs**—the core concepts that are the basic elements in a stress-reduction or anxiety-reduction program.

TABLE 14.4. "THE FIVE Rs": CORE CONCEPTS USED IN THE REDUCTION OF ANXIETY OR STRESS

Recognition of the causes and sources of the threat or distress; education and consciousness raising
Relationships identified for support, help, reassurance
Removal from or of the threat or stressor; managing the stimulus
Relaxation through techniques, such as meditation, massage, breathing exercises, or imagery
Reengagement through managed reexposure and desensitization

From Shader RI. Stress, fear, and anxiety. In: Tupin JP, Shader RI, Harnett DS, eds. *Handbook of clinical psychopharmacology.* Northvale, NJ: Aronson, 1988:73–96, with permission.

Meditation techniques are currently popular, and these may be beneficial to some stress-prone or potentially anxious persons. Many variations exist (see Appendix IV). Most meditation techniques share common elements: (a) a focusing chant or mantra that distracts one from preoccupying thoughts and feelings, (b) deep rhythmic (usually abdominal) breathing that emphasizes a prolonged expiratory phase, and (c) muscle relaxation. For more information on stress reduction or meditation, the interested reader is encouraged to consult relevant references. Many factors influence people's choices of interventions and treatments. Table 14.5 lists some of the factors affecting both the choice and outcome of interventions for stress and of treatments for anxiety states and disorders.

For task-related or occupation-related stress, developing approaches that reduce stress is often possible. Table 14.6 lists one such effective strategy ("**LESS STRESS**"). Simple physical exercises that can be done in the workplace are also useful. These primarily involve relaxing tense muscles of the head, neck, or shoulders by stretching and relaxing the affected muscles in an alternating manner (e.g., squeezing a tennis ball to relieve writer's cramp).

III. Diagnostic Features of Anxiety Disorders
A. Generalized Anxiety Disorder

This syndrome is broadly recognized as being responsive in varying degrees to pharmacotherapy with benzodiazepines, azapirones (e.g., **buspirone**), SSRIs, or the mixed monoamine reuptake inhibitor **venlafaxine**. Unrealistic or excessive anxiety or worry about life circumstances characterizes the

TABLE 14.5. SOME FACTORS AFFECTING THE CHOICE AND OUTCOME OF THERAPEUTIC INTERVENTIONS

Acuteness or chronicity of the disorder
Severity of impairment of functioning from the disorder
Availability, beliefs, and attitudes of supportive persons or systems
Cultural expectations or sanctions
Personal beliefs about, attitudes toward, and past experiences with issues, such as self-help and the use of medications
Awareness of the treatment outcomes of other patients (i.e., what helped)
Attitudes and beliefs of primary care physicians and other clinicians and other referral sources
Availability of alternative therapies and the skills and reputations of various practitioners
Logistics of getting to various treatment settings
Time requirements of various interventions (i.e., time per treatment, duration of treatment)
Costs of various interventions
Nature of the coverage provided by third-party payers

TABLE 14.6. "LESS STRESS": A TASK-RELATED STRESS-REDUCTION APPROACH

List goals, both short and long range; eliminate those not attainable
Establish a hierarchy of tasks based on realistic time requirements and priorities
Subdivide remaining tasks into manageable units or projects
Start with achievable (doable) tasks; starting with the hardest task may promote procrastination
Simplify your work environment; avoid clutter, have good lighting
Tell yourself that saying "no" to additional work is okay when you are already doing more than you can handle
Remember to interrupt stressful periods with breaks for relaxation strategies (e.g., take 6–10 deep breaths, trying to fill the chest, while sitting in a relaxed way and having adequate support for your arms, shoulders, and neck)
Envision (in conjunction with the above relaxation strategy and with your eyes closed) your favorite place, trying to capture the sounds, smells, sights, and textures of the place
Share and discuss your situation with others
Structure nonwork hours to provide for adequate exercise, distraction, nutrition, and sleep

From Shader RI. Fear, stress, and anxiety. In: Tupin JP, Shader RI, Harnett DS, eds. *Handbook of clinical psychopharmacology*. Northvale, NJ: Aronson, 1988:73–96, with permission.

syndrome. Specific identifiable symptoms that reflect, for example, motor tension, autonomic hyperactivity, or excessive vigilance are also present (Table 14.7). The diagnosis of GAD requires that the specific or general symptoms are not attributable to a mood or psychotic disorder or that they are not secondary to a medical condition, such as hypoxia, thyrotoxicosis, pheochromocytoma, caffeinism, stimulant abuse, or alcohol or substance withdrawal (Table 14.3). Readers familiar with the DSM, 3rd edition, (-III) and the DSM, 3rd edition, revised, (-III-R) will likely note that the accompanying features of GAD emphasized in the DSM-IV have been reduced in number from 18 to 6 and that they are less dominated by manifestations of autonomic nervous system overactivity.

TABLE 14.7. DIAGNOSTIC FEATURES OF GENERALIZED ANXIETY DISORDER

Excessive worry (apprehensive expectation) or anxiety that is difficult to control voluntarily and that is focused on a variety of experiences or situations must have been present on a majority of days for a minimum of 6 months. The subjective cause for the worry or anxiety should not be limited to the features of an axis 1 disorder (e.g., having panic attacks in panic disorder, becoming contaminated in obsessive-compulsive disorder). At least three of the six symptoms that follow must also be present on a majority of days in this period and must not be secondary to the use of medications or abusable substances or to a medical condition. Similarly, these symptoms should not be present as a feature of a mood, psychotic, or pervasive developmental disorder. These symptoms and the worry or anxiety must be of sufficient magnitude to cause marked distress or a significant impairment of social or occupational functioning.
1. Nervousness, restlessness, feeling keyed up or on edge
2. Easy fatigability
3. Concentration difficulties or having one's mind go blank
4. Irritability
5. Muscle tension
6. Sleep difficulties, especially difficulty falling or staying asleep

From the American Psychiatric Association. *Diagnostic and statistical manual of mental disorders*, 4th ed. Text revision. Washington, D.C.: American Psychiatric Association, 2000, with permission.

Patients presenting in primary care settings frequently do not meet the full syndromal criteria for GAD, and their clinicians often rely on the qualitative features of GAD in reaching a working diagnosis. In some rural areas and in certain cultures or subpopulations, patients use unique or limited descriptors for their anxiety (Table 14.1). Such patients may be no less ill or no less in need of treatment than those meeting the formal diagnostic criteria for GAD. (*Note:* Complaints of some degree of worry can be elicited from 70% to 90% of patients seeking any form of medical attention; most of these patients need attention given to the concerns underlying their worries, and they do not require specific forms of antianxiety interventions.)

When GAD was first codified in DSM-III, the time requirement for diagnosis was 1 month of continuous or persistent symptoms. In DSM-III-R, this was lengthened to 6 months, and more emphasis was placed on worry as a cardinal manifestation. The 6-month requirement has been maintained in DSM-IV. Again, patients with symptoms lasting weeks to less than 6 months are as much in need of relief as those who technically qualify for the GAD diagnosis. None of the current diagnostic systems distinguishes worry about the future (e.g., "I am afraid this plane will crash") from past-oriented worry (e.g., "I am worried that what I said offended him"). This distinction may have treatment implications as worries about the future are more susceptible to reassurance, whereas past-focused worries may reflect greater contributions from factors such as low self-esteem, guilt, or depression.

B. Panic Disorder

PD is a diagnostic subtype that has been recognized for almost two decades. The central clinical feature of PD is the spontaneous panic attack, a discrete period usually lasting 5 to 30 minutes of intense fear or discomfort that does not occur in association with a specific anxiety-provoking situation (i.e., it appears to come "out of the blue"). This is sometimes problematic because an incomplete or hurried history-taking may lead the clinician to miss the precipitants. Panic attacks are experienced as anxiety carried to its extreme; they frequently occur when patients find themselves restricted in either their freedom of movement or access to help. The sense of terror in panic attacks can be so severe that the patients appear disorganized, disoriented, and depersonalized. Patients fear that they will suffocate, "go crazy," or die. These fears can be so extreme that they lead to a variety of avoidance and escape behaviors. Some patients abuse **alcohol** and sedative-hypnotics in their efforts to contain their fears.

Spontaneous attacks occur more frequently when a susceptible person is subjected to increased stress. Panic attacks arouse about one-third of patients from sleep when their carbon dioxide levels are increasing. PD patients have a greater likelihood of having experienced early separations and losses, including deaths, than do patients with major depressive disorder. Nevertheless, PD and major depressive disorder are highly comorbid. The modal age at onset for PD is in the mid-20s.

Current criteria for the diagnosis of PD are given in Table 14.8. Specific symptoms generally are associated with panic attacks, and the disorder is not secondary to a medical condition. PD may exist with or without **agoraphobia**, a state characterized by a fear of being in places or situations from which escape might be difficult or embarrassing or in which help might not be available in the event of a panic attack. The afflicted person usually stays at home and restricts travel, or he or she only ventures away from home or familiar places when accompanied by a known companion. The anxiety experienced by agoraphobic patients may be so severe that they will not leave home even to shop for food or other necessities. Many agoraphobic patients cannot even get to their clinicians' offices without accompaniment.

Although agoraphobia is considered a diagnosis in DSM-IV, viewing it as an adaptation or coping response to the panic attacks is also possible. By staying at home or leaving only with familiar persons, patients reduce their stress and thereby raise their thresholds for the emergence of panic attacks.

TABLE 14.8. DIAGNOSTIC FEATURES OF PANIC DISORDER

The essential feature of panic disorder (PD) is the panic attack, a period of intense fear, dysphoria, and physical discomfort lasting 5–30 minutes.[a] These panic attacks must be recurrent and at least some must occur spontaneously (i.e., unexpected, uncued), whereas others may be situational (i.e., cued). They must not be secondary solely to medications or substance abuse or to a medical condition. At least one of the panic attacks must have been followed by at least 1 month of anticipatory anxiety about further attacks; worry about dire outcomes, such as dying or "going crazy;" or clinically significant secondary behavior changes (e.g., various avoidance behaviors[b]). The panic attacks in PD must include at least 4 of the 13 symptoms that follow:

1. Palpitations, tachycardia
2. Sweating
3. Tremor, shaking
4. Nausea, abdominal distress
5. Numbness, paresthesias
6. Chills, hot flushes
7. Dizziness, faintness, unsteadiness
8. Chest discomfort or pain
9. Choking sensations
10. Shortness of breath, fear of smothering
11. Derealization, depersonalization
12. Fear of dying (e.g., from a heart attack)
13. Fear of losing control or "going crazy"

[a]In DSM-IV, peak intensity must be reached in 10 minutes.
[b]In DSM-IV, PD is classified as occurring "Without Agoraphobia" or "With Agoraphobia."
From the American Psychiatric Association. *Diagnostic and statistical manual of mental disorders,* 4th ed. Text revision. Washington, D.C.: American Psychiatric Association, 2000, with permission.

The degree of avoidance behavior can range from mild, in which a relatively normal life-style can be pursued despite the need to endure some distress, to severe, in which the patient is completely housebound. Some patients experience agoraphobia without a history of PD. This subgroup has epidemiologic features similar to those observed among patients experiencing panic attacks. Agoraphobia occurring without prior panic attacks is sometimes classified as a form of social phobia. This latter group includes mostly women; the onset is typically gradual with symptoms beginning most often between very late adolescence and the mid-30s.

In most PD patients, panic attacks can be reproduced after the administration of such diverse agents as intravenous **sodium lactate, doxapram,** or **isoproterenol**; oral **caffeine, *m*-chlorophenylpiperazine,** or **yohimbine**; or the inhalation of **marijuana** or of more than 4% to 5% **carbon dioxide**. Such exposures can sometimes be used for diagnostic clarification.

C. **Specific and Social Phobias**

1. **Specific phobia**. One formal definition of specific phobia is given in Table 14.9. This phobic presentation was called simple phobia in DSM-III and DSM-III-R. Many, but not all, specific phobias begin in childhood (e.g., bugs, thunder) and disappear spontaneously. Occasionally, childhood phobias have a symbolic or psychodynamic significance (e.g., the latency-age boy whose sudden fear of policemen reflects his ambivalence about his punitive father). Some patients develop their phobias in late adolescence or early adulthood (e.g., claustrophobia, fears of going into the water). Phobias that develop later in life are less likely to disappear spontaneously. Although most specific phobias are not treated, those severe enough to warrant a diagnosis could benefit from treatment. Treatment usually consists of any of a variety of cognitive-behavioral

TABLE 14.9. DIAGNOSTIC FEATURES OF SPECIFIC PHOBIA

Specific phobia is a persistent and intense situational or context-dependent anxiety in which the threat (object, situation) is known and exposure to it immediately triggers anxiety. The patient understands that the anxiety is excessive, but he or she finds avoidance preferable to encountering the threat, even though the avoidance and anticipatory anxiety interfere with functioning or cause marked distress. The following five types are currently codified in the *Diagnostic and Statistical Manual of Mental Disorders,* 4th ed.:
  Animal type
  Blood, injection, injury type
  Other type (e.g., avoidance of situations that may lead to an illness, irrational avoidance of certain foods may fit here)
  Natural environment type (e.g., heights, water)
  Situational type (e.g., elevators, enclosed spaces)

From the American Psychiatric Association. *Diagnostic and statistical manual of mental disorders,* 4th ed. Text revision. Washington, D.C.: American Psychiatric Association, 2000, with permission.

strategies that combine education and understanding with some form of learned relaxation techniques and graded contact with the avoided situation or object (imagery usually precedes actual exposure). Brief pharmacotherapy with anxiolytics or β-adrenergic receptor antagonists can sometimes be beneficial to ease the patient into the early stages of exposure. See Chapter 21 for a discussion of phobias in youth.

2. **Social phobia.** This phobia, which is also called **social anxiety disorder**, is considered in Table 14.10. Some degree of social phobia can be quite common in postpubertal females and in males beyond their mid-20s. In severe cases of social phobia, patients will go to great lengths to avoid the contexts in which they anticipate humiliation or embarrassment: for example, they will not eat or sign their names in front of others, and some men will not urinate at a public urinal. Although cognitive-behavior therapies (CBTs) can help some patients, many can benefit from pharmacotherapy (e.g., the use of an SSRI, such as **paroxetine**, currently approved for social anxiety disorder). Other agents, such as **venlafaxine XR**, have been used with some success as well. Rarely, the use of an MAOI, such as **phenelzine** or **isocarboxazid**, may be indicated. At least one trial supports the use of the anticonvulsant and γ-aminobu-

TABLE 14.10. DIAGNOSTIC FEATURES OF SOCIAL PHOBIA OR SOCIAL ANXIETY DISORDER

Social phobia is a persistent and intense situational (e.g., social situations, performance) anxiety in the presence of strangers or in the context of scrutiny by others. Such patients anticipate humiliation or that they will act in embarrassing ways, and they find avoidance preferable even though they know their concerns are excessive or unreasonable and that their avoidance and anticipatory anxiety interfere with functioning or cause marked distress. Entering or enduring these contexts is sometimes accomplished, but the individual experiences intense anxiety, discomfort, and distress. When a medical condition is present, the social or performance anxiety must not be secondary to it (e.g., worry about stuttering or trembling). The *Diagnostic and Statistical Manual of Mental Disorders,* 4th ed. recognizes a **generalized type,** in which pervasive anxiety about most social situations is present.

From the American Psychiatric Association. *Diagnostic and statistical manual of mental disorders,* 4th ed. Text revision. Washington, D.C.: American Psychiatric Association, 2000, with permission.

tyric acid analogue **gabapentin**. Several as yet unmarketed agents may also be effective in social anxiety disorder; one promising agent is **pregabalin**, another γ-aminobutyric acid analogue also under study for seizure control and reduction of neuropathic pain. Combining behavioral therapy and pharmacotherapies can be highly effective.

D. Posttraumatic Stress Disorder

Current criteria for PTSD are given in Table 14.11. Why some people can experience extreme trauma and appear to emerge unscathed and others cannot or why some who are traumatized will develop immediate symptomatology and others may show a delayed onset or may only show a response when the trauma has been repeated remains unclear. War victims with this disorder have received the most attention; until recently, much less attention had been paid to those who suffered from early physical or sexual abuse, rape (see Chapter 27), kidnapping, or exposure to natural disasters.

TABLE 14.11. DIAGNOSTIC FEATURES OF POSTTRAUMATIC STRESS DISORDER

Posttraumatic stress disorder (PTSD)[a] follows exposure to a traumatic and stressful event in which the patient (a) experienced, witnessed, or was confronted by actual or threatened death or serious injury or a threat to his or her own or another's physical integrity (e.g., rape) and (b) felt intense fear, anxiety, helplessness, or horror. The resulting symptomatology is sufficiently severe to cause marked distress or impairment of functioning, and, even when the patient is removed from the event, it is persistently reexperienced for at least 1 month in at least one of the following five ways:

1. Recurrent, intrusive, and distressing recollections (e.g., images, thoughts, perceptions).
2. Recurrent and distressing dreams involving the event.
3. Reliving the event or feeling as if it is recurring (e.g., illusions, flashbacks, hallucinations).
4. Intense anxiety and distress triggered by reminders or internal cues that resemble or symbolize the event.
5. Physiologic (autonomic nervous system-mediated) changes triggered by reminders or internal cues that resemble or symbolize the event.

The patient experiences a general numbing of responsiveness and avoids reminders and stimuli identified with the trauma; this is manifested for at least 1 month by at least three of the seven symptoms that follow:

1. Avoidance of thought, feelings, or discussions linked to the trauma.
2. Avoidance of people, places, or activities that prompt recollections of the trauma.
3. Impaired or no recall of an important aspect of the trauma.
4. Markedly diminished interest or involvement in significant experiences.
5. Estrangement or detachment from others.
6. Restricted range of affect (e.g., absence of loving feelings).
7. Sense of a bleak, unfulfilled, or foreshortened future (e.g., expects an early death or failing relationships).

For at least 1 month, the patient experiences increased arousal that is manifested by at least two of the five symptoms that follow:

1. Difficulty falling or staying asleep
2. Irritability or outbursts of anger
3. Exaggerated startle response
4. Difficulty concentrating
5. Hypervigilance

[a]The *Diagnostic and Statistical Manual of Mental Disorders*, 4th ed, (DSM-IV) classifies PTSD as **Acute** (i.e., symptom duration of less than 3 months), **Chronic**, or **With Delayed Onset** (i.e., at least 6 months after the trauma). DSM-IV also contains an **Acute Stress Disorder** diagnosis for a more muted pattern of symptoms that follows the trauma by less than 4 weeks and lasts from 2 days to no more than 4 weeks.
From the American Psychiatric Association. *Diagnostic and statistical manual of mental disorders*, 4th ed. Text revision. Washington, D.C.: American Psychiatric Association, 2000, with permission.

A tendency may appear in some situations for the individual to claim causality that links (or blames) current distress or suffering to past experiences that may be unrelated or that may be the product of distorted memories of these experiences. Some caution may be appropriate, and not all connections should be taken at face value.

Although patients with PTSD share enough common features so that the disorder was recognized and defined, their treatment is most likely to be effective when it is individualized. Some need to be seen in groups and to hear from others before they can speak about their own experiences or begin to trust others. Others may need an individual therapist who can establish a trusting relationship and who can then help the patient acknowledge what happened, how they felt (e.g., they may have felt both shame and excitement; personal values may have been violated), and what their role, if any, may have been (personal accountability). Rebuilding self-esteem, personal pride, and self-control or mastery and working through any guilt are also essential. When and how to involve any available family members also requires thoughtful judgment. For these reasons, at the present time, the treatment of PTSD is best entrusted to clinicians with considerable experience in this area. Pharmacotherapy can sometimes be quite effective. **Sertraline** is approved for PTSD by the United States Food and Drug Administration (FDA). Other SSRIs may be helpful (see Chapter 27). When these agents are not effective, an MAOI (e.g., **phenelzine**) can be tried if the clinician is experienced with its use. Case reports and a few small sample studies have shown some improvement after the administration of **valproic acid** or **carbamazepine**, of **clonidine** as an adjunctive therapy to TCAs, or of β-adrenergic receptor antagonists. Benzodiazepines, such as **alprazolam** and **clonazepam**, have also provided some symptom relief; sometimes they are coprescribed with an SSRI or an MAOI. (*Note:* Careful monitoring is advisable when using benzodiazepines in this population, because some degree of unpredictable disinhibition may occur.)

IV. Prevalence and Consequences

Population-based surveys of the American population identify a 1-year prevalence rate for all anxiety disorders as being in the range of 5% to 15% for the adult population. This rate reflects persons meeting full syndromal criteria; the prevalence rates for those with a few symptoms or subsyndromal presentations would obviously be much higher.

A. Generalized Anxiety Disorder

For GAD, which is three to four times more prevalent than PD, the 1-year prevalence estimates are in the 2.5% to 6.5% range. A frequently quoted figure is 64 per 1,000. In one major study, the lifetime prevalence for GAD in patients not meeting criteria for any other comorbid psychiatric disorder was 0.5%, which is quite low. A slight male predominance for GAD is seen. GAD is more concordant in monozygotic twins (40% to 50%) than in dizygotics (4% to 15%). About 80% of patients will have symptoms when examined 3 years later, and about 50% will relapse within a few months after an effective pharmacotherapy is discontinued. About one-fourth of the male relatives of GAD patients misuse alcohol. Most GAD patients are never treated; about one-fourth have subsequent panic attacks, and over half later meet criteria for major depressive disorder. The prognosis for GAD is worse when symptoms such as depersonalization, agitation, and syncope are prominent.

B. Panic Disorder

The lifetime prevalence of PD is in the range of 1% to 3.5%. It is two to four times higher in women than it is in men. Most studies suggest a genetic component. As was noted earlier, the modal onset is in the mid-20s, and about three-fourths meet PD criteria by the age of 30.

C. Other Disorders

Estimates here are highly variable. About 5% to 12.5% in the aggregate meet criteria for all other anxiety disorders. The 1-year prevalence rate for

PTSD is often given as 1%, but this figure would change greatly in years in which many unnatural or natural disasters occurred.

V. Chronicity and Morbidity

Both GAD and PD are typically chronic illnesses. In some patients, these illnesses follow a periodic course characterized by remissions and exacerbations. In many instances, recurrence of symptomatology is triggered by situational stress. A frequent pattern for both disorders is a more or less continuous or unrelenting course. Although these disorders are frequently viewed as minor or trivial illnesses by many clinicians and third-party payers, the available data do not support this perspective. Some patients do maintain reasonable functioning despite continuing or intermittent distress. However, a substantial proportion is seriously impaired or is even disabled by the illness. About 15% of PD patients have chronic and disabling symptoms. Family and social dysfunction, financial dependency or economic loss due to impaired work function, and the perception of poor physical health are all identified correlates. GAD and PD patients use emergency departments and other health care facilities at increased rates, and they are more likely to use or abuse cigarettes, alcohol, or illegal drugs than is an age-matched general population sample. Anxiety is associated with significantly increased rates of mortality from all causes. PD by itself is associated with increased occurrence of suicidal ideation, as well as of actual suicide attempts.

VI. General and Nonpharmacologic Treatment Considerations

Based on behavioral studies with animals, one may argue that some drug treatments for anxiety work by lessening learned (acquired) avoidance responses or by diminishing arousal and anticipatory responses to external or imagined danger or unpleasant situations. Decrements in anticipatory anxiety should be accompanied by a reduction in avoidance behaviors. Although avoidance and escape can be adaptive at times, for many people an appropriate reduction of anxiety could facilitate making better use of information, insights, or relationships in preparation for coping with stress or anxiety. Because some degree of arousal or anxiety is essential to promote effective coping strategies and learning, reducing the anxiety too much could be counterproductive. Once the anxiety is manageable, the patient can be helped to develop some perspective about the causes; manifestations (symptoms); and consequences, including the unwanted effects on relationships. The anxious patient can also learn whether any secondary gain comes from the anxiety (e.g., does it get others to act in a more thoughtful, caring, or giving manner?).

A. Therapeutic Listening

The clinician must learn not to become anxious when listening to patients' stories. The history-taking should permit the clinician to listen for any material suggesting that the patient becomes anxious about impulses that are forbidden or unacceptable or about painful memories or feelings that are threatening to emerge. Sometimes the sharing of memories, feelings, or impulses with a nonanxious, noncritical clinician will suffice to reduce anxiety. When the clinician does choose to offer a behavioral intervention or to prescribe medication, this should never be done as a substitute for empathic involvement.

B. Cognitive-Behavior Therapy

Most CBTs are based on the assumption that anxiety that does not arise solely as a manifestation of a medical condition reflects faulty or exaggerated appraisal of a threat or of one's appropriately aroused state; the degree of danger in the environment is misperceived, or one's own coping abilities are underestimated. Under these conditions, the apprehension and helplessness lead to a state of self-focused attention that amplifies and negatively interprets the inner physiologic sensations. Concomitant hypervigilance further narrows the attention, disrupts the concentration, or produces deteriorated performance and less successful coping and mastery.

CBTs try to restore mastery and coping by increasing lost self-confidence and overcoming demoralization, decreasing physical tension, decreasing avoidance, and breaking through negative feedback. Even something as simple as worry beads can be understood as a way of shifting focus from one's inner negative experiences into a calming ritual. Breathing exercises reestablish control and slow the heart rate. Education about the disorder is also an important component of many CBTs. Patients who recognize a panic attack for what it is and who know that it will end and that they will not "go crazy" or have a heart attack can reduce the likelihood of an uncontrollable escalation of symptomatology. Collecting more facts about fear-inducing situations, considering various options and alternatives for action when symptoms appear, and doing behavioral homework all can help. With few exceptions (see Chapter 27), no particular form of CBT is consistently more effective than another for any specific disorder. A flexible approach to the nonpharmacologic aspects of the care of anxious patients is essential.

VII. A Comment on the Prevalence of Pharmacotherapy

Data on psychotropic drug use in the United States fail to support the popular perception of Americans as excessive and inappropriate users of anxiolytic medications. Among adults identified as having enough symptomatology to warrant an intervention, only about one in four actually receives medication. Most antianxiety agent users take their medications as prescribed or use less. The typical use patterns are intermittent or occasional, or they last for relatively short periods of time. Only about 15% of all users of anxiolytic medications take medication continuously for over a year. During a typical 1-year interval, the overall prevalence of any use of an antianxiety agent, regardless of frequency or duration, for all diagnoses, including sleep and convulsive disorders, is estimated at 10% to 11% of the adult population. This puts Americans somewhere in the middle of the usage range among industrialized nations. Reliable data also indicate that anxiolytic users usually have significant levels of emotional distress and appropriate diagnoses. The prevalence of anxiolytic use has actually decreased somewhat over time. On balance, most data suggest that Americans use antianxiety agents conservatively and appropriately.

VIII. Pharmacotherapy

A. When to Treat

Approximately 50% of GAD patients will have prominent somatic distress that is referred to the cardiovascular, gastrointestinal, or another organ system. Therefore, the fact that most benzodiazepines and other sedative-hypnotics are prescribed by nonpsychiatric clinicians is not surprising. Most of these patients first undergo a medical evaluation for diseases other than anxiety; generally, no identifiable abnormality is revealed. Patients with symptoms consistent with a diagnosis of GAD or PD not secondary to some other cause should be considered for an initial trial of nonpharmacologic treatment, provided that their symptoms can be tolerated long enough for these alternatives to have time to work. Some approaches are short-term counseling or psychotherapy, various CBTs, reduction or elimination of **caffeine** intake or **alcohol** use, stress management techniques, physical exercise, or meditation. In many health care settings and rural areas, nonpharmacologic options for the treatment of anxiety may not be available at all. In such settings, pharmacotherapy may be the only appropriate option.

The decision to use a benzodiazepine or any other medication should be based on a risk-benefit assessment that weighs the degree of emotional distress and functional disability, the hazards of medication, the potential future hazards of nontreatment, and the probability of success of pharmacotherapy. Table 14.12 lists all the agents currently approved by the FDA for the range of anxiety disorders. Subsequent tables provide additional information.

B. Choosing a Specific Medication for GAD

1. **Benzodiazepines** as a class continue to be commonly prescribed anxiolytics in the United States. Table 14.13 lists the benzodiazepines currently marketed in the United States. Specific preferences, both of the patients and the prescribing clinicians, within this class have changed over the last decade. Until the early 1980s, **diazepam** was the most

TABLE 14.12. CURRENTLY USED UNITED STATES FOOD AND DRUG ADMINISTRATION APPROVED ANXIOLYTICS FOR GENERALIZED ANXIETY DISORDER, NONPSYCHOTIC ANXIETY, "PSYCHONEUROTIC" ANXIETY, OR UNSPECIFIED ANXIETY[a]

Class (Most Common American Trade Name)	Typical Starting Dosage in mg (and Range)[b]
Benzodiazepines[c]	
Alprazolam (Xanax)	0.25 (0.25–4)
Chlordiazepoxide (Librium)	10 (5–100)
Clorazepate (Tranxene)	7.5 (7.5–60)
Diazepam (Valium)	2 (2–40)
Lorazepam (Ativan)	1 (1–10)
Oxazepam (Serax)	10 (10–90)
Selective serotonin reuptake inhibitors (SSRIs)	
Paroxetine[d,e] (Paxil)	10 (10–60)
Sertraline[d] (Zoloft)	25 (25–200)
Conventional antipsychotic agents	
Prochlorperazine (Compazine)[f]	5 (5–20)
Trifluoperazine (Stelazine)[f]	1 (1–6)
Antihistamines	
Hydroxyzine (Atarax, Vistaril)[g]	25 (25–200)
Other agents	
Buspirone[h]	5 (5–50)
Doxepin	10 (10–75)
Venlafaxine XR (Effexor XR)[e]	37.5 (37.5–225)

[a]Obsessive-compulsive disorder is not considered in this table (see Chapter 6).
[b]Ranges may vary for specific indications; based on the authors' clinical experience.
[c]Other benzodiazepines are available elsewhere.
[d]Other SSRIs may be beneficial.
[e]Only agents with specific generalized anxiety disorder (GAD) indication.
[f]Use should be for no longer than 12 weeks.
[g]Short-term treatment of anxiety; available as tablets, capsules, syrup, or suspension.
[h]For anxiety; for children, capsules may be opened and mixed with applesauce.

widely prescribed benzodiazepine anxiolytic and was in fact one of the most frequently prescribed drugs in the world. **Diazepam** is the prototype of the longer half-life accumulating benzodiazepines. Multiple daily doses result in the accumulation of diazepam and its major metabolite **desmethyldiazepam** due to the long elimination half-life of both of these compounds. Potential benefits of this type of profile include the possibility of sustained drug effects throughout the day even with infrequent dosing, as well as a relatively low likelihood of rapid-onset discontinuation phenomena if treatment is abruptly stopped. Possible disadvantages include the potential for an increase in the sedative, performance-impairing, and amnestic effects that develop over time as a consequence of drug accumulation.

The introduction of **alprazolam** in the early 1980s shifted prescribing patterns; by 1988, **alprazolam** was the most commonly prescribed anxiolytic in the United States. (*Note:* In 1992, **alprazolam** was the third most frequently used medication among all types of medications.) Because of its short to intermediate half-life, it has a low potential for accumulation or for producing cumulative sedation with multiple doses. However, multiple daily doses are usually needed to achieve a sustained

TABLE 14.13. BENZODIAZEPINE ANTIANXIETY (ANXIOLYTIC) AGENTS

Parent Drug	Typical Daily Range[a] (mg)	Effective Half-Life	Active Metabolites
Chlordiazepoxide (Librium and others)	15–100	Long	Desmethylchlordiaz-epoxide Demoxepam Desmethyldiazepam
Diazepam (Valium and others[b])	4–40	Long	Desmethyldiazepam
Oxazepam (Serax)	30–120	Short	None
Clorazepate[c] (Tranxene)	15–60	Long	Desmethyldiazepam
Lorazepam (Ativan and others)	2–6	Short to intermediate	None
Alprazolam (Xanax)	0.75–4 (for anxiety) 1.5–10 (for panic disorder)	Short to intermediate	None
Clonazepam (Klonopin)	0.5–4[d]	Intermediate to long	None

[a]Given as the usual adult dosage range. Lower doses recommended for elderly or debilitated patients.
[b]Also available in sustained-release as Valrelease (15 mg capsules).
[c]Precursor or prodrug for desmethyldiazepam.
[d]Clonazepam is United States Food and Drug Administration approved for the treatment of panic disorders.

effect, and discontinuation phenomena are more likely to occur after the abrupt discontinuation of treatment.

This shift in prescribing patterns stems from a combination of accumulating scientific data, clinician preferences, and marketplace forces. Throughout the past 15 to 20 years, **lorazepam** has continued to be prescribed at relatively steady rates, although it is used less frequently than **alprazolam** and **diazepam**. Oxazepam; chlordiazepoxide; and **clorazepate**, a prodrug for **desmethyldiazepam**, are much less frequently prescribed. In recent years, **clonazepam** use for GAD has increased steadily, even though its FDA-approved indication is PD.

For the treatment of GAD, the benzodiazepines listed in Tables 14.12 and 14.13 are consistently more effective than a placebo during short-term outpatient treatment. Long-term efficacy has never been unequivocally established. Some research (e.g., discontinuation or naturalistic studies) and patient reports are consistent with long-term benefit. The increment in therapeutic response that is attributable to a benzodiazepine compared with that of a placebo is variable from study to study because high placebo response rates are often observed in controlled trials. As one might expect, controlled trials comparing specific benzodiazepines with each other fail to demonstrate any consistent differences in efficacy within the class. The available scientific data indicate that the proper and thoughtful use of any of these benzodiazepines has an approximately equal likelihood of producing a reasonable therapeutic benefit in the treatment of patients with GAD. No evidence indicates that either the response to treatment or the potential hazards of these medications will be different for patients fulfilling formal diagnostic criteria for anxiety disorder than for those with anxiety as identified by primary care physicians and other clinicians using less formal and more qualitative diagnostic features.

That many clinicians avoid the use of benzodiazepines for a variety of both rational and nonevidence-based reasons should be noted. Their drugs of choice for initiating treatment are the SSRIs and other antidepressants.

2. Only one **SSRI, paroxetine**, has received FDA approval for use in GAD on the basis of controlled trials. In the authors' experience, all SSRIs can be effective in specific patients. The SSRIs are preferred by some clinicians and many patients because of concerns about the abuse potential, anterograde memory loss, and possible addiction liability of benzodiazepines in some patients. Although this could be a concern for particular patients, this issue needs to be balanced against the weight gain, sedation, and sexual side effects experienced by some patients on SSRIs. Because SSRI use may be accompanied by a slow onset of action and an initial incremental increase in anxiety, some clinicians may start a benzodiazepine, such as **lorazepam** or **clonazepam**, concurrently with the SSRI for the first 4 to 6 weeks and may then discontinue the benzodiazepine using a gradual tapering procedure (see Chapter 9). Because discontinuation reactions can occur with some SSRIs, (especially **paroxetine**), the SSRI should be gradually tapered when stopping the drug is indicated. **Paroxetine** is an inhibitor of cytochrome P-450 (CYP) 2D6, and it may inhibit its own metabolism (see Chapter 29).

3. **Venlafaxine XR**, a sustained-release preparation that is an inhibitor of both serotonin and norepinephrine presynaptic transporters, is also FDA approved for use in GAD. Reminding patients not to divide, chew, or crush these capsules is important. When discontinuing the use of this medication, the recommendation is that a tapering process should be followed, rather than abruptly discontinuing its use. Hypertension can be a problem for some patients on **Venlafaxine XR**, and blood pressure should be monitored, at least during the initial weeks of treatment and with subsequent dosage increases. Tremor can also occur. **Venlafaxine XR** is unique in that its beneficial effects are supported by a controlled trial that lasted for 26 weeks.

4. **Buspirone**, an azapirone anxiolytic, is also effective in GAD, but the response rates are more variable and the onset of action is slower for some patients (i.e., up to 2 to 3 weeks) compared with that of the benzodiazepines. When **buspirone** is effective for a particular patient, it offers some advantages, such as less potential for dependence and little, if any, memory or motor impairment. Some data suggest that **buspirone** may be most helpful in patients whose worries focus on the past, in those with minimal to mild concomitant depressive symptoms, or in those who do not welcome the mild sedation that is produced by benzodiazepines.

5. **Doxepin**[2] has demonstrated effectiveness in some GAD patients, even those who have not yet shown any concurrent depressive symptoms. It is FDA approved for symptoms of anxiety.

6. **Barbiturates**, such as **amobarbital**, **butabarbital**, and **phenobarbital**, are not particularly efficacious for GAD or any other anxiety disorder. However, they are the least expensive antianxiety agents; some increase in their use has occurred in states controlling and regulating benzodiazepine use. Because barbiturates produce generalized central nervous system (CNS) depression and, in many patients, an unacceptable amount of sedation, their use involves considerable risk, particularly in patients who may overdose. Intentional overdosage is frequently lethal. Barbiturates induce hepatic microsomal enzymes, and dependence and tolerance can occur (see Chapter 9).

7. **Propanediols**, such as **meprobamate**, were popular for the treatment of anxiety in the late 1950s and early 1960s. Controlled trials did not

---

[2]**Doxepin** is sometimes particularly helpful for patients with pruritus as one of their anxiety complaints. **Doxepin** has strong antihistaminic actions; consistent with this property, it is quite sedating. **Doxepin** is marketed in a topical form for pruritus. **Doxepin** is a CYP 2D6 inhibitor.

support their use in any specific anxiety disorder. **Meprobamate** has significant addiction potential, and completed suicides have occurred with some frequency. Drowsiness and ataxia are common unwanted effects. Unfortunately, **meprobamate** use has slightly increased in states regulating the use of benzodiazepines.

8. **Antipsychotic agents** are also occasionally prescribed for the treatment of GAD-like states in nonpsychotic patients. Their major use is in states of acute psychotic terror, but they may be helpful in certain anxious and agitated elderly patients showing signs of delirium or dementia, particularly when irascibility and aggression are part of the clinical picture. Some nonpsychotic anxious patients occasionaly find antipsychotic agents beneficial, although trying other agents first is usually preferable. Examples include (a) patients whose anxiety is associated with a high degree of distractibility; (b) those with racing thoughts, periods of thought blocking, or both; (c) those with strong imaginations, considerable magical thinking, and occasionally poor reality testing; and (d) those for whom other antianxiety regimens have been successful. Although some of these patients may seem psychotic, many show no further evidence of disorganization or decompensation.

When antipsychotic regimens are selected for nonpsychotic patients, the dosages should be kept as low as possible; for example, **prochlorperazine** (5 to 10 mg per day) or **trifluoperazine** (1 to 2 mg per day) should be given for no more than 12 consecutive weeks, usually in a single bedtime dose. Unwanted effects even at low dosages, however, typically make the use of antipsychotic agents undesirable (e.g., drowsiness, ataxia, dry mouth, blurred vision, postural hypotension, weakness, and feelings of unreality). Extrapyramidal side effects and tardive dyskinesia are less common at low dosages and with short durations of use, but they may still occur.

No published experience with the use of atypical antipsychotic agents in GAD exists at this time, and no agent has FDA approval for this indication.

9. **Antihistamines** are still prescribed by some clinicians. Some antihistamines have weak nonspecific CNS effects; most are also anticholinergic. **Hydroxyzine** is the most commonly used drug within this group. It may have a special usefulness in patients with anxiety-related pruritic dermatoses. **Hydroxyzine** is usually prescribed at oral dosage levels of 25 to 200 mg per day.

10. **β-Adrenergic receptor antagonists** may reduce symptoms, such as tachycardia, palpitations, tremor, and hyperventilation, but they are not effective in GAD. β-Adrenergic receptor antagonists may, however, be of some use in social phobia. The most commonly studied drug of this class is **propranolol**. Its use is contraindicated in patients whose cardiac compensation depends on sympathetic stimulation. It is also contraindicated in patients with obstructive lung diseases and asthma, and it should be used with caution in patients with diabetes mellitus. The key to using β-adrenergic receptor antagonists is to prescribe them at an appropriate dose and for a sufficient duration so that β-receptor antagonism will be achieved. Oral dosages of 30 to 120 mg per day in three to four divided doses are typically used.

Atenolol at 25 to 50 mg per day is another alternative. It is preferred by some clinicians because it has fewer CNS side effects (e.g., depressed mood) than does **propranolol**. Clinicians prescribing these agents should be alert to their potential to cause or exacerbate symptoms of depression.

C. **Choosing a Specific Medication for Panic Disorder** (Table 14.14)

1. **Antidepressants**. Moderate to longer term pharmacotherapy of PD patients may be quite satisfactory with SSRIs; **paroxetine** and **sertraline** have FDA approval for PD. Other agents, such as **imipramine** and MAOIs like **phenelzine**, have been successfully used in PD. These agents may be most beneficial for blocking further panic attacks; they are

TABLE 14.14. UNITED STATES FOOD AND DRUG ADMINISTRATION APPROVED AGENTS FOR THE TREATMENT OF PANIC DISORDER

Class	Typical Mean Daily Dosage in mg (Range)[a]
Benzodiazepines	
Alprazolam	4 (2–10)
Clonazepam	2 (0.5–4)
Selective serotonin reuptake inhibitors	
Paroxetine	40 (10–60)
Sertraline	75 (25–200)

[a]Based on the authors' clinical experience.

not effective acutely (i.e., they are not effective during a panic attack). The dosage requirements for all of these are variable. Occasional patients respond to doses as low as 10 mg per day of **paroxetine** or even as little as 10 mg per day of **imipramine** when enough time (sometimes up to 6 weeks) is allowed for determining whether that dosage level will be effective. Troublesome side effects generally are more common with all these antidepressants than they are with the benzodiazepines.

2. **Benzodiazepines**. These are effective agents for both the reduction of any anticipatory anxiety and for acute care in PD. Approaches to initiating benzodiazepine therapy in PD are derived from clinical experience and common sense rather than from well-established scientific guidelines. Based on factors such as age, gender, body size, and prior medication experience, a dosage at the low end of the usual effective range is chosen and is titrated upward every few days until therapeutic benefit is achieved or side effects supervene. When side effects are encountered at a given dose, further dosage increments can be delayed, or the dose can be somewhat reduced. Many patients who experience drowsiness or other sedative side effects early in the course of therapy will report that these symptoms diminish with continued therapy. This is attributable to adaptation or tolerance. In most patients, a daily dosage can be found that produces significant clinical improvement with either no sedative side effects or with side effects mild enough to be tolerated.

Most of the published experience and research in the treatment of PD has focused on **alprazolam**; its efficacy has been shown to be significantly greater than a placebo in reducing the frequency and severity of panic attacks and associated anticipatory anxiety and avoidance behavior. The published documentation with **clonazepam** is more limited; however, both are FDA approved for PD. Limited data suggest that other benzodiazepine derivatives, such as **diazepam** and **lorazepam**, may have comparable efficacy in specific patients.

For **alprazolam**, enough data exist to recommend using plasma **alprazolam** levels for titrating therapy. Steady-state levels of less than 20 ng per mL are associated with little or no improvement in PD patients; levels in the range of 20 to 40 ng per mL are generally associated with clear benefit in terms of global clinical improvement and reduction of specific symptoms of anxiety. Some data suggest that levels in excess of 40 ng per mL may be required for the suppression of both spontaneous and precipitated panic attacks, but this is not clearly established. Increments of 1 mg per day of **alprazolam** appear to raise plasma levels by about 10 ng per mL; 1 mg three times a day could be expected to result in steady-state levels of 30 ng per mL, a concentration that is likely to be beneficial in PD. The maximum recommended dose is 10 mg per day, although some patients occasionally benefit from and tolerate higher doses (Table 14.14). An extended release form of **alprazolam** was recently approved for use in the United States. Many clinicians find it to be clinically comparable with the immediate release agent **clonazepam**.

For other benzodiazepines, no clear dose-response or concentration-response relationships have been established. However, a few plasma level ranges associated with usual therapeutic doses can be identified as follows: for **diazepam**, 300 to 1,000 ng per mL each of **diazepam** and its metabolite **desmethyldiazepam**; for **clorazepate**, 600 to 1,500 ng per mL of **desmethyldiazepam**; and for **lorazepam**, 20 to 80 ng per mL of **lorazepam**. Even when clear therapeutic ranges are not available, benzodiazepine plasma level monitoring may still be useful in some clinical situations in patients with PD. For example, a patient with poor therapeutic response might be either an intrinsic nonresponder to typical drug concentrations (i.e., steady-state plasma levels are in the "usual" range) or a person with rapid metabolism or questionable adherence (i.e., low or zero plasma levels are found). Similarly, treatment of a patient with a symptom such as fatigue, which could be attributable either to the underlying disease or to the medication, could be assisted by plasma level monitoring. An extremely high steady-state plasma level would suggest a drug-related side effect, whereas a low level would suggest the persistence of original symptoms due to undertreatment.

    3. Anticonvulsants. **Valproate** and **gabapentin** have shown evidence of efficacy in PD. However, data are not sufficient at the present time to recommend their use.

D. Duration of Medication Use

    1. GAD. GAD is a chronic illness. Nevertheless, a patient's need for the medication should be periodically reassessed. Some patients with GAD have persistent symptoms, and, in order to live productive and more comfortable lives, these individuals need more or less indefinite treatment. Continuing an antidepressant-based regimen (e.g., an SSRI or **venlafaxine XR**) for at least several years to promote a symptom-free period of stability seems reasonable. Then, a well-planned taper should be considered to determine the value of more extended treatment. In most instances, benzodiazepine use should not be continued without interruption. Periodic reassessment of the need for medication makes both clinical and medicolegal sense. At about 4-month to 6-month intervals, gradual tapering of the medication dosage can be initiated. Some patients will reach zero dosage without the recurrence of symptoms; others will experience a recurrence during or after the taper period. Medication can then be reinstituted when enough emotional distress is seen to warrant restarting treatment. A strategy of periodic discontinuation may reveal the subgroup of benzodiazepine-responsive patients whose anxiety is persistent and for whom chronic therapy may be uniquely beneficial. At the present time, the size of this group is unknown, and no criteria exist to identify these patients.

    2. Panic disorder. Similar issues pertain to PD. In this condition, however, treatment is often initiated with a combination of a benzodiazepine and an antidepressant. The benzodiazepine can usually be tapered after 4 to 6 weeks, and treatment with the antidepressant alone is usually sufficient. After several years of stability, a planned tapered discontinuation should be considered.

E. Side Effects

Side effects **caused** by a medication must be clearly distinguished from unrelated effects occurring while a medication is being taken and from symptoms of the underlying disorder.

    1. Benzodiazepines. An expected consequence of benzodiazepine use is nonspecific CNS depression or sedation. The intensity and time course of sedation produced by single doses of any benzodiazepine depend on the magnitude of the dose, the resulting plasma and brain concentrations, and the degree of receptor occupancy. Sedation should be the most common and predictable side effect for all benzodiazepines.

a. **Sedation** may be revealed through the patient's reports of fatigue, tiredness, drowsiness, or sleepiness. Patients may also report difficulties with concentration or in staying awake, problems with visual accommodation, the feeling of having their thought processes slowed down, or ataxia and difficulties with balance. Controlled psychomotor testing procedures can be used to document a slowing of psychomotor performance speed, reaction time, or impairment of coordination.

b. **Anterograde amnesia** appears to be another consequence of nonspecific CNS depression. Patients may have impairment of information acquisition, impairment of storage of recently acquired information, or both. Patients typically report a partial or complete failure to recall information that has been acquired or acts that have been performed after their last dose.

Both of these effects are temporary and reversible, and they will diminish and disappear as the drug is eliminated from the body and cleared from the brain. No consistent evidence indicates that one benzodiazepine differs from another in its capacity to produce such dose-dependent and concentration-dependent sedative effects. Some studies suggest that the emergence of daytime drowsiness is more likely to occur during treatment with long half-life accumulating benzodiazepines than it is with short half-life nonaccumulating compounds. However, this is not a constant finding. The clinical consequences of sedative side effects during repeated administration of benzodiazepines are partly counterbalanced by the development of tolerance to these effects. Tolerance reflects an intrinsic change in receptor sensitivity that occurs as a consequence of continued drug exposure. In clinical terms, patients frequently report a diminution or disappearance of sedative effects despite the continued use of the medication. (*Note:* Tolerance to nonspecific sedative effects of benzodiazepines is not accompanied by tolerance to their antianxiety effects.)

c. Seemingly **paradoxical effects** of benzodiazepines have received attention in the lay media that is vastly out of proportion to their incidence and clinical importance. Very rarely, benzodiazepine users report experiencing increased feelings of anger or hostility, feelings that are the opposite of the usual and expected calming effects of these drugs. From one perspective, such effects would not always be paradoxical—they could represent the consequences of anxiolytic effects in persons having feelings of anger that were previously held in check by their anxiety. A drug-induced reduction of anxiety could facilitate the release or expression of any suppressed anger. To date, this effect has been demonstrated only rarely, and it has been seen principally in controlled laboratory studies in which feelings of anger or hostility are measured by rating scales or psychologic tests. Any assumption that these laboratory findings extend to the occurrence of antisocial expressions of anger or hostility, such as aggressive or assaultive behavior, has not been proved. No documented medical or scientific evidence indicates that benzodiazepine use directly or reproducibly impairs impulse control or conscience or leads to aggressive or self-destructive acts. Similarly, no evidence appears to indicate that benzodiazepine use is causally related to the occurrence of psychotic behavior, delusions, hallucinations, or depersonalization.

d. **Discontinuation syndrome** is the term applied to the clinical worsening that results from stopping benzodiazepines. At least three distinct syndromes can be identified, and distinguishing among these is clinically important.

(1) **Recurrence**. Because benzodiazepines do not cure GAD, PD, or insomnia, the symptoms of these chronic conditions can be expected to recur in most patients after treatment discontinuation. The symptoms should resemble those for which the drug was originally given. Recurrence of symptoms may be rapid once treatment is stopped, but, in most patients, they reappear relatively slowly.

(2) **Rebound**. The rebound syndrome is similar or identical in character to the original disorder for which the benzodiazepine was prescribed; however, it is transiently more intense than the premorbid condition. Rebound anxiety and insomnia have been clearly established as possible consequences of benzodiazepine discontinuation, particularly after stopping benzodiazepines with short half-lives. Rebound phenomena usually last only a few days after discontinuation; they may be followed by the recurrence of the underlying disorder. (*Note:* Rebound does not imply physical dependence.)

(3) **Withdrawal**. The occurrence of an objective autonomic withdrawal syndrome implies some degree of physical dependence. Withdrawal is likely to include psychologic and physiologic symptoms, such as increased anxiety, fearfulness, easy startling, hyperacusis, increased heart rate and blood pressure, and insomnia. As Chapter 9 discusses, the benzodiazepine withdrawal syndrome is self-limited, and complete recovery from all manifestations should occur. (*Note:* Recurrence of the underlying disorder may follow a withdrawal syndrome.)

Although these three syndromes can be distinguished in concept, they may be difficult to distinguish in clinical practice, particularly when they occur simultaneously or sequentially in the same patient.

e. **Short half-life benzodiazepines** should be tapered when discontinuing their use as abrupt discontinuation of short half-life benzodiazepines is associated with an increased likelihood of discontinuation syndromes of relatively rapid onset. That short half-life benzodiazepines should be tapered rather than abruptly stopped is now well recognized.

Many tapering schemes have been used with success. One example is the "quarter per week" approach in which the daily dose is reduced by 25% once a week. For example, a patient taking 4 mg per day of **alprazolam** would reduce the daily dose to 3 mg in week 1, 2 mg in week 2, and 1 mg in week 3 and would then discontinue it completely in week 4. Flexibility and close monitoring are essential during the taper period. In some patients, the final phase of the taper (i.e., 1 mg down to zero) may be difficult; in these patients, it must be extended in duration and may then be undertaken in even smaller decrements.

2. **SSRIs**. The side effects of SSRIs are generally tolerable. Among the most common initial side effects are nausea, diarrhea, insomnia or nervousness, and sometimes sedation. Sexual dysfunction can be quite troublesome. Weight gain with extended use can also be problematic. Discontinuation syndromes are also noted with agents without active metabolites. Paroxetine is associated with the highest incidence of discontinuation reactions. Tapering of SSRIs is advisable. Chapter 18 contains more information on the side effects of SSRIs and other antidepressants

IX. **Anxiety Disorders Association of America (ADAA)**

The Anxiety Disorders Association of America (ADAA) provides advocacy and support for improved care, education, and research in the area of anxiety disorders. The ADAA can be reached by mail at Anxiety Disorders Association of America, 11900 Parklawn Drive, Suite 100, Rockville, MD 20852 (United States); by telephone at 301-231-9350; or on their website at *http://www.adaa.org/*.

X. A Categorization of Phobias

The following website can be consulted for the accepted names of various phobias: *http://www.health.discovery.com/stories/phobias/phobias.html.*

ADDITIONAL READING

American Psychiatric Association. Practice guidelines for the treatment of patients with panic disorder. *Am J Psychiatry* 1998;155:1–34.

Angst J, Vollrath M. The natural history of anxiety disorders. *Acta Psychiatr Scand* 1991;84:446–452.

Ballenger JC, Wheadon DE, Steiner M, et al. Double-blind, fixed-dose, placebo-controlled study of paroxetine in the treatment of panic disorder. *Am J Psychiatry* 1998;155:36–42.

Barlow DH. *Anxiety and its disorders.* New York: Guilford, 1988.

Barlow DH, Gorman JM, Shear MK, et al. Cognitive-behavioral therapy, imipramine, or their combination in panic disorder. *JAMA* 2000;283:2529–2536.

Beck AT, Emery G, Greenberg R. *Anxiety disorders and phobias.* New York: Basic Books, 1985.

Beck AT, Sokol L, Clark DA, et al. A crossover study of focused cognitive therapy for panic disorder. *Am J Psychiatry* 1992;149:778–783.

Black DW, Wesner R, Bowers W, et al. A comparison of fluvoxamine, cognitive-therapy, and placebo in the treatment of panic disorder. *Arch Gen Psychiatry* 1993;52:44–50.

Borkovec TD, Inz J. The nature of worry in generalized anxiety disorder: predominance of thought activity. *Behav Res Ther* 1990;28:153–158.

Brown TA, Barlow DH. Long-term outcome of cognitive behavioral treatment of panic disorder. *J Consult Clin Psychol* 1995;63:754–765.

Butler G, Fennell M, Robson P, et al. A comparison of behavior therapy and cognitive behavior therapy in the treatment of generalized anxiety disorder. *J Consult Clin Psychol* 1991;59:167–175.

Charney D, Drevets W. The neurobiological basis of anxiety disorders. In: Davis KL, Charney D, Coyle JT, et al., eds. *Neuropsychopharmacology: the fifth generation of progress.* Philadelphia: Lippincott Williams & Wilkins, 2002:901–930.

Ciraulo DA, Antal EJ, Smith RB, et al. The relationship of alprazolam dose to steady-state plasma concentrations. *J Clin Psychopharmacol* 1990;10:27–32.

Cowley DS. Alcohol abuse, substance abuse, and panic disorder. *Am J Med* 1992;92:41S–48S.

Croft-Jeffreys C, Wilkinson G. Estimated costs of neurotic disorder in UK general practice 1985. *Psychol Med* 1989;19:549–558.

Cross-National Collaborative Panic Study, Second Phase Investigators. Drug treatment of panic disorder: comparative efficacy of alprazolam, imipramine, and placebo. *Br J Psychiatry* 1992;160:191–202.

Curran HV. Benzodiazepines, memory and mood: a review. *Psychopharmacology* 1991;105:1–8.

DeMartinis N, Rynn M, Rickels K, et al. Prior benzodiazepine use and buspirone response in the treatment of generalized anxiety disorder. *J Clin Psychiatry* 2000;61:91–94.

Dietch JT, Jennings RK. Aggressive dyscontrol in patients treated with benzodiazepines. *J Clin Psychiatry* 1988;49:184–188.

Eaton WW, Kessler RC, Wittchen HU, et al. Panic and panic disorder in the United States. *Am J Psychiatry* 1994;151:413–420.

Fried R. *The hyperventilation syndrome.* Baltimore: Johns Hopkins, 1987.

Gelenberg AJ, Lydiard RB, Rudolph RL, et al. Efficacy of venlafaxine extended-release capsules in nondepressed outpatients with generalized anxiety disorder. *JAMA* 2000;283:3082–3088.

Ghoneim MM, Mewaldt SP. Benzodiazepines and human memory: a review. *Anesthesiology* 1990;72:926–938.

Greenblatt DJ, Miller LG, Shader RI. Benzodiazepine discontinuation syndromes. *J Psych Res* 1990;24:73–79.

Greenblatt DJ, Shader RI. *Benzodiazepines in clinical practice.* New York: Raven, 1974.

Greenblatt DJ, Shader RI, Abernethy DR. Current status of benzodiazepines. *N Engl J Med* 1983;309:354–358,410–416.

Hindmarch I, Kerr JS, Sherwood N. The effects of alcohol and other drugs on psychomotor performance and cognitive function. *Alcohol Alcoholism* 1991;26:71–79.

Katon WJ, von Korff M, Lin E. Panic disorder: relationship to high medical utilization. *Am J Med* 1992;92:78–118.

King DJ. Benzodiazepines, amnesia, and sedation: theoretical and clinical issues and controversies. *Hum Psychopharmacol* 1992;7:79–87.

LeCrubier Y, Bakker A, Dunbar G, et al. A comparison of paroxetine, clomipramine and placebo in the treatment of panic disorder. Collaborative Paroxetine Panic Study Investigators. *Acta Psychiatr Scand* 1997;95:145–152.

Lepola UM, Wade AG, Leinonen EV, et al. A controlled, prospective, 1-year trial of citalopram in the treatment of panic disorder. *J Clin Psychiatry* 1998;59:528–534.

Lucki I, Rickels K, Geller AM. Chronic use of benzodiazepines and psychomotor and cognitive test performance. *Psychopharmacology* 1986;88:426–433.

Lydiard RB, Lesser IM, Ballenger JC, et al. A fixed-dose study of alprazolam 2 mg, alprazolam 6 mg, and placebo in panic disorder. *J Clin Psychopharmacol* 1992;12:96–103.

Mavissakalian M, Perel JM. Clinical experiments in the maintenance and discontinuation of imipramine therapy in panic disorder with agoraphobia. *Arch Gen Psychiatry* 1992;49:318–323.

Mellinger GD, Balter MB, Uhlenhuth EH. Prevalence and correlates of the long-term regular use of anxiolytics. *JAMA* 1984;251:375–379.

Mental, behavioral, and developmental disorders. In: *International classification of statistical diseases and related health disorders,* tenth revision. Vol 1. Geneva: World Health Organization, 1992:311–387.

Modigh K, Westberg P, Ericksson E. Superiority of clomipramine over imipramine in the treatment of panic disorder: a placebo-controlled trial. *J Clin Psychopharmacol* 1992;12:251–261.

Murphy SM, Owen R, Tyrer P. Comparative assessment of efficacy and withdrawal symptoms after 6 and 12 weeks' treatment with diazepam or buspirone. *Br J Psychiatry* 1989;154:529–534.

Nair NP, Bakish D, Saxena B, et al. Comparison of fluvoxamine, imipramine, and placebo in the treatment of outpatients with panic disorder. *Anxiety* 1996;2:21–32.

Pande AC, Davidson JR, Jefferson JW, et al. Treatment of social phobia with gabapentin: a placebo-controlled study. *J Clin Psychopharmacol* 1999;19:341–348.

Pohl RB, Wolkow RM, Clary CM. Sertraline in the treatment of panic disorder: a double-blind multicenter trial. *Am J Psychiatry* 1998;155:1189–1195.

Pollack MH, Matthews J, Scott EL. Gabapentin as a potential treatment for anxiety disorders. *Am J Psychiatry* 1998;155:992–993.

Rapee RM, Barlow DH, eds. *Chronic anxiety.* New York: Guilford, 1991.

Reich J. The epidemiology of anxiety. *J Nerv Ment Dis* 1986;174:129–136.

Rickels K, DeMartinis N, Aufdembrinke B. A double-blind, placebo-controlled trial of abercanil and diazepam in the treatment of patients with generalized anxiety disorder. *J Clin Psychopharmacol* 2000;20:12–18.

Rickels K, Schweizer E. Panic disorder: long-term pharmacotherapy and discontinuation. *J Clin Psychopharmacol* 1998;18:12S–18S.

Rickels K, Schweizer E, Case WG, et al. Long-term therapeutic use of benzodiazepines. I. Effects of abrupt discontinuation. *Arch Gen Psychiatry* 1990;47:899–907.

Romach MK, Somer GR, Sobell GR, et al. Characteristics of long-term alprazolam users in the community. *J Clin Psychopharmacol* 1992;12:316–332.

Rosenbaum JF, Moroz G, Bowden CL. Clonazepam in the treatment of panic disorder with and without agoraphobia. *J Clin Psychopharmacol* 1997;17:390–400.

Roy-Byrne PP, Cowley DS, eds. *Benzodiazepines in clinical practice: risks and benefits.* Washington, D.C.: American Psychiatric Press, 1991.

Roy-Byrne PP, Stang P, Witchen HU, et al. Lifetime panic-depression comorbidity in the National Comorbidity Survey. *Br J Psychiatry* 2000;176:229–235.

Rudolph RL, Entsuah R, Chitra R. A meta-analysis of the effects of venlafaxine on anxiety associated with depression. *J Clin Psychopharmacol* 1998;18:136–144.

Schneier FR, Leibowitz MR, Davies SO, et al. Fluoxetine in panic disorder. *J Clin Psychopharmacol* 1990;10:119–121.

Shader RI. Stress, fear, and anxiety. In: Tupin JP, Shader RI, Harnett DS, eds. *Handbook of clinical psychopharmacology*. Northvale, NJ: Aronson, 1988:73–96.

Shader RI, Dreyfuss D, Gerrein JR, et al. Sedative effects and impaired learning and recall following single oral doses of lorazepam. *Clin Pharmacol Ther* 1986;39:526–529.

Shader RI, Goodman M, Gever J. Panic disorders: current perspectives. *J Clin Psychopharmacol* 1982;2:2S–10S.

Shader RI, Greenblatt DJ. Some practical approaches to the understanding and treatment of symptoms of anxiety and stress. In: Berger PA, Keith H, Brodie H, eds. *American handbook of psychiatry*. Vol. 8. New York: Basic Books, 1986:597–619.

Shader RI, Greenblatt DJ. Use of benzodiazepines in anxiety disorders. *N Engl J Med* 1993;328:1398–1405.

Snaith P, Owens D, Kennedy E. An outcome study of a brief anxiety management programme: anxiety control training. *Irish J Psychol Med* 1992;9:111–114.

Spiegel DA, Bruce TJ. Benzodiazepines and exposure-based cognitive behavior therapies for panic disorder. *Am J Psychiatry* 1997;154:773–781.

Stein MB, Liebowitz MR, Lydiard RB, et al. Paroxetine treatment of generalized social phobia (social anxiety disorder): a randomized controlled trial. *JAMA* 1998; 280:708–713.

Uhlenhuth EH, Balter MB, Ban TA, et al. International study of expert judgment on therapeutic use of benzodiazepines and other psychotherapeutic medications. IV. Therapeutic dose dependence and abuse liability of benzodiazepines in long-term treatment of anxiety disorders. *J Clin Psychopharmacol* 1999;19:23S–29S.

Van Ameringen M, Mancini C, Streiner DL. Fluoxetine efficacy in social phobia. *J Clin Psychiatry* 1993;54:27–32.

van Vliet IM, den Boer JA, Westenberg HG, et al. A double-blind comparative study of brofaromine and fluvoxamine in outpatients with panic disorder. *J Clin Psychopharmacol* 1996;16:299–306.

Wincor MZ, Munjack DJ, Palmer R. Alprazolam levels and response in panic disorder: preliminary results. *J Clin Psychopharmacol* 1991;11:48–51.

Woods JH, Katz JL, Winger G. Benzodiazepines: use, abuse, and consequences. *Pharmacol Rev* 1992;44:151–347.

Woods JH, Katz JL, Winger G. Use and abuse of benzodiazepines: issues relevant to prescribing. *JAMA* 1988;260:3476–3480.

Worsening C, Lavori PW. Excess mortality among 3302 patients with "pure" anxiety neurosis. *Arch Gen Psychiatry* 1991;48:599–602.

Zajecka J, Tracy KA, Mitchell S. Discontinuation symptoms after treatment with serotonin reuptake inhibitors: a literature review. *J Clin Psychiatry* 1997;58:291–297.

15. TREATMENT OF TRANSIENT INSOMNIA

Richard I. Shader
David J. Greenblatt

Insomnia has different meanings to different people. For example, the term can refer to difficulty falling asleep because of preoccupations with worries (ruminations) or because of pain or discomfort (e.g., gastrointestinal reflux disease); waking with a full bladder and not being able to fall back to sleep readily; feeling too activated to fall asleep because of the ingestion of **caffeinated** beverages too close to bedtime; or waking at 5 a.m. with a sense of dread after a mere 3 hours of sleep, as sometimes occurs in disorders of mood. From an adaptive or coping perspective, insomnia simply means not getting enough restorative sleep. When total sleep time is even transiently insufficient, the consequences for daytime functioning can be clinically significant, including impaired concentration and memory, irritability, drowsiness or falling asleep without warning, or altered reaction times. A workable but nonspecific definition of insomnia is *a subjective description of a person's difficulty with falling asleep or a lack of restorative or restful sleep in spite of ample time and opportunity to sleep.*

Insomnia can be subdivided in many ways. Some commonly accepted but clearly arbitrary dichotomies are (a) primary (i.e., intrinsic; likely of unknown origin) and secondary (i.e., extrinsic; likely from some determinable cause, such as worry, pain, or noise); (b) short term (less than 3 weeks) or long term (longer than 3 weeks); (c) the further subdivision of short term into transient (typically less than 4 nights) and short term (4 to 21 nights); and (d) short term and situational versus chronic. Most clinicians also find that separating out sleep-onset insomnia (i.e., problems with falling asleep) from sleep-maintenance insomnia (i.e., difficulties with staying asleep) is useful. Another important form is the early morning awakening that is common in major depressive episodes (see Chapter 18). A good example of transient insomnia is the nonrestorative sleep that is commonly experienced by hospitalized patients whose sleep is interrupted by a variety of factors, including noise, intravenous lines, light, pain, and fear. Inadequately treated chronic pain is a frequent cause of insomnia.

In the United States, about 80 million adults are currently estimated to have problems with sleep. About one-third of the persons with insomnia complain that their sleep problem is persistent (chronic) or that it recurs frequently (episodic), and almost two-thirds say that their sleep is disturbed at least two nights per week. About 40% of American adults say that their impaired sleep interferes with their daily activities. Disturbed sleep is particularly frequent in the elderly and in patients suffering from psychiatric disorders. About half of patients with schizophrenia have insomnia. The estimate for patients with major disorders of mood is even higher—about 75%. These estimates delineate the breadth of the population complaining of sleep disturbances; they do not address the issues of etiology or treatability.

This chapter focuses on the assessment and treatment of transient insomnia.

I. Evaluation, Diagnosis, and Sleep Hygiene

Careful evaluation and accurate diagnosis are critical first steps in responding to patients' sleep complaints. For example, some patients with daytime drowsiness, irritability, and depression are actually showing the daytime manifestations of a nocturnal problem, such as the alpha intrusions of fibromyalgia, obstructive or central sleep apnea, familial akathisia (restless leg syndrome), or nocturnal myoclonus. Treating any underlying cause (e.g., implementing continuous positive airway pressure for obstructive apnea or providing antidepressant therapy for those whose sleep difficulty is secondary to depression) is clearly more appropriate than is using sedative-hypnotic agents that, for some, may actually worsen the problem. Furthermore, some sleep problems that occur reflect grief reactions; phase-shift problems, such as jet lag (time zone changes) or shift work; separation anxiety; or behavioral conditioning. For example, some patients say they only have trouble sleeping when away from home. Others sleep well when they are not at home; they have difficulty sleeping at home because the bed or bedroom at home has become linked through conditioning to disquieting experiences, such as arguments or unwanted sexual experiences, or to moods, such as resentment or fear. Many complaints about disturbed sleep reflect lifestyle or stress problems. Women report a higher prevalence of disturbed sleep than men do. Further review, however, is beyond the scope of this chapter's coverage of insomnia.

Careful history-taking is essential to elicit situational causes that the patient may be ignoring. The patient may benefit from looking at the factors that he or she can change to promote better sleep hygiene. Often patients are helped simply by hearing from the clinician that missing a few nights of sleep will not be harmful. Suggesting that they read a book, listen to restful music, or watch a movie on television instead of focusing on the fact that they are not sleeping may allow the patient to have a less distressed reaction to the loss of sleep. Some data also suggest that picturing a peaceful and quiet scene (e.g., an isolated beach) is more effective than the customary advice to visualize and count sheep. If no daytime napping is occurring, the patient may soon become tired enough to resume a normal sleep pattern. Many patients will also benefit from simple suggestions about altering their before-sleep behaviors (Table 15.1).

Polysomnographic investigation is not indicated for the typical transient sleep disturbances usually seen by clinicians.

II. "Sleeping Pills"

In the United States, about 15% of all persons with sleep complaints use either prescription or over-the-counter sleep remedies. With short-term use, the benefits from pharmacotherapy are usually manifested as shortening of the latency to persistent sleep or as an increase in the total time asleep; the former occurs more frequently than the latter. Although effective sleeping pills may provide these very real short-term benefits for some people, more controversy is seen with regard to the general long-term use of hypnotic agents. Some, but not all, studies suggest that some degree of tolerance typically develops after weeks or a few months of nightly use. Abrupt discontinuation of short half-life hypnotic agents, which either deliberately or inadvertently happens all too often (e.g., when a patient is admitted to a hospital and does not disclose a history of use), can result in transient rebound insomnia or a withdrawal (abstinence) syndrome when prior use has been prolonged or when in it has occurred at high doses. About 30% of insomniacs use **alcohol** as a hypnotic (see section II.A.4).

A. Self-Prescribed Treatments

1. **Over-the-counter remedies** are the most widely used agents for inducing sleep. They typically contain **diphenhydramine** (e.g., Compoz, Dormin, Miles Nervine, Nytol, Sominex) or some other **antihistamine** (e.g., **chlorpheniramine, doxylamine** [e.g., Unisom Nighttime Sleep-Aid]) with sedating properties (Table 15.2). The resulting sedation or drowsiness may produce enough relaxation to promote sleep, but this effect may often be more subjective and indirect, rather than having a direct effect on sleep architecture. Their effectiveness has not been established by a sufficient number of carefully controlled clinical trials. Compliance with over-the-counter remedies, in general, is higher than with prescribed hypnotics. However, because antihistamines are not short acting, many people complain of next-day drowsiness or "thick-headedness," a "hangover," impaired coordination, reduced physical dexterity, or delayed reaction time. During sleep, **diphenhydramine** may increase motor activity. Anticholinergic effects, including dry mouth, urinary retention or difficulty urinating (hesitancy), or confusion, also may occur; these unwanted effects pose particular problems for the elderly, especially for men with prostatic hypertrophy. Tolerance to the sedating properties of **antihistamines** usually develops within days to weeks. Antihistamines should also be avoided in patients with

TABLE 15.1. HELPFUL HINTS FOR BETTER SLEEP

Do not go to bed to try to sleep when you are not tired.

Avoid evening naps.

Pain interferes with sleep. If possible, take an appropriate medication to reduce any physical pain you may be having.

Eat selectively. Being hungry when you go to bed may disrupt your sleep. Avoid a heavy meal too close to bedtime. Avoid caffeine and other methylxanthines (e.g., chocolate, colas, coffee, tea) after 4 p.m. A warm noncaffeinated beverage and a small carbohydrate snack before bedtime may be soothing, and they may enhance drowsiness.

Exercise at least two to three times per week. Avoid vigorous and sustained exercise close to bedtime (i.e., within the 2–3 hours before trying to go to sleep). A short early evening walk or bicycle ride may be relaxing.

Try to keep stress and conflict out of the bedroom; whenever possible, resolve the stresses of that day and enter the bedroom with a clean slate.

Enhance relaxation whenever possible (e.g., a warm unhurried bath; a massage; comforting sexual experiences; meditation; reading a good, but not too exciting, book). Try deep breathing methods (e.g., abdominal breathing in which slow inhalation is linked to the downward movement of the diaphragm and slow exhalation is linked to the upward movement of the diaphragm). Do this for 10 breaths, working to slow your breathing rate progressively. Repeat as necessary while trying to relax the rest of your body. Focus on a relaxing image and try to capture the whole scene including scents and temperature.

Develop comfortable and easily doable nighttime rituals or routines. Try to go to bed at a consistent time. Darken the room whenever possible.

If you do not fall asleep after a half hour or so, read a book or watch a pleasant television program for awhile. With this in mind, watching the late (e.g., 11 p.m.) news is probably not a good habit. When possible, leaving the bedroom if you do not readily fall asleep and returning only when you feel tired may be better. Keep your arising time as regular as possible as well.

Keep the room temperature comfortable for you. A hot room may increase awakenings (>24°C [75°F]), and a cold room may promote an increase in unpleasant dreams (<12°C [54°F]). Some fresh air may be helpful. Humidify your bedroom if it is too dry.

Try to use a supportive, preferably firm, mattress and pillows of comfortable thickness and density. Sometimes an adjustable bed should be considered because having the knees bent may decrease lower back muscle strain and pain.

Avoid noise, unless it is a form of "white" noise that is soothing to you.

For most people, alcohol use when kept to a minimum (i.e., one to two drinks with dinner) does not disrupt sleep. Alcohol use of any amount close to bedtime may be disruptive to the sleep of some.

TABLE 15.2. SOME OVER-THE-COUNTER SLEEP AIDS[a] COMMONLY AVAILABLE IN THE UNITED STATES

Product Name	Active Ingredient[b]
Benadryl	Diphenhydramine
Compoz	Diphenhydramine
Sleepinal	Diphenhydramine
Sominex	Diphenhydramine
Miles Nervine Nighttime Sleep-Aid	Diphenhydramine
Nytol	Doxylamine
Nytol QuickCaps	Diphenhydramine
Unisom	Doxylamine
Unisom SleepGels	Diphenhydramine

[a]Other sedating antihistamines include triprolidine, clemastine, and promethazine.
[b]Various strengths and formulations contain between 25 and 50 mg of the active antihistamine.

glaucoma or asthma. Some agents, such as **doxylamine**, may be dangerous during pregnancy.

Remembering that antihistamines may also be present in combination products, such as Alka-Seltzer PM, Aspirin Free Excedrin PM, Extra Strength Bayer PM Caplets, and Extra Strength Tylenol PM Gelcaps, is important.

2. **L-Tryptophan** was used, usually on a nonprescription basis, to help with sleep-onset insomnia until contamination problems led to its withdrawal from the market in the United States and many other countries in 1990. (*Note:* Some dietary supplements and enteral nutrition products may contain **L-tryptophan**.) Although the available data on the efficacy and safety of this drug are neither extensive nor conclusive, the clinical consensus is that **L-tryptophan** is a weakly effective hypnotic agent without significant risks in the absence of contaminants. The eosinophilic-myalgia syndrome reported with its use has been linked to a contaminant in the manufacturing process. No acceptable reformulation has been introduced into the market in the United States. The folk remedy of warm milk with crackers before bedtime probably has its basis in the facilitation of **L-tryptophan** absorption from milk by the accompanying carbohydrate or through mediation by cholecystokinin. Some people believe that the soporific effects of **L-tryptophan** seen after eating turkey or bananas are also predictable.

3. **Melatonin** is a naturally occurring pineal gland peptide hormone. When purified or synthesized and taken orally, it alters circadian rhythms, lowers the core body temperature, and reduces daytime alerting phenomena originating in the suprachiasmatic nucleus. Although it has been found to be effective for the treatment of insomnia in a number of populations and settings, the results are inconsistent and some degree of controversy remains about its efficacy and long-term safety. One factor that may influence efficacy studies has been a lack of information about dose-response relationships. Efficacy has been reported with doses as low as 0.3 mg at bedtime. Others believe that 6 mg is the necessary dose. The authors have had some inconsistent success with **melatonin** for the treatment of transient insomnia at doses of 6 mg per night.

Some data suggest that the endogenous **melatonin** levels increase in patients receiving monoamine oxidase inhibitors or selective serotonin reuptake inhibitors and that they decrease during the use of some β-adrenergic receptor antagonists (e.g., **atenolol, propranolol**).

Side effects attributed to **melatonin** use include pruritus, tachycardia, headache, and daytime drowsiness.

4. **Alcohol** is probably even more frequently used to induce sleep than are over-the-counter remedies. What most **alcohol** users do not realize, however, is that, although **alcohol** may promote sleep onset, it then fragments the subsequent sleep architecture. This means that most **alcohol**-induced sleep will not be as restorative as unaided sleep is. Many persons who consume **alcohol** at bedtime sleep quite deeply and soundly for a few hours but then awaken; they are then unable to fall back to sleep. **Alcohol** use may pose additional risks for those who are sleep deprived. For example, in a driving simulation test conducted after a night of sleep deprivation, volunteers performed poorly after the ingestion of small amounts of **alcohol**, some at levels that were insufficient to result in detectable blood **alcohol** levels.

5. **Kava**, as **kavalactones** and **kavapyrones**, is sometimes used as a sleep aid. Called the "intoxicating pepper" by the sea-going James Cook, **kava** is derived from the roots of a shrub (*Piper methysticum*) grown on some South Pacific islands. **Kava-kava** is called **kavain** in some other countries. A typical dose of **kavalactones**—15 have been isolated and 6 are thought to be γ-aminobutyric acid (GABA)ergic—is 200 to 500 mg. Curiously, despite its putative GABAergic mode of action, **kava** is not thought to potentiate the sedative effects of **alcohol**.

As the controlled or long-term assessment of **kava** is insufficient at this time, it cannot be endorsed as either an effective or safe substance; more rigorous trials are being conducted currently. Some side effects attributed to its use include headache, gastrointestinal distress, fatigue, and so-called **kava** dermopathy (a fish scale–like change in the skin seen in some persons after chronic use). *Recently, the United Kingdom Medicines Control Agency advised prudence regarding kava-kava use and recommended discontinuation of products containing kava-kava because of serious adverse hepatic events. Switzerland has discontinued sales of these products, and Germany and the Food and Drug Administration in the United States are reviewing data at the time of the writing of this chapter. At least one case on file at the United States Food and Drug Administration involved hepatic failure requiring liver transplantation.*

6. **Valerian** was described by Samuel Taylor Coleridge as "a gentle thing, beloved from pole to pole." It is approved by the German Commission E as a prescription sleep aid. Many varieties of **valerian** exist, and, as with many herbal extracts, standardization problems and inconsistent potency are rampant. Some of **valerian's** sleep-inducing activity is attributed to **valerenic acid** and various **valpotriates**. Dosages usually range from 300 to 900 mg. Side effects are not common at these dosage levels; headache, gastrointestinal distress, and palpitations have been noted. Tolerance, physical dependence, and withdrawal reactions have not been substantiated. Systematic assessments of efficacy and safety that meet American research design standards are still lacking.

7. **Aromatherapies** are also available. One such product simply called SLEEP (by Essence of Vali) contains lavender flowers, cedar wood, marjoram leaves, and ylang-ylang petals. The manufacturer's recommended strategy is to place a few drops of the oil on the corner of the pillowcase or on a separate cloth that is placed under the pillowcase. Curiously, this product contains a warning cautioning against use during pregnancy or in persons treated for low blood pressure.

B. **Prescription Medications**

1. **Benzodiazepines** are more consistently effective than self-prescribed treatments. They shorten sleep latency, decrease stage 1 sleep, and increase stage 2 sleep. Slow-wave sleep (stages 3 and 4) generally is reduced. Patients believe that their sleep experience is more restorative. Five benzodiazepines are currently marketed as hypnotics in the United States (Table 15.3). No convincing evidence that is currently available consistently distinguishes among them in terms of efficacy or safety with proper usage (i.e., dosages, dosing intervals, and duration of use). Some differences among the benzodiazepines have been suggested on the basis of stage 3 and stage 4 effects and possible variations in receptor binding,

TABLE 15.3. BENZODIAZEPINE RECEPTOR AGONISTS MARKETED IN THE UNITED STATES AS HYPNOTICS

Generic Name	Trade Name	Dosage Strength(s) (mg)	Relative Duration of Action
Triazolam	Halcion and generics	0.125, 0.25	Short
Zolpidem	Ambien	5, 10	Short
Zaleplon	Sonata	5, 10	Short
Temazepam	Restoril and generics	7.5, 15, 30	Intermediate
Estazolam	ProSom	1, 2	Intermediate
Flurazepam	Dalmane and generics	15, 30	Long
Quazepam	Doral	7.5, 15	Long

but no basis for any clinically relevant variability has been established. Data suggest that all currently marketed benzodiazepines bind to cortical (ω_1, ω_2), cerebellar (ω_1), and spinal (ω_2) benzodiazepine receptor sites on $GABA_A$-chloride channels.

Any benzodiazepine, including those not marketed as hypnotics, could be used to induce sleep as long as an appropriate dose is chosen. The basic issues are rapidity of absorption from the gastrointestinal tract, rapid uptake into the brain, adequate duration of action, duration of activity of any active metabolites, and the elimination of the parent compound and any active metabolites at a rate that significantly reduces brain concentrations before the patient awakens the next morning. From this perspective, one can imagine the possibility that certain agents would be good for sleep-onset problems and that others might be good for maintaining sleep. Problems with benzodiazepines when they are used in appropriate dosages and for brief courses (e.g., a few nights to several weeks) are infrequent. Unfortunately, some patients mix benzodiazepines and **alcohol**, which can enhance the sedation or adverse effects from both and can produce, for example, excessive and prolonged sedation, dizziness, or falls. Cross-tolerance among benzodiazepines and between benzodiazepines and **alcohol** has not been adequately clarified, even though benzodiazepines are successfully used in the treatment of **alcohol withdrawal** (see Chapter 12). Some problems seen shortly after starting a patient on a new benzodiazepine hypnotic may actually reflect a withdrawal syndrome from a prior benzodiazepine, particularly if the former was a shorter half-life type, or from **alcohol** that was abruptly stopped.

Rebound insomnia is common with abrupt discontinuation after several nights of use of shorter half-life benzodiazepine hypnotics, and some patients find that this seems worse than their original problem. Rebound insomnia may in fact be more marked or exaggerated than the original insomnia problem. However, it rarely lasts for more than a few nights, and it generally can be avoided either by dose tapering rather than by abrupt stoppage or by using lower dosages during treatment. Individual susceptibility to rebound insomnia is variable. Some evidence suggests that the likelihood of rebound is greater in those who experience a greater hypnotic efficacy.

Some patients receiving shorter half-life benzodiazepines complain of increased wakefulness during the terminal hours of sleep (i.e., the last 2 to 3 hours). This is similar to what may happen when **alcohol** is used as a hypnotic. Another concern experienced by some patients taking shorter half-life benzodiazepines is increased daytime anxiety, particularly during the morning.

Benzodiazepines are relatively safe when they are used as directed. A small proportion of patients, usually persons who have a tendency to abuse other substances, becomes involved in dosage escalation and abuse. Daytime drowsiness may be a problem, particularly with longer-acting benzodiazepines (Table 15.4). Falls[1] occur and confusion may develop, particularly in the elderly. Anterograde amnesia is not uncommon, particularly with **triazolam** or in phase-shifted persons. Any consideration of comparative safety claims among benzodiazepines must take into consideration dosage, the activity of the metabolites, the timing of use, age, and concomitant diagnoses.

2. **Chloral hydrate** is viewed by many clinicians as an obsolete agent. However, it is reasonably effective in dosages of 0.5 to 1.5 g (Table 15.5). The elimination half-life of 6 to 8 hours for its active metabolite, **trichloroethanol**, is consistent with a minimal likelihood of next-day

---

[1]Factors increasing susceptibility to falls include impaired visual contrast sensitivity, decreased visual acuity, and decreased sensation in the legs. In addition, sedative-hypnotic use may augment any existing decrements in reaction time, muscle strength, or postural stability.

TABLE 15.4. SOME UNWANTED EFFECTS COMMON TO MOST BENZODIAZEPINE RECEPTOR AGONIST SEDATIVE-HYPNOTIC AGENTS[a]

Motor impairment and falls
Anterograde impairment of memory and new learning (recall)
Discontinuation syndromes (e.g., rebound insomnia, withdrawal reactions)
Tolerance and physical dependence
Respiratory depression
Interactions (additive or synergistic) with alcohol (ethanol)
Architecture of sleep altered
Daytime drowsiness and other carryover effects

[a]The unwanted effects have been ordered to produce the mnemonic MAD TRIAD.

TABLE 15.5. SOME NONBENZODIAZEPINE RECEPTOR AGONIST SEDATIVE-HYPNOTIC AGENTS AVAILABLE BY PRESCRIPTION IN THE UNITED STATES

Generic Name	Trade Name	Dosage Range (mg)	Class
Butabarbital	Butisol	50–100	III
Phenobarbital	Luminal	100–300	IV
Mephobarbital	Mebaral	32–400	IV
Chloral hydrate	Noctec	500–1,500	IV
Meprobamate	Miltown Equanil	400–1,600	IV
Hydroxyzine hydrochloride	Atarax	50–400	—
Hydroxyzine pamoate	Vistaril	50–400	—

performance impairment. In many clinical drug studies, particularly those of antidepressants, it is used for the initial 7 to 10 days to give the patients some relief while the study drug begins to become effective. This is actually an arbitrary decision, because little research has been done on the molecular basis of **chloral hydrate's** mode of action or on its interactions with study drugs. **Chloral hydrate's** drawbacks include a narrow therapeutic index (toxic dose to therapeutic dose), gastric irritation leading to nausea and vomiting, and gastric necrosis with high dosages. As with other sedative-hypnotics, dependence and tolerance may develop. It may also displace other drugs from their protein-binding sites, and, during prolonged dosage, it may be a hepatic microsomal enzyme-inducing agent.

3. **Zolpidem**, an imidazopyridine compound, is currently the most widely prescribed hypnotic in the United States. Although it is promoted as a nonbenzodiazepine, its activity is based on its binding to central (ω_1) **benzodiazepine receptors**. The assumption made is that the more restricted binding of **zolpidem** confers a more limited range of unwanted effects. To some extent, this is borne out by clinical experience, but more time and data across a spectrum of dosages in different age groups are needed before adequate comparisons can be made.[2] **Zolpidem's** half-life typically is 2.5 to 3 hours. **Zolpidem's** hypnotic activity can be reversed by the benzodiazepine antagonist **flumazenil** (Romazicon). Based on its

[2]One recent case-control study among elderly patients who had undergone hip fracture surgery found that **zolpidem** use was associated with a twofold increase in the risk for these fractures compared with that of control subjects. This risk compares with an approximately 1.5-fold increase for those taking benzodiazepines in this same age group (Wang et al.). A study from Australia reports experiences including visual hallucinations, confusion, and depression (Adverse Drug Reactions Advisory Committee. Seeing things with zolpidem. *Australian Adverse Drug Reactions Bulletin* 2002;21:3.).

extensive use, **zolpidem** appears to have a somewhat reduced likelihood of producing tolerance or withdrawal syndromes. Its abuse potential also seems lower than that seen with some benzodiazepines, but it does have some cross-tolerance with **alcohol** at higher than standard hypnotic dosages. See Table 15.3 for available dosage forms. The use of lower dosages is usually important for elderly patients. Rebound insomnia has been reported with its discontinuation.

4. **Zaleplon** is another nonbenzodiazepine that acts by binding to central (ω_1) benzodiazepine receptors; its hypnotic effects can also be antagonized by **flurazepam**. **Zaleplon** is classified as a pyrazolopyrimidine compound (Table 15.3 details the available dosage forms). The usual starting dose in adults is 10 mg; 5 mg is a typical dose for the elderly. Although it is currently less popular in the United States than **zolpidem**, it is similar in most respects; one notable difference is its even shorter elimination half-life, which is approximately 1 to 2 hours. Some clinicians find this quality useful for patients who awaken during the middle of the night and who want to fall asleep again. Many clinicians limit the consecutive nights of use to two to three nights, which is then followed by an interruption in use of one to several nights. Rebound insomnia has been reported with discontinuation.

5. A variety of **other prescription hypnotics**, particularly oral hypnotic agents, remains available, including the barbiturates (e.g., **butabarbital** [intermediate duration of action], **mephobarbital** [because of long duration of action it is used mainly for anxiety]) and **meprobamate** (Table 15.5). These agents do not have either efficacy or safety profiles that are comparable with those of the **benzodiazepines, zolpidem,** or **zaleplon**. Their use is not encouraged by the authors, even though health care cost pressures and other forces have led to a resurgence in their use in some locations.

6. **Trazodone**, a triazolopyridine compound marketed as an antidepressant, is frequently used as a hypnotic. Given in doses of 25 to 150 mg at bedtime, it appears to be effective as a hypnotic for many patients. One of **trazodone's** common uses is to counter the insomnia associated with selective serotonin reuptake inhibitor use. Daytime drowsiness can usually be minimized by choosing the lowest effective hypnotic dose. Tolerance development is not common, so **trazodone** is frequently used for patients with chronic insomnia. Because anticholinergic side effects and postural hypotension are not common with its use, **trazodone** has some advantages over other sedating antidepressants.

7. **Other sedating antidepressants** are still used by some clinicians in small doses (i.e., 25 to 50 mg); these include sedating antidepressants, such as **amitriptyline** or **trimipramine**. These may be appropriate alternatives, especially for patients with depression, but the risks from the antiadrenergic and anticholinergic properties of these agents must also be considered.

III. **Suggested Guidelines for Prescribing Medications**
   Universally accepted guidelines for the dosing and duration of use for hypnotics are not established. Both must be individualized, with the goal of finding the lowest dose and minimizing the duration to the shortest possible. Generally, between one and three tablets or capsules per night of the lowest dosage strength is appropriate. Short-term treatment (i.e., one to two nights to 1 to 2 weeks) is reasonable for most patients. However, some patients with chronic insomnia may benefit from longer term use, as long as the prescribing clinician provides careful monitoring. Because no criteria are presently available to identify this subpopulation, considering several short-term trials, with gradual tapering at the end of each period and a drug-free interval between each period, seems reasonable for establishing the patient's need for, and the appropriateness and value of, continued therapy. The drug-free time interval between the initial periods should be from 1 to 3 weeks, depending on the half-lives of

the agent and its active metabolites and the rapidity of the taper schedule. Reevaluation of such a patient's continued need for hypnotic medication at 3-month to 6-month intervals is also reasonable. Because the elderly are particularly susceptible to falls or confusion from hypnotic use, using the lowest available dosage strength is advisable.

When insomnia is of the primary and chronic form, controversy exists about continuous long-term use of hypnotics. Although many patients do benefit from long-term use, to establish whether the occurrence of rebound insomnia or withdrawal has been the deciding factor in convincing the patient of the continued value of the hypnotic agent is important.

For those individuals who hope to benefit from behavioral or nonpharmacologic approaches to their insomnia, prescribing hypnotics two to three times per week while they are working out such modifications may be beneficial. For patients with chronic, persistent, sleep-maintenance insomnia, some evidence exists that suggests that cognitive-behavior therapy is more helpful than either muscle relaxation exercises or a sham form of behavior therapy. Unfortunately, the comparative benefits of cognitive-behavior therapy as compared with the use of hypnotic agents and of the combined use of cognitive-behavior therapy and hypnotic agents has been insufficiently studied.

IV. Overdosage and Abuse of Sedative-Hypnotics
These important topics are covered in Chapters 3, 9, 11, and 12.

V. Internet Sites
Some useful sites for persons with sleep disorders include *http://www.sleepfoundation.org/* and *http://www.nhlbi.nih.gov/about/ncsdr/*. These sites provide facts about research, contact telephone numbers, a sleep diary for tracking actual sleep patterns that can be helpful to both clinicians and patients, and other useful information.

ADDITIONAL READING

Akerstedt T. Sleepiness as a consequence of shift work. *Sleep* 1988;11:17–34.

Aldrich MS. Automobile accidents in patients with sleep disorders. *Sleep* 1989; 12:487–494.

Andrade C, Srihari BS, Reddy KP, et al. Melatonin in medically ill patients with insomnia: a double-blind, placebo-controlled study. *J Clin Psychiatry* 2001;62:41–45.

Attenburrow ME, Cowen PJ, Sharpley AL. Low dose melatonin improves sleep in healthy middle-aged subjects. *Psychopharmacology* 1996;126:179–181.

Balderer G, Borbély AA. Effect of valerian on human sleep. *Psychopharmacology* 1985;87:406–409.

Balter MB, Uhlenhuth EH. The beneficial and adverse effects of hypnotics. *J Clin Psychiatry* 1991;52:16–23.

Biondi F, Casadei GL. Results of a multicenter trial with the hypnotic zolpidem in 1152 insomniac patients. *Curr Ther Res Clin Exp* 1994;55:262–274.

Boonen G, Häberlein H. Influence of genuine kavapyrone enantiomers on the GABA binding site. *Planta Med* 1998;64:504–506.

Brzezinski A. Melatonin in humans. *N Engl J Med* 1997;336:186–195.

Chase JE, Gidal BE. Melatonin: therapeutic use in sleep disorders. *Ann Pharmacother* 1997;31:1218–1226.

Clark NA, Alexander B. Increased rate of trazodone prescribing with bupropion and selective serotonin-reuptake inhibitors versus tricyclic antidepressants. *Ann Pharmacother* 2000;34:1007–1012.

Darcourt G, Pringuey D, Sallière D, et al. The safety and tolerability of zolpidem—an update. *J Psychopharmacol* 1999;13:81–93.

Dement WC. The proper use of sleeping pills in the primary care setting. *J Clin Psychiatry* 1992;53:50–56.

Dement WC, Mitler MM. It's time to wake to the importance of sleep disorders. *JAMA* 1993;269:1548–1550.

Dolberg OT, Hirschmann S, Grunhaus L. Melatonin for the treatment of sleep disturbances in major depression. *Am J Psychiatry* 1998;155:1119–1121.

Drake CL, Roehrs TA, Mangano RM, et al. Dose-response effects of zaleplon as compared with triazolam (0.25 mg) and placebo in chronic primary insomnia. *Hum Psychopharmacol* 2000;15:595–604.

Edinger JD, Wohlgemuth WK, Radtke RA, et al. Cognitive behavioral therapy for the treatment of chronic primary insomnia. *JAMA* 2001;285:1856–1864.

Ford DE, Kamerow DB. Epidemiologic study of sleep disturbances and psychiatric disorders: an opportunity for prevention? *JAMA* 1989;262:1479–1484.

Gallup Organization. *Sleep in America*. Princeton, NJ: National Sleep Foundation, 1991.

Garfinkel D, Laudon M, Nof D, et al. Improvement in sleep quality in elderly people by controlled-release melatonin. *Lancet* 1995;346:541–544.

Gillin JC, Spinweber CL, Johnson LC. Rebound insomnia: a critical review. *J Clin Psychopharmacol* 1989;9:161–172.

Greenblatt DJ, Harmatz JS, Zinny MA, et al. Effect of gradual withdrawal on the rebound sleep disorder after discontinuation of triazolam. *N Engl J Med* 1987; 317:722–728.

Greenblatt DJ, Miller LG, Shader RI. Neurochemical and pharmacokinetic correlates of the clinical action of benzodiazepine hypnotic drugs. *Am J Med* 1990;88:18S–24S.

Guro-Razuman S, Anand P, Hu Q, et al. Dermatomyositis-like illness following kava-kava ingestion. *J Clin Rheumatol* 1999;5:342–345.

Hedner J, Yaeche R, Emilien G, et al. Zaleplon shortens subjective sleep latency and improves subjective sleep quality in elderly patients with insomnia. *Int J Geriatr Psychiatry* 2000;15:704–712.

Hughes RJ, Sack RL, Lewy AJ. The role of melatonin and circadian phase in age-related sleep-maintenance insomnia: assessment in a clinical trial of melatonin replacement. *Sleep* 1998;21:52–68.

Jacques CH, Lynch JC, Samkoff JS. The effects of loss of sleep on cognitive performance of resident physicians. *J Fam Pract* 1990;30:223–229.

Kuhlmann J, Berger W, Podzuweit, et al. The influence of valerian treatment on reaction time, alertness and concentration in volunteers. *Pharmacopsychiatry* 1999;32:235–241.

Langer S, Mendelson W, Richardson G. Symptomatic treatment of insomnia. *Sleep* 1999;22:S437–S445.

Lauber JK, Kayten PK. Sleepiness, circadian dysrhythmia, and fatigue in transportation system accidents. *Sleep* 1988;11:503–512.

Pittler MH, Ernst E. Efficacy of kava extract for treating anxiety: systematic review and meta-analysis. *J Clin Pharmacol* 2000;20:84–89.

Roehrs T, Beare D, Zorick F, et al. Sleepiness and ethanol effects on simulated driving. *Alcohol Clin Exp Res* 1994;18:154–158.

Sack RL, Lewy AJ, Hughes RJ. Use of melatonin for sleep and circadian rhythm disorders. *Ann Med* 1998;30:115–121.

Salzman C, Fisher J, Nobel K, et al. Cognitive improvement following benzodiazepine discontinuation in elderly nursing home residents. *Int J Geriatr Psychiatry* 1992;7:89–93.

Shader RI, Greenblatt DJ, Balter MB. Appropriate use and regulatory control of benzodiazepines. *J Clin Pharmacol* 1991;31:781–784.

Soldatos CR, Dikeos DG, Whitehead A. Tolerance and rebound insomnia with rapidly eliminated hypnotics: a meta-analysis of sleep laboratory studies. *Int Clin Psychopharmacol* 1999;14:287–303.

Thase ME. Antidepressant treatment of the depressed patient with insomnia. *J Clin Psychiatry* 1999;60:28–31.

Tsutsui S. A double-blind comparative study of zolpidem versus zopiclone in the treatment of chronic primary insomnia. *J Int Med Res* 2001;29:163–177.

Walsh JK, Mahowald MW. Avoiding the blanket approach to insomnia: targeted therapy for specific causes. *Postgrad Med* 1991;90:211–224.

Wang PS, Bohn RL, Glynn RJ, et al. Zolpidem use and hip fractures in older people. *J Am Geriatric Soc* 2001;49:1685–1690.

Wright SW, Lawrence LM, Wrenn KD, et al. Randomized clinical trial of melatonin after night-shift work: efficacy and neuropsychologic effects. *Ann Emerg Med* 1998;32:334–340.

16. BEREAVEMENT REACTIONS AND GRIEF

Richard I. Shader
Wayne A. Ury

Death is inevitable, and losses are a part of life; so, too, are grief and bereavement. Family members and others touched by a loss may need to go through these processes to move on with their lives. Bereavement and grief are central to "letting go." In providing bereavement care, a key clinical issue is distinguishing what is normal and painful from that which is dysfunctional or illness, yet realizing that both require care, social support, and someone who will listen. Physicians, nurses, social workers, and other health care providers regularly encounter bereavement and grief; it is an integral part of caring for patients and their families. They encounter sorrow in the survivors of their patients; in their patients who are survivors; and in themselves when they lose people important to their lives, including patients. Death and grief are issues with which they need to be familiar and that they should be able to address in the clinical setting. To help others, clinicians need to be aware of their own reactions to people who are in grief and of their own concerns about death and dying.

The terms **bereavement** and **grief** are generally used interchangeably. Technically, **bereavement** refers to the experience of a loss through death, whereas **grief** refers to the feelings (e.g., the emotional suffering) and the behaviors (e.g., crying) associated with loss. Based on the attachments people normally form throughout life, grief and bereavement are the expected consequences of the death of a significant person, whether that individual is loved or not. Also included, however, are significant losses, such as those of a pet, of physical function, or of a part of the body (e.g., stroke, mastectomy); a new diagnosis that results in the loss of the ability to perform certain tasks or that makes giving up work or other activities that are an important part of a person's identity necessary; important relationships (e.g., divorce) or even jobs; a familiar home; or one's community. Therefore, grieving may occur not only with the death of another person but also with a loss of function or one's sense of self. Because more is known about grief as it relates to death, the sections below are focused accordingly.

Given the number of people who die each year and the average size of an American family, a reasonable estimate is that 7 to 9 million Americans experience the death of a family member in any year. Some estimates suggest that, across all demographic groups, at least 5% of all children lose one or both parents by the age of 15. Grief and bereavement are normal aspects of life and the life cycle, but, in certain instances, abnormalities in behavior and social or occupational function can occur. Clinicians need to recognize and to distinguish the sometimes subtle differences between normal grief, abnormal grief, and depression, a distinction that may not always be straightforward.

In normal grief and bereavement (see section I), the bereft person is significantly distressed, but he or she is still able to function. Over time, the distress and sadness gradually resolve. Grief and bereavement become abnormal (see section III) when the mourner suffers from clinical depression or some other form of psychopathologic response. In some instances of abnormal grief, significant occupational, family, or social dysfunction results from the bereavement process. In normal grief, social and, in some circumstances, psychologic support help the bereaved to return gradually to a place where he or she can move on with life. In abnormal grief, an appropriate intervention with psychologic or psychiatric care, social support, or spiritual resources is necessary.

Table 16.1 contrasts some of the features that may differentiate an episode of normal bereavement from an episode of major depressive disorder (MDD) (see Chapter 18). In addition to these features, the *Diagnostic and Statistical Manual of Mental Disorders,* 4th edition, points out that any hallucinatory experiences occurring during normal grief must be confined to thinking that one hears the voice of or transiently sees the image of the deceased. Any guilt should be limited to feelings about actions taken or not taken by the survivor at the time of death. The *Diagnostic and Statistical Manual of Mental Disorders,* 4th edition, classifies bereavement as an additional con-

TABLE 16.1. BEREAVEMENT VERSUS MAJOR DEPRESSIVE DISORDER

Uncomplicated Bereavement	MDD
Should follow a recent major loss	May be unrelated to loss
Self-esteem changes not typically seen	May develop feelings of worthlessness
Social and occupational functioning mildly and transiently impaired	Significant impairment is common
Assessment of lost person is realistic	Lost person typically is idealized or distorted
Any neurovegetative features are transient	Prolonged neurovegetative features
Acute distress usually subsides in 6–12 weeks	Persistent distress
Suicidal thoughts are rare or typically uncommon	Suicidal thoughts and plans are not transient, and they may include fantasies of "rejoining" the lost one

Abbreviation: MDD, major depressive disorder.

dition that may be the focus of clinical attention. A coding category of **bereavement** can be added to other diagnoses.

I. Normal Grief

Commonly, acute grief can be expected to last days to weeks, perhaps with recurrence on anniversaries of important losses. When grief is uncomplicated, it typically proceeds in the following three phases: initial numbness and shock; waves of sadness and weeping along with altered sleep, appetite, and ability to concentrate; and resolution or acceptance—an awareness that life will go on. During the second phase, transient feelings of guilt or self-blame (e.g., "I should have done more"); blaming of others; or anger at fate, one's God or other deities, the person who died, or those who tried to help, including the treating physician, may be present. Some observations of bereaved persons suggest that one's first experience with loss is often the most difficult to endure and that how it progresses and resolves may set the tone for how future losses are handled.

Any feelings of guilt and anger should be short-lived, but they may return. Typically, grief then gradually fades over a period of several months, coming back only with "reminders" of past shared experiences or when the individual encounters events or things that were special to, or shared with, the deceased. Grief can also be anticipatory, as with a loved one or friend who has an inoperable or untreatable illness, such as human immunodeficiency virus infection or cancer.

II. The Mourning Period

Customarily, acute grief is followed by a mourning period lasting 6 to 12 months or even up to 3 or more years. During this time, the bereaved person comes to terms with the painful feelings of loss and the changes in life that occur as a result of the loss. The process of "working through" a loss typically involves a number of steps that are listed in Table 16.2. These steps can be remembered by the mnemonic **AFTER**. Although these steps are commonly seen, tremendous variability in the time frame, experience, and process of mourning is observed. Therefore, the clinician needs to consider and address the needs of each person.

Mourning is also a social process. Most societies and cultures have rituals to aid mourners. Considering the potential social and psychologic benefits that religion or ritual can provide to certain individuals is important. A significant loss can trigger a questioning of religious beliefs that may even cause a worsening of depressive symptoms. For some, their congregation or a religious leader can provide social support during the period of grief and mourning. One's religious community may even be able to provide individuals who will visit those in mourning, as well as meals or aid with transportation.

TABLE 16.2. TYPICAL STEPS IN THE MOURNING PROCESS

Accepting the loss and its finality
Feeling and experiencing the full range and intensity of the emotions stirred up by the loss
Taking up life again and planning for life without the deceased (the lost person, pet)
Engaging and investing in new relationships (new job or pet, etc.)
Retaining "a place in one's heart" for the deceased (lost person or pet) and remembering him or her; death does not diminish the importance of significant relationships

These steps have been phrased as the mnemonic **AFTER** to aid in remembering them.

Although normal mourning can last up to 3 or more years, many bereaved persons believe that something must be wrong when their loss-related distress lasts so long. Sometimes well-meaning family, friends, and physicians "push" them to get beyond the mourning period sooner than may be natural. Observers may react with impatience rather than tolerance, or they may mistake prolonged normal mourning for pathologic grief. Family and close friends, as identified by the mourner, need to be educated by the health care provider or the mourner about how long mourning can last. They need to know that a normal mourning process can include feeling sad on anniversaries or birthdays, occasional periods of crying, and occasional displays of mourning and sadness that occur after the mourning period appears to have passed, as long as the mourner is functioning adequately in daily life and the pattern of symptoms seen in abnormal grief is not present.

Normal grieving is also not accompanied by drug or alcohol abuse; a prolonged period of social isolation after the death; loss of interest in hobbies, work, or intellectual pursuits; or problems with occupational functioning that do not remit. A prolonged pattern of any of the above signs requires further professional evaluation. If a practitioner is unable to evaluate or to address these concerns, a consultation or referral should be initiated. Possible sources of referral include psychologists, psychiatrists, social work therapists, bereavement counselors, or other persons trained to do bereavement counseling.

Recent data suggest that the mourning period may be associated with increased vulnerability to and morbidity from a variety of illnesses. This has been hypothesized to be the result of the stress of loss and readjustment or to secondary alterations in immunologic function. The first year after a significant loss may be a particularly vulnerable time for elderly widowers. They may suffer social isolation and despair, and they are at high risk for alcoholism, depressive disorders, and suicide. A recent study suggests that depression and weight loss are more likely to occur among those spouses who did not actively participate as caregivers before a death. For those spouses strained by the caregiver role, the death itself did not appear to increase their overall distress. Instead, the surviving spouses reduced their health risk behaviors (e.g., skipping their own medical checkups, getting insufficient rest). Those who live alone or who do not eventually remarry are at especially high risk. However, in general, remarriage shortly after a loss may compromise the resolution of grief, and those counseling the bereaved may wish to convey this perspective.

III. Abnormal Grief

Grief can become prolonged or pathologic. It may also merge into or trigger a major depressive episode. Some degree of sadness, despair, or unhappiness is to be expected in all normal grieving, but these feelings should gradually resolve. Depression *per se* should be suspected when the symptoms and signs persist or intensify (e.g., transiently disrupted sleep becomes a persistent pattern of early morning awakening). In normal grief, a bereaved person may transiently fear losing his or her mind, or he or she may have brief (i.e., minutes to a few days after the funeral) thoughts of or impulses toward self-harm or suicide. In depression, such thoughts or impulses are likely to persist or intensify, and they interfere with social, occupational, or physical functioning.

When suicidal ideation, slowed speech or motor movements, or agitation persist for more than a few days after a death, an abnormal reaction to grief, including the possibility of MDD, should be considered; immediate evaluation is then necessary. When neurovegetative symptoms (e.g., sleep or appetite disturbances) persist or social and occupational functions do not begin to return to normal after approximately 2 months, the possibility of a major depressive episode should be considered, and an evaluation by an experienced psychiatrist or psychologist should be conducted or obtained. In 15% to 20% of those who grieve after a loss, clinically significant depression may be present 1 year later.

Grief can also be intensified or unresolved in other ways. The grieving person (a) may deny the loss or feel despairing helplessness; (b) may pine for the deceased or lost person, a preoccupation that blocks engagement with others and getting on with life; (c) may avoid experiences, people, and things linked to the deceased; (d) may identify with the deceased (e.g., taking on some characteristics or even symptoms); (e) may overidealize the deceased; or (f) may suffer nightmares and social withdrawal suggestive of a posttraumatic stress reaction.

Grief may be especially painful when parents lose children, including adult children; spouses or life partners die; or children lose parents. Table 16.3 lists categories of people in whom complicated or dysfunctional grief may be more likely to occur. Patients with a history of mental illness often have difficulty with grief and mourning. Clinicians may wish to consider all these aspects when they are trying to identify risk factors in their patients.

IV. Treatment Considerations

A. Social Support

People who are experiencing grief should be urged to have a friend or relative move in with them for at least the first few days after a death. When this is not possible, sleeping at the house of a relative or friend may be a wise alternative. This is not a good time to be isolated, but it is also not a good time to rush into other relationships or to make other major changes or moves. Relatives or friends can often be helpful by assisting with funeral and burial arrangements. Through its sense of community, religious rituals that aid in coping with grief, organized programs, and networks of volunteers, the mourner's place of worship can also be an invaluable resource. Some funeral homes now provide grief counseling or have arrangements for referrals.

B. Clinician Support and Counseling

Physicians and other appropriately licensed clinicians should encourage and support an open discussion of the feelings of loss and sadness, as well as of the individual's "positive" and "negative" feelings about the deceased person. When involvement in bereavement rituals seems appropriate, they should also encourage this, especially with those that are consistent with, and supported by, one's religious (e.g., wake, "sitting shiva") community or

TABLE 16.3. PERSONS AT RISK FOR DYSFUNCTIONAL GRIEF

People vulnerable to affective disorders, such as depression
Survivors of multiple losses
People who were overdependent on or ambivalent about the lost or deceased person
People who have inadequate support systems
Survivors who feel significant guilt
People who had major losses in early childhood
Survivors who are primarily concerned with their own feelings and needs (i.e., narcissism)
People who have been recent substance abusers
Parents who have lost a child, including miscarriage, infant death, and sudden infant death syndrome
People who lose someone through unanticipated or societally stigmatized death (e.g., some suicides, some human immunodeficiency virus-related deaths)

cultural background. People sometimes feel helped if they are encouraged to find their own rituals. Physicians and other clinicians also need to remind the bereaved that grief is often recurrent or cyclical and that it is not simply a linear process that goes from sorrow to recovery. Many clinicians fail to consider that helping a patient with his or her grief may be difficult if the patient has not previously experienced concern and a caring attitude from the clinician.

C. Sedative-Hypnotic Medications

Transient and judicious use of a **sedative-hypnotic medication** may be considered, but requests for prolonged use should lead to the consideration of some form of unresolved grief or the emergence of depression. When making the clinical judgment of whether to use a sleep-promoting agent, the treating physician also has to consider and balance a number of different and sometimes conflicting issues.

Short-acting rapid-onset benzodiazepines (e.g., **triazolam**) or other agents that bind to these same receptors (e.g., **zolpidem, zaleplon**) are good choices when a short-term pharmacologic treatment of insomnia (see Chapter 15) is indicated. Because **diphenhydramine** or sedating antidepressants (e.g., **trazodone, amitriptyline**) that are sometimes used to help with insomnia have a high rate of unwanted effects (e.g., anticholinergic side effects, daytime sedation, difficulties with concentration), their use can be problematic and it should be avoided.

The sedative-hypnotic agent chosen should be used for a brief period (typically up to a maximum of 2 weeks). Requests for prolonged use or the presence of a sleep problem that does not improve with medication should lead to the consideration of some form of pathologic grieving or MDD.

An important caveat is to ensure that one does not block or delay the grieving process by prescribing medications that may interfere with it. Similarly, because many sedative-hypnotics can impair memory for new learning to some degree at or near doses that are close to those that are effective for the desired target (e.g., the induction of restorative sleep) or because they may have next-day carryover effects on motor performance, the benefit from sedative-hypnotics also may carry some potential of side effects. Physicians should be concerned that, in some high-risk patients (e.g., an older male with a drinking history who will now be alone), the availability of sedative-hypnotics could contribute to the lethality of a suicide attempt by overdose. On the other hand, grief is an acute stress, and the stress *per se* along with its sequelae (e.g., insomnia, daytime fatigue, irritability) may take its toll in the form of medical illness, somatization, depression, and significant anxiety. One could also argue that persistent insomnia is a physiologic response resulting from the loss and suffering and thus medical treatment (medication) is indicated.

Two additional considerations are also present. First, some bereaved respond to the act of giving them something for relief, so over-the-counter products, such as **acetaminophen**, combined with a low dose of an antihistamine, may be sufficient. Second, the use of alcohol to promote sleep should be discouraged because its use may lead to fragmentation of sleep and increased daytime difficulties.

D. Antidepressants

Antidepressants probably have only a limited role to play in managing acute grief. Their preventative use early in the grieving process is most likely to benefit patients with a history of MDD or other affective disorders. For this latter group, intervention with an antidepressant may reduce the likelihood of a transition from grief to depression and may thereby facilitate the resolution of the grief and may lessen the morbidity associated with depression (e.g., excessive emotional pain and impaired quality of life). Making the decision to initiate antidepressant therapy is not always straightforward because having and tolerating some degree of emotional pain is part of the normal grieving process and its resolution. When a clinician is uncertain about the use of antidepressants, a psychiatrist with pharmacologic and bereavement experience should be consulted.

When grief triggers an episode of MDD (see Chapter 18) or persisting depressive symptoms (sometimes called minor depression), antidepressants should be given serious consideration. Positive results have been reported in preliminary studies of **paroxetine, nortriptyline,** and sustained-release **bupropion.** Because many patients who require an antidepressant have taken one before, reinstituting one they are familiar with and that they have benefitted from is the best starting point. When pharmacologic treatment is chosen, the antidepressant doses used to treat a major depression should be instituted, and the patient should have frequent appointments (i.e., every 1 to 2 weeks) to identify and treat side effects, to provide support, and to assess the treatment response. Unfortunately, many people either who are at high risk for depression or who develop significant depressive or anxiety symptoms will decline the offered antidepressant treatment. In these instances, follow-up appointments should be scheduled, and the physician should again try to prescribe medication for the clinically depressed mourner or to work out a referral for grief work or targeted cognitive-behavior therapy.

E. Psychotherapy and Self-Help Groups

Counseling or psychotherapy is of benefit to the bereaved with symptoms serious enough to merit antidepressant treatment; it should therefore be offered as adjuvant therapy. Referral to a psychiatrist or another appropriately trained mental health specialist should be considered for those with prolonged or complicated grief. Patients who decline pharmacologic treatment should be strongly encouraged to engage in grief counseling or psychotherapy with a psychologist, psychiatrist, or licensed therapist. Counseling or psychotherapy may also benefit those in whom normal mourning and grief are prolonged or in which their daily activities are particularly impaired.

The therapist to whom the patient is referred should have familiarity and experience in dealing with grief and bereavement. Another option is a grief counselor who is trained in and who specializes in this type of counseling. Even if the patient agrees to psychotherapy or grief counseling, the primary health provider should also see him or her for frequent regular visits (every 1 to 2 weeks) because this provides short-term and long-term support.

Therapy for these patients addresses their feelings of helplessness and dependency; their numbness, avoidance, or persistent denial; or their feelings of being overwhelmed and traumatized. Some degree of transient emotional withdrawal may be necessary and may facilitate the mourner's ability to carry on. In addition to providing support and encouragement during the exploration of feelings about the deceased, including the negative feelings, the therapist also emphasizes regaining autonomy and achieving self-acceptance and a feeling of wholeness. Each person has to establish a new relationship with the lost one in his or her own way. Some characterize this process as internalizing the loss; perhaps, it may be more simply stated as finding "a place in one's heart" for him or her.

Many neonatal intensive care units provide grief work for parents, and they can help with referrals to groups for parents who have lost newborns or older children. Other self-help groups include those for widows or widowers, parents of deceased children, or women who have undergone a mastectomy. They can provide support, an opportunity to share the grief experience, information about other resources in the community, and perspective. Self-help groups are not a form of medical treatment because they are not monitored by a health provider; therefore, they should not be considered as an alternative to psychotherapy or grief counseling.

V. Special Considerations for Children and Young Teens

Some children can be too young to understand death and its consequences, and some older adolescents may be unwilling to share with or expose their grief to adults. Grief work can only be done by a child who is developmentally "ready" and who is given the time and support to do so. Children less than 2 years of age have no frame of reference for death, so they experience only abandonment; children from about 2 years of age to about 6 or 7 may think of death as similar to a prolonged sleep (i.e., death is impermanent). Young children may temporarily lose developmental gains and may blame themselves for the death. They may also use play as a way of expressing their feelings. Older children (7 to 11 years of age) gradually become aware of the finality of death, but they may believe that some people are immortal. An understanding of children's developmental capacities, temperament, and coping styles will help any adult who has to inform a child about a death, and it may help to guide any decisions about participation in organized bereavement rituals. For example, for a 7 year old who is accompanied by a trusted person to leave a "special picture" or some other personal memento for the lost loved one at the grave site or some other meaningful place may be appropriate. Similarly, for some grieving adolescents, having a few close friends sit with them during a service may be even more beneficial than sitting with the family would be. Children may also reexperience their losses as time goes by, as their development progresses, and as important life events are encountered that bring up the absence of the deceased. As with adults, distinguishing between normal grief and abnormal grief or childhood depression may not be easy. For the latter two outcomes, a referral for counseling to a child or adolescent mental heath clinician is generally indicated. Table 16.4 outlines some of the features that might be of aid in deciding when a referral is in order. Those wishing for more understanding of childhood and adolescent depression should consult Chapter 21.

VI. **Additional Issues**

Several trends that have occurred in recent years may affect the mourning process. Among these are the increasingly frequent choice of cremation, a movement away from open caskets, and the specification in living wills of preferred approaches to the way one's death should be managed (e.g., end of life care, organ or body donation, burial procedures, rituals). Life-prolonging treatments may also permit some grieving to take place well before death occurs. How these changes and experiences alter the mourning experience for a given individual may vary from comfort and relief that is found in following the wishes of those who have died to distress, guilt, and even conflict among survivors who may prefer not to follow these wishes. Concerned clinicians need to be aware of these differing perspectives and outcomes and to find ways to be supportive.

TABLE 16.4. FEATURES THAT MAY DISTINGUISH NORMAL FROM ABNORMAL GRIEF IN CHILDREN

Normal Grieving	Abnormal Grieving
Initial shock or avoidance	Persistent belief that the deceased still lives
Transient crying or irritability	Persistent anger or depressed mood or wish to join the deceased
Transient disobedience or "perfect" behavior	Persistent changes in behavior
Increased clinging	Persistent separation anxiety
Transient problems with sleep	Persistent sleep problems
Temporary "regression" in developmental skills	Persistent "regression"
Transient lack of interest in peers or school	Persistent difficulties with peers or school
For adolescents, an increased need for and desire to be with peers	Antisocial behaviors

ACKNOWLEDGMENT

We thank Jessica R. Oesterheld, M.D., for her help with our understanding of children and death, and Sandra L. Bertman, Ph.D., for her perspective that death does not diminish the importance of special relationships.

ADDITIONAL READING

Alexander DA. Bereavement and the management of grief. *Br J Psychiatry* 1988; 153:860–864.

Attig T. *How we grieve: relearning the world.* New York: Oxford University Press, 1996.

Bertman SL. *Facing death: images, insights, and interventions.* New York: Hemisphere, 1991.

Bornstein PE, Clayton PJ. The anniversary reaction. *Dis Nerv Syst* 1972;33:470–472.

Clayton P, Desmarais L, Winokur G. A study of normal bereavement. *Am J Psychiatry* 1968;125:168–178.

Clayton PJ, Herjanic M, Murphy GE, et al. Mourning and depression: their similarities and differences. *Can Psychiatr Assoc J* 1974;19:309–312.

Jacobs SC, Kasl SV, Ostfeld AM, et al. The measurement of grief: bereaved vs nonbereaved. *Hospice J* 1986;2:21–35.

Jacobs SC, Kim K. Psychiatric complications of bereavement. *Psychiatric Ann* 1990;20:314–317.

Levav I, Friedlander Y, Kark JD, et al. An epidemiologic study of mortality among bereaved parents. *N Engl J Med* 1988;319:457–461.

Levy B. A study of bereavement in general practice. *J R Coll Gen Pract* 1976;26: 329–336.

McHorney CA, Mor V. Predictors of bereavement depression and its health services consequences. *Med Care* 1988;26:882–893.

Nuss WS, Zubenko GS. Correlates of persistent depressive symptoms in widows. *Am J Psychiatry* 1992;149:346–351.

Osterweiss M, Solomon F, Green M, eds. *Bereavement: reactions, consequences and care.* Washington, D.C.: National Academy Press, 1984.

Parkes CM. *Bereavement: studies of grief in adult life.* New York: International University Press, 1972.

Parkes CM, Weiss RS. *Recovery from bereavement.* New York: Basic Books, 1983.

Pasternack RE, Reynolds CF III, Schlernitzauer M, et al. Acute open-trial nortriptyline therapy for bereavement-related depression in late life. *J Clin Psychiatry* 1991;52:307–310.

Piper E, Ogrodniczuk JS, Azim HF, et al. Prevalence of loss and complicated grief among psychiatric outpatients. *Psych Serv* 2001;52:1069–1074.

Raphael B. *The anatomy of bereavement.* New York: Basic Books, 1983.

Reynolds CF, Miller MD, Pasternack RE, et al. Treatment of bereavement-related major depressive episodes in later life: a controlled study of acute and continuation treatment with nortriptyline and interpersonal psychotherapy. *Am J Psychiatry* 1999;156:202–208.

Sahler OJ. The child and death. *Pediatr Rev* 2000;21:350–357.

Sanders CM. Risk factors in bereavement outcome. *J Social Issues* 1988;44:97–111.

Schulz R, Beach SR, Lind B, et al. Involvement in caregiving and adjustment to death of a spouse. *JAMA* 2001;285:3123–3129.

Webb N, ed. *Helping bereaved children: a handbook for practitioners.* New York: Guilford, 1993.

Zisook S, Paulus M, Shuchter SR, et al. The many faces of depression following spousal bereavement. *J Affect Disord* 1997;45:85–95.

Zisook S, Shuchter SR. Major depression associated with widowhood. *Am J Geriatr Psychiatry* 1993;1:316–326.

Zisook S, Shuchter SR, Irwin M, et al. Bereavement, depression and immune function. *Psychiatry Res* 1994;52:1–10.

Zisook S, Shuchter SR, Pedrelli P, et al. Bupropion sustained release for bereavement: results of an open trial. *J Clin Psychiatry* 2001;64:227–230.

Zygmont M, Prigerson HG, Houck PR, et al. A post hoc comparison of paroxetine and nortriptyline for symptoms of traumatic grief. *J Clin Psychiatry* 1998;59:241–245.

Helpful Books for Grieving Parents or Children

Buscaglia L. *The fall of Freddie the leaf.* Thorofare, NJ: Slack, 1982.

Fitzgerald H. *The grieving child—a parent's guide.* New York: Simon & Shuster, 1992.

Maning D. *Don't take my grief away from me.* Oklahoma City, OK: In-Sight Books, 1979.

Mellonie B, Ingpen R. *Lifetimes—the beautiful way to explain death to children.* Toronto: Bantam Books, 1983.

Schaefer D, Lyons C. *How do we tell the children?* New York: Newmarket Press, 1993.

17. ASSESSMENT AND TREATMENT OF SUICIDE RISK

Richard I. Shader

As with other human behaviors, suicide, whether attempted or completed, can reflect many disparate determinants. By far the most important of these is depression. In states of depression, self-inflicted death is usually experienced as a **release** or **relief** from hopelessness or despair; a struggle that feels as if it cannot be favorably resolved; an intolerable dissatisfaction with oneself; overwhelming or intractable pain, especially when it is chronic; an incurable or stigmatizing illness, such as cancer or human immunodeficiency virus infection; old age; or a sense of a bleak and barren future. Such hopelessness and despair were poignantly captured in James Forrestal's suicide note (May 22, 1949), when he quoted the Chorus from Sophocles' *Ajax*, "Better to die, and sleep the never waking sleep, than linger on and dare to live, when the soul's life is gone." Suicide can also be a **response** to the disordered thinking of a psychotic decompensation, particularly in patients suffering from depression or schizophrenia who may hear a voice directing them to die or saying that they do not deserve to live, or the result of a drug-induced (e.g., **alcohol**) or toxic state, which may result in stepping out of a window and falling or jumping to one's death in a false belief that one can walk on air or fly. Although self-immolation is much less frequent, nevertheless it is a well-known **religious**, nationalistic, or political phenomenon (a psychotic condition may cause some of these acts but may not be recognized). Some even see suicide as a means of **rebirth**. Suicide can also be experienced as **revenge** (e.g., "You'll be sorry when I'm dead") or as an attempt at **reunification** with a lost loved one. A few clinicians and ethicists use the term **rational suicide** for deaths involving unremitting pain and suffering that is not relieved by treatment or for which no treatment exists and in which no treatable mood disorder is present (see Chapters 18 and 19).

Precise incidence, prevalence, and other risk estimates for suicide are always difficult to establish. Because of the obvious difficulties in determining whether some deaths are accidental or if they are suicide or homicides (e.g., automobile accidents, poisonings, impulsive actions by adolescents who are neither depressed nor psychotic), available statistics likely underestimate the frequency of suicide. Population demographics and treated-prevalence figures for various illnesses also change, as do usage patterns and availability of **alcohol** and potentially lethal drugs (both licit and illicit). Working estimates of 25,000 to 35,000 suicide deaths per year appear to be reasonable. This figure is sometimes expressed as 10 to 13 deaths from suicide per year per 100,000 in the general United States population. The rates are about 18.6% for all men and 34.1% for men over 65; the comparable figures for women are 4.4% and 4.7%, respectively. Comparable figures for white males versus African-American males are 20.3% and 36.6% and 10.2% and 11.6%, respectively. About 10% of patients who have been diagnosed with schizophrenia will commit suicide, most likely when they are still young; when they are without strong supports from family, friends, or a job; or soon after a hospitalization that has not meaningfully changed their status.[1] About 10% of patients who have been hospitalized for a mood disorder will also die from suicide. About 90% of suicide victims have a diagnosable psychiatric disorder, either as a current diagnosis or as one that can be made in retrospect, at the time of death. Suicide coupled with homicide occurs at an approximate rate of 0.2 to 0.3 per 100,000 person-years in the United States.

Firearms and explosives are by far the most frequently recorded means of suicide (57%); rates of suicide rise and fall to some extent based on the availability of firearms. Hanging, strangulation, and suffocation are less common, but these exceed the number of suicides linked to ingestions of solid or liquid poisons. All other methods are comparatively infrequent. Crashing a motor vehicle is estimated at 0.4%; this

---

[1]Recent data suggest that the use of clozapine may significantly reduce suicide rates in schizophrenic patients.

229

is obviously a difficult figure to establish because some single car deaths may be ruled accidental or **alcohol** related.

Physician-assisted suicide has received much attention in recent years. Because of the legal, moral, and philosophical issues involved in physician-assisted death, this topic deserves extensive discussion and is beyond the scope of this chapter.

I. Mental Status Examination Questions About Suicide

Just as vital signs are an elemental part of a physical examination, in the mental status examination or psychiatric interview, an assessment of suicidal risk is fundamental. Questioning should not be restricted to patients who appear depressed. Because suicidal impulses may wax and wane and as they may be more or less evident, continuing reassessment may also be required for some patients. Inquiry about suicidal concerns and impulses can be conducted systematically, progressing from more general to more specific questions in the following manner:

"Are you happy (or satisfied) with your life?"
"How often does it really get you down?"
"How depressed do you feel?"
"Do you ever want to die?"
"Do you ever think about suicide?"
"What was going on in your life when you were thinking about dying?"
"Were there particular things upsetting you that connect to your wanting to die?"
"Do you think about injuring or killing yourself?"
"Do the feelings and thoughts last very long?"
"Has anyone close to you ever attempted suicide or succeeded?"
"Do you think about acting on your feelings?"
"Do you have a plan?"
"Were you ever on the verge of trying to kill yourself but then changed your mind before you acted on your feelings?"
"Did you ever try to kill yourself?"
"Did you ever start to kill yourself and then change your mind once you had started to do so?"
"Are there any guns, pills, or poisons in your house?"
"Do you have any reasons that would stop you, such as loved ones or religious beliefs?"

The answers to these questions reflect the level of the motivation and intent of the potentially suicidal patient and the existence of a means or plan. **Clinical experience does not support the fear that asking about suicide will put the idea into anyone's mind.**

The assessment of an individual patient's potential for suicide is complex and difficult. Observation of the patient for facial, postural, and other nonverbal clues is important, as is questioning family members or other informants about their sense of the patient's suicide potential. Attention must be paid to what is said (and what is **not**), to what has happened (or **not** happened), to who is available to the patient (giving particular attention to patients who believe **no one** is available or who have just lost or been separated from their latest or only caring relationship); and to what has been done (or **not** done). The melange of suicidal variants—attempts, failed attempts, attempts during which the patient changed his or her mind, manipulative gestures, thoughts, preoccupations and obsessive ruminations, and the act *per se*—must be sorted out. Examples are the hurt and angry young child who says, "You'll be sorry when I die myself;" the young woman who tries to hold onto her lover by ingesting a nonlethal dose of **aspirin**; the recently widowed 60-year-old man who wants to die; the middle-aged man who shoots himself when he learns that he has an inoperable carcinoma; and perhaps even the persistent smoker who somewhat jokingly says, "I wonder why I'm paying someone to kill me."

Learning how patients feel about **the future** is important. Do they have an orientation toward the future? Do they entertain realizable goals and realistic expectations, or are they setting themselves up for disappointment and loss?

Assessment must be a continuing process, and one must remain alert to new stresses in patients' lives and to changes in patients' available interpersonal and material resources.

No single sign or set of signs is a reliable indicator of suicide potential. Attention must be paid to patients' appearance, mood, and thought content and to the overall significance of biographic elements (e.g., the fact that a patient is known to have recently put his or her affairs in order[2] may be a clue to a plan for suicide). As was noted earlier, the recognized incidence of suicide is likely an underestimate that ignores the suicidal implications of numerous automobile accidents, home fires, and so on. At least transient suicidal thoughts are reported in some surveys to occur in about 15% to 20% of the general population. The following section details specific factors that may increase the clinician's index of suspicion. Assessing risk is often straightforward; predicting action is not. One should understand that risk factors and markers may not be identical for suicide attempters and completers. The high rate of false positives with many of these variables helps to explain why clinicians have difficulty predicting suicide.

II. **Biographic Risk Factors Relevant to Suicide Assessment**
    A. **History of Previous Attempts**
        1. **A pattern of repeated threats or attempts is common**. Depending on samples and methods of study, between 20% and 60% of patients who complete suicide have tried before. Attempts involving violent means (e.g., gunshots, hanging) or overdoses in the context of angry or hostile feelings are likely to be repeated. Failed attempts (i.e., the attempter expected to succeed) are more likely to be repeated and to lead to death than are manipulative attempts or gestures (i.e., the attempter did not expect to die and hoped the act would change the responses of others). So-called **aborted** attempts (i.e., the individual's intent was serious, but a change of mind immediately before the attempt halted the attempt) are common among those who make further attempts and those who succeed; aborted attempts are a clinically meaningful risk factor. Known attempts are about 10 times more frequent than completed suicides.
        2. **Those who have attempted suicide before are more likely to die than are the nonattempters**.
        3. **Second attempts commonly come within 3 months after the first attempt**.
    B. **Emotional and Diagnostic Factors**
        1. **Depression** (e.g., grief, hypochondriasis, insomnia, guilt) is a major factor in suicides, as are **hopelessness** and **impulsivity**. The presence of acute anxiety, especially panic attacks, and anhedonia (decreased capacity to experience pleasure and gratification) may be particularly ominous. The clinician should remember that having an unhappy or sad mood about having an illness is not equivalent to having a mood disorder and that mood disorders may be masked and that these may present as somatization. Suicidal thoughts occur for varying durations and in varying intensity, and they form in almost all patients suffering from major depressive disorder (see Chapter 18).
        2. **Psychosis**, particularly with associated terror, suspiciousness, persecutory delusions, or hallucinations urging suicide or reasons for dying, may motivate suicide attempts. Patients with psychotic depressions and young catatonic patients are especially high-risk groups (see Chapters 18, 19, and 20).
        3. **Borderline Personality Disorder (BPD)** patients, particularly during the first and second decades of life, are a high-risk group. The presence of recurrent suicidal behavior, gestures, or threats is one of the diagnostic criteria for the diagnosis of BPD in the *Diagnostic and Statistical Manual of Mental Disorders,* 4th edition.

---

[2] Some examples are the writing of or changes in a last will or testament, buying a burial plot, or making a plan for the disposition of one's remains or effects.

4. **Acute and chronic alcoholism**, other forms of drug dependency, and toxic delirium predispose some patients to self-destructive acts.
5. **For women of childbearing age**, postpartum months and the premenstrual week are times of higher risk.

C. Occupational Status
1. **The unemployed and the unskilled** have higher suicide rates than do those who are skilled and employed.
2. **By profession**, higher suicide rates occur in policemen, musicians, dentists, insurance agents, farmers, physicians (especially psychiatrists, ophthalmologists, and anesthesiologists), air traffic controllers, and lawyers.
3. **A sense of failure** in fulfilling one's occupational role (e.g., in a job or as a wife or mother) is a common factor in suicides.

D. Marital Status and Other Supports
   Single (never married) persons are at greatest risk for suicide, followed by persons who are widowed, separated and divorced, married without children, and married with children. Those who live "all alone in the world" or who feel alone (they are with no one who cares or they have no one to care about) and those who have recently **lost a loved one or failed in a love relationship**, particularly within the preceding 6 months to 1 year, must always be considered serious suicide risks. The **anniversary of the loss of a loved one** can be a particularly high-risk time.

E. Gender
1. **Men commit suicide** more frequently than women, perhaps up to three times as often. Probably those at highest risk for suicide are men over 75 and the middle-aged male with a recent life crisis (e.g., a health problem, such as myocardial infarction, carcinoma, or kidney disease; a **major financial setback**; a significant loss of a loved one) who makes use of **alcohol** and who tends to deny depression.
2. **Women attempt suicide** more often (from two to four times) than men do.
3. **Gay, lesbian, and bisexual youth** in the United States and in some other countries are at higher risk for suicide attempts than are other youth of comparable socioeconomic status. Some surveys suggest that the risk is highest among effeminate gay male youth.

F. Age
1. **Suicides may occur in the young**, but they are less common before adolescence. Over a quarter of a million high school students per year from 15 to 19 years of age make suicide attempts requiring medical attention. In this age cohort, girls attempt suicide more often than boys do, and the highest suicide attempt rate is found among teenaged girls of Hispanic origin (just over one in seven or about 15%). For the same age group, rates for white and African-American girls are about 10% and 8%, respectively.

   A particularly high-risk situation involves the linkage of guns, alcohol, adolescent boys, and impulsivity. The suicide rate in the United States for white adolescent and young adult males from the ages of 15 to 24 years, although it was considerably lower than the rate for older men, increased alarmingly from the 1960s to the mid-1990s. Recent data suggest that this trend is now stabilizing and is possibly reversing.

   About 12% of adolescent and young adult deaths in the United States are from suicide. In recent years, suicide has been the third highest cause of death among African-American males from the ages of 15 to 24 years, resulting in rates ranging from 16 to 18.5 per 100,000 persons. Firearms were the method of death in almost three out of four suicides in 15-year-old to 19-year-old white and African-American males.

2. **The frequency of suicide increases with age** for men from about the beginning of the fifth decade until the seventh decade. Some data suggest that suicide rates may now be increasing in the cohorts of those 75 years

of age and older. Only about one in seven men in this age cohort who commit suicide will have had contact with a mental health professional, a fact consistent with the observation that the elderly make less use of mental health services than younger adults do. Recent estimates are that white men over the age of 64 have a suicide rate that ranges from 35 to 45 deaths per 100,000. For white women, this age cohort rate ranges from 5 to 7.5 per 100,000.

   3. **In women, the frequency of suicide increases** from the beginning of the fifth decade and peaks between 55 and 65 years of age.
G. **Family History and Religion**
   Completed and attempted suicides are more common among people with a family history of attempts or suicides and among those with a close friend who committed suicide. Suicide rates tend to be low for persons from families that are Roman Catholic or Moslem.
H. **Health Factors**
   Patients who have undergone recent surgery are at special risk, as are patients with intractable pain, chronic or protracted diseases, terminal illnesses, or incurable or stigmatizing illnesses. Although persons with human immunodeficiency virus infections have a 30-fold to 40-fold increase in suicide rates compared with age-matched and gender-matched control subjects, this increment appears to be proportionate to their greater levels of major depressive disorder as compared with control subjects. Non–central nervous system cancer patients have suicide rates that are increased by two to four times over control subjects. Some data indicate that many illnesses directly affecting the brain, such as human immunodeficiency virus infection, Huntington disease, and epilepsy, are associated with increased suicide rates, thus suggesting that loss of restraint mechanisms may be involved.
I. **Help Seeking**
   Although, in general, most persons who commit suicide have sought medical or psychiatric care within the year preceding the attempt, help seeking is not always a reliable indicator. One study of suicides among college students found that none had sought help nor had they appeared depressed to those who knew them. About half of high school suicide victims seek help before making an attempt.
J. **Race**
   Within the United States, recorded suicide rates are higher, in general, for whites than for nonwhites. Young African-American males have a higher than expected rate of suicide. Similarly, rates are higher than expected for Native Americans and Eskimos.
K. **Geographic Location and Seasonal Variation**
   In the United States, suicide rates are highest in Alaska, yet overall they are higher in urban areas than in rural settings. More suicides occur in the spring and summer, perhaps because people feel despair when the change of seasons does not bring relief from their winter depression or doldrums. Despite impressions to the contrary, no consistent evidence suggests a higher rate of suicide during the Christmas holidays. Methods of suicide may also vary by geography; in Hong Kong, for example, where many people live in tall buildings, jumping from a rooftop or window is the most common means reported.
L. **Medication and Substance Abuse**
   Certain medications, such as reserpine and estrogen-containing oral contraceptives, may worsen mood disorders and may contribute indirectly to suicidal thoughts and acts. Various licit and illicit substances may increase suicide risk (e.g., **alcohol** through disinhibition and **lysergic acid diethylamide [LSD]** through toxic false beliefs).
M. **Suicide After Homicide**
   Suicides following homicidal acts usually occur shortly after the homicide. Circumstances and motives vary, but dominant patterns include spousal murder for reasons of jealousy or failing health and the killing of

TABLE 17.1. SOME MYTHS ABOUT SUICIDE

Myth	Comment
People who talk about suicide are not serious risks.	Most suicide victims communicate their plan or distress before death.
Suicide is an impulsive act with little warning and few clues.	As was noted above, some form of communication is common.
Suicidal persons are rarely indecisive or ambivalent.	People who attempt suicide usually seek comfort or help before they act on their self-destructive impulses.
Suicidal tendencies or behaviors are inherited.	Although some people who attempt suicide have a relative or friend who has attempted or succeeded at suicide, suicide does not appear to be an inherited predisposition or trait.
The risk of suicide is short-lived, and it usually is over when signs of improvement appear.	Improvement may be deceptive, and it may reflect the person's calm from having made a plan; a return of some energy may also give the patient enough energy to act; the postattempt period can be a vulnerable time.

From Schneidman ES, Farberow NL. *Some facts about suicide.* Washington, D.C.: United States Government Printing Office, 1961, with permission.

one's children, the killing of one's entire family, and retaliation against another family member related either to suspected infidelity or to self-proclaimed altruism.

N. Suicide Notes

The content of a note written during a failed or aborted attempt may provide clues as to the seriousness of the attempt. However, notes may also be written in attempts that are manipulative or that are a cry for help. When pens are used, finding ink on the correct writing hand of the deceased may be an important forensic clue.

O. Myths

Table 17.1 lists some commonly held myths about suicide that should be understood by clinicians.

III. Biologic Markers for Suicide

Although results from studies of the biologic basis for suicide vary considerably, some trends and generalizations are informative. People who commit suicide may have reduced concentrations of 5-hydroxyindoleacetic acid and serotonin in some brain regions, such as the brainstem. Reduced imipramine binding (or affinity) in brain tissue has also been observed. Reduced concentrations of 5-hydroxyindoleacetic acid in the cerebrospinal fluid have been found in some suicide attempters (e.g., in patients with unipolar major depressive disorder, personality disorders, and schizophrenia). In addition, some data suggest increased hypothalamic-pituitary-adrenal axis activity, including increased 24-hour urinary excretion of cortisol in this vulnerable group. A number of authors have suggested that, taken together, these findings may identify patients who are emotionally overwhelmed and vulnerable, as reflected by the overactivity of the hypothalamic-pituitary-adrenal axis, or those who are prone to impulsivity, as reflected in the low cerebrospinal fluid 5-hydroxyindoleacetic acid levels. When these alterations coincide with disordered mood, the potential for suicide may be high. These findings also point to a consistency between attempters and completers with regard to altered serotonin system functioning.

These and other lines of evidence have converged in ways that lead some experts to conclude that both suicidal behavior and major depression are independently related to alterations in serotonergic function and regulation (Mann et al., 2001). Additional findings that support this assessment are altered kinetics for ligand binding to the serotonin transporter on platelets and reduced ligand binding to 5-hydroxytryptamine-1A (5-HT$_{1A}$) receptors in the prefrontal cortex; these changes occur independently of diagnosis. Moreover, a correlation is seen between blunted prolactin increases in response to oral fenfluramine and the occurrence and lethality of past suicide attempts in patients with major depression.

Twin and adoption studies also suggest genetic determinants for suicidal behavior, in both attempts and deaths. Possibly involved candidates that are supported by preliminary findings but that require further study are the genes for the 5-HT$_{1B}$ and 5-HT$_{2A}$ receptors, tryptophane hydroxylase, the serotonin transporter, and monoamine oxidase. One recent study revealed an elevation in RNA editing at a locus in the 5-HT$_{2C}$ receptor in the postmortem prefrontal cortex tissue of patients with major depression or schizophrenia who committed suicide; the comparator tissue was taken from "psychiatrically normal" persons who died in accidents or from homicide.

IV. Treatment

The proper assessment and treatment of suicide risk are extremely critical aspects of medical practice. Unfortunately, assessment of suicide risk and treatment planning can be influenced by the varied reactions of clinicians to suicidal patients. A few clinicians, for example, imply or openly state that they cannot take responsibility for someone else's life. This attitude often confuses the clinician's feelings of helplessness, anger, disappointment, and rejection with the civil liberties arguments or philosophical positions about individuals' rights. Important realizations are that, in all states, **suicide has legal implications** and that commitment laws may allow the hospitalization of people who are considered a danger to themselves.

Although this approach is not widely accepted, a few clinicians use a **bantering** interview style with suicide attempters, as a way to try to minimize or undercut the seriousness of the attempt; some restrict the bantering approach to those who have made repeated attempts. This controversial therapeutic style assumes a consciously manipulative aspect to the attempt. In the view of the author, *the risks of adopting this approach outweigh any possible benefits.*

Some clinicians hospitalize suicide attempters, and then they are reluctant to discharge them because they feel uncertain about judging their patients' freedom from suicidal impulses. In this era of managed care, keeping patients for more than limited stays as inpatients is particularly difficult. When a clinician feels unable to assess a patient's status, consultation with the ward team or other clinicians is essential.

Although offering guidelines for the treatment of individual patients is beyond the scope of this chapter, consideration of aspects of one approach to treatment may be helpful. The author approaches most suicidal patients with a bias based on clinical experience—**most suicidal patients change their minds**. When patients have suicidal thoughts or behavior associated with major depressive disorder, effective treatment of the depression usually is sufficient. However, the clinician should keep in mind the fact that for currently available antidepressants to work rapidly is unusual.[3] For acute exacerbations of suicidal feelings, the only effective treatment with a rapid onset of action is electroconvulsive therapy (see Chapter 24).

For suicidal behavior secondary to the hallucinations or delusions of schizophrenia, adequate treatment of the psychosis should be effective. Patients with BPD who have intense dysphoria may respond to treatment with monamine oxidase inhibitors or **fluoxetine** or to another specific selective serotonin reuptake

[3] Prescribing clinicians should keep in mind the potential for serious or even fatal overdosage with any antidepressants they prescribe; adjusting the number of pills dispensed and the timing and number of refills must be a consideration. The clinician should also remember that the tricyclic antidepressants and monamine oxidase inhibitors have a higher risk for more serious overdose consequences than the selective serotonin reuptake inhibitors and other newer agents do.

inhibitor. Some clinicians believe that the early increases in anxiety or the occasional occurrence of akathisia that is associated with some selective serotonin reuptake inhibitors may pose special difficulties for the impulsive suicidal patient with a low tolerance for frustration or added distress. This concern must be weighed against data that show reductions in suicidal feelings in placebo-controlled studies of selective serotonin reuptake inhibitors. Because impulsivity is a central feature in many patients with BPD, the risks of medication use must be considered along with any potential benefits. The recently widowed patient may be helped to grieve (see Chapter 16) and may find support and companionship with others who are successfully handling widowhood.

With each suicidal patient, however, the aim is to come to understand and to have the patient understand why he or she wants to die, what might help to make life more worthwhile, and what adaptations can be made that would diminish the thought that suicide is the only or best solution. Some key elements in working with suicidal patients are (a) sympathetic listening, or being open to hearing their often ambivalently expressed cries for help and their deep despair or loneliness; (b) understanding and managing one's own countertransference reactions, such as helplessness, anger, or rejection; and (c) **taking all threats of suicide seriously**.

Providing **a safe, nonrejecting environment** is also important; this can range from helping a patient reveal feelings and impulses to family and friends so that they will spend more time with the patient to hospitalization with continuous observation. All obvious means of suicide should be removed from a patient's living areas, including, but not limited to, medications, poisons, knives, ropes, belts, shoelaces, and guns (*note:* separating bullets from guns is not sufficient). With the patient's permission, family members or close friends should be contacted and should be allowed to be involved in aftercare when this is assessed to be appropriate. Establishing a clear plan for the family or close friends to follow if the patient's condition worsens is important (see below).

Hospitalization, preferably voluntarily, should always be considered. The decision to hospitalize is based on an assessment of many factors, including the severity of the patient's stated suicidal thoughts and plans, the depth of any concomitant depression, the degree of available family or peer support, the presence of current and recent substance abuse, the presence of other comorbid medical complications or psychiatric disorders, or the presence of clear impulsivity with the availability of lethal means (Table 17.2).

TABLE 17.2. SOME IMPORTANT FACTORS INFLUENCING THE DECISION TO HOSPITALIZE PERSONS THREATENING OR PREOCCUPIED WITH SUICIDE

Social isolation, particularly when previously important persons are dead or are no longer available.

Lack of alliance with the treating clinician.

A clear plan has been made.

Psychosis, especially with hallucinations telling the patient to die, calling for a reunion with a lost loved one, or indicating that God wants this to happen.

History of prior attempts or when the previous (most recent) attempt was **serious and planned**.

A sense that suicide is the only available solution.

Recurrent or persistent suicidal ideation, despite therapeutic interventions, positive responses from significant others, or positive or beneficial changes in external factors or conditions.

Depression, especially when delusions of guilt are present, evidence indicating that rage has been turned inward exists, or excessive self-recriminating thinking or self-blame is present.

These factors have been ordered by the mnemonic **SLAPHARD** to facilitate learning. This ordering is not intended to convey any ranking of their comparative importance.

Once in the hospital, the patient's accessible environment may again require attention to minimize self-destructive opportunities. Sharp objects, belts, shoelaces, and other objects that could be used for self-harm must be removed because the patient may have picked these up in anticipation of being hospitalized. Safety screens for hospital windows must not be overlooked. Appropriate interpersonal and somatic therapies should be tried, while retaining the awareness that any improvement in a patient's mood may reflect his or her decision to try again. Continued support and involvement during this phase are essential. When one takes the crucial risk of reducing suicide precautions and permitting the patient more freedom, the timing of the shift must include a consideration of the amount of improvement in the patient's suicidal thoughts, depressed mood, or withdrawal; evidence of an orientation toward the future; and a sense that the patient is engaged with the staff in some form of therapeutic alliance. Family members, friends, and other key persons in the patient's life should be involved, when appropriate (within the constraints of confidentiality), so that the patient does not return to the same circumstances that contributed to his or her decision to die.

Before discharge, working out a plan for follow-up care with the patient is important. Planning should take into consideration the fact that some patients feel less suicidal when a therapist temporarily fills some void; this can lead to a reemergence of suicidal impulses when treatment termination or interruption is discussed. The plan for follow-up care should be explicit, with thoughtful preparation for any transition to a new therapist or to the referring therapist. Discharge assessment should include an estimate of the patient's capacity for self-care. The quality, absence, instability, or uncertainty of available object relationships must be considered; a component of treatment planning should include helping the patient to develop positive relationships. Group therapy or the involvement of community resource persons, such as a teacher, family member, physician or other trained clinician, or clergyman, may be beneficial. The benefits of a longer hospital stay (when this is actually possible) must be weighed against any other issues (e.g., regression, interruption of work or family ties, costs of continued care). Long-term planning must address the possibility of further suicide attempts.

A second bias has emerged from the author's clinical experience—**those suicidal patients who do not change their minds will usually find a way**. Clinicians can delay death and can provide an opportunity for the patient to improve from a particular episode of depression, demoralization, grief, or psychosis. Some patients, however, find life so empty or painful that a second chance to them means a second chance to die, not a second chance to find something to live for or to have time to work out their disappointment in themselves. A word of **caution** is in order—*clinicians must not let their own feeling that they would not want to live under a particular set of conditions dictate their care of the patient.* For example, avoiding the influence of one's own personal feelings about the value and meaning of life can be especially difficult when a clinician is treating a patient with inoperable and painful metastatic carcinoma.

Finally, some clinicians have had positive experiences with the use of formal **"no suicide contracts."** In the author's view, the use of a contract may be reasonable when the patient is assessed as low risk, he or she has available people to call or stay with for support, and he or she has some stated reasons for wanting to live and when an alliance exists with the treating clinician. That a patient who refuses to discuss or sign a contract may be at high risk is also likely. In any contract, the patient must agree, preferably in writing and signing it in the presence of a witness, not to act on any self-destructive feelings when the wish to die becomes strong and to call the treating clinician **and** 911, a suicide or crisis hotline, a local emergency department, or a designated support person—a person stipulated in the contract, along with that person's telephone number(s). The contract must also give the designated person the right to call the treating clinician or any other backup resources if the patient's condition worsens; the treating clinician must also have the right to call the designated person or the police if the patient fails to keep a scheduled appointment. In effect, the patient is agreeing to contain any suicidal impulses in between specified appointments or to call to arrange for a more immediate appointment. In the author's experience most impulsive, psychotic, substance abusing, or markedly depressed patients cannot be expected to do this, even when they agree to do so. That **no suicide contracts** have no legal standing must be remembered.

V. **Comment and Caveats**

Suicidal patients should be viewed as medical emergencies; treatment and program planning must recognize the need for 24-hour services. Suicide is a frequent basis for malpractice actions against psychiatrists. Careful documentation is essential, including recognition of the risk and past and present treatment and prevention efforts. The jeopardy for psychiatrists and other clinicians and their suicide-prone patients has increased in recent years with the higher threshold for hospitalization and the shortened lengths of stay that have resulted from managed care plans and increasing hospital costs. For example, the author has been consulted about managed care reviewers who have stated without seeing the patient that the suicidal concerns or behaviors of a patient were either not acute enough to require hospitalization or too chronic to benefit from hospitalization.

In the event of a suicide, immediate **notification of one's malpractice insurance carrier** is essential. An important early concern may be the issue of talking to the patient's family or to other staff. Unfortunately, the medicolegal aspects of suicide can become complicated when dealing with surviving family members. A delicate balance must be achieved between any natural desire to comfort the family, to help them understand, or to share one's own emotional responses and respecting the deceased patient's right to confidentiality. For a family to be irrational, to view the clinician as responsible for the death, and to interpret any caring responses as a manipulation to avoid a suit is also not uncommon. For clinicians and families to remember that suicide may be inextricably linked to certain disorders or to patients' responses to their suffering is not easy.

Many clinicians and other staff are devastated by the suicide of a patient. Although some may try to continue as if nothing has happened, the suicide will likely have an impact on the clinician's care of other patients, as well as on the self-concepts, self-esteem, and interpersonal lives of those involved. Review and supervision from a trusted and knowledgeable colleague can be beneficial to individual clinicians. Formal review in the form of a psychologic postmortem can also be useful for staff involved in the patient's care. The timing of such reviews may be affected by risk management and malpractice issues.

One possible method of suicide prevention or reduction—limiting the widespread availability of handguns—should be supported by clinicians. For clinicians to check for and urge the removal of lethal methods of suicide from their high risk patients is not sufficient (*note:* locking gun cabinets or separating guns from bullets is not sufficient): the participation of both them and their professional organizations in raising awareness among families, teachers, and other members of the community about the role of handguns and in encouraging injury prevention education is also essential.

VI. **Useful Online Information**

The American Association of Suicidology (AAS; see *http://www.suicidology.org/*) trains and certifies suicide hotline counselors and provides other valuable information on its website. For 24-hour nationwide hotline access, call 1-800-SUICIDE (1-800-784-2433) or visit the website (*http://www.suicidehotlines.com/*). Facts and statistics can be found at *http://www.nimh.nih.gov/research/suifact.htm* and at the AAS website.

ADDITIONAL READING

American Academy of Child and Adolescent Psychiatry. Practice parameter for the assessment and treatment of children and adolescents with suicidal behavior. *J Am Acad Child Adolesc Psychiatry* 2001;40:24S–51S.

Åsberg M, Schalling D, Träskman-Bendz L, et al. Psychobiology of suicide, impulsivity, and related phenomena. In: Meltzer HY, ed. *Psychopharmacology: the third generation of progress*. New York: Raven Press, 1987:655–668.

Barber ME, Marzuk PM, Leon AC, et al. Aborted suicide attempts: a new classification of suicidal behavior. *Am J Psychiatry* 1998;155:385–389.

Blumenthal SJ. Youth suicide: the physician's role in suicide prevention. *JAMA* 1990;264:3194–3196.

Dublin LJ. *Suicide*. New York: Ronald Press, 1963.

Durkheim E. *Le suicide*. Glencoe, IL: Free Press, 1950.

Ertugrul A. Clozapine and suicide. *Am J Psychiatry* 2002;159:323–324.

Farberow NL, Schneidman ES. *The cry for help*. New York: McGraw-Hill, 1961.

Hoyert D, Kochanek K, Murphy S. Deaths: final data for 1997. *Natl Vital Stat Rep* 1999; 47:1–104.

Joe S, Kaplan MS. Firearm-related suicide among young African-American males. *Psych Serv* 2002;53:332–334.

Kaplan MS, Geling O. Firearm suicides and homicides in the United States: regional variations and patterns of gun ownership. *Soc Sci Med* 1998;46:1227–1233.

Ludwig J, Cook PJ. Homicide and suicide rates associated with implementation of the Brady Handgun Violence Prevention Act. *JAMA* 2000;284:585–591.

Mann JJ, Brent DA, Arango V. The neurobiology and genetics of suicide and attempted suicide: a focus on the serotonergic system. *Neuropsychopharmacology* 2001;24: 467–477.

Marzuk PM, Leon AC, Tardiff K, et al. The effect of access to lethal methods of injury on suicide rates. *Arch Gen Psychiatry* 1992;49:451–458.

Marzuk PM, Tardiff K, Hirsch CS. The epidemiology of murder-suicide. *JAMA* 1992; 267:3179–3183.

Meltzer H. Clozapine and suicide. *Am J Psychiatry* 2002;159:323–324.

Meltzer HY, Okayli G. Reduction of suicidality during clozapine treatment of neuroleptic-resistant schizophrenia: impact on risk-benefit assessment. *Am J Psychiatry* 1995;152:183–190.

Motto JA, Bostrom AG. A randomized controlled trial of postcrisis suicide prevention. *Psych Serv* 2001;52:828–833.

Munro J, O'Sullivan D, Andrews C, et al. Active monitoring of 12,760 clozapine recipients in the UK and Ireland: beyond pharmacovigilance. *Br J Psychiatry* 1999; 175:576–580.

Murphy S. Deaths: final data for 1998. *Natl Vital Stat Rep* 2000;48:1–100.

Niswender CM, Herrick-Davis K, Dilley GE, et al. RNA editing of the human 5-HT$_{2C}$ receptor: alterations in suicide and implications for serotonergic pharmacology. *Neuropsychopharmacology* 2001;24:478–491.

Reid WH, Mason M, Hogan T. Suicide prevention effects associated with clozapine therapy in schizophrenia and schizoaffective disorder. *Psych Serv* 1998;49:1029–1033.

Schneidman ES, Farberow NL. *Clues to suicide*. New York: McGraw-Hill, 1957.

Sernyak MJ, Desai R, Stolar M, et al. Impact of clozapine on completed suicide. *Am J Psychiatry* 2001;158:931–937.

Shaffer D, Craft L. Methods of adolescent suicide prevention. *J Clin Psychiatry* 1999;60:70–74.

Walker AM, Lanza LL, Arellano F, et al. Mortality in current and former users of clozapine. *Epidemiology* 1997;8:671–677.

18. APPROACHES TO THE TREATMENT OF DEPRESSION

Ronald W. Pies
Richard I. Shader

The basic features of single or recurring episodes of clinically significant depression, which hereafter will be called major depressive disorder (MDD) have been recognized since the time of Hippocrates. Ironically, the "humoral" notions about the etiology of depression put forward by Hippocratic-era writers have striking resemblances to contemporary theories of neuroendocrine and neurotransmitter dysfunction in mood disorders. Although the lifetime expectancies vary somewhat because of the survey methodologies used, the lifetime expectancy for developing MDD is about 12% for women and 6% for men. With anxiety disorders, MDD is among the most common psychiatric disorders seen in adults. Some episodes of MDD may be triggered by traumatic life events like losses or disappointments; once triggered, however, the mood disturbance and other features of this disorder may become autonomous, just as they are in spontaneously occurring episodes (i.e., those that appear to arise "out of the blue"). MDD is not simply a severe form of unhappiness or despair, nor is it synonymous with grief (see Chapter 16) or demoralization. Given the morbidity and mortality of MDD, which are nearly comparable with those of chronic cardiovascular disease, the recognition and vigorous treatment of this disorder are critical. Recent data suggest that depression is second only to ischemic heart disease in its total disease burden.

Despite the prevalence of MDD, better public and professional educational programs, and improvement in screening procedures for depression, the rate of outpatient treatment in the United States was only 2.33 per 100 persons in 1997. Although this rate shows a dramatic increase from 1987 (0.73 per 100 persons), most people in the United States who are depressed do not receive treatment.

Because of important similarities in clinical presentation and treatment, MDD and dysthymic disorder are considered together in this chapter.

I. Clinical Features of Major Depressive Disorder and Dysthymic Disorder
A. Major Depressive Disorder

A variety of research and clinical criteria has been proposed to define MDD. In the typical patient, however, the clinical presentation is quite characteristic. Central features are a loss of interest, satisfaction, or pleasure in almost all activities that lasts at least 2 weeks; some degree of appetite and sleep disturbance; decreased energy, concentration, or libido; low self-esteem or excessive guilt; and recurrent thoughts of death or suicide. Psychomotor agitation or retardation is usually observed. Psychotic features that are either mood congruent or incongruent may also be present. Some clinicians argue that MDD with psychotic features is a distinct clinical entity because it usually does not respond to classic antidepressant therapy when given alone. In a more severe form of MDD that is sometimes called **melancholia**, neurovegetative features such as weight loss or early morning awakening are especially prominent. The essential features of MDD are summarized in Table 18.1.

In addition to these typical features, MDD patients may reveal "atypical" signs and symptoms (see section VIII). Some patients, particularly adolescents and the elderly, may not report and may even deny subjective feelings of depression. Instead, depression may be manifested as behavioral disturbances, such as delinquency in adolescents, or as multiple vague somatic complaints. Crying spells or tearfulness are common. Some patients, however, may report being on the verge of tears or being unable to cry despite feelings of deep sadness or despair. Great variability in the nature of the appetite or sleep disturbance in MDD is observed. Many patients report loss of appetite and weight; others, often those with atypical features, may report

TABLE 18.1. DIAGNOSTIC FEATURES OF MAJOR DEPRESSIVE DISORDER

At least five of the symptoms that follow must be present nearly every day during a period lasting at least 2 weeks. The appearance of these symptoms (a) must not be secondary to substance or medication use (e.g., prednisone), to an underlying medical condition such as hypothyroidism, or to uncomplicated bereavement; (b) must represent a change from antecedent functioning; and (c) must cause marked distress or significant impairment of social or occupational functioning. **At least one of the five symptoms should be a loss of interest or pleasure or a depressed mood that persists for the majority of the day.**

Depressed mood (or irritability in children or adolescents) manifested by subjective report (e.g., sadness or emptiness) or the observations of others (e.g., tearfulness)

Markedly diminished interest or pleasure in almost all activities or observations made by others of significant apathy

Significant change in appetite or weight (typically more than 5% of body weight in 4 weeks) in the absence of planned weight loss or gain

Insomnia or hypersomnia

Psychomotor agitation or retardation

Fatigue or loss of energy

Feelings of worthlessness, excessive or inappropriate guilt, or loss of self-esteem

Indecisiveness or diminished ability to think or concentrate

Recurrent thoughts of death or suicidal ideas without a specific plan, a specific plan for suicide, or an actual attempt

From the American Psychiatric Association. *Diagnostic and statistical manual of mental disorders,* 4th ed. Text revision. Washington, D.C.: American Psychiatric Association, 2000, with permission.

excessive eating and weight gain. Similarly, although early morning awakening is the classic complaint, some patients with MDD will report excessive sleep or daytime somnolence. In the *Diagnostic and Statistical Manual of Mental Disorders* (DSM), 4th edition, the term major depressive episode can be used to describe either an episode of MDD or the depressed phase of bipolar disorder (see Chapter 19); no symptomatic differences are outlined. Many clinicians, however, have noted the predominance of hypersomnia (excessive sleeping), psychomotor retardation, and weight gain in patients who are in the depressed phase of bipolar (versus unipolar) disorder. These features overlap with patterns seen in some patients with atypical depression (AD) or seasonal affective disorder (SAD) (see section VIII).

Importance is often attached to the "autonomy" versus the "reactivity" of the patient's mood. Patients with the most severe forms of MDD often show nearly complete autonomy of mood (i.e., no mood elevation even in the presence of marked psychosocial stimulation, support, or reward). Other depressed patients (see section VIII.A) are markedly, albeit transiently, responsive to admiration, attention, or other "ego boosts." The presence of psychotic features in MDD generally predicts a more disabling episode and a slower recovery than those seen in nonpsychotic MDD patients; however, eventual recovery appears equally likely in both groups. Delusional features are often of the paranoid or "nihilistic" variety (e.g., fixed and exaggerated ideas of worthlessness, guilt, or bodily decay). The prototypical patient may believe that he or she is "the greatest sinner of all time" or that his or her body is being eaten away by worms "because I'm so evil." Such delusions are often deemed "mood congruent" because they resonate with the patient's depressive affect. The significance of so-called mood-incongruent delusions is not yet clear; some overlap with schizoaffective disorder (see Chapters 19 and 20) may be present in such patients. As has been noted, the presence of psychotic features in MDD usually suggests the need for different or additional treatment modalities (see also section VII.B.6).

B. Dysthymic Disorder

Dysthymic disorder (Table 18.2) may be to MDD what cyclothymia is to bipolar disorder—an attenuated, although perhaps more chronic, form or presentation of the illness. For many years, terms such as "neurotic depression" or "chronic characterological depression" were applied to patients who are now diagnosed with dysthymic disorders. These earlier terms did not provide useful operational definitions, and their prognostic implications were never established. Dysthymic disorder is a chronic disturbance involving depressed mood (or irritability in children) most of the time for at least 2 years (or 1 year in children or adolescents). During these periods of depressed mood, some or all of the following features are present: poor appetite or overeating; insomnia or hypersomnia; low energy or fatigue; low self-esteem; poor concentration or difficulty making decisions; and feelings of hopelessness. Unlike MDD, dysthymic disorder may lead to only mild or moderate impairment in social and occupational functioning; however, its chronicity may predispose the individual to substance abuse, possibly as an attempt to self-treat the experiences of dysphoria and distress. Patients with dysthymic disorder do not show the profound neurovegetative signs seen in MDD: rarely is severe weight loss or psychomotor change seen. Suicidality and psychotic features are not common in uncomplicated dysthymic disorder; either, however, may be present in patients with dysthymic disorder who have superimposed or concomitant MDD ("double depression").

Dysthymic disorder is subclassified as either **primary** or **secondary** and as either **late onset** or **early onset**. In primary dysthymic disorder, the mood disturbance must not be linked to a preexisting, chronic, non–mood disorder (e.g., other axis I or axis III pathology). Early-onset dysthymic disorder begins before the age of 21. Some evidence seems to suggest that early-onset primary-type dysthymic disorder may be a distinct clinical entity.

II. Prevalence, Demographics, and Comorbidity of Major Depressive Disorder and Dysthymic Disorder

A. Major Depressive Disorder

Although the prevalence of bipolar disorder is roughly the same in men and women, most studies find that MDD is approximately twice as preva-

---

TABLE 18.2. DIAGNOSTIC FEATURES OF DYSTHYMIC DISORDER

Depressed mood (or irritability in children or adolescents) must be present on the majority of days for at least 2 years as noted by self-report or the observations of others. During this 2-year interval, no symptom-free periods should last more than 2 months. At least three of the symptoms that follow should be present for most of the day during periods of depressed mood, and accompanying episodes of major depressive disorder (MDD), mania, or hypomania should not be present. As with MDD, these symptoms must not be secondary to substance or medication use, an underlying medical condition, or unresolved bereavement.

1. Low energy, fatigue, or chronic tiredness
2. Social withdrawal
3. Loss of interest or enjoyment in sex or other pleasurable activities
4. Feelings of inadequacy, loss of self-esteem or self-confidence, or self-deprecation
5. Decreased effectiveness or productivity at school, work, or home or less active or talkative
6. Poor concentration, difficulty making decisions, or poor memory
7. Feelings of hopelessness, pessimism, or despair
8. Pessimism about the future, feelings of guilt, brooding about past events, or self-pity
9. Irritability or excessive anger

From the American Psychiatric Association. *Diagnostic and statistical manual of mental disorders,* 4th edition. Text revision. Washington, D.C.: American Psychiatric Association, 2000, with permission.

lent in women as in men. Worldwide surveys report prevalence rates of 4.7% to 25.8% for women and of 2.1% to 12.3% for men. The large multicenter Epidemiological Catchment Area study in the United States found the lifetime risk for major depressive episodes (per the DSM, 3rd edition [-III]) to be from 4.9% to 8.7% in women and from 2.3% to 4.4% in men. Most cross-national data suggest that these differences are not an artifact of differential treatment-seeking behavior but rather that they are a consequence of biologic and developmental differences between men and women; cross-national studies find the lifetime prevalence rates to be from 4.4% to 18% for major depressive episodes. Evidence from the mid-1980s suggests that race and social class do not appreciably affect the risk for DSM-III–defined depression. However, one reanalysis suggests that poverty (as defined by federal guidelines) does increase the risk for major depressive episodes. Although a major depressive episode or MDD can occur at any age, data from the Epidemiological Catchment Area study show that the highest lifetime prevalence is in the age cohort of 25 to 44 years. Data from the Cross-National Collaboration Group and other surveys suggest that more recent birth cohorts are at increased risk for major depression.

B. Dysthymic Disorder

The lifetime prevalence of dysthymic disorder is roughly 3% in the United States, making this a common psychiatric disorder. Cross-national data yield similar lifetime prevalence rates of 3.1% to 3.9%. Dysthymic disorder appears to be about twice as frequent in adult women as in men, but it is distributed equally in children. In one study, 65% of patients with dysthymia (the DSM-III, revised, term for dysthymic disorder) and 59% of patients with major depression received at least one additional axis I diagnosis, usually of social phobia or generalized anxiety disorder. Just over 10% of patients with dysthymia received additional diagnoses of **alcohol** abuse or dependence. This study points out the vexing problem of comorbidity in patients with mood disorders, as well as the risks of associated substance abuse. Dysthymic disorder and MDD also frequently occur together. The genetics, epidemiology, course, and treatment of patients with comorbid axis I disorders may differ, depending on which disorder developed first (e.g., did the major depression precede or follow the onset of panic disorder?). See the Additional Reading for more detailed discussions of comorbidity.

III. Etiology of Major Depressive Disorder and Dysthymic Disorder

A. Psychosocial Theories

No single psychodynamic or cognitive theory of depression has been verified by systematic research; however, each theory may contribute to the clinician's understanding and treatment of depressed people. Psychoanalytic formulations have evolved primarily from the work of Freud and Abraham. Freud believed that, in "melancholia" (as opposed to normal "mourning" or grief), hostile feelings previously directed against the lost person become directed at the self, which, through introjection, has incorporated the lost person. The commonly used formulation of "anger turned inward" to explain depression stems from Freud's view. Abraham believed that early and repeated disappointments in childhood predisposed the individual to later depression in the face of similar stressors. The ego, according to Abraham, "retreats" or regresses from its maturely functioning state.

Cognitive theories of depression have evolved, guided principally by the work of Beck and Ellis, and these are now generally accepted and widely taught. The cognitive model views depression as the consequence of irrational or negative thinking. The depressed person is seen as the victim of his or her own internal "propaganda" (i.e., irrational or self-defeating statements that distort reality). Thus, the depressed patient may espouse beliefs, such as "If I am not perfect in everything I do, I am no good." Therapy with these patients tries to correct this faulty mode of thinking (see section VII.A.3).

A variety of psychosocial factors is correlated with the onset of depression, particularly in women. These include the absence of close interpersonal ties, marital discord and separation, the absence of employment outside the home, the loss of one's mother before the age of 11, more than three children under the age of 14 at home, and recent death or illness in the family. Ethnic and cultural factors may also shape the symptomatic presentation of depression; for example, African Americans with mood disorders appear to be more likely than whites to have hallucinations or delusions even after socioeconomic status has been considered.

Although psychodynamic theories are not based on reproducible data, these theories suggest that primary dysthymic disorder results from some as yet ill-defined problem in personality or ego development that culminates in difficulty adapting to adolescence and young adulthood. Chronic stress and acute loss may also predispose the individual to dysthymic disorder. As was noted above, secondary dysthymic disorder may develop as a consequence, feature, or complication of both psychiatric and medical disorders like anorexia nervosa, somatization disorder, or rheumatoid arthritis, or it may be present as an independent comorbid condition.

B. Biologic Theories

A large number of biochemical and neuroendocrine studies of depression have accrued over the past 50 years. Nevertheless, no single biologic theory accounts for all of the amassed data. Epidemiologic studies clearly suggest that both bipolar disorder and MDD have familial and genetic components as both generally "breed true" (i.e., if one monozygotic twin has unipolar illness, the other twin, if affected, is likely to have unipolar illness). However, some twin pairs follow a unipolar–bipolar pattern, suggesting that both disorders may be associated with a common element in their genetic vulnerability. In general, association and linkage studies have not demonstrated a single-gene susceptibility for MDD. That MDD is a heterogeneous condition encompassing several subtypes seems likely. The prevalence of unipolar depression ranges from 11% to 18% in relatives of MDD patients, a rate that is threefold higher than that seen in control subjects.

A number of biologic hypotheses have been offered to explain MDD. About 40 years ago, a relatively simple deficiency hypothesis attributed depression to low levels of one or more monoamines, usually serotonin (5-HT) or norepinephrine (NE). This model is clearly inadequate; it cannot account even for the time course of response to antidepressant treatment. Much of the evidence today points to a complex interplay of neurobiologic factors, including compromised neurons affected by insufficient amounts of nerve growth factors (e.g., brain-derived nerve growth factor), altered concentrations of relevant precursors for neurotransmitter synthesis from diet or other reasons, relative amounts of neurotransmitter in the synaptic cleft, the sensitivity of numerous postsynaptic receptors, the feedback sent to the presynaptic neuron via autoreceptors, and altered second-messenger systems. Recently, interest has been focused on the role of cyclic adenosine monophosphate (AMP), cyclic AMP response element binding protein, and a cyclic AMP response element binding protein–regulated gene that codes for *brain-derived neurotrophic factor*. Some have suggested that *up-regulation of the cyclic AMP and brain-derived neurotrophic factor systems* may provide a model of antidepressant action and perhaps of depression as well. For example, many effective antidepressant treatments increase the expression of brain-derived neurotrophic factor in the hippocampus. Despite this focus on gene activation, continued interest in the role of altered neuronal receptors in depression is seen.

Evidence derived from *in vitro* studies suggests that most, but not all, effective antidepressants down-regulate postsynaptic β-adrenergic receptors over a period of 1 to 3 weeks, corresponding to the time course of drug effect. The situation is undoubtedly more complicated, however, because the 5-HT system is intimately linked to the down-regulation of β-adrenergic receptors. Modest evidence also indicates that the α_2-adrenergic autoreceptor that normally mediates inhibition of NE release may be overactive in some depressed patients. This could lead to deficient release of NE. Although this might suggest a critical "noradrenergic" mechanism in depression, the situation is undoubtedly more complicated because, as noted, the down-regulation of β-adrenergic receptors is intimately linked to the 5-HT system.

Of all the hypotheses put forth to date to explain MDD, the most robust involves 5-HT dysregulation, regardless of its cause. Numerous studies support the association of low 5-HT function with the presence of MDD. Both reduced reuptake of presynaptic 5-HT and antagonism at or down-regulation of postsynaptic 5-HT$_{2A}$ receptors appear to be involved in the mechanism of action of most effective antidepressants. **Nefazodone**, for example, appears to act primarily as a 5-HT$_{2A}$ receptor antagonist.

Cholinergic overactivity has also been linked to depression, a hypothesis consistent with the euphoric "buzz" that some patients experience from the overuse of anticholinergic agents.

Neuroendocrine factors have also been implicated in MDD. As with neuro-transmitter findings, separating cause from effect is difficult. About 50% of MDD patients before treatment will show elevated 24-hour plasma concentrations of cortisol; a similar percentage (although not necessarily the same patients) will show early escape of cortisol secretion after suppression by the ingestion of dexamethasone (an "abnormal dexamethasone suppression test [DST]"). Recently, the role of *corticotropin-releasing factor* has been scrutinized because corticotropin-releasing factor hypersecretion may contribute to depressive symptoms. A blunted thyroid-stimulating hormone response to the administration of thyroid-releasing hormone has also been observed in about 25% of patients with MDD. Some data suggest that reduced thyroid-stimulating hormone responses in women are associated with the presence of suicidality, agitation, or concomitant panic attacks. Whether these various abnormalities are markers for MDD or are instead integral reflections of its pathophysiology is not yet clear. Finally, a number of sleep abnormalities have been linked to major depression, including decreased rapid eye movement latency and increased rapid eye movement density in the first half of sleep. The traditional interpretation was that changes in sleep architecture or physiology were secondary to the underlying depression; however, the effectiveness of sleep deprivation as a temporarily helpful treatment suggests that abnormal sleep may itself induce or contribute to depression.

The pathophysiology of dysthymic disorder is even more murky. Some primary dysthymic disorder patients with a positive family history of major depression and decreased rapid eye movement latency may share pathophysiologic mechanisms with MDD.

IV. Prognosis and Course
A. Major Depressive Disorder
Ambiguities in the usage of terms such as "remission," "relapse," and "recurrence" have made definitive comment about the prognosis and course of MDD difficult. Some generalizations from the literature are as follows: (a) about 50% of patients who recover from an initial episode of MDD will have at least one subsequent episode; (b) patients with two or more past episodes of MDD have roughly a 75% chance of another recurrence; and (c) although a given episode of MDD usually responds well to short-term treatment, about 30% will show only partial recovery and about 20% will have a chronic course. Historical, psychosocial, and biologic risk factors for relapse or recurrence of MDD are summarized in Table 18.3.

B. Primary Dysthymic Disorder
This condition usually has an insidious onset and a chronic course, often evolving into a superimposed episode of MDD. Alternatively, dysthymic disorder may be seen as the residuum of an episode of MDD. "Pure" dysthymic disorder, which is uncomplicated by short-lived bouts of more severe affective symptomatology, appears to be uncommon in clinical practice. A small

TABLE 18.3. RISK FACTORS FOR RECURRENCE OF MAJOR DEPRESSIVE DISORDER

Historical or Clinical	Psychosocial	Biologic
Antecedent history of relapse or recurrence Severity of index episode Comorbid dysthymic disorder ("double depression") Comorbid nonaffective psychiatric disorders	Marital discord Inadequate emotional support Cognitive vulnerability to stressors	Persistently abnormal DST Shortened rapid eye movement latency

Abbreviation: DST, dexamethasone suppression test.
From Thase ME. Relapse and recurrence in unipolar major depression: short-term and long-term approaches. *J Clin Psychiatry* 1990;51:51–57, with permission.

percentage of dysthymic disorder patients will go on to develop hypomanic or manic episodes. The prognosis of secondary dysthymic disorder seems to depend on the course of the primary underlying disorder.

V. Evaluation and Diagnosis

A. Adjunctive Psychologic Testing

A variety of objective and projective tests may support the diagnosis of MDD. On the Minnesota Multiphasic Personality Inventory, scale 2 (i.e., depression) is consistently elevated in patients with chronic MDD, and some evidence indicates that this elevation is correlated with an increased risk of suicide. On the Wechsler Adult Intelligence Scale-Revised, the classic depressive pattern is reflected by an overall performance score that is significantly lower than the verbal score. Depressed patients often "give up" on items or answer "I don't know." On the Rorschach test, long reaction times to the cards are typical; chromatic color responses are diminished, as one might expect. On the thematic apperception test, patients typically give short stereotyped responses that amount to mere descriptions of the cards. Several useful scales for MDD and other mood disorders have been developed. The Zung Depression Scale is a self-report scale consisting of 20 items, each with a four-point severity rating. The Zung Depression Scale assesses affective, psychic, and somatic features of depression. The Beck Depression Inventory is also a self-report scale, but it may emphasize asthenia (lack of drive, pep, or energy) more than depression in some populations. Results using self-report scales depend heavily on the motivation of the patient and the tester. The Schedule for Affective Disorders and Schizophrenia developed by Spitzer et al. in 1978 is a highly detailed 78-page protocol that assesses both present and historic functioning. It is used primarily in research settings along with clinician-rated measures of morbidity, such as the Hamilton Depression Rating Scale and the Montgomery Åsberg Depression Rating Scale. In contrast, the Zung and Beck scales are most often used as screening devices.

B. Adjunctive Biologic Testing

1. **Neuroendocrine studies**. Despite the volumes of data amassed in this area, no "blood test" exists for MDD as yet. During the 1980s, the DST seemed promising as a simple test; subsequent research and clinical experience have substantially diminished this initial optimism. Abnormal DSTs (nonsuppression) may occur in a variety of medical and neuropsychiatric conditions, such as Cushing syndrome, pregnancy, nondepressed bulimia nervosa, Alzheimer disease, and alcoholism. That the DST can serve even as a validating criterion for MDD is by no means

clear. Nevertheless, an abnormal DST may be predictive of clinical course and outcome. More specifically, when an abnormal DST precedes the onset of an episode of MDD, its normalization may herald clinical recovery. A persistently abnormal DST despite apparent recovery can be an ominous sign and can be predictive of rapid relapse.

Thyroid abnormalities, often of a subclinical nature, are seen in a substantial subgroup of depressed patients. The maximum thyroid-stimulating hormone response to thyroid-releasing hormone is diminished or blunted in about one-fourth of depressed patients; however, abnormal responses may also be seen in manic or mixed bipolar disorder patients. The thyroid-releasing hormone stimulation test may be helpful in distinguishing MDD from so-called reactive or neurotic depressions, many of which fall into the category of dysthymic disorder. These conditions typically do not show a blunted thyroid-stimulating hormone response. Other neuroendocrine probes for MDD are under investigation (e.g., growth hormone response to a variety of stimuli, such as **clonidine** and **desipramine**, may be diminished in MDD).

2. **Other biologic studies**. A number of studies using positron emission tomography or other imaging techniques suggest both functional and structural abnormalities in MDD. Positron emission tomographies of MDD patients may show a decreased ratio of caudate-to-hemisphere metabolism when compared with patients with bipolar disorder or with normal control subjects. This may suggest a role for the dopamine system in a subgroup of MDD patients. In a magnetic resonance imaging study of elderly patients with MDD, greater cortical and subcortical atrophy, as well as increased basal ganglia pathology, was seen in these patients compared with age-matched control subjects. Some functional neuroimaging data point to *abnormal prefrontal cortical and limbic function* in depression, suggesting that improved mood is associated with increases in prefrontal and anterior cingulate metabolism.

VI. **Differential Diagnosis of Major Depressive Disorder and Dysthymic Disorder**
  A. **Medical Conditions**
   A plethora of medical conditions may present with symptoms suggesting MDD, dysthymic disorder, or both. Some of the most common of these are shown in Table 18.4.

   In a study of 755 patients seen by the psychiatric consultation-liaison service in one general hospital, nearly 40% of depressed patients had a diagnosis of "organic mood disorder" (i.e., secondary mood disorder). The most frequent causes or precipitants were stroke, Parkinson disease, lupus cerebritis, and human immunodeficiency virus infection. Hypothyroidism and multiple sclerosis also accounted for a substantial number of cases. Somewhat surprisingly, medications accounted for only about 7% of cases. As might be expected, **propranolol** and corticosteroids were implicated. Clues to a secondary etiology for an episode of MDD include onset after age 45, negative

TABLE 18.4. SOME MEDICAL CONDITIONS AND MEDICATIONS ASSOCIATED WITH DEPRESSIVE SYMPTOMS

Use of certain antihypertensive agents, such as α-methyldopa, reserpine, and propranolol
Use of certain steroids, especially corticosteroids (e.g., prednisone), progesterone, estrogens
Immune and collagen-vascular disorders, such as multiple sclerosis, systemic lupus erythematosus, and rheumatoid arthritis
Treatment with interferons β-1a or α-2b
Other central nervous system pathology (e.g., Parkinson disease, Huntington disease, stroke, subdural hematoma)

family history of mood disorders, marked weight loss, accompanying signs of delirium or dementia, and absence of any evident psychosocial precipitant. (*Note:* The presence of a seemingly obvious precipitant such as the death of a spouse **does not** eliminate secondary organic factors as causes of the depression.)

Since the introduction of the cytokine immunomodulator **interferon-β1a** for the treatment of relapsing forms of multiple sclerosis, both depression and suicidal ideation and attempts that seem attributable to the treatment agent have been observed. This is a somewhat unusual finding because both the underlying disease and the treatment can produce the same psychiatric manifestations. Depression has also been found to be more common among patients being treated with **interferon-α2b** for malignant melanoma. An intriguing study has shown that pretreatment with the selective serotonin reuptake inhibitor (SSRI) **paroxetine** at about 30 mg per day reduces both the likelihood of a depressive episode and the severity of any depression that has occurred.

B. Other Psychiatric Disorders

A number of other psychiatric conditions may be mistaken for MDD or dysthymic disorder. Among the most important are normal bereavement and grief (see Chapter 16), various personality disorders (see Chapter 13), adjustment disorder with depressed mood, schizoaffective disorder (see Chapters 19 and 20), depression secondary to schizophrenia (see Chapter 20), and anxiety disorders (see Chapter 14) or somatoform disorders (see Chapter 4). Many patients with MDD will have comorbid axis I or II disorders. The chief differences between MDD and normal bereavement and grief are summarized in Table 16.1. However, these are, at best, crude guidelines; in some cultures, normal mourners may have a variety of depressive symptoms, including visual images of the deceased, persisting for more than a year after a loved one's death.

Among the personality disorders that may be confused with MDD or dysthymic disorder are borderline, narcissistic, avoidant, dependent, and obsessive-compulsive personality disorders. However, in such disorders, evidence of nearly lifelong impairment consistent with the supervening personality disorder criteria is usually seen. (*Note:* Sometimes, chronically depressed patients develop secondary alterations of personality that make differential diagnosis very difficult.)

Schizoaffective disorder is a poorly understood condition that is, in all likelihood, a rather heterogeneous collection of disorders. An apparent kinship seems to exist between the so-called bipolar type schizoaffective disorder and classic bipolar disorder. By contrast, the depressed type of schizoaffective disorder probably overlaps with patients with MDD and psychotic or delusional features, schizophrenia with intercurrent depression, and "true" schizoaffective disorder of a genetically distinct type. In practice, many patients diagnosed with schizoaffective disorder receive pharmacotherapies quite similar to those used in either bipolar disorder or MDD with psychotic features.

Secondary depression also presents complex diagnostic and treatment issues. Ideally, one tries to tease out the primary condition by carefully examining the longitudinal development of symptoms. For example, did the patient first develop panic attacks, followed months later by symptoms of MDD, or did the reverse occur? Similarly, a depressed patient with an antecedent history of deteriorating psychosocial function, ideas of reference, auditory hallucinations, and thought process abnormalities is most likely suffering from schizophrenia with secondary depression, a condition with different treatment implications than those for MDD with psychotic features. Such temporal distinctions are not always possible, and treatment often proceeds empirically and is directed against specific target symptoms. The relationship between depressive and anxiety disorders is discussed in section VIII.A.

VII. Treatment of Major Depressive Disorder and Dysthymic Disorder

A. Psychosocial Approaches

Some have said that there are as many psychotherapies for depression as there are psychotherapists. However, most approaches fall into one of the following four main categories: psychodynamic, experiential-expressive, cognitive-behavior, or interpersonal. These approaches are not mutually exclusive, nor do they necessarily rule out conjoint pharmacotherapy. No single approach has been demonstrated to be superior to the others, although cognitive-behavior and interpersonal approaches have been subjected to, and bolstered by, a number of reasonably well-controlled outcome studies. Although some writers distinguish cognitive from behavioral approaches, the former quite often include elements of the latter (e.g., cognitive therapists often give patients "homework assignments" or encourage *in vivo* exposure to troublesome situations). The converse, however, is not necessarily true.

1. **Psychodynamic therapies**. Belak elucidated the basic principles for brief psychodynamically oriented therapy for nonpsychotic depression. His approach, however, often evolves into longer term treatment. The following ten main problem areas are considered:

   Self-esteem;
   Punitive "superego" demands;
   Aggression against the self;
   Feelings of loss;
   Feelings of anger and disappointment;
   Feelings of having been deceived in relationships;
   Unmet dependency needs ("oral demands");
   Narcissism;
   Denial of hidden rage;
   Overall "object relations," including the patient's transference to the therapist and others.

   Classically conducted psychoanalysis is not appropriate for the treatment of severe depression, especially when psychotic features are present.

2. **Experiential-expressive therapies**. These therapies for depression have their roots in the work of Rogers, Maslow, and Peris. The emphasis is on the release of "pent-up" emotions, a "here-and-now" focus, and an empathic understanding on the part of the therapist. In general, little emphasis is placed on probing early experiences or the unconscious. Few well-controlled studies supporting this approach in the treatment of MDD have been conducted.

3. **Cognitive-behavior therapies**. Pioneered by Beck and Ellis, these therapies focus on the "preconscious" "irrational" ideas often espoused by depressed patients, as noted in section III.A. Treatment manuals for cognitive therapy have been developed that facilitate comparative outcome studies, if not therapeutic flexibility. Most studies of depression (variously defined) have shown cognitive or cognitive-behavioral approaches to be superior to minimal-treatment or no-treatment control subjects and perhaps to some psychodynamic approaches. A number of studies have found cognitive therapy to be comparable to or even superior to pharmacotherapy, but most of these studies have methodologic flaws, including generally inadequate pharmacotherapy and patient selection that excludes those with marked to severe pathology.

4. **Interpersonal therapy**. Developed by Klerman et al., interpersonal therapy assumes that depression occurs in an interpersonal context. Treatment is directed at helping the patient deal more effectively with current interpersonal problems, improve social functioning, communicate more effectively, and express painful affects. Little emphasis is given to early developmental experiences, unconscious mechanisms, or personality reconstruction. A manual of interpersonal therapy is also

available. A few controlled studies have shown interpersonal therapy to be comparable with pharmacotherapy for certain symptom areas such as social functioning.

Neurovegetative complaints appear to be more responsive to properly chosen pharmacotherapies than to any of the currently practiced psychosocial therapies. A number of studies suggest that the optimal treatment of MDD involves the combination of pharmacotherapy with an effective form of psychotherapy delivered by a skilled clinician.

B. Somatic Approaches

1. **Tricyclic antidepressants (TCAs).** TCAs were the mainstay in the treatment of MDD for over 30 years. Despite the introduction of many "new and improved" medications, none has shown consistently superior efficacy to the original TCAs. Nevertheless, few clinicians would claim that TCAs are the drugs of first choice for MDD in most depressed patients, except for when cost issues are placed ahead of overall tolerability. SSRIs, which primarily block the presynaptic 5-HT transporter and generally lack direct effects on other receptors, are the most frequently used of the alternatives to TCAs; they appear to offer some advantages in their patterns and intensity of side effects when compared with the TCAs. Given the moderately improved side-effect profile and greatly reduced toxicity of newer antidepressants, today most clinicians begin a depressed patient on either an SSRI or one of the newer non-TCA agents (see section VII.B.3). However, because the TCAs are used in refractory MDD, usually as adjunctive agents, this group of medications is considered here in detail.

The TCAs and the some of their other pharmacologic properties are summarized in Table 18.5. These agents may be viewed along a continuum of additional effects (usually called side effects) that may help guide the clinician in choosing the agent. Often, these predictable side-effect profiles are what determine the choice of TCA, because all of these agents appear to be equally effective on a population basis in the treatment of MDD. This means that approximately equal efficacy is observed when these agents are prescribed to randomly chosen groups of patients; individual patients, however, may respond preferentially to a specific TCA. In addition to the patient's specific symptom pattern, other factors involved in selecting a particular TCA may include the patient's previous response to TCAs and the responses of any affected family members to TCAs. Despite much hope and effort, little evidence exists

TABLE 18.5. COMPARATIVE QUALITIES OF SOME TRICYCLIC ANTIDEPRESSANTS

	Anticholinergic	Sedative	Cardiovascular[a]
Tertiary amines			
Amitriptyline	4	4	3
Imipramine	2	2.5	2
Doxepin	2.5	4	2.5
Clomipramine	2.5	3	2.5
Trimipramine	2.5	3	2
Secondary amines			
Desipramine	1	1	1.5
Nortriptyline	1.5	2	1.5
Protriptyline	3	0.5	1.5

Numbers are on a scale of 0 to 4, representing the following: 0, none; 1, minimal; 2, moderate; 3, substantial; 4, strong or marked.
[a]"Cardiovascular" represents an estimated proportional summation of hypotension, tachycardia, and conduction abnormalities. All values are approximations based on *in vitro* and clinical data.

to indicate that the unique neurochemical profile of a given TCA (e.g., the degree to which it inhibits presynaptic transport of NE, 5-HT, or dopamine) predicts anything about its efficacy in a specific patient.

The neurochemical basis for TCA side effects is not precisely known, but some of the following generalizations derived from *in vitro* and clinical studies can be made: (a) tertiary amine TCAs (e.g., **amitriptyline, imipramine**) tend to have greater sedative, anticholinergic, and hypotensive effects than do secondary amines (e.g., **desipramine, nortriptyline**); (b) the sedative and weight-promoting effects appear to be related to their affinity for the H_1 (histamine) receptor and perhaps to effects on the $5\text{-}HT_{2C}$ receptor; (c) their orthostatic hypotensive propensity is modestly related to their affinity for the α_1-adrenergic receptor; (d) cardiac conduction abnormalities may be related to the presence and amount of hydroxy metabolites, especially in the elderly; and (e) sexual dysfunction, although extremely complex, may be mediated by their 5-HT properties. Considering the following four prototypical TCAs may be helpful for anchoring oneself: **desipramine, amitriptyline, nortriptyline**, and **imipramine**.

a. **Desipramine** is the least sedating and the least anticholinergic of the TCAs. Indeed, some patients may complain of agitation or insomnia with **desipramine**, at least during the first few weeks of treatment. Patients with depression and accompanying panic attacks seem especially sensitive to these effects. **Desipramine**, like all the TCAs, has some cardiovascular side effects stemming from at least the following three mechanisms: α-adrenergic receptor antagonism leading to postural hypotension; vagolytic effects leading to tachycardia; and **quinidine**-like properties, which are shared with all class 1A antiarrhythmic agents, leading to various conduction abnormalities. Among the TCAs, however, **desipramine** is the least likely to provoke anticholinergic effects, such as dry mouth, constipation, blurred vision, and urinary retention. At therapeutic concentrations, its cardiovascular effects are relatively benign, although it may be associated with a higher than expected frequency of falls. **Desipramine** is not likely to be the TCA of choice for the extremely agitated patient with severe insomnia; for such a patient, a more sedating agent might be subjectively preferable, at least during the initial weeks of treatment. However, no compelling evidence exists indicating that the long-term outcome depends on matching the agent to the symptom picture; even in agitated insomniac patients, remission would be expected with **desipramine** in just as many cases as if **amitriptyline** were used. Presumably, a period of 3 to 6 weeks may be required for any TCA to modify the pathology underlying the depression; any earlier improvement may be due to nonspecific sedating effects.

b. **Amitriptyline**, the most anticholinergic and perhaps the most sedating TCA, is on the other end of the side-effects continuum. (*Note:* Some data suggest that **doxepin** and **trimipramine** are comparable in their sedating effects.) **Amitriptyline** is often associated with peripheral anticholinergic complaints, as well as with some central complaints, such as confusion, memory impairment, and delirium. In comparison with other TCAs, **amitriptyline** has a high incidence of cardiovascular effects, including postural hypotension. Sexual side effects, such as retrograde ejaculation, impotence, and anorgasmia, are also comparatively more frequent, although these can occur with any TCA (even though SSRIs cause even more sexual side effects than does amitriptyline). **Amitriptyline** would rarely be the TCA of choice, for example, in an elderly patient with bladder dysfunction, first-degree atrioventricular block, mild dementia, and psychomotor slowing or lethargy. **Amitriptyline** might be selected for an extremely agitated younger adult patient with severe initial (sleep-onset) insomnia; however, even in such a patient, the anticholinergic side effects of this agent may prohibitively limit the necessary dosage increases. Despite these putative limitations, some primary care physicians use low-dose **amitriptyline** regimens because its sedative properties are seen as beneficial for any concomitant insomnia, agitation, or anxiety. Because it also has some effects on somatic pain and in the prevention of migraine, **amitriptyline** is popular among some clinicians.

    c. **Nortriptyline** is in the middle of the continuum of TCA side effects. Although **nortriptyline** is an active metabolite of **amitriptyline**, it is less anticholinergic and less sedating than **amitriptyline**; it is also less agitating and activating than **desipramine**. In this sense, **nortriptyline** is seen by some clinicians as the TCA for the "average" patient with MDD. It also has a fairly benign cardiovascular profile, and it is often recommended for the elderly patient with MDD. Even in elderly patients with mild conduction abnormalities, nortriptyline usually does not cause significant orthostatic (postural) hypotension. However, dosing with **nortriptyline** is more complicated than with other TCAs, because it is unique among the TCAs in having a fairly well-defined therapeutic window (i.e., in its concentration-response curve, levels above and below which it is less likely to be efficacious do exist). Most studies support 50 to 150 ng per mL as the optimal range for plasma levels of **nortriptyline**.

    d. **Imipramine** is often chosen as an effective prototypical comparator TCA in research trials. As the first TCA introduced in the mid-1950s, it has been subjected to the most scrutiny. Its side-effect profile is midway between that of **amitriptyline** and that of **nortriptyline**. It is slightly less sedating and less anticholinergic than **amitriptyline** and is slightly more so than **nortriptyline**. Postural hypotension is not uncommon with **imipramine**; its other cardiovascular effects are less severe than those seen with **amitriptyline**.

    e. TCAs may have **additional side effects**, such as tremor; excessive sweating; edema; skin rash; exacerbation of narrow-angle glaucoma; and behavioral complications, such as mania or psychosis. TCAs lower the seizure threshold, so they must be used cautiously in patients with a family or personal history of seizure disorder. (*Note:* The cumulative yearly incidence of TCA-related seizures is only about 0.3%.) TCAs can interact with a variety of other medications (see Chapter 29). Finally, TCAs may be very toxic when taken in overdoses; for example, even a 3-week supply (3,000 mg) of **amitriptyline** may be fatal if it is ingested all at once (see Chapter 3).

2. Some guidelines for prescribing TCAs

    a. **Principles**. A few principles involved in the prescription and monitoring of the TCAs deserve emphasis.

        (1) **Dose range**. For the prototypical patient, a total daily dose of 175 to 300 mg for **imipramine** or its equivalent is usually required. One rule of thumb for **imipramine** is to attempt to reach 3.5 mg per kg per day, unless significant improvement or side effects occur at lower doses.

        (2) **Plasma levels**. Many clinicians attempt to use plasma levels to guide dosing, even though therapeutic ranges have not been unequivocally established. Once enough time has elapsed to reach steady state, a level in the putative therapeutic range may provide a degree of assurance that the drug was ingested, absorbed, and metabolized as expected. Modest evidence does indicate that most TCAs need to reach plasma levels of at least 100 ng per mL of the parent compound to achieve a full thera-

peutic effect. Some patients may respond at lower concentrations, whereas others may not respond until 250 to 300 ng per mL has been reached or slightly exceeded (e.g., patients on **imipramine, desipramine,** or **doxepin**). **Nortriptyline,** with its putative therapeutic window, is an exception. **Amitriptyline,** which is partially metabolized to **nortriptyline,** may have an upper limit of effectiveness in some patients.

(3) **Monitoring for side effects.** Excessively high plasma TCA levels may be associated with increased adverse reactions, such as seizures and cardiotoxicity. With respect to the latter, obtaining baseline and follow-up electrocardiograms is a good practice in patients over the age of 50 or in those with a known history of cardiovascular disease. Because certain conduction abnormalities in children (e.g., congenitally long QT intervals [see Chapter 21]) and young adults may be subclinical, a few clinicians recommend obtaining a baseline electrocardiogram on all patients placed on TCAs. Certainly patients with first-degree or second-degree atrioventricular block should be monitored closely and perhaps should be treated with a non-TCA. Checking the patient's vital signs periodically is also a good medical practice.

(4) **Duration.** TCAs usually should be prescribed at tolerated therapeutic doses for a minimum of 6, and perhaps up to 18, months after recovery from an episode of MDD; the old practice of tapering down to a maintenance dose as soon as the patient recovers has been linked to higher relapse rates.

b. **Side effects.** Treating TCA-related side effects can be difficult; sometimes, a difference of 10 to 20 mg in the daily TCA dose can markedly affect the patient's tolerance of the drug. For any TCA-related side effect, dose reduction is a reasonable first step. Unfortunately, some patients are so sensitive to the anticholinergic, hypotensive, or "libidolytic" effects of the TCA that dose reduction alone will not suffice. Dry mouth, constipation, and other anticholinergic side effects may be helped by advising the patient to increase water intake and dietary fiber. Urinary retention will sometimes require the addition of **bethanechol** (50 to 150 mg per day), which may also ameliorate dry mouth and constipation to some degree, to the therapeutic regimen. (*Note:* The clinician must rule out bladder obstruction before prescribing this agent.) Stool softeners, such as **docusate sodium** (100 mg, once to three times per day), may be helpful. Some clinicians recommend the use of fluoride lozenges for dry mouth. Postural hypotension may respond to a variety of interventions, including salt tablets, modest amounts of caffeine, or pressure (TEDS) stockings. In resistant cases, the mineralocorticoid **fludrocortisone** may be helpful in doses of about 0.4 mg per day.

c. **Duration of MDD (recurrence versus relapse).** The term "relapse" generally implies a worsening of an ongoing episode of depression; "recurrence" refers to the occurrence of a new episode. An arbitrary but common convention holds that worsening that occurs within 6 months after remission constitutes a relapse; worsening occurring thereafter is considered a recurrence. The highest rate of relapse occurs in the first few months after remission from an episode of MDD; the probability of relapse declines steadily during the course of the prospective follow-up. Patients with residual symptoms at the time of withdrawal of antidepressant medication have a higher rate of relapse than do patients who manifest no such symptoms. In terms of interval-specific probabilities of recovery from MDD, about 60% of patients will recover after 6 months. Of those not recovered by 6 months, about 30% can be expected to recover within the next 6 months. Of those not recovered by 1 year, about 15% will recover in the next 6 months. Among those not recovered by 18 months, only 10% will remit in the next 6 months. Thus, the likelihood of recovery decreases substantially the longer that a patient remains depressed after initially entering treatment. The reader should note that most data of this type are derived from university medical centers; therefore, they may not generalize to other populations of depressed patients. Some evidence suggests that the duration of MDD episodes tends to remain constant or to lengthen slightly with each recurrence; the length of the preceding episode may serve as the lower estimate for the duration of the next one.

d. **Prevention of relapse and recurrence: the role of lithium**. Results from a National Institute of Mental Health collaborative study suggest that discontinuation of antidepressant therapy is "safe" only after the patient has been free of significant symptoms for at least 16 to 20 weeks and that focusing on mild and severe symptoms is critical in reaching this decision. The National Institute of Mental Health study, based on its inclusion criteria, also incorporated patients with bipolar disorder. Both TCAs and **lithium** are effective in preventing recurrence of MDD, but TCAs appear to be more effective, especially for the prevention of severe episodes. Between 10% and 15% of patients initially diagnosed as having MDD will have a subsequent manic episode. When a high suspicion of latent or "undeclared" bipolar disorder is present, some clinicians advocate the addition of **lithium** to the TCA regimen. Factors suggesting a higher likelihood of bipolar disorder include an early age at onset of depression (under 25), a family history of bipolar disorder, a family history of affective disorder in consecutive generations, and the presence of atypical signs and symptoms.

3. **Non–monoamine oxidase inhibitors (MAOIs), non-TCAs ("heterocyclics")**. This "nongroup," which is sometimes called the "heterocyclics," includes a wide array of agents, some of which are not cyclic in structure. Included in this grouping are the infrequently used tetracyclic **maprotiline**, the triazolopyridines **trazodone** and **nefazodone**, and the aminoketone **bupropion**. Their properties are summarized in Table 18.6.

TABLE 18.6. COMPARATIVE SIDE EFFECTS OF SOME NON-MONOAMINE OXIDASE INHIBITOR, NONTRICYCLIC, OR "HETEROCYCLIC" ANTIDEPRESSANTS

	Anticholinergic	Sedative	Cardiovascular
Maprotiline	1.5	2.5	1
Trazodone	1	4	2
Fluoxetine[a]	+/−	1	+/−
Paroxetine[a]	0.5	1	+/−
Sertraline	+/−	1	+/−
Bupropion[a]	+/−	1	+/−
Venlafaxine[a]	+/−	2	1
Mirtazapine	1	3.5	1
Nefazodone	+/−	2	1

Numbers are on a scale of 0 to 4, representing the following: 0, none; 1, minimal; 2, moderate; 3, substantial; 4, strong or marked; +/−, negligible.
[a]These agents also come in extended-release, sustained-release, or controlled-release formulations. Pharmacokinetic differences from the immediate release product result in reduced adverse effects for some patients.

a. **Maprotiline**, a compound that primarily inhibits the presynaptic transport of NE, appears to be as effective as the TCAs, but it also seems to have a somewhat higher incidence of seizures and skin rashes. It is less sedating than **doxepin** and also somewhat less anticholinergic. Seizures are especially common with **maprotiline** overdose. In general, **maprotiline** has few advantages over the TCAs or SSRIs, and it is infrequently prescribed as a first-line agent.

b. **Trazodone** is a proserotonergic antidepressant that is also an antagonist at several 5-HT$_1$ and 5-HT$_2$ receptor subtypes. Its primary side effects are sedation, dizziness, and gastrointestinal complaints. Even though **trazodone** is not strongly anticholinergic *in vitro,* some patients complain of dry mouth, which perhaps is a result of its α_1-adrenergic receptor antagonist actions. Unlike some TCAs, **trazodone** usually does not promote substantial weight gain. Although it does not typically cause cardiac conduction abnormalities, **trazodone** has been linked with ventricular arrhythmias in a few instances. Nevertheless, **trazodone** appears to be significantly safer than the TCAs when it is taken in overdose. One rare but potentially dangerous side effect is priapism. Although this may occur in only about 1 in 7,000 men who take **trazodone**, permanent damage to the penis can occur when medical or surgical intervention is not given promptly. Other sexual side effects, including both anorgasmia and increased libido, have also been reported. Some studies suggest that **trazodone** is less consistently effective than are the standard TCAs. One possible explanation for this is the formation of significant amounts of its metabolite metachlorophenylpiperazine when **trazodone** doses exceed about 250 mg per day; metachlorophenylpiperazine has anxiogenic properties that may undermine the parent compound's antidepressant effect.

Trazodone is most frequently prescribed as a "piggyback" medication for sleep-onset insomnia in patients taking SSRIs or MAOIs. Evidence indicating that **trazodone** may increase deep sleep while preserving normal sleep architecture in healthy nondepressed adults does exist. **Trazodone** is also finding occasional use as an antiaggression agent in agitated demented patients.

c. **Nefazodone** is structurally similar to **trazodone**, but it was developed to have less α_1-adrenergic receptor antagonism. It also lacks clinically significant anticholinergic and antihistaminic effects. It blocks presynaptic 5-HT transport, and it is a postsynaptic 5-HT$_{2A}$ receptor antagonist. It is rapidly absorbed and has a high first-pass metabolism involving cytochrome CYP 3A4 oxidative pathways for which it is both a substrate and an inhibitor. The parent compound has a half-life of 2 to 4 hours; it has at least three metabolites that contribute to its clinical actions, including small amounts of metachlorophenylpiperazine. **Nefazodone** appears to be a broadly effective antidepressant.

In contrast to other antidepressants, **nefazodone** produces minimal or no suppression of rapid eye movement sleep; it does not appear to cause priapism, even though this unwanted effect is associated with **trazodone**. Side effects, such as nausea, dry mouth, somnolence, dizziness, and constipation, have been observed, but they occur less often than with the TCAs. Sexual side effects are less common than they are with SSRIs. That a **black box** warning was added to the labeling for **nefazodone** because of rare cases of life-threatening hepatic failure should be noted. (*Note:* The estimated rate is 1 per 250,000 to 300,000 patient-years resulting in transplantation or death; the true rate is unknown.) Twice a day dosing is recommended (100 mg, twice a day, for the initial dose; reaching 400 mg per day after 1 week; 600 mg per day is often considered its maximum dose).

d. **Bupropion** is a nonsedating antidepressant that appears to inhibit the presynaptic dopamine transporter. It bears some structural and functional similarity to **amphetamine**. **Bupropion** has little, if any, anticholinergic activity; it does not promote weight gain; and it appears to have few cardiovascular side effects. It seems to be well tolerated in elderly patients with heart disease; in one study, it did not prolong cardiac conduction, exacerbate ventricular arrhythmias, or induce higher degrees of atrioventricular block. Lower doses of bupropion are usually indicated for the elderly, particularly to avoid the mild confusional states that sometimes occur with its use. Sexual dysfunction, an unwanted effect that is fairly common with SSRIs, is not common with **bupropion**; its prodopaminergic action may have a potentiating effect on erectile function. When **bupropion** was first studied, it appeared to have a more pronounced effect on the seizure threshold than the TCAs did. The usual figure quoted was a cumulative yearly seizure incidence of about 0.4% for **bupropion** versus that of about 0.2% for TCAs. (*Note:* In doses above 600 mg per day, the **bupropion** rate rose to about 0.6%.) However, a 102-site study of **bupropion** at doses of up to 450 mg per day involving more than 3,000 patients showed a seizure rate of 0.24% during an 8-week treatment phase and a rate of 0.4% for the entire study period. The overall seizure rate of 0.36% was interpreted as comparable with other antidepressants. The daily dose of **bupropion** should not exceed 450 mg, and it should be administered in divided doses of no more than 150 mg. A slow-release form of **bupropion (bupropion-SR)** may be administered on a twice daily basis; at steady-state, 150 mg twice a day of the slow-release form is bioequivalent to 100 mg three times a day of regular **bupropion**. The seizure risk for the slow-release preparation appears to be about 0.1% in the dosage range of 100 to 300 mg per day. (*Note:* Some data suggest that **maprotiline** [at greater than 150 mg per day], **amoxapine** [at greater than 300 mg per day], and **clomipramine** [at greater than 250 mg per day] may also enhance seizure risk.)

Because **bupropion** is sometimes given along with SSRIs, any inhibition by the SSRI of the hepatic clearance of **bupropion** must be considered, and appropriate dosage reductions must be made. Because **bupropion** appears to potentiate dopamine function, one might expect it to induce psychosis in predisposed individuals; case reports support this possibility, but no convincing evidence exists to indicate that **bupropion** is more likely to induce psychosis than is any other antidepressant. Some reports suggest that secondary brain syndromes or psychosis associated with **bupropion** tend to occur in patients with bipolar disorder or in those with premorbid psychotic features. Some data suggest that plasma levels of **bupropion** in the range of 10 to 19 ng per mL yield better responses than levels above 30 ng per mL.

e. **Buspirone**, an anxiolytic that first introduced a group of 5-HT_{1A} partial agonists known as the azapirones, may also have antidepressant properties. In doses of 40 to 60 mg per day, **buspirone** appears to be safe and effective when compared with a placebo.

f. **Venlafaxine**, a phenethylamine derivative, is a racemic mixture with the active metabolite, O-desmethylvenlafaxine. Together they inhibit presynaptic transporter mechanisms for both NE and 5-HT (i.e., **venlafaxine** is a reuptake blocker for both neurotransmitters). It is relatively free of antimuscarinic, antihistaminic, and α_1-adrenergic receptor antagonist properties. **Venlafaxine** has comparable efficacy with TCAs and SSRIs at doses of 75 to 375 mg per day; a modal dose is 250 mg per day in tablet form. Nausea, drowsiness, dizziness, dry mouth, and sweating are its most common side effects; all of these probably affect between 10% and 35% of patients. However, an extended-release capsule formulation, **venlafaxine XR**, is better tolerated and is now more widely used than the immediate release formulation. Elevated blood pressure that is probably related to its presynaptic adrenergic effects may be a concern for some patients (e.g., when dosage exceeds 200 mg per day [or lower in elderly patients]).

g. **Mirtazapine** is a novel agent that effectively facilitates both noradrenergic and serotonergic transmission. It antagonizes the α_2-adrenergic receptors that normally reduce NE outflow; thus, it "releases" the noradrenergic neuron from its autoreceptor, leading to increased NE outflow. By also antagonizing α_2-adrenergic *heteroreceptors* located on *serotonergic* nerve terminals, it leads to increased 5-HT output as well. Because **mirtazapine** blocks 5-HT$_{2A/C}$ and 5-HT$_3$ receptors, its serotonergic effect may be more selectively directed at 5-HT$_{1A}$ receptors, the activation of which is thought to have antidepressant and anxiolytic effects. Moreover, the lack of 5-HT$_{2A/C}$ and 5-HT$_3$ activation seems to reduce the typical serotonergic side effects, such as sexual dysfunction and gastrointestinal complaints (its 5-HT$_{2C}$ receptor antagonism may, however, contribute to weight gain in some patients). The main side effects associated with mirtazapine are *somnolence, increased appetite, weight gain,* and *dizziness.* Some clinicians advocate beginning with 30 mg per day (versus 15 mg per day), based on the theory that the increased noradrenergic effects will counteract some of mirtazapine's sedating antihistaminic effects. However, patients react quite individually to this agent, and, for many, 15 mg at bedtime is a reasonable initial regimen. Premarketing reports of agranulocytosis associated with mirtazapine have not proved to be a significant clinical problem.

h. **Duloxetine** is a recent addition to the non-SSRI, non-TCA pool of antidepressants. It affects reuptake of both 5-HT and NE and lacks affinity for muscarinic and histaminergic receptors. Some data suggest that it has higher binding affinity for these transporters than does **venlafaxine**. Clinical trials using doses in the range of 20 to 60 mg twice daily suggest that its efficacy is greater than that of a placebo in nonpsychotic MDD. More experience is needed with this agent to assess its place in the current armamentarium of antidepressants.

i. **Reboxetine** is a selective noradrenergic agent that is awaiting release. Although its comparative advantages are not yet clear, **reboxetine** is expected to be useful in patients in whom serotonergic agents either have been ineffective or are poorly tolerated (e.g., those with SSRI-related sexual dysfunction or gastrointestinal complaints). On the other hand, one might anticipate less robust effects for comorbid conditions, such as obsessive-compulsive disorder, premenstrual dysphoric disorder, or other conditions, that appear to benefit from a proserotonergic agent.

4. **SSRIs.** At the present time, SSRIs are the most commonly used and most widely accepted antidepressants in the United States. Although some clinicians have individual preferences for particular agents and some patients may tolerate one SSRI better than another, the only study that examined their comparable effectiveness in primary care settings found them to be quite comparable. This study examined 573 adults who were randomly assigned to **fluoxetine, paroxetine,** or **sertraline.** These SSRIs are relatively specific inhibitors of the presynaptic 5-HT transporter; this group also currently includes **citalopram**. In addition, the S enantiomer of **citalopram, escitalopram,** is also marketed in the United States for depression. Another SSRI, **fluvoxamine,** is also marketed in the United States, but it does not carry an indication for MDD.

The pharmacokinetic properties and dosages of these agents are shown in Table 18.7.

All the SSRIs have a similar side-effect profile as follows: gastrointestinal distress, loose stools or diarrhea, sexual dysfunction (in men, mainly ejaculatory delay), tremor, and increased sweating. Dry mouth and constipation are somewhat more common with **paroxetine**. Either excitation or somnolence may occur; in one study, **sertraline**-associated insomnia or somnolence occurred in 17.5% and 14.5% of patients, respectively. However, these values were not significantly greater than those that were seen with the placebo. It appears that **citalopram, sertraline**, and **paroxetine** may be somewhat less likely than **fluoxetine** to cause psychomotor agitation. SSRIs also differ in their hepatic microsomal enzyme-inhibiting effects (see Chapter 29). The SSRIs should not be considered any more homogeneous as a group than the TCAs are. They may even have different effects on certain aspects of central nervous system function (e.g., **paroxetine's** effect on the sleep electroencephalogram is opposite to those of **fluoxetine** and **fluvoxamine**). **Paroxetine** appears to be more likely than the other SSRIs to produce a discontinuation syndrome in some patients after abrupt cessation of its use. Because other SSRIs may also cause this withdrawal problem, tapering is a better strategy than is abrupt withdrawal.

The SSRIs may be especially useful in patients who cannot tolerate TCA side effects, in the elderly, and perhaps in depressed patients with panic attacks or atypical features. They are far less toxic than the TCAs in overdose, and preliminary evidence suggests that at least one of the SSRIs, **paroxetine**, is less likely than **clomipramine**, a TCA mainly used in the treatment of obsessive-compulsive disorder (see Chapter 6); **amitriptyline**; or **imipramine** to induce mania in patients with bipolar disorder. Recent evidence has cast doubt on whether the SSRIs as a group are less likely than other antidepressants to induce "switching" in bipolar patients.

Fluoxetine has evoked more interest and emotion than has any other antidepressant in recent years. **Fluoxetine** and other SSRIs appear to be as effective as TCAs in controlled trials in outpatients with MDD. **Fluoxetine** appears to be associated with less weight gain than that seen with the TCAs, MAOIs, and **paroxetine**. Some patients may even lose 2 or 3 pounds during the first few months of taking **fluoxetine**. However, some patients taking any SSRI for 6 months or more report

TABLE 18.7. SOME SELECTIVE SEROTONIN REUPTAKE INHIBITOR PHARMACOKINETIC AND DOSAGE DATA

	Mean $T_{\frac{1}{2}}\beta$	Active Metabolite	Daily Dose Range[a] (mg)	Active Metabolite $T_{\frac{1}{2}}\beta$
Citalopram	1.5 d	—	20–40	—
Escitalopram	1.5 d	—	10–30	—
Fluoxetine[b]	2–3 d	Norfluoxetine	5–80	5–9 d
Fluvoxamine	15 h	—	25–300	—
Paroxetine[c]	1 d	—	20–50	—
Sertraline	1 d	Desmethylsertraline	25–250	2–4 d

Abbreviation: $T_{\frac{1}{2}}\beta$, terminal half-life.

[a]Based on manufacturer's recommendation and the authors' clinical experience; activity may be prolonged in the elderly; $\frac{1}{2}$ to $\frac{1}{3}$ of the usual adult dosage may be indicated for some agents in the elderly. The elimination half-life ($T_{\frac{1}{2}}\beta$) may also be prolonged for some agents in patients with hepatic disease.

[b]An extended-release once-a-week formulation (90 mg/wk) is available.

[c]A controlled-release once-a-day formulation is available.

bothersome weight gain. When *premorbid weight* is used as the baseline, however, many patients taking **fluoxetine** (and perhaps other SSRIs) appear to be simply regaining the weight lost during their depressive episode. **Fluoxetine** and other SSRIs can cause not only sexual dysfunction in men but also anorgasmia in women (the latter complaint may be more prevalent than was initially reported; it may possibly affect as many as 20% to 50% of patients). **Fluoxetine** differs from other SSRIs in that it is marketed in capsules of 10 or 20 mg, rather than as tablets, and in a liquid preparation. A preparation is available for the treatment of premenstrual dysphoric disorder. (*Note:* This formulation is called Sarafem rather than Prozac.) **Fluoxetine** is also the first SSRI to be available as a generic.

Titration of the dose may be particularly important for patients either with panic attacks alone or with depressive symptoms, because some of these patients may be exquisitely sensitive to the activating effects of SSRIs. One such SSRI side effect, **akathisia**, may be associated with considerable distress and even suicidal ideation. Contrary to exaggerated stories in the lay press, no convincing evidence indicates that fluoxetine or any other SSRI is more likely to be associated with an increased incidence of suicide when compared with other antidepressants or a placebo. (*Note:* When TCAs are ingested during an intentional overdose, there is a higher rate of death.) Some patients, particularly the elderly, may do best on doses of 5 to 10 mg per day of **fluoxetine** or its equivalent. Some clinicians use initial doses of 1 to 2.5 mg per day of **fluoxetine** or its equivalent in depressed patients with concomitant panic attacks. On the other hand, other patients clearly fare best on 40 to 80 mg per day of **fluoxetine** or its equivalent, and they tolerate these amounts without difficulty. Because SSRIs are sometimes activating and as they are capable of causing insomnia early in treatment, prescribing many of them as a single dose in the morning is a common practice. For **sertraline**, morning or evening dosing appears comparable. Given the long half-life of **fluoxetine**—the parent compound and its principal metabolite **norfluoxetine** have elimination half-lives of 1 to 3 days and 7 to 9 days, respectively—intermittent dosing (i.e., every 2 or 3 days) may make pharmacokinetic sense for some patients. This also raises the issue of the clinical need for a once a week formulation. A 90 mg, once weekly **fluoxetine** capsule that is available appears to be clinically comparable for most patients on the immediate formulation at 20 mg per day.

A controlled-release formulation of **paroxetine** (paroxetine CR) is available in the following three strengths: 12.5 mg, 25 mg, and 37.5 mg. It uses a polymeric matrix to release the tablet's contents over a 4-hour to 5-hour time period. Its enteric coating delays the onset of drug release until the tablets have reached the small intestine. Limited evidence suggests that the controlled-release formulation may be associated with less nausea in the first week of treatment.

As was noted earlier, some patients who experience SSRI-associated insomnia may benefit from the addition of a small dose of **trazodone** or **doxepin** at bedtime. **Trimipramine**, another highly sedating TCA, can also be used. SSRIs should not be coadministered with MAOIs because a "serotonin syndrome" can result from the combination; a 5-week washout of **fluoxetine** is suggested before initiating MAOI therapy, whereas 2 weeks should be sufficient for the other SSRIs.

5. **MAOIs**. For many years, the MAOIs were shunned by some psychiatrists as either dangerous or ineffective. In actuality, the MAOIs can be both safe and effective when used in the right way and for the right patient. Essentially, the currently available MAOIs are most appropriate for patients with atypical features and for those who have not responded to the classic antidepressants. AD is discussed in more detail in section VIII.A;

it is a mood disorder characterized by depression admixed with prominent anxiety, especially phobic or panic symptoms. Reversed neurovegetative signs are particularly common. The latter include increased appetite and weight gain, hypersomnia, and reversed diurnal variation in which mood worsens in the evening rather than in the morning. Notwithstanding the utility of MAOIs in AD, many patients with more typical depression may also respond to these agents.

As Table 18.8 shows, MAOIs may be classified in several ways. The mitochondrial enzyme monamine oxidase (MAO) catabolizes catecholamines and serotonin. MAO occurs in two forms, A and B; and MAOIs may be more or less selective for either. MAO-A acts most selectively on the substrates 5-HT and NE, and it is found mainly in the gut and liver, as well as in the brain. MAO-B acts most selectively on phenylethylamine and benzylamine and predominates in the brain. Dopamine is a substrate for MAO-B, as well as for MAO-A. All currently marketed MAOIs (**phenelzine, tranylcypromine**, and **isocarboxazid**) are nonselective.

So-called irreversible MAOIs, such as **phenelzine, isocarboxazid**, and **L-deprenyl** (more recently renamed **selegiline**), bind tightly to their target enzyme, and they are not readily displaced. Reversible MAOIs are readily displaced by tyramine and other pressor amines found in various foods and beverages. The clinical importance of selective or reversible MAOIs lies mainly in their reduced likelihood of causing the "cheese reaction" in response to exogenous tyramine or other pressor amines. **L-Deprenyl** is relatively MAO-B selective at low concentrations, typically 10 mg per day; and it is thought to act primarily in the brain. (*Note:* **L-Deprenyl** is metabolized to **methamphetamine** and **amphetamine**.) At low concentrations, it does not interfere with MAO-A's metabolism of tyramine in the gastrointestinal tract. The reversible MAO-A inhibitors **moclobemide** and **brofaromine** (not yet marketed in the United States) appear to be particularly safe in the event of tyramine ingestion. They are displaced from the enzyme by the tyramine; the tyramine is then metabolized.

These theoretic issues notwithstanding, the MAOIs that are currently available and are indicated for use in depression are the three nonselective inhibitors **phenelzine, isocarboxazid**, and **tranylcypromine**. (*Note:* **Tranylcypromine** is a partially reversible inhibitor; MAO activity returns in about 7 to 10 days, rather than the 2 to 3 weeks needed for **phenelzine** or **isocarboxazid**.) The usual starting doses for these agents are as follows: **tranylcypromine**, 10 to 20 mg per day; **phenelzine**, 15 to 30 mg per day; and **isocarboxazid**, 20 to 30 mg per day. Elderly patients may require downward adjustment, as may others

TABLE 18.8. SOME MONOAMINE OXIDASE INHIBITORS

	Chemical Class	Specificity	Reversibility
Phenelzine	Hydrazine	Nonselective	Irreversible
Tranylcypromine	Nonhydrazine	Nonselective	Irreversible[a]
Isocarboxazid	Hydrazine	Nonselective	Irreversible
Selegiline (L-deprenyl)	Nonhydrazine	MAO-B[b]	Irreversible
Meclobemide[c]	Nonhydrazine	MAO-A	Reversible
Brofaromine[c]	Nonhydrazine	MAO-A	Reversible

[a] Usually reversible after 7–10 days rather than after 2–3 weeks.
[b] At greater than 10 mg/d, selegiline usually loses its specificity.
[c] Not currently marketed in the United States.
Abbreviation: MAO, monoamine oxidase.

who encounter side effects even at these low starting doses. Up to 6 weeks may be required for a robust clinical response to occur; the onset of action may be more rapid with **tranylcypromine**. The upper daily dosage ranges for **tranylcypromine**, **phenelzine**, and **isocarboxazid** are 60, 90, and 50 mg, respectively. Higher doses are occasionally required for some resistant patients.

Aside from the cheese reaction, the main unwanted effects of MAOIs are insomnia, orthostatic hypotension, weight gain, sexual dysfunction, dry mouth, constipation, delayed micturition, nausea, and swelling or edema. Daytime drowsiness is occasionally reported, as are myoclonic twitches, sweating, chills, flushing, and restlessness. Disinhibition or hypomania may be seen, but the MAOIs appear to be less likely than the TCAs to precipitate mania in patients with bipolar disorder. A relatively infrequent neuropathy secondary to MAOI-induced vitamin B_6 deficiency has been reported. This condition is readily treated with oral vitamin B_6 (pyridoxine), 50 to 100 mg per day. Although hepatic toxicity is uncommon, it may be seen with the hydrazine-type MAOIs (i.e., **phenelzine** and **isocarboxazid**). Cardiac conduction abnormalities are relatively rare with the MAOIs, which gives them an edge over the TCAs. Some clinicians prefer MAOIs for elderly patients who have various degrees of atrioventricular block. Nonadherence and "dropout" are fairly common with the MAOIs, probably due to their high frequency of side effects. With **phenelzine**, insomnia, daytime somnolence, dry mouth, impaired sexual function, and orthostatic hypotension may be seen in up to 20% of patients. Both preparing the patient for such side effects and treating those that occur are important. Strategies for side effects treatment should begin with dosage reduction; other techniques are summarized in Table 18.9. Time alone may be sufficient to reduce some unwanted effects (e.g., **phenelzine**-induced anorgasmia may diminish after 2 to 4 months).

The most feared event with the MAOIs is the hypertensive response triggered by tyramine ingestion or the concomitant administration of certain sympathomimetic agents (e.g., indirect-acting drugs, such as **ephedrine** or L-**dopa**). In clinical practice, serious reactions of this type are infrequent. Although this habit is not to be encouraged, many patients test the dietary restrictions by ingesting one of the prohibited foods; they report either no reaction or only a bad but tolerable

TABLE 18.9. TREATING SELECTED MONOAMINE OXIDASE INHIBITORS' SIDE EFFECTS

Side Effect	Some Treatment Strategies
Hypotension, dizziness	Increased salt intake; TEDS stockings; fludrocortisone (0.2 mg per day); T_3 or T_4; tranylcypromine least associated with postural hypotension
Insomnia	Addition of trazodone (25–50 mg h.s.); benzodiazepines; "paradoxical" bedtime dosing; for tranylcypromine, consider less-stimulating MAOI
Weight gain	Dietary counseling (e.g., decreasing sweets, fats); increased daily aerobic exercise
Sexual dysfunction	For delayed ejaculation or anorgasmia, try switching to another MAOI after 1 to 2 week washout; bethanechol or cyproheptadine before intercourse

Abbreviations: h.s. at bedtime; MAOI, monoamine oxidase inhibitor; T_3, triiodothyronine; T_4, thyroxine; TEDS, pressure.

headache. Moreover, about 30% of hypertensive crises in MAOI-treated patients cannot be ascribed to antecedent dietary factors; some reactions have no clear precipitating factor. Nevertheless, severe hypertensive crises that, on rare occasions, lead to death have been reported; providing the patient with a clear but realistic set of precautions is important. Prototypical dietary guidelines are summarized in Table 18.10. Probably the most important food items to avoid are those whose taste is enhanced by aging or fermentation (e.g., aged cheese of any type) and any spoiled foods. Patients should be warned that the tyramine content of foods varies from sample to sample, country to country, and even region to region. If a suspicious food is to be eaten, a small amount should be tried first, and the patient should then wait at least 2 hours before consuming any more. If a hypertensive episode does occur, it will usually start within 2 hours after tyramine ingestion; it will begin as a severe throbbing temporooccipital headache that is accompanied by marked palpitations and is followed by flushing, sweating, nausea, and vomiting. If untreated, this state may progress to cerebral hemorrhage. (*Note:* Young adults with occult circle of Willis aneurysms may be at particular risk.) Informing the patient of this reaction and advising him or her to seek immediate attention at an emergency department if such a reaction occurs are crucial.

Some clinicians provide patients with one or two tablets of the calcium channel blocker **nifedipine**, 10 mg, to bite and then swallow in the event of a cheese reaction. Although it is usually effective, **nifedipine** can provoke excessive hypotension in some patients. A reasonable plan may be to advise the patient to take the **nifedipine** and then to call 911

TABLE 18.10. SOME DIETARY RESTRICTIONS WITH MONOAMINE OXIDASE INHIBITORS

Foods to Avoid	Usually Safe Foods	Foods Unlikely to Pose Problems When Eaten in Moderation
Aged or matured cheeses; this includes cooked foods containing these cheeses	Cottage, cream, ricotta, or farmer's cheeses	Yogurt or sour cream that has been properly refrigerated
Beer (especially tap and unpasteurized), red wine, sherry, liqueurs	Vodka, gin, dry white wines	Other alcoholic drinks, including bottled or canned beer if the
Fermented (dry) sausage, beef or chicken liver, smoked or pickled fish, caviar	All fresh meats or fish Banana pulp Shelled beans	quantity is limited to less than 12 oz/d and the beer is not con-
Canned or overripe figs, whole bananas, banana peel fiber		sumed rapidly Other fruit, if not overripe
Fava or broad bean pods		Avocado, New Zealand
Yeast or protein extracts (e.g., marmite), some fermented soy products, sauerkraut		spinach Some soy sauces, yeast-containing breads, soy milk Chocolate, caffeine-containing drinks

From Folks D. Monoamine oxidase inhibitors: reappraisal of dietary considerations. *J Clin Psychopharmacol* 1983;3:249–252, with permission.

or to proceed immediately to an emergency department. **Phentolamine** (typically 5 mg either intramuscularly or intravenously) or **phenoxybenzamine** (orally or parenterally) are the usual drugs administered in emergency departments (see Chapter 3).

Patients taking **selegiline** in doses of no more than 10 mg per day do not need to adhere to the "MAOI diet"; however, the main active metabolites of **L-deprenyl**, **amphetamine** and **methamphetamine** may have dopaminergic actions of their own, including some pressor effects. In addition to the prohibited foods, numerous drugs and medications can interact adversely with MAOIs. The most severe drug–drug reaction is that which occurs between MAOIs and **meperidine**; a single dose of the latter can provoke fatal hyperthermia. (*Note:* **Dextromethorphan** can also provoke this reaction, and it should be avoided.) In general, sympathomimetic agents, such as **phenylephrine**, **ephedrine**, and **phenylpropanolamine**, should be avoided; antihistamines are usually safe in moderation. The adverse interaction between the SSRIs and MAOIs has already been noted. **Buspirone** also has proserotonergic properties; it probably should not be combined with MAOIs. A washout of at least 2 weeks should occur before changing from one MAOI to another, because hypertensive reactions have been observed with abrupt switching. An up-to-date manufacturer's product brochure should be consulted for a complete list of drug–drug interactions for a particular MAOI.

6. **Treatment of MDD with psychotic features**. Despite early controversy over the effect of TCAs in psychotic depression, most studies to date support the conclusion that TCAs alone (and by inference, "heterocyclics" alone) are not especially effective when psychotic features, such as somatic delusions, are present. Most studies suggest that only about 25% to 30% of patients with psychotic features respond well to TCAs alone, compared with the typical response rates of 65% to 70% in nonpsychotic MDD patients. MAOIs or SSRIs given alone produce similar outcomes. The best pharmacologic approach to psychotically depressed patients is probably a combination of an atypical antipsychotic agent and an antidepressant, either an SSRI (e.g., **sertraline**, **citalopram**) or a non-TCA, non-SSRI agent (e.g., **venlafaxine**). Although few controlled studies of such combined regimens have been conducted, one report found the combination of **citalopram** (20 to 40 mg per day) and **haloperidol** (4 to 9 mg per day) to be useful in seven patients with MDD with psychotic features. Preliminary evidence suggests that atypical antipsychotic agent monotherapy (eg., **risperidone, quetiapine, olanzapine**) may be useful in some patients. However, electroconvulsive therapy (see Chapter 24) may be the treatment of choice.

The clinician should keep in mind that some TCAs or SSRIs and some antipsychotic agents may inhibit each other's metabolism, thus resulting in higher than expected levels of each. Lower doses of each agent may sometimes be necessary to avoid anticholinergic or parkinsonian side effects. Some clinicians have had good results with **thiothixene** (10 to 30 mg per day) and **nortriptyline** (at doses producing nortriptyline plasma levels of about 80 ng per mL). Some evidence suggests that atypical antipsychotic agents may be useful in patients with schizoaffective illness, some of whom are psychotically depressed.

Valproic acid, carbamazepine, and **lithium** may all be useful in some patients with MDD with psychotic features, perhaps primarily in those who have bipolar features.

7. **Refractory MDD and augmentation**. "Refractory" or "treatment-resistant" MDD may be related to inadequate antidepressant dosing,

duration of treatment, or plasma levels or some combination of these factors. In some cases, plasma antidepressant levels may be within the putative therapeutic range, but they are inadequate for the particular patient. Although specific blood levels of non-TCAs (e.g., SSRIs) are less clearly linked with therapeutic effects, a *negligible* SSRI blood level may point to *noncompliance, poor drug absorption,* or *"hypermetabolism."* Once dosing problems have been considered, the clinician should next reconsider the diagnosis (i.e., has a concomitant or comorbid medical, substance abuse, or personality disorder been overlooked?). The patient who is truly refractory to antidepressant monotherapy may benefit from a number of potentiating or "switching" strategies, depending on whether the patient has had a partial response or no response to the agent. In general, *complete nonresponders* to an adequate trial of one agent should be *switched* to a second agent. Although most clinicians seem to favor switching to a new chemical class (e.g., from an SSRI to **bupropion**), some consider changing from one SSRI to another to be a rational alternative. Indeed, response to one SSRI does not necessarily predict the response to another. In contrast, *partial responders* may benefit from *augmentation* of the original agent. Most clinicians wait about 4 weeks before beginning an augmentation strategy. For details on switching and augmentation strategies, the reader is referred to a useful supplement of the *Journal of Clinical Psychiatry* (2000;61[Suppl. 12]). The patient who is truly refractory to TCAs given alone may benefit from a number of potentiating strategies (Table 18.11).

Probably the most robust of these approaches is the addition of **lithium** to a TCA or an SSRI. (*Note:* Most augmentation strategies noted for TCAs may also apply to SSRIs [see sections VII.B.3 and VII.B.4].) Clinical improvement may occur within 2 to 3 days, even at "subtherapeutic" **lithium** doses (e.g., 600 mg per day). Other patients may require several weeks at conventional levels of **lithium** (0.5 to 0.9 mEq per L) for improvement.

Thyroid hormone may also be used to potentiate TCAs; for this purpose, **triiodothyronine** is considered by many clinicians to be superior to **thyroxine**. However, few "head-to-head" comparisons of the use of thyroxine with that of triiodothyronine for this purpose have been conducted. The addition of stimulants such as **methylphenidate** or **pemoline** may also be helpful. (*Note:* Tolerance to stimulants may develop in some patients after a few weeks; some clinicians prefer to taper and discontinue the stimulant once improvement has occurred.) The addition of an MAOI to a TCA, which was long regarded by many clinicians as taboo, may have significant benefits for some patients. Unfortunately, research data demonstrating the efficacy and safety of this combination are limited. The risk of TCA–MAOI combinations is primarily that of

---

TABLE 18.11. SOME WAYS TO POTENTIATE THE THERAPEUTIC ACTIONS OF TRICYCLIC ANTIDEPRESSANTS[a]

Concomitant use of one or more of the following:
Lithium
Thyroid hormone
Antipsychotic agents, generally in the presence of delusional features
Monamine oxidase inhibitors (with extreme caution)
Selective serotonin reuptake inhibitors

---

[a] Potentiation should always be selective, and it should be undertaken with caution to avoid potentially harmful drug interactions or enhanced side effects.

inducing a "serotonin syndrome" of hyperthermia, delirium, and myoclonus, not of the occurrence of hypertension (i.e., the cheese reaction associated with excess tyramine). Limited evidence implicates **imipramine** as being the drug that is most likely to cause problems when used in combination with an MAOI. The best approach to combination therapy is to begin the TCA and MAOI together, using small doses of each, or to add a small amount of the MAOI (e.g., 5 mg per day of **tranylcypromine**) to ongoing TCA therapy.

Some clinicians suggest that small doses of TCAs (e.g., **desipramine**, 10 to 30 mg per day) can be used as an augmentation strategy to enhance the efficacy of SSRIs in the treatment of MDD. The potential for drug interactions exists with these combinations; particular caution is indicated when **desipramine** and **paroxetine** are combined (see Chapter 29).

8. **Antidepressants for dysthymic disorder**. Few placebo-controlled studies of antidepressant therapy in pure dysthymic disorder have been conducted. As was noted earlier, dysthymic disorder often coexists with MDD or other axis I disorders. To date, studies examining various forms of chronic low-grade depression generally suggest that antidepressants are helpful. Some patients with dysthymic disorder overlap with atypical depressive patients. Others may have a "characterologic" (axis II) overlay that reduces the effectiveness of antidepressants; however, one should *never* assume that chronically depressed individuals are "just axis II" and that therefore they are unworthy of a vigorous antidepressant trial. Furthermore, some data suggest that some dysthymic patients may require more than 3 months of treatment before they show an adequate response to the SSRI.

VIII. Atypical, Seasonal, and Other Variant Forms of Depression
A. Diagnostic Considerations

The term "**atypical depression**" has been used in a variety of ways, and it may be misleading in an important sense—patients with putatively atypical features are actually common in clinical practice. However, such patients share many clinical features with a variety of diagnostic groups, including patients with panic disorder, SAD, bipolar II disorder (i.e., MDD with hypomanic episodes), and borderline personality disorder (BPD). One possible set of criteria for AD is given in Table 18.12. Other classifications emphasize the features of reactive mood disturbance (nonautonomy); hyperphagia or binge eating (especially on carbohydrates or sweets); hypersomnolence; and interpersonal difficulties, such as rejection and criticism

---

TABLE 18.12. A PROTOTYPICAL CRITERIA SET FOR ATYPICAL DEPRESSION[a]

Reactive (nonautonomous) mood disturbance, lability, dysphoria, or rejection or criticism sensitivity
Prominent anxiety (e.g., separation anxiety, panic attacks)
Histrionic features (e.g., overly dramatic responses to frustration, change, or loss)
Phobic features
Marked fatigue (e.g., inertia, lethargy, heaviness in the legs or arms)
Reversed neurovegetative features (e.g., mood is typically worse in the afternoon than in the morning, increased rather than decreased appetite [self-soothing eating], weight gain rather than weight loss)
Initial (sleep-onset) insomnia often combined with hypersomnolence
Adequate premorbid personality
Psychosomatic complaints or hypochondriasis

---

[a] In the *Diagnostic and Statistical Manual of Mental Disorders*, 4th ed., "with atypical features" is a term that can be used to modify major depressive disorder, dysthymic disorder, or bipolar disorders.

sensitivity. Many of these features are found in patients with **hysteroid dysphoria** (HD), a group described by Liebowitz and Klein. HD patients tend to be "attention junkies" who have exquisitely fragile self-esteem, as well as a tendency to overeat and oversleep when depressed. This picture is strikingly similar to the "winter-depressive" category of SAD described by Rosenthal et al. These latter patients, in turn, are often women with bipolar II disorder.

Given the diverse criteria for AD, its prevalence is difficult to establish. The prevalence of HD features, one possible prototypical AD subset, may be high. One study found that 6 of 18 depressed inpatients met HD criteria; most of the patients meeting HD criteria also met criteria for BPD, thus suggesting some overlap between AD, HD, and BPD. (*Note:* These data could also suggest that HD and BPD features may alter the threshold for hospitalization of depressed patients in some settings.) In another study of AD patients helped by **isocarboxazid**, the author concluded that his patient sample was typical of depressed outpatients.

The prevalence of SAD is estimated to be 5% for the general population; it may be as high as 38% in patients with recurring depression. Some data suggest that 20% to 25% of bipolar disorder patients may show seasonal mood fluctuations. About 75% of SAD patients meet the criteria for bipolar II disorder, and 15% to 20% meet the criteria for bipolar disorder. The hyperphagia (often with carbohydrate craving) and hypersomnolence seen in "winter-type" SAD suggest some commonality with AD. One population study in Fairbanks, Alaska suggested that about 9% and 19% of the sample met criteria for SAD or subsyndromal SAD, respectively, and concluded that one in four persons is affected by the seasonal changes found at that latitude.

One could view the aggregate of patient subtypes discussed in this section as being subsumed by a Venn diagram of three overlapping circles labeled AD, SAD, and bipolar II disorder. Many patients with low lethality "borderline" features (e.g., mood lability, disturbed interpersonal relationships, binge eating, and stimulant abuse) will also overlap with these patient types. Many "neurotic" features, including obsessive-compulsive, hysterical conversion, and hypochondriacal traits, have also been viewed as atypical or "masked" forms of depression. Of interest is the fact that the *International and Statistical Classification of Diseases and Related Health Problems,* tenth revision, contains the category mixed anxiety and depressive disorder. Patients with this diagnosis are primarily seen in primary care settings.

The relationships among anxiety, depression, and AD continue to be discussed. Despite comorbidity and overlapping symptoms, reasonable evidence exists to justify separating these disorders. Symptoms such as depressed mood, early morning awakening, and psychomotor retardation delineate patients whose future decompensations will most likely meet MDD criteria, whereas compulsive features, panic attacks, and agoraphobia are more closely associated with anxiety disorders.

B. Treatment Considerations

The heterogeneity of AD precludes any single drug of choice. A patient who has hypersomnia, hyperphagia, and carbohydrate craving when depressed but who also has hypomanic periods may do best on **lithium**, which perhaps may be combined with an MAOI, SSRI, or **bupropion** during the individual's depressed phases. **Bupropion** and **tranylcypromine** may have particular value in "winter-type" SAD, according to some authors. A patient with true SAD might benefit from phototherapy, although various antidepressants and **lithium** have been used successfully in SAD. A patient with BPD might benefit from any one of several pharmacologic approaches, including the use of low-dose antipsychotic medication (see Chapter 13). AD remains a diagnosis in search of a pharmacospecific treatment.

Given these complexities, how should the clinician proceed when faced by an AD patient who does not appear to fit into either the bipolar II disorder or SAD subtype? The presence of anxiety or panic attacks does not consistently predict a good response to an MAOI, such as **phenelzine**, or to an SSRI (as compared with **imipramine** or a placebo). Preferential response to an MAOI or SSRI seems to be more closely related to the presence of mood reactivity, reversed neurovegetative patterns, or hysteroid dysphoric features. Because weight gain is often a problem in such patients, some clinicians choose **tranylcypromine** rather than **phenelzine**, even though most of the studies to date have used **phenelzine**. In AD patients who lack panic attacks or features of HD, looking closely at the symptom dimensions can be helpful (see Chapter 13). For the lethargic hypersomniac group, treatment with a nonsedating antidepressant, such as **desipramine**, **protriptyline**, or **bupropion**, is reasonable, although controlled trials with these are lacking. Some data suggest that mixed anxious-depressed patients or those with psychosomatic complaints may also respond well to **bupropion**. **Bupropion** does not seem to be useful, however, for depressed patients with concomitant panic attacks. The 5-HT$_{IA}$ partial agonist **buspirone** may provide relief to some patients with MDD with significant concomitant anxiety (i.e., with Hamilton Anxiety Rating Scale scores greater than 17). However, in one such study, **buspirone** (40 to 60 mg per day) worked best in patients with MDD with melancholia or in those who were more symptomatic. Because AD patients are often conceptualized as nonmelancholic (e.g., lacking profound weight loss, autonomy of mood, mood worsening in the morning), this study could also be construed as being unsupportive of **buspirone's** efficacy in AD. On the other hand, if one conceptualizes AD as a form of anxious depression, these data could support the usefulness of **buspirone**. **Buspirone** was also considered effective in patients suffering from irritability; mild secondary symptoms of depression; and interpersonal sensitivity—symptoms consistent with, but not specific for, AD.

Some AD patients with impulsive features and histories of substance abuse resemble patients with borderline personality disorder (BPD). Some evidence suggests that **fluoxetine** and other SSRIs may be helpful in BPD (see Chapter 13). That some AD patients with "borderline features" would also respond well to **fluoxetine** or other SSRIs is plausible. Some clinicians support this use, but no controlled studies using well-defined AD patients have been published. A recent multicenter study of 395 outpatients with MDD that remitted with **fluoxetine** treatment failed to find evidence of **fluoxetine's** efficacy in *maintaining remission* for patients with atypical symptoms. This study's authors concluded that **fluoxetine** may not be as effective as the MAOIs for the treatment of AD.

Patients with SAD probably constitute a special subgroup of patients with AD. Phototherapy using bright full-spectrum artificial light is often considered the treatment of choice, but controlled studies versus MAOIs, SSRIs, **bupropion**, or other agents have not been published. Despite theories linking SAD with alterations in melatonin metabolism or sleep–wake cycle shifts, no treatment specifically addressing these putative abnormalities has been demonstrated to be superior to the standard treatment alternatives. Whether the timing of phototherapy (e.g., morning or midday) makes any difference is also not clear; patients appear to do equally well with either. Many SAD patients with clear bipolar features merit a trial on **lithium**, possibly in combination with phototherapy. Such patients would also be expected to do better with MAOIs, SSRIs, or **bupropion** than with the TCAs because these appear less likely to induce mania.

IX. Depression in the Elderly

Faced with a variety of socioeconomic stressors, losses, health problems, and age-associated changes in organ system functioning (e.g., increased brain MAO activity, increased subcortical white matter pathology, and decreased brain choline acetyltransferase activity), the elderly may be at particular risk for depressive symptomatology. Data on age-related prevalence rates for MDD, however, are ambiguous. Prevalence rates vary from 1% to 10% for persons over 65 years of age. Recent data suggest that, in age cohorts over the age of 65, prevalence rates of 1% to 2% are the norm, a rate much lower than that seen in younger groups. Suicide rates, however, are higher in the elderly (45 per 100,000) compared with the general population (13 per 100,000) (see Chapter 17). The prevalence of syndromes other than MDD, such as mixed anxiety-depression and dysphoric-dysthymic states, is higher in the elderly; and they are estimated to affect about 25% of persons over age 65. Depression in the elderly may also be more difficult to detect, and "masked depressions" are not infrequent (i.e., depression presenting as apathy or somatic complaints). The elderly are said to complain less of guilt and to have more depression-based cognitive decrements (see Chapter 5), compared with that seen in younger adults. Some depressed elderly are written off as mere hypochondriacs. Many medications taken by older persons may cause secondary depressions, and hypothyroidism and stroke-related depressions are more common among the elderly.

Treatment of depression in the elderly requires a biopsychosocial approach. Family involvement, when it is possible, is important; and short-term cognitive behavioral psychotherapies can be useful. Despite much commentary to the contrary, no single antidepressant of choice exists for the elderly. As was discussed earlier (see section VII.B), the classical tertiary amine TCAs have unwanted properties that can be particularly problematic for the elderly (e.g., constipation, urinary retention, blurred vision, and postural hypotension). The non-TCA agents, such as **bupropion**, the MAOIs, or the SSRIs, may be better tolerated than the tertiary amine TCAs; unfortunately, they have not yet been evaluated in large-sample trials in the elderly. **Trazodone** has some popularity, but it may be associated with hypotension and rarely with ventricular arrhythmias. Studies of SSRIs in depressed cardiac patients, most of whom are elderly, have generally been favorable. Although **mirtazapine**-related orthostatic hypotension is unusual, somnolence and dizziness are common, and they merit conservative dosing in debilitated elderly patients. On the other hand, some medically ill elderly patients with significant weight loss might benefit from **mirtazepine's** weight-promoting effects. Many clinicians claim a preference for **nortriptyline** or an MAOI, such as **phenelzine** or **tranylcypromine**. Stimulants, such as **methylphenidate**, may be effective, especially for short-term use.

When prescribing drugs for the elderly, the wise approach is to "start low and go slow." One-third to one-half of the typical adult dose is generally used. (*Note:* Individual variation in dose requirements is significant in the elderly; plasma levels can be useful when available, particularly because other agents taken by the elderly may affect drug levels.) For the most part, elderly and younger adult patients appear to require comparable antidepressant blood levels; however, the elderly may achieve these same levels at lower doses. On the other hand, at least one study examining **nortriptyline** doses and plasma levels in frail elderly nursing home residents suggested that the optimum plasma level for these patients may be somewhat lower than that of younger populations (42 to 111 ng per mL versus 50 to 150 ng per mL).

X. Herbal or "Over-the-Counter" Antidepressants

A great deal of interest for these diverse agents has been expressed, but, unfortunately, little systematic research has been conducted. Herbal and over-the-counter agents touted as antidepressants include, but are not limited to, *S*-adenosyl-L-methionine (SAMe), dehydroepiandrosterone, inositol, St. John's wort (*Hypericum perforatum*), various amino acids and vitamins, and omega-3 fatty acids. Although a complete review of this topic is beyond the scope of this chapter, the reader is directed to the recent reviews referenced. In brief, only modest and sometimes controversial evidence exists for antidepressant effects with SAM-e, St. John's wort, and perhaps dehydroepiandrosterone and inositol. Few rigorously designed, long-term, controlled studies of these agents are available. The evidence to date suggests a possible role for SAM-e and St. John's wort in mild nonpsychotic MDD. How well these agents work compared with newer antidepressants used at clinically meaningful doses is still not clear. Furthermore, each of these nonprescription agents—contrary to the popular image of "organic" or "natural" remedies—may have significant neuropsychiatric side effects, including the induction of mania or other systemic effects (e.g., the induction of the gastrointestinal track transporter protein p-glycoprotein by St. John's wort).

XI. The Depressed Suicidal Patient
The depressed patient who is suicidal is a medical emergency. Chapter 17 discusses the evaluation and treatment of the suicidal patient.

XII. National Depressive and Manic Depressive Association (NDMDA)
The NDMDA is an important lay (consumer) organization whose membership is drawn from patients, family members, and interested professionals. They provide support and information to patients and their families, and they actively advocate for improved care, education, and research. NDMDA, which is based in Chicago, can be reached at 1-800-82-NDMDA.

ADDITIONAL READING

Akiskal HS. Dysthymic disorder: psychopathology of proposed chronic depressive subtypes. *Am J Psychiatry* 1983;140:11–20.

Akiskal HS. New insights into the nature and heterogeneity of mood disorders. *J Clin Psychiatry* 1989;50:6–10.

Amsterdam J, ed. *Refractory depression*. New York: Raven Press, 1991.

Angst J. The course of monopolar depression and bipolar psychoses. *Psychiatr Neurol Neurochir* 1973;76:489–500.

Bonomo V, Fogliani AM. Citalopram and haloperidol for psychotic depression. *Am J Psychiatry* 2000;157:1706–1707.

Boulenger JP, Lavalée YJ. Mixed anxiety and depression: diagnostic issues. *J Clin Psychiatry* 1993;54:3–8.

Bruce ML, Takeuchi DT, Leaf PJ. Poverty and psychiatric status: longitudinal evidence from the New Haven Epidemiologic Catchment Area Study. *Arch Gen Psychiatry* 1991;48:470–474.

Bymaster FP, Dreshfield-Ahmad LJ, Threlkeld PG, et al. Comparative affinities of duloxetine and venlafaxine for serotonin and norepinephrine transporters in vitro and in vivo, human serotonin receptor subtypes, and other neuronal receptors. *Neuropsychopharmacology* 2001;25:871–880.

Caine ED, Lyness JM, King DA. Reconsidering depression in the elderly. *Am J Geriatr Psychiatry* 1993;1:4–20.

Cornelius JR, Soloff PH, Perel JM, et al. A preliminary trial of fluoxetine in refractory borderline patients. *J Clin Psychopharmacol* 1991;11:116–120.

Danish University Antidepressant Group. Paroxetine: a selective serotonin reuptake inhibitor showing better tolerance, but weaker antidepressant effect than clomipramine in a controlled multicenter study. *J Affect Disord* 1990;18:289–299.

Demitrack MA. Can monoamine-based therapies be improved? *J Clin Psychiatry* 2002;63:14–18.

Dewan MJ, Pies RW. The difficult-to-treat patient with depression. In: Dewan M, Pies R, eds. *The difficult to treat psychiatric patient*. Washington, D.C.: American Psychiatric Press, 2001:81–114.

Duman RS. Novel therapeutic approaches beyond the serotonin receptor. *Biol Psychiatry* 1998;44:324–335.

Fabre LF. Buspirone in the management of major depression: a placebo-controlled comparison. *J Clin Psychiatry* 1990;51:55–61.

Fogelson DL, Bystritsky A, Pasnau R. Bupropion in the treatment of bipolar disorders: the same old story? *J Clin Psychiatry* 1992;53:443–446.

Goodnick P. Blood levels and acute response to bupropion. *Am J Psychiatry* 1992; 149:399–400.

Harnett DS. The difficult to treat psychiatric patient with co-morbid medical illness. In: Dewan M, Pies R, eds. *The difficult to treat psychiatric patient*. Washington, D.C.: American Psychiatric Press, 2001:325–358.

Janicak PG, Pandey GN, Davis JM, et al. Response of psychotic and nonpsychotic depression to phenelzine. *Am J Psychiatry* 1988;145:93–95.

Joffe R. Triiodothyronine potentiation of fluoxetine in depressed patients. *Can J Psychiatry* 1992;37:48–50.

Kocsis JH, Klein DN. *Diagnosis and treatment of chronic depression.* New York: Guilford Press, 1995.

Kroenke K, West SL, Swindle R, et al. Similar effectiveness of paroxetine, fluoxetine, and sertraline in primary care. *JAMA* 2001;286:2947–2955.

Liebowitz MR, Klein DF. Hysteroid dysphoria. *Psychiatric Clin North Am* 1979; 2:555–575.

Mann JJ, Aarons SF, Frances AJ, Brown RD. Studies of selective and reversible monoamine oxidase inhibitors. *J Clin Psychiatry* 1984;45:62–66.

McGrath PJ, Stewart JW, Petkova E, et al. Predictors of relapse during fluoxetine continuation or maintenance treatment of major depression. *J Clin Psychiatry* 2000; 61:518–524.

Musselman DL, Lawson DH, Gumnick JF, et al. Paroxetine for the prevention of depression induced by high-dose interferon alpha. *N Engl J Med* 2001;344:961–966.

National Institute of Mental Health. *The impact of mental illness on society.* NIH publication no. 01-4586. Bethesda, MD: National Institute of Mental Health, 2001.

Nelson JC. Augmentation strategies in depression 2000. *J Clin Psychiatry* 2000; 61:13–19.

Olfson M, Marcus SC, Druss B, et al. National trends in the outpatient treatment of depression. *JAMA* 2002;287:203–209.

Osser DN. A systematic approach to the classification and pharmacology of nonpsychotic major depression and dysthymia. *J Clin Psychopharmacol* 1993;13:133–144.

Pies R. Atypical depression. In: Tupin JP, Shader RI, Harnett DS, eds. *Handbook of clinical psychopharmacology,* 2nd ed. Northvale, NJ: Aronson, 1988:329–356.

Pies R. The diagnosis and treatment of subclinical hypothyroid states in depressed patients. *Gen Hosp Psychiatry* 1997;19:344–354.

Pitsikas N. Duloxetine Eli Lilly & Co. *Curr Opin Investig Drugs* 2001;1:116–121.

Quitkin FM, Harrison W, Stewart JW, et al. Response to phenelzine and imipramine in placebo nonresponders with atypical depression. *Arch Gen Psychiatry* 1991; 48:319–323.

Rosenthal NE, Sack DA, Gillin JC, et al. Seasonal affective disorder. *Arch Gen Psychiatry* 1984;41:72–80.

Rundell JR, Wise MG. Causes of organic mood disorder. *J Neuropsych Clin Neurosci* 1989;1:396–400.

Salzman C, Schneider L, Lebowitz B. Antidepressant treatment of very old patients. *Am J Geriatr Psychiatry* 1993;1:21–29.

Shader RI. Current clinical applications of monoamine oxidase inhibitors: issues and concerns. In: Shader RI, ed. *MAOI therapy.* New York: Audio Visual Medical Marketing, 1988:5–30.

Shader RI, Fogelman SM, Greenblatt DJ. Epiphenomenal, causal, or correlational—more on the mechanism(s) of action of antidepressants. *J Clin Psychopharmacol* 1998;18:265–267.

Thase ME. Relapse and recurrence in unipolar major depression: short-term and long-term approaches. *J Clin Psychiatry* 1990;51:51–57.

Thase ME, Entsuah AR, Rudolph RL, et al. Remission rates during treatment with venlafaxine or selective serotonin reuptake inhibitors. *Br J Psychiatry* 2001; 178:234–241.

Thase ME, Greenhouse JB, Frank E, et al. Treatment of major depression with psychotherapy or psychotherapy-pharmacotherapy combinations. *Arch Gen Psychiatry* 1997;54:1009–1015.

Waalinder J, Feighner JP. Novel selective serotonin reuptake inhibitors, part 1. (Academic highlights). *J Clin Psychiatry* 1992;53:107–112.

Wong AH, Smith M, Boon HS. Herbal remedies in psychiatric practice. *Arch Gen Psychiatry* 1998;55:1033–1043.

Zajecka JM. Clinical issues in the long-term treatment with antidepressants. *J Clin Psychiatry* 2000;61:20–25.

19. APPROACHES TO THE TREATMENT OF MANIC-DEPRESSIVE STATES (BIPOLAR DISORDERS)

Richard I. Shader

Descriptors such as bipolar or manic-depressive evoke the image of patients whose moods regularly alternate between "up," excessively happy, or "high" periods and "down," excessively depressed, or "low" periods. In fact, alternating episodes rarely occur, and manic shifts probably account for less than 15% of all episodes in this diagnostic group. Manic and depressive states have been described for many centuries, but the notion of manic-depressive illness *per se* was not proposed until the middle of the 19th century by Falret (*la folie circulaire*) and Baillarger (*la folie a double forme*). Later, Kraepelin added impetus to its recognition as a distinct disorder when he separated it from schizophrenia by pointing out its episodic course and the importance of abnormal moods, which stood in contrast to the thought disturbance of schizophrenia. In 1957, Leonhard further subdivided manic-depressive illness by separating patients with mania and depression (bipolar) from those with depression or mania alone (monopolar, unipolar).

I. General Diagnostic Considerations

Both subtle and significant changes and controversies have occurred as the diagnostic criteria for manic-depressive illness and bipolar disorder (BD) have evolved into their current iteration in the *Diagnostic and Statistical Manual of Mental Disorders*, 4th edition (DSM-IV).

Bipolar I disorders describe those disorders in which at least one manic, hypomanic (with at least one previous manic), or mixed manic and depressive episode clearly is or has been present. Bipolar I disorder presenting solely or even mostly as recurrent manic episodes is extremely rare. This author has seen patients with episodic paranoia, and he believes that they may actually represent this otherwise underrecognized diagnostic subgroup.

Bipolar II disorder describes patients with at least one depressive and one hypomanic episode when no manic episode is or has been present. A diagnosis of **BD, not otherwise specified** is recommended when the mania, depression, or hypomania appears to be solely secondary to a medical condition, such as multiple sclerosis or hyperthyroidism; to substance use (e.g., amphetamines, **cocaine**); or to treatment with antidepressants (e.g., monamine oxidase inhibitors), electroconvulsive therapy (ECT), sympathomimetic amines, decongestants, or corticosteroids. Curiously, some patients with secondary presentations (e.g., during **prednisone or cocaine** use) may be manic in one episode and paranoid in another.

Cyclothymic disorder (CyD) is another currently recognized mood disorder. Its relationship to BD corresponds to the relationship between major depressive disorder (MDD) and dysthymic disorder in many ways (see Chapter 18). Limited data suggest that cyclothymic personality, a diagnostic predecessor of CyD, occurs more often in relatives of BD patients than it does in the relatives of normal control subjects or in patients with MDD. To meet criteria for CyD, patients must have numerous bouts of hypomanic behaviors or symptoms and depressed mood, including anhedonia, for a minimum of 2 years (*note:* for at least 1 year in youth). Obviously, these descriptive criteria for CyD are both arbitrary and time bound. For example, a patient with muted mood shifts during the year before a consultation likely has CyD, even though the 2-year requirement has not yet been met. Some of these patients may later go on to have full-blown BD. DSM-IV contains a requirement that the symptom intensity or frequency is such that it interferes with functioning or relationships. Many people known for their sustained, optimistic, energetic, and sometimes driven approaches to life would technically qualify as having CyD if this requirement were not present.

The following subsections consider specific types of episodes in BD.

A. Depressive Episodes

As Chapter 18 noted, the clinical features of a **depressive episode** (see Table 18.1) are the same in the DSM-IV for both MDD and BD, even though many clinicians recognize differentiating characteristics. Among characteristics of BD are earlier age at onset, shorter episode duration, and a greater likelihood of hypersomnia, rather than the reduced sleep and early morning awakening common to MDD depressive episodes. As is discussed below, treatment response also differs; **lithium** is more effective in BD depressive episodes than it is in MDD depressive episodes. Depressive episodes of BD most commonly begin in the fall or winter. Most serious postpartum depressions turn out to be episodes of BD.

An important finding from a cohort study conducted in Pittsburgh was a suicide attempt rate of 46.3% during depressive episodes in patients with BD; the comparable rate for patients with manic episodes was 13.4%.

B. Manic Episodes

Table 19.1 lists the clinical features of a **manic episode**. Manic episodes vary considerably in their intensity both within the same patient over time and among patients. Onset may be rapid and acute (hours to days) or subacute (over a few weeks), and episodes commonly begin in the spring. The durations are also variable; at least 1 week is required by current convention. Before effective therapies were available, some patients had episodes lasting 4 to 13 months, and for approximately four discrete manic episodes to occur within a decade was not unusual. Some episodes appear to occur in re-

---

TABLE 19.1. DIAGNOSTIC FEATURES OF A MANIC EPISODE

At least three of the following symptoms must be present during an episode of elevated (e.g., excessively optimistic, cheerful, or joyous), expansive, or irritable[a] mood that is present persistently for at least 1 week. (*Note:* Less than 1 week is sufficient if hospitalization was necessary or if effective treatment was quickly initiated.) The mood alteration must be of sufficient severity to cause marked impairment of functioning or to elicit actions from others to control harm to self or others and it must not be secondary[b] to an underlying medical condition (e.g., multiple sclerosis), substance use (e.g., **cocaine**, amphetamines), or treatment (e.g., antidepressants, electroconvulsive therapy, corticosteroids).

*I*ncreased, subjectively experienced high levels of energy and goal-directed activity (either socially, at school or work, or sexually); psychomotor agitation

*R*acing thoughts, flight of ideas, or copious thoughts appear to be crowding out others

*I*ncreased and more rapid speech, more talkative than usual, or feeling pressure to keep talking

*S*leep need decreased (e.g., feels rested even after 2–3 hours of sleep)

*D*istractibility and impaired concentration (e.g., attention is easily shifted by seemingly irrelevant or unimportant external stimuli)

*O*verly involved in hedonistic (pleasurable) activities having a high potential for unwanted or painful outcomes (e.g., unrestrained, impulsive, extravagant, or irrational spending or business investments; sexual indiscretions)

*G*randiosity; inflated self-confidence, self-importance, or self-esteem

---

The author believes that treatment planning and response rates are not altered by the adoption of these additional requirements. Remembering these criteria may be facilitated by the mnemonic **IRIS DOG**.

[a] In *Diagnostic and Statistical Manual of Mental Disorders*, 4th edition, Text revision, (DSM-IV-TR), 4 symptoms are required when the mood disturbance is limited to irritability.

[b] In DSM-IV, when the mood disturbance appears to result solely from a medical condition, substance use, or a treatment, the appropriate diagnosis is "Bipolar Disorder, not otherwise specified."

From the American Psychiatric Association. *Diagnostic and statistical manual of mental disorders*, 4th ed. Text revision. Washington, D.C.: American Psychiatric Association, 2000, with permission.

sponse to external stressors (e.g., the loss of a significant person in one's life); others seem to develop spontaneously.

Up to 50% of acute manic episodes involve some psychotic features. Some data suggest that the earlier the onset of BD, the greater the likelihood is of psychotic features during the course of the disorder. For example, both mood-congruent (e.g., "I am the Messiah") and mood-incongruent (e.g., "God made me strike him") delusions and behaviors may occur. The distinction between congruence and incongruence is often difficult to establish in mania; the idea that God was behind an action, which is a delusion of being controlled, may reflect a sense of being singled out (i.e., exaggerated self-importance). A patient with schizophrenia or MDD with psychosis who says the same thing probably does not feel special in a positive or grandiose sense to God.

Humor is often noted during manic episodes. It is frequently contagious, but it may be caustic or hostile. Manic patients are frequently intrusive, frenetic, or labile in mood. Some are violent; violence is generally seen only during periods of extreme and untreated symptomatology or when the individual misinterprets the intentions of others in a crowded, noisy, or otherwise overstimulating environment.

C. Hypomanic Episodes

Table 19.2 lists the clinical features of a **hypomanic episode**. Although the intensity of the elevated or irritable mood during a hypomanic episode is by definition less extreme than it is in mania, more lability and volatility may be seen, perhaps as a consequence. Some clinicians believe that patients are more likely to attempt suicide, for example, when they are hypomanic rather than when they are manic. Efforts to initiate any therapeutic intervention during an episode of hypomania are likely to be unsuccessful.

TABLE 19.2. DIAGNOSTIC FEATURES OF A HYPOMANIC EPISODE

At least three of the following symptoms must be present during an episode of elevated (e.g., excessively optimistic, cheerful, or joyous), expansive, or irritable[a] mood that is present persistently for at least 4 days and that is distinctly different from one's characteristic nondepressed mood. The mood alteration (a) must be reflected in an unequivocal change in functioning that is not severe enough to cause marked impairment of functioning or hospitalization; (b) must be readily apparent to others; and (c) must not be secondary to an underlying medical condition (e.g., multiple sclerosis), substance use (e.g., **cocaine**, amphetamines), or treatment (e.g., antidepressants, electroconvulsive therapy, corticosteroids).

More rapid speech, more talkative than usual, or feels pressure to keep talking
Inflated self-confidence or self-esteem, grandiosity, or excessive self-importance
Decreased sleep (e.g., feels rested even after 2–3 hours of sleep)
Flight of ideas, feels subjectively that thoughts are racing, or copious thoughts appear to be crowding out others
Activity is increased and goal-directed (either socially, at school or work, or sexually), subjectively experienced high energy level, or psychomotor agitation
Distractibility (e.g., attention is too easily shifted to seemingly irrelevant or unimportant external stimuli)
Excessive involvement in pleasurable (hedonistic) activities having a high potential for unwanted or painful consequences (e.g., unrestrained, impulsive, extravagant, or irrational spending or business investments; sexual indiscretions)

The author believes that treatment planning and response rates are not altered by the adoption of this additional requirement. Remembering these criteria may be facilitated by the mnemonic **MID FADE**.

[a]In *Diagnostic and Statistical Manual of Mental Disorders*, 4th edition, four symptoms are required when the mood disturbance is limited to irritability.

From the American Psychiatric Association. *Diagnostic and statistical manual of mental disorders*, 4th ed. Text revision. Washington, D.C.: American Psychiatric Association, 2000, with permission.

Most patients like their hypomanic phases (e.g., they enjoy their sense of freedom or their increased productivity or creativity), and their behavior is rarely disruptive enough for others to become involved in trying to bring about treatment.

D. Rapid-Cycling Mania

DSM-IV offers a course-specifying option **"with rapid cycling"** for patients having more than three episodes of mood cycling within a year. This modifier can be applied to both bipolar I and bipolar II patients. As the phrase is used in the DSM-IV, "with rapid cycling" then refers solely to the course and frequency and not to the severity of the moods. Up to 20% of BD patients exhibit rapid cycling; frequency estimates depend in part on whether duration criteria for manic, hypomanic, or depressive episodes are required or whether CyD patients are included. Patients who cycle rapidly probably do not represent a homogeneous subgroup. Some patients have frequent episodes from the very beginning; others cycle more rapidly only after many years of untreated cycling. In at least some patients, antidepressant therapy or the use of psychostimulants may also possibly be a contributing factor.

E. Mixed Mania and Dysphoric Mania

In the DSM-IV, one subcategory under bipolar I disorder is **"with most recent episode mixed."** This refers to patients who meet criteria for both manic and depressive episodes at some time during the day for at least 7 consecutive days. Many clinicians view the diagnosis of mixed mania as overlapping considerably with the unofficial diagnosis of **dysphoric mania**. One literature review of patients with these diagnoses suggests that dysphoric mania appears in about one-third of BD patients, that a mixed symptom presentation is not limited to any specific stage of BD, and that both shorter and longer term outcomes are less optimistic than they are for unmixed episodes.

II. Genetic, Epidemiologic, Course, and Other Considerations

BD represents about one-fifth of all mood disorders; most patients have their first full episode between 15 and 24 years of age. The Pittsburgh cohort study of 2,308 patients with BD found the mean age at onset to be 19.8 years (median, 17.5 years), a figure close to the commonly stated age of 21 years. The mean age at onset for MDD is about 27 years. The ratio of women to men is approximately equal, although some studies suggest that BD is slightly more common in women. These observations are in contrast to the ratio of 2 or 3 to 1 for women to men in MDD. When BD appears for the first time in a patient over the age of 60, it is likely to be secondary to an eventually identifiable medical condition (e.g., a lesion in the right temporal lobe). Lifetime prevalence rates for BD are estimated at 1.2%; the corresponding figure for MDD is 4.4%. Cross-national data yield lifetime prevalence rates of 0.6% to 3.3% for BD. Some data suggest that the lifetime prevalence rate for bipolar I disorder is slightly higher than that for bipolar II disorder (i.e., 0.8% vs. 0.5%). The 1-year prevalence rate for manic or hypomanic episodes is estimated to be 3.0%.

Twin studies support a genetic vulnerability or predisposition to BD. No single genetic model is accepted; a multifactorial polygenetic model seems most likely. Concordance rates for BD in monozygotic twins are 65% to 80%, whereas the rates in dizygotic twins are approximately 20%. Family studies also suggest that BD is familial; BD is more common among the first-degree relatives of BD patients than it is among control subjects, but MDD is even more common among these same relatives. Adoption studies are not conclusive. The Pittsburgh cohort study found BD in 54% of family members of patients with BD, whereas 52.1% had relatives with MDD. Some authorities believe that a 2-threshold genetic model is needed to characterize the relationship between MDD and BD.

As is noted above, most serious postpartum depressive and psychotic disturbances are episodes of BD. The risk of a postpartum episode is about 1 per 1,000 deliveries. Infanticide occurs during 3% to 4% of these episodes. Postpartum BD episodes generally respond well to standard interventions, such as **lithium**, mood-stabilizing anticonvulsants, antipsychotic agents, and ECT.

It is not uncommon for a period of 3 to 5 years of euthymic functioning to occur between the first and second episodes of BD. This interval usually shortens over time. Concomitant problems with substance misuse or abuse are common in bipolar I patients in the United States.

III. General Treatment Considerations

Most BD patients are treated on an outpatient basis. To accomplish this successfully, involvement of key relatives or reliable and responsible friends is often necessary. Because most BD patients enjoy their highs, they cannot be counted on to seek treatment when their symptomatology begins to escalate. Family members or significant others need to understand the nature and course of BD and its treatment. Anticipating potentially disastrous outcomes and having contingency plans in place whenever possible are essential. For example, if overspending is characteristic of the episodes, limits may need to be placed on bank accounts or credit cards. If hospitalization may be required, a plan for getting the patient to the hospital must already be formulated, because the patient's cooperation is unlikely if he or she has become overexcited and hostile or suicidal. During a manic episode, most patients have little or no insight into either their condition or their negative effects on others; manic denial is almost invariable.

For those patients with access to and an interest in psychotherapy, benefit can be achieved through a cognitive-behavioral approach that pays attention to issues, such as adherence, denial, autonomy or dependency, impact on significant others, and real or symbolic losses. For some, a psychoeducational component that ascertains patients' beliefs about their disorder and that provides clarifications and information about the nature, course, and genetic transmission of BD can be helpful. Family therapy should also include a psychoeducational component, strategies to promote adherence, methods of relapse prevention, and attention to eliciting early signs of pending decompensations. Psychotherapies may be particularly helpful for those BD patients who have episodes that seem to be precipitated by external stresses or that include behaviors that are disruptive to the family. Friends can serve as an early warning system when arrangements have been made in advance. They can also be helpful with regard to issues of treatment and medication compliance.

Hospitalization is often required for patients in the advanced stages of a manic episode. Reducing external stimulation through the use of quiet rooms or even seclusion rooms (see Chapter 25) can be extremely beneficial, particularly in the hours before medications become effective. Physical restraints (see Chapter 26) at times may be indicated to protect the patient from self-injury or from harming others. In implementing these, involving only trained staff and following all guidelines and regulations regarding the use of restraints and seclusion are essential.

IV. Psychopharmacologic Treatments

Although **lithium** carbonate is the mainstay of the treatment of BD for many, but not all, clinicians, it is not often the best approach to treating an acute manic episode. Although **lithium** treatment may be initiated, it may not be effective during the acute or dysphoric manic episodes or symptoms, or the symptoms may be too extreme to be able to wait for **lithium** to take effect. Beginning concomitant use of an antipsychotic agent (e.g., **olanzapine**, **haloperidol**, **mesoridazine**) or a benzodiazepine (e.g., **clonazepam**, **lorazepam**) is often necessary to achieve a more prompt response. Parenteral forms of these five agents are available. Loading doses of **valproate** are also an option.

When antidepressants are necessary during depressive episodes, a variety of different antidepressants can be added; some antidepressants, like the selective serotonin reuptake inhibitors (SSRIs) and **bupropion**, are thought to cause fewer switches into mania than do others, such as **imipramine** and monamine oxidase inhibitors. Among the currently marketed antidepressants, **imipramine** is associated with more switches into mania than other agents are. Monamine oxidase inhibitors tend to do this somewhat less frequently, and these are considered by some clinicians to be especially useful in the treatment of depressive episodes in

BD. Short-term treatment is not recommended. Relapses within 12 months are to be expected.

For rapid-cycling patients or those with mixed or dysphoric mania, mood-stabilizing anticonvulsants or **clozapine** may be preferable to **lithium**. These agents are considered in the following sections.

A. Lithium Salts

Curiously, in 1949, the year Cade reported on the specific value of **lithium carbonate** in the treatment of mania, the *Journal of the American Medical Association* published several articles on severe and sometimes fatal **lithium** poisoning from the use of **lithium chloride** as a table salt substitute. Fortunately, the significance of Cade's work was recognized by Schou in Denmark. He and his colleagues undertook the further development of **lithium carbonate** as the earliest cornerstone in the treatment of manic-depressive illness. Their work contributed to its eventual marketing in the United States in 1970 for the treatment of acute mania and to its expanded indication in 1974 for prophylaxis against recurrences of mania. (*Note:* United States Food and Drug Administration (FDA)-approved indications for **lithium** salts do not mention depressive episodes.)

The exact mechanisms of **lithium's** actions in BD are not known. It is a ubiquitous agent that has such diverse effects as (a) altering sodium transport; (b) modest but consistent proserotonergic properties, including sensitization of postsynaptic hippocampal CA_3 receptors; (c) augmentation of acetylcholine synthesis and tone in the cortex; (d) reduction of presynaptic (exocytotic) release of norepinephrine and dopamine, perhaps by increasing intraneuronal metabolism of catecholamines; (e) attenuation of circadian rhythms; (f) actions on G-protein–coupled second-messenger systems; and (g) reduction of phosphoinositol turnover through the inhibition of the phosphatase that generates inositol from inositol phosphate.

1. **Preparations, pharmacokinetics, and dosing**. Lithium carbonate is rapidly absorbed from the gastrointestinal tract, and it reaches peak concentrations in 1 to 6 hours. Absorption is generally complete within 8 hours. **Lithium citrate**, a formulation that is not always readily available, is absorbed even more rapidly. **Lithium** concentrates in saliva, the thyroid gland, and bone. It may remain in the bone for years. Although measuring red blood cell concentrations of **lithium** is by no means routine, these intracellular levels may correlate better with **lithium's** effects than do serum concentrations. Three percent to 5% of **lithium** is eliminated in sweat; this irritates the skin of some patients, which may be particularly problematic for patients with psoriasis.

Based on the pharmacokinetics of immediate release forms of **lithium**, twice-daily dosing has been its traditional pattern of use. However, clinical use data suggest that renal complications are reduced by using single bedtime doses, particularly when higher range dosing is required. Compliance is also improved by implementing this bedtime regimen. Some clinicians prefer sustained-release preparations. In this author's experience, the latter reduce the appearance of gastrointestinal complaints and tremor by reducing peak concentrations; however, their use prolongs the kidney's exposure to the drug. The author prefers sustained-release preparations only for patients requiring 450 to 900 mg of **lithium** per day.

Table 19.3 describes the brand names, dosage strengths, and forms of **lithium carbonate** and **lithium citrate** currently available in the United States. Considerable variability has been observed in serum concentrations produced by various generic preparations; this probably reflects variations in particle size and excipients.

2. **Monitoring**. Until the patient is stabilized, a flexible approach to the frequency of determining serum **lithium** concentrations, such as one that is responsive to the patient's need for dosage adjustments (e.g., the degree of clinical improvement; the presence of side effects; risk situations, such as diarrhea and vomiting), seems appropriate. Once stabilization is achieved,

TABLE 19.3. SOME FORMS AND BRAND NAMES OF LITHIUM

Lithium carbonate[a]
Lithium citrate[b]
Lithotabs
Lithonate[c]
Eskalith
Lithobid[d]
Eskalith CR[e]

---

[a]Generic forms available in 300 mg uncoated tablets; 150 mg, 300 mg, or 600 mg gelatin capsules; and 125 or 500 mg as powder. The molecular weight of lithium is 73.89 g/mol.
[b]Generic syrups available as well; 8 mEq of lithium per 5 mL is equivalent to 300 mg of carbonate.
[c]Capsules (300 mg).
[d]Sustained-release tablets (300 mg).
[e]Sustained-release tablets (450 mg).

intervals of up to 3 months can be considered. Considerable interindividual variation in effective serum concentrations for **lithium** are seen. The range for most patients during an episode is 0.3 to 1.2 mEq per L. The lower part of this range may be adequate for many elderly patients and for some stabilized patients. For patients who respond at low **lithium** concentrations (e.g., 0.3 to 0.5 mEq per L), monitoring intervals of 6 to 12 months are sometimes appropriate. For patients requiring sustained concentrations above 1.2 mEq per L, chart documentation should include an indication that the treating clinician is aware that these are higher than typical levels and should provide the reasoning behind using such levels. Obtaining a consultation from an experienced psychopharmacologist may be prudent.

Once pre-**lithium** baseline levels have been established for the following parameters, thyroid functioning (thyroid-stimulating hormone and thyroxine levels, antithyroid antibodies) and renal functioning (e.g., blood urea nitrogen and creatinine levels) should be monitored at least yearly; more frequent monitoring may be indicated depending on the values obtained or the patient's clinical condition. Some physicians believe that a yearly assessment of creatinine clearance is appropriate.

3. **Discontinuation**. Most patients who respond to **lithium** tolerate its chronic use (i.e., continuous use for decades) once their individual dosage needs have been established. In patients with recurrent episodes, **lithium** discontinuation typically (i.e., about 50% of the time) results in the reappearance of symptoms within 6 months. When **lithium** is discontinued after many years for whatever reason and symptoms recur, it has been observed that some patients may not benefit from reexposure to **lithium** to the same degree as they did during their earlier treatment with it. These patients may even become less responsive to any other currently available therapies. This lack of effectiveness and possible refractoriness has led some authorities on **lithium** use to recommend that it not be discontinued in patients who benefit from and are well maintained on continuous **lithium** treatment. For this reason the author does not recommend **lithium** "holidays." Discontinuation during pregnancy is generally advocated, even though many apparently healthy children have been born to women taking **lithium**. (*Note:* Although associated with maternal first trimester use of **lithium**, Ebstein anomaly, a tricuspid valve malformation, is probably less common than was previously thought. Data also suggest that, in children identified as having this problem, **lithium** exposure was not a major risk factor.)

The "off-label" use of **lithium** to modify premenstrual mood lability and irritability is sometimes successful. Because some SSRIs have premenstrual dysphoric disorder as an approved indication, it may be prudent to try an SSRI alone first, before **lithium** is used adjunctively or by itself. Dosing is usually 300 to 600 mg per day (typically at bedtime) for 10 days before the onset of menstruation. This intermittent usage pattern has not yet been shown to cause treatment refractoriness in premenstrual dysphoric disorder patients.

4. **Side effects and toxicity.** Some of **lithium's** more common side effects are nausea, loose stools or diarrhea, thirst, polyuria, metallic taste, headache, and tremor; the latter is responsive to **propranolol** (20 to 80 mg per day; **atenolol** at 25 to 50 mg per day is an alternative). Some patients also complain of cognitive dulling. Most of **lithium's** side effects can be ameliorated by dosage reduction. Because most of **lithium's** minor side effects are associated with its peak levels, taking the drug after meals or at bedtime or using sustained-release preparations may improve its tolerability. **Lithium citrate** use is associated with fewer unwanted gastrointestinal effects.

Hypothyroidism is found in 5% to 30% of **lithium**-treated patients after 6 to 18 months of continuous use. It appears to occur more frequently in women and in rapid-cycling patients. In patients with Hashimoto thyroiditis, **lithium** may aggravate or cause hypothyroidism. The author regularly screens patients for antithyroid antibodies to identify patients with subclinical Hashimoto thyroiditis.

When **lithium** reaches toxic concentrations, confusion, restlessness, lethargy, and slurred speech are frequently seen. Stupor and coma may follow. The elderly are particularly susceptible to **lithium** toxicity. The treatment of **lithium** toxicity and overdosage is considered in Chapter 3.

Chronic use of **lithium** is sometimes associated with neurotoxicity. Acute overdosage is a more infrequent cause. Risk factors for neurotoxicity during chronic **lithium** administration include diabetes insipidus, thyroid dysfunction, impaired renal function, and advanced age. Agents that impair **lithium** clearance (e.g., **aspirin**) may also contribute to neurotoxicity.

5. **Drug interactions.** Only two interactions will be considered in this section; Chapter 29 reviews some of **lithium's** important interactions with other drugs. In treatment-resistant depressions, SSRIs are not infrequently combined with **lithium**; some patients have been reported to show signs of a toxic serotonin syndrome from this combination (see Chapter 3). Of greater concern is the interaction between **lithium** and the thiazide diuretics (e.g., **hydrochlorothiazide**). This combination can lead to decreased renal clearance of **lithium** and increases in serum levels that, if they are high enough, may cause **lithium** toxicity. **Potassium**-sparing diuretics (e.g., **amiloride**, **triamterene**) are usually safer to use when these agents need to be prescribed together. The safety of loop diuretics (e.g., **furosemide**) and carbonic anhydrase inhibitors (e.g., **acetazolamide**) with **lithium** is ambiguous because contradictory observations have appeared in the literature. A **potassium**-sparing diuretic alone or in combination with a thiazide diuretic is sometimes added to **lithium** to reduce **lithium**-induced polyuria or nephrogenic diabetes insipidus. Another option is switching to a mood-stabilizing anticonvulsant.

B. **Mood-Stabilizing Anticonvulsant Agents**

The discussion of these agents also covers selected benzodiazepines.

1. **Valproate.** A **divalproex sodium** delayed release tablet formulation has FDA approval for the treatment of mania associated with BD. An extended release version (500 mg) that is currently approved for use in migraine headaches is used by some clinicians to support adherence. A carboxylic acid derivative, **valproate** enhances γ-aminobutyric acid (GABA) activity, increases **potassium** conductance, and appears to block N-methyl-D-aspartate receptor-mediated (i.e., calcium channel) depolarization. Cross-tolerance between **valproate** and **carbamazepine** is seen

on amygdala-kindled seizures, even though **valproate** has little affinity for peripheral-type benzodiazepine receptors. Some data suggest that **valproate** may desensitize GABA autoreceptors. How these and other actions of **valproate** contribute to its antimanic effects is not known.

Valproate is reasonably effective in acute mania, and it sustains its antimanic effectiveness during chronic administration. **Valproate** also appears to work well in rapid-cycling patients and in patients with mixed or dysphoric mania. Table 19.4 lists the forms of **valproate** currently marketed in the United States. Concentration-response relationships for **valproate** are not strong; a range of 50 to 125 µg per mL is often cited for the serum concentration of **valproic acid**. Starting doses depend on the severity, and they can range from 500 to 1,500 mg per day (divided doses). Longer term use is typically in the range of 1,000 to 2,000 mg per day. For acutely manic patients, some clinicians advocate beginning with a loading dose of 30 mg per kg per day and decreasing to 20 mg per kg per day once improvement is noted.

Common side effects include nausea, anorexia, and other gastrointestinal effects; sedation; propranolol-responsive tremor; and ataxia. The enteric-coated **divalproex sodium** formulation is preferred by many clinicians because it may produce fewer gastrointestinal side effects. Reversible asymptomatic liver transaminase elevation is not uncommon; rare cases of idiosyncratic hepatic toxicity have been fatal. Increased appetite and accelerated hair loss are seen in some patients; some data suggest that concomitant daily use of a multivitamin preparation containing **selenium** and **zinc** may be beneficial. Acute pancreatitis can occur; the development of polycystic ovaries has also been noted.

Some clinicians choose **valproate** formulations instead of **carbamazepine** because **valproate** use is associated with fewer drug interactions.

2. **Carbamazepine.** This agent, an iminostilbene, resembles tricyclic antidepressants in its structure but it has a carbamyl side chain that conveys anticonvulsant effects. These appear to be mediated at least in part through its GABA-linked calcium channel blocking at the so-called peripheral or

TABLE 19.4. VALPROATE PREPARATIONS

Brand Name, Form (Strengths)	Preparation	Time to Peak Serum Concentration (h)[a]
Depakene, capsules (250 mg)	Valproic acid	1–2
Depakene, syrup (250 mg/5 mL)	Sodium valproate	1–2
Depakote, delayed-release tablets (125, 250, 500 mg)[b]	Divalproex sodium	3–8
Depakote, sprinkle capsules (125 mg)	Divalproex sodium coated particles in capsules	[c]
Depakote ER, extended release[d] (500 mg)	Divalproex sodium	—
Depacon, injectable (100 mg/mL i.v. use)	Sodium valproate	—

Abbreviation: i.v., intravenous.
[a]Measured in serum as valproic acid.
[b]This is the only formulation specifically marketed for the treatment of manic symptoms in bipolar disorder.
[c]Compared with divalproex sodium tablets, sprinkle capsules have earlier onset and slower rate of absorption, with slightly lower peak serum concentrations.
[d]Marketed for migraine headache prophylaxis.

$GABA_B$-benzodiazepine receptor and via its α_2-adrenergic receptor agonist properties (see section IV.D.1), as well as by way of its membrane-stabilizing effects. **Carbamazepine** appears to act preferentially in limbic brain areas. Although its mood-stabilizing and antimanic properties are not FDA approved, **carbamazepine** use in BD is somewhat common, especially as a prophylactic agent for **lithium** nonresponders and in rapid-cycling patients. **Carbamazepine** is sometimes used concurrently with **lithium** and other agents. Onset of action is variable, and it may take from 3 to 15 days.

Although a concentration-response range has not been established for the use of **carbamazepine** in BD, plasma levels in the range of 4 to 12 μg per mL appear to be appropriate for many patients. These levels are typically achieved with dosages between 100 and 1,600 mg per day; this wide and variable range reflects **carbamazepine's** nonlinear kinetics (i.e., induction of its own oxidative metabolism). Orally administered, **carbamazepine** is slowly absorbed, and it has poor water solubility. **Carbamazepine** use is not infrequently associated with benign neutropenia; very rare and sometimes fatal cases of agranulocytosis and aplastic anemia have occurred. Earlier concerns about its hematopoietic toxicity arose when it was coprescribed with other antiepileptic agents. Therefore, regular monitoring of both plasma levels and complete blood counts is recommended. **Carbamazepine's** most common unwanted effects include ataxia, headache, lightheadedness, rash, and sedation.

Carbamazepine is an inducer of cytochrome P-450 (CYP) 2D6 (see Chapter 29) hepatic microsomal enzymes (e.g., it will probably lower levels of **haloperidol**), but the principal pathway (CYP 3A4) in its own metabolism is likely inhibited by CYP 3A family-metabolized drugs, such as **verapamil, ritonavir, ketoconazole, erythromycin,** or **nefazodone**. Its major active metabolite is a 10,11-epoxide; increased amounts of this metabolite contribute significantly to **carbamazepine's** toxicity. Increased levels of this metabolite occur, for example, with coadministration of **phenobarbital** (i.e., from enzyme induction). **Valproate**, by inhibiting an epoxide hydroxylase, also increases the levels of this **carbamazepine** metabolite.

   3. **Other anticonvulsants**. Modest support is found for the use of two additional agents in BD. **Lamotrigine**, which shares some mechanisms of action with **carbamazepine** (e.g., blockade of neuronal sodium channels, decreased release of excitatory amino acids), can be of benefit for the depressed phase in some patients with BD. Its antidepressant effects are more consistent than its antimanic effects. **Topiramate** appears to have a degree of antimanic effects, and it may reduce cycle frequency. **Topiramate** blocks AMPA glutamate receptors, and it is a carbonic anhydrase inhibitor; this latter property may contribute to the formation of renal calculi. The bulk of present evidence does not support benefits from the use of **gabapentin** in BD; dosage could be a factor.
   4. **Clonazepam and lorazepam**. Although all benzodiazepines are $GABA_A$ agonists and have sedative and anticonvulsant properties, **clonazepam** and **lorazepam** enjoy greater popularity in the treatment of manic symptomatology. Both are relatively free from drug interactions other than potentiated sedation, and neither has active metabolites. Benzodiazepines are often preferred for the treatment of secondary mania (i.e., from medical conditions, medications, or abusable substances) and for patients who develop extrapyramidal side effects from the use of antipsychotic agents. **Clonazepam's** half-life $(t_{1/2}\beta)$ (18 to 50 hours) and duration of action are somewhat longer than those of **lorazepam** $(t_{1/2}\beta = 8$ to 24 hours). **Clonazepam** reaches **peak blood levels** somewhat faster than **lorazepam** (1 to 2 vs. 1 to 6 hours). Oral dosage ranges for **clonazepam** and **lorazepam** are 1.5 to 20 and 2 to 10 mg per day, respectively. Both agents act more rapidly than **lithium** does, and they are sometimes combined with **lithium** or other antimanic

agents. **Lorazepam** is also used intramuscularly (1 to 5 mg every 2 hours), either alone or in combination with **haloperidol** (1 to 5 mg). The most common side effect of **lorazepam** or **clonazepam** is **sedation**; because of its longer duration of action, **clonazepam** use is more likely to be associated with unwanted daytime drowsiness. Anterograde memory impairment is not uncommon from both agents at the higher dosage ranges that are used to treat manic excitement (see Chapter 14).

C. Antipsychotic Agents

1. **Olanzapine and haloperidol.** All classes of antipsychotic agents have been used in acute mania; their efficacy is thought to be related to their dopamine-2 receptor antagonism.

   Olanzapine has specific FDA approval for use in acute manic episodes associated with BD. Initial dosing is usually in the range of 5 to 15 mg per day (maximum recommended dose of 20 mg per day). Short-term use (i.e., up to 3 to 4 weeks) is generally recommended. **Olanzapine's** clearance is increased by activities (e.g., cigarette smoking) or agents (e.g., **omeprazole**) that induce CYP 1A2. A tablet that dissolves in the mouth without additional fluids is also available (**Zydis**). Either can be used with **lithium** to treat the patient before **lithium** becomes effective.

   Although **haloperidol** is not FDA approved for this use, it is used in some settings for the treatment of manic symptomatology. **Haloperidol** is given either orally or intramuscularly (2 to 40 mg per day), and it has a half-life of about 18 hours. Intramuscular **haloperidol** dosing (1 to 5 mg every 2 to 6 hours) is sometimes used with **lithium**. **Haloperidol** is sometimes combined with **lorazepam** when greater sedation is required. Extrapyramidal side effects are problematic with **haloperidol** (see also Chapter 20). The markedly reduced likelihood of extrapyramidal side effects associated with **olanzapine**, its FDA approval for the short-term treatment of acute manic episodes associated with BD, and its availability in oral (10 to 20 mg per day) and intramuscular (2.5 to 15 mg per day) forms are key factors in its increasing usage. Drowsiness and weight gain are more common with **olanzapine** than they are with **haloperidol**.

2. **Mesoridazine.** **Mesoridazine** (75 to 300 mg per day) is an option used by some clinicians; it is also the principal active product of **thioridazine** metabolism. In contrast to **thioridazine**, **mesoridazine** can also be given intramuscularly (12.5 to 50 mg every 6 hours). Its half-life is highly variable, ranging from 1 to 3 days. As with **haloperidol** and **olanzapine**, **mesoridazine** is often combined with **lithium** in the initial days of treatment. Extrapyramidal side effects are rare, and the pigmentary retinopathy observed with high-dose **thioridazine** is not reported with comparable doses of **mesoridazine**; **mesoridazine** is twice as potent as **thioridazine**. Prolongation of the cardiac QT interval and an associated risk for ventricular tachyarrhythmias limit the value of both **thioridazine** and **mesoridazine** in current practice.

3. **Risperidone.** This agent has also been reported to be useful for the treatment of acute manic symptomatology in BD patients, and many clinicians suggest its use. Unfortunately, adequate trials have not yet been published.

4. **Pimozide.** **Pimozide** (2 to 20 mg per day) is an unusual antipsychotic agent that also has calcium channel blocking properties. Some clinicians, particularly in Europe, have found it useful for treating acute mania; this is not an FDA-approved indication. Sedation and anticholinergic side effects are common, and dose-dependent prolongation of the QTc interval and other electrocardiographic changes should be expected. Cardiac arrhythmias that have included rare instances of fatal tachydysrhythmias have been reported. Pretreatment and follow-up electrocardiograms are essential to good patient care; these may be difficult to obtain in the acutely manic patient. Because a warning about associated hepatic injury was added to **pimozide's** product labeling,

pimozide use in BP is now rare. **Pimozide** reaches peak blood levels slowly, and it has a long elimination half-life of 1.5 to 2.5 days (see also Chapters 4 and 7).

5. **Clozapine**. This atypical antipsychotic agent has shown effectiveness, typically in the range of 250 to 800 mg per day, in case and small series reports describing the treatment of patients with dysphoric mania (*note:* this is not an FDA-approved indication). It has a relatively short half-life that averages about 8 hours. Some patients do well on **clozapine** alone, whereas others require concomitant medications (e.g., **valproate, lithium**). Close monitoring for granulocytopenia is essential; this need is magnified when combination therapies are used because many of the possible adjunctive agents have their own effects on the hematopoietic system (see also Chapter 20).

D. **Cardiovascular Agents with Mood-Stabilizing Properties**
1. **Clonidine**. This α_2-adrenergic receptor partial agonist is sometimes helpful in manic patients through its reduction of central sympathetic outflow (*note:* this is not an FDA-approved indication for its use) (see also Chapter 10). It also has peripheral presynaptic α_2-adrenergic agonist activity, and clonidine lowers blood pressure by reducing norepinephrine release. It is rapidly absorbed orally, and it quickly reaches adequate central nervous system concentrations. The dosage range is 0.2 to 1.2 mg per day. At higher doses, decreases in blood pressure are observed. In addition to hypotension, dry mouth and drowsiness are common unwanted effects. Any depressive symptoms that are present may worsen with its use. **Clonidine** should be used only when standard approaches have failed; close monitoring of the patient is essential.

2. **Calcium channel blocking agents**. Verapamil (240 to 400 mg per day) and **diltiazem** (150 to 300 mg per day) may have some effectiveness in reducing manic symptomatology (*note:* these are not FDA-approved indications for their use). Supporting their possible usefulness is the observation that cerebrospinal fluid levels of calcium are low during manic episodes and high during depressive episodes. **Verapamil** has weak anticonvulsant properties, and both agents increase synaptic calcium levels. Neither is a first-line treatment for mania; their use should be considered only when standard treatments have not been effective. **Verapamil** use has been associated with increased depression and anxiety in some patients.

V. **Electroconvulsive Therapy**
ECT is discussed in Chapter 24. Although most clinicians and patients prefer pharmacotherapies, considerable data exists that supports the greater efficacy of ECT as compared with **lithium** in the earliest days of severely manic decompensations. Chapter 24 notes the possibly unique role for ECT as a comparatively safe and effective treatment for BD episodes during pregnancy.

VI. **Comment**
Patients with bipolar I disorders are somewhat less prevalent than those with some of the other major mental disorders; their impact, however, is far from inconsequential. On the positive side, many of these patients are exceptionally creative and energetic, and they have made singular contributions to society in areas such as the arts, politics, sciences, and business. On the negative side, the costs to society of squandered talents and dollars, lost days from work, family disruptions, suicides, hospitalizations, and the like from the large numbers of untreated patients are enormous. No more than one-fourth of these patients receive adequate treatment at the present time. Much work has to be done to find ways to engage these patients in treatment and to improve their compliance. More consistently effective and safer agents are also needed. Finally, the roles of kindling phenomena and sensitization—the effects of untreated or inadequately treated episodes or discontinuations of treatment on subsequent episode severity, frequency and duration, and treatment refractoriness—must be better understood.

VII. Treatment Algorithms

Appendix VII contains useful information about algorithms for BD.

ADDITIONAL READING

Anand A, Verhoeff P, Seneca N, et al. Brain SPECT imaging of amphetamine-induced dopamine release in euthymic bipolar patients. *Am J Psychiatry* 2000;157:1108–1114.

Appelbaum PS, Shader RI, Funkenstein HH, et al. Difficulties in the diagnosis of lithium toxicity. *Am J Psychiatry* 1979;136:1212–1213.

Baastrup PC. The use of lithium in manic-depressive psychosis. *Compr Psychiatry* 1964;5:396–408.

Baastrup PC, Schou M. Lithium as a prophylactic agent: its effects against recurrent depression and manic-depressive psychosis. *Arch Gen Psychiatry* 1967;16:162–172.

Begley CE, Annegers JF, Swann AC, et al. The lifetime cost of bipolar disorder in the US. *Pharmacoeconomics* 2001;19:483–495.

Berk M, Ichim L, Brook S. Olanzapine compared to lithium: a double-blind randomized controlled trial. *Int Clin Psychopharmacol* 1999;14:339–343.

Bowden CI, Calabrese JR, McElroy SL, et al. A randomized placebo-controlled 12-month trial of divalproex and lithium in treatment of outpatients with bipolar disorder. *Arch Gen Psychiatry* 2000;57:481–489.

Cade JF. Lithium—past, present and future. In: Johnson FN, Johnson S, eds. *Lithium in medical practice*. Baltimore: University Park Press, 1978:5–16.

Cade JF. Lithium salts in the treatment of psychotic excitement. *Med J Australia* 1949;2:349–352.

Calabrese JR, Keck PE Jr, McElroy SL, et al. A pilot study of topiramate as monotherapy in the treatment of mania. *J Clin Psychopharmacol* 2001;21:340–342.

Calabrese JR, Markovitz PJ, Kimmel SE, et al. Spectrum of efficacy of valproate in 78 rapid-cycling bipolar patients. *J Clin Psychopharmacol* 1992;12:53S–56S.

Carlson GA, Bromet EJ, Sievers S. Phenomenology and outcome of subjects with early- and adult-onset psychotic mania. *Am J Psychiatry* 2000;157:213–219.

Chouinard G. Clonazepam in acute and maintenance treatment of bipolar affective disorder. *J Clin Psychiatry* 1987;48[Suppl]:29–36.

Clothier J, Swann AC, Freeman T. Dysphoric mania. *J Clin Psychopharmacol* 1992;12:13S–16S.

Colom F, Viete E, Martinez-Aran A, et al. Clinical factors associated with treatment noncompliance in euthymic bipolar patients. *J Clin Psychiatry* 2000;61:549–555.

Dunner DL. Mania. In: Tupin JP, Shader RI, Harnett DS, eds. *Handbook of clinical psychopharmacology*, 2nd ed. Northvale, NJ: Aronson, 1988:97–109.

Frye MA, Ketter TA, Kimbrall TA, et al. A placebo-controlled study of lamotrigine and gabapentin monotherapy in refractory mood disorders. *J Clin Psychopharmacol* 2000;20:607–614.

Gerner RH, Stanton A. Algorithm for patient management of acute manic states: lithium, valproate, or carbamazepine? *J Clin Psychopharmacol* 1992;12:57S–63S.

Goodwin FK, Jamison KF. *Manic-depressive illness*. New York: Oxford University Press, 1990.

Grunze H, Erfurth A, Amann B, et al. Intravenous valproate loading in acutely manic and depressed bipolar I patients. *J Clin Psychopharmacol* 1999;19:303–309.

Grunze HC, Normann C, Langosch J, et al. Antimanic efficacy of topiramate in 11 patients in an open trial with an on-off-on design. *J Clin Psychiatry* 2001;62:464–468.

Hurowitz GI, Liebowitz MR. Antidepressant-induced rapid cycling: six case reports. *J Clin Psychopharmacol* 1993;13:52–56.

Keck PE Jr, Strakowski SM, Hawkins JM, et al. A pilot study of rapid lithium administration in the treatment of acute mania. *Bipolar Disord* 2001;3:68–72.

Kupfer DJ, Frank E, Grochocinski VJ, et al. Demographic and clinical characteristics of individuals in a bipolar disorder case registry. *J Clin Psychiatry* 2002;63:120–125.

Leonhard K. *Aufteilung der Endogenen Psychosen*. Berlin: Akademie-Verlag, 1957.

Licht RW. Drug treatment of mania: a critical review. *Acta Psychiatr Scand* 1998;97:387–397.

Meehan K, Zhang F, David S, et al. A double-blind comparison of the efficacy of intramuscular injections of olanzapine, lorazepam, or placebo in treating acutely agitated patients diagnosed with bipolar mania. *J Clin Psychopharmacol* 2001;21:389–397.

Milkowitz D. Psychotherapy in combination with drug treatment for bipolar disorder. *J Clin Psychopharmacol* 1996;16:56S–66S.

Mitchell PB, Wilhelm K, Parker G, et al. The clinical features of bipolar depression: a comparison with major depressive disorder patients. *J Clin Psychiatry* 2001;62: 212–216.

Modell JG, Lenox RH, Weiner S. Inpatient clinical trial of lorazepam in the management of manic agitation. *J Clin Psychopharmacol* 1985;5:109–113.

Oakley PW, Whyte IM, Carter GL. Lithium toxicity: an iatrogenic problem in susceptible individuals. *Austr N Z J Psychiatry* 2001;35:833–840.

Pande A, Crockatt J, Janney C, et al. Gabapentin in bipolar disorder: a placebo-controlled trial of adjunctive therapy. *Bipolar Disord* 2000;2:249–255.

Post RM, Leverich GS, Altshuler L, et al. Lithium-discontinuation–induced refractoriness: preliminary observations. *Am J Psychiatry* 1992;149:1727–1729.

Sachs GS, Printz DJ, Kahn DA, et al. The expert consensus guideline series: medication treatment of bipolar disorder 2000. *Postgrad Med* 2000;Spec No:1–104.

Santos AB, Morton WA. More on clonazepam in manic agitation. *J Clin Psychopharmacol* 1987;7:439–440.

Schou M. Normothymics, "mood-normalizers": are lithium and the imipramine drugs specific for affective disorders? *Br J Psychiatry* 1964;109:803–809.

Segal J, Berk M, Brook S. Risperidone compared with both lithium and haloperidol in mania: a double-blind randomized controlled trial. *Clin Neuropharmacol* 1998;21: 176–180.

Shader RI, Jackson AH, Dodes LM. The antiaggressive effects of lithium in man. *Psychopharmacologia* 1974;40:17–24.

Small JG, Klapper MH, Kellams JJ, et al. Electroconvulsive treatment compared with lithium in the management of manic states. *Arch Gen Psychiatry* 1988;45:727–732.

Suppes T, McElroy SL, Gilbert J, et al. Clozapine in the treatment of dysphoric mania. *Biol Psychiatry* 1992;32:270–280.

Tohen M, Jacobs TG, Grundy SL, et al., for the Olanzapine HGGW Study Group. Efficacy of olanzapine in acute bipolar mania: a double-blind, placebo controlled study. *Arch Gen Psychiatry* 2000;57:841–849.

Tohen M, Zarate CA Jr. Antipsychotic agents and bipolar disorder. *J Clin Psychiatry* 1998;59:38–48.

Young RC, Biggs JT, Ziegler VE, et al. A rating scale for mania: reliability, validity and sensitivity. *Br J Psychiatry* 1978;133:429–435.

20. APPROACHES TO THE TREATMENT OF SCHIZOPHRENIA

Richard I. Shader

For more than 100 years, extensive efforts have been made to define or classify schizophrenia as an illness or group of illnesses. At the present time, a reasonable consensus about clinical phenomenology and descriptive diagnostic criteria has been reached, but the etiology and pathobiology remain obscure. Fortunately, most clinicians have little difficulty reaching diagnostic agreement about patients deemed to be suffering from schizophrenia; inevitably, though, some patients do appear for whom a diagnostic consensus is difficult to reach. These less easily categorized patients are sometimes given other diagnoses, including borderline or schizotypal personality disorder (see Chapter 13), delusional disorder (see Chapter 4), bipolar disorder (see Chapter 19), latent schizophrenia, pseudoneurotic or pseudopsychopathic schizophrenia, and even psychotic depression. The misguided tradition of categorizing schizophrenia as a **functional** illness prevailed for much of the 20th century and contributed to an underinvestment in research and to some continuing confusion about nosology and treatment. **Functional** suggests to many an exclusively interpersonal, social, or intrapsychic origin for this group of disorders. The sections that follow should make apparent the fact that schizophrenia represents a heterogeneous group of disorders with multiple etiologies linked to one or more forms of genetically based vulnerabilities and to some as yet unspecified environmental mishaps or trauma (e.g., inadequate nutrition during pregnancy from a local famine, exposure to influenza virus during gestation or perinatally).

I. Symptoms and Diagnostic Considerations

In 1896, Emil Kraepelin organized the observations of previous workers (e.g., Morel, Hecker, and Kahlbaum) and developed the concept of dementia praecox, which he saw as a peculiar pathologic condition of the internal connections of the personality that resulted in a disturbed emotional and volitional life. In 1911, Eugen Bleuler extended these efforts and offered the concept of a group of schizophrenias characterized by disturbances of thinking, feelings, and relationships to the external world. He isolated the following four fundamental diagnostic criteria, sometimes called The 4 "A"s: loosening of *a*ssociations, inappropriate *a*ffects, *a*utistic thoughts, and *a*mbivalence. These four features overlap to some extent with the following 6 "A"s that characterize the so-called **negative** symptoms of schizophrenia: *a*logia, *a*ffective blunting (flattening), *a*nhedonia, *a*sociality, *a*volition, and *a*pathy. Many clinicians consider these features, in the aggregate, to be the core impairments in schizophrenia and believe that they do not receive adequate emphasis in the current diagnostic schema, the *International Statistical Classification of Diseases and Related Health Problems,* tenth revision, (ICD-10) and the *Diagnostic and Statistical Manual of Mental Disorders,* 4th edition (DSM-IV). Some clinicians and researchers prefer to emphasize alterations in selective attention, information processing, or cue response (e.g., if the word "dog" had been misheard or misprocessed as "frog," "green" as an association would not be loose).

In the 1930s, Kurt Schneider elaborated a phenomenologic definition of the schizophrenias. He asserted the primacy of 11 empirically determined first-rank symptoms that he considered pathognomonic of schizophrenia. Some research has challenged their specificity to schizophrenia (e.g., some of these symptoms are not uncommon in bipolar disorder) and thereby their value in assessing prognosis. However, Schneider's approach is useful for organizing some of the disparate experiences patients report. As Table 20.1 illustrates, Schneider's symptoms are grouped into five broad categories. These symptoms are central to the so-called **positive** symptoms of schizophrenia.

In 1958, K. Conrad focused attention on the time course and differing stages of symptom appearance. Table 20.2 lists his notions about progressive stages.

TABLE 20.1. SCHNEIDER'S FIRST-RANK SYMPTOMS OF SCHIZOPHRENIA

Thought broadcasting—the sense that one's thoughts are escaping aloud from one's head

Experiences of alienation—the sense that one's thoughts, impulses, and actions are not one's own but that they come from an external source

Experiences of influence—the sense that one's thoughts, feelings, and actions are being imposed by some external force or agency to which one must passively submit

Delusional perceptions—the organization of real perceptions in a private way, often leading to fixed beliefs that are in conflict with reality

Auditory hallucinations—hearing clearly audible voices coming from outside one's head, commenting on one's actions or speaking one's thoughts; these voices must consist of more than one-word or two-word phrases, unintelligible mumbling sounds, whispers, or the like

From Schneider K. *Clinical psychopathology*. New York: Grune & Stratton, 1959, with permission.

Few patients actually articulate a progressive decompensation; nevertheless, this conceptualization may help the clinician appreciate the importance of course to the diagnosis of schizophrenia, as well as the existential distress that some patients experience in the early stages of illness.

Course, other historical data, and specific symptom requirements may help separate schizophrenia from toxic or other causes of schizophrenia-like presentations or from the affective psychoses. DSM-IV criteria for schizophrenia require the consideration of course variables in conjunction with particular positive or negative symptoms. A listing of some positive and negative symptoms seen in schizophrenia is provided in Table 20.3.

That the symptoms observed at any given point in time will depend on many factors, including when in the course of the illness a patient is seen, past or present treatments, and the type and prognosis of the patient's illness, should be apparent to the reader. Diagnosis also must take into account whether or not the patient is psychotic at the time of observation; the presence of other etiologic factors (e.g., toxic conditions due to **cocaine** or amphetamines); a past history of alterations in mood, behavior, perceptions, thought, and present mental status; and social and cultural expectations (e.g., a belief in voodoo could significantly influence the assessment).

TABLE 20.2. CONRAD'S PROGRESSIVE STAGES OF SCHIZOPHRENIA

Trema
    Patients experience a loosening or lack of coherence between their sense of their inner and outer worlds; the patient has a feeling of loss of freedom, a sense that the environment has changed (i.e., a form of depersonalization), or a feeling of inability to communicate.
Apophany
    The loosening and lack of coherence to the sense of the inner and outer worlds is so extensive that the inseparable can now seem separate, resulting in delusional and paranoid experiences.
Apocalypse
    Complete breakdown of the sense of coherence and a fragmentation of psychic life and the sense of self (fragmentation of the ego) is present
Consolidating and residual stages

From Fish F. A neurophysiological theory of schizophrenia. *J Ment Sci* 1961;107:828–838, with permission.

TABLE 20.3. SOME POSITIVE AND NEGATIVE SYMPTOMS OF SCHIZOPHRENIA

Positive Symptoms	Negative Symptoms
Conceptual disorganization	Anhedonia
Delusions	Apathy
Excitement	Avolition
Grandiosity	Blunted or flattened affect
Hallucinations	Emotional withdrawal
Hostility	Inappropriate affect
Suspiciousness (ideas of reference)	Lack of spontaneity
Uncooperativeness	Poor abstract thinking
	Poverty of thought (alogia)
	Social withdrawal (asociality)

A. Schizophrenia

The following is a description of schizophrenia that draws on the author's clinical experiences and on the DSM-IV and ICD-10 (Table 20.4). Schizophrenia is the diagnostic concept used to classify a group of psychotic patients who, at some points in time, suffer from a defect state characterized by apathy, avolition, asociality, affective blunting, and alogia. They also have alterations in thoughts, percepts, mood, and behavior—subjective experiences of disordered thought are manifested in disturbances of concept formation that sometimes lead to misinterpretations of reality; delusions, particularly of influence and ideas of reference; and hallucinations, particularly of voices repeating the patient's thoughts or commenting on his or

TABLE 20.4. DIAGNOSTIC CRITERIA FOR SCHIZOPHRENIA[a]

During a period lasting at least 6 months, various prodromal or residual symptoms must be continuously present, including negative symptoms (e.g., alogia, affective blunting, anhedonia, asociality, apathy, avolition) or from the list that follows at least two attenuated symptoms (e.g., odd beliefs and/or delusions, perceptual distortions and/or hallucinations). During this same period, an active phase lasting at least 1 month (less if effective treatment has been initiated) must occur that is characterized by at least two of the following symptom areas:
1. Delusions
2. Hallucinations
3. Disorganized thought or speech (e.g., incoherence, blocking, derailment)
4. Disorganized or catatonic behavior
5. Negative symptoms (see above)
During a significant proportion of these months, these symptoms must be associated with deteriorated functioning (self-care, work, school, or relationships) that is noticeably below levels existing before the onset of this period of symptomatic illness. Both the symptoms and associated dysfunction must not be part of or secondary to a medical condition, substance use, medication, or schizoaffective or mood disorder.

[a]In the *Diagnostic and Statistical Manual of Mental Disorders,* 4th edition, further classification is according to course (e.g., continuous, episodic) and type: **disorganized** (e.g., disorganized speech and behavior, flat or inappropriate affect), **catatonic** (e.g., immobility [catalepsy or stupor], excessive internally driven motor activity, negativism or mutism, stereotypies or mannerisms, echolalia or echopraxia), **paranoid** (e.g., delusions or hallucinations, not consistent with catatonic or disorganized types), **undifferentiated** (i.e., not consistent with the above three types), or **residual** (i.e., continuous evidence of the disorder, but the patient no longer meets full criteria).
From the American Psychiatric Association. *Diagnostic and statistical manual of mental disorders,* 4th ed. Text revision. Washington, D.C.: American Psychiatric Association, 2000, with permission.

her thoughts and actions. Mood changes include ambivalence, constriction, or inappropriateness of feeling and loss of empathy with others; behavior may be withdrawn, regressive, or bizarre. These alterations usually occur in a setting of clear consciousness; disorientation and amnesia typically are absent.

Central to this characterization is the concept of a disorder of thought. This may be manifested in the inappropriate rate, flow, or content of thinking or communication. It may be evident in the supervening style of the thinking process and the associated verbal productions. Typical **manifestations of disordered thought processes in schizophrenia** arranged according to the mnemonic "B/NOT/MVP/DDT" are as follows:

- **B**locking, often associated with the subjective feeling of not being in control of one's own thoughts;
- **N**eologisms, new personal language;
- **O**verinclusive thinking in which usual conceptual boundaries are lost or blurred;
- **T**hinking that is overly personalized and not abstract;
- **M**uteness;
- **V**erbigeration (the senseless repetition of words and phrases, seen particularly in chronic patients);
- **P**rivate logic;
- **D**ifficulties in generalizing correctly and in seeing similarities and differences;
- **D**ifficulties in separating relevant from irrelevant and in screening out the irrelevant;
- **T**hings may be seen as identical because they share a common or similar property.

B. Schizoaffective Disorder

Clinicians often see psychotic patients who reveal delusions, hallucinations, and disordered thoughts but who also appear elated or depressed. When depressive symptoms are prominent, such patients are classified as **depressive type** in the DSM-IV. Patients with the **depressive type** must be differentiated from patients with psychotic depressions whose delusions usually involve guilt or bizarre somatic concerns (e.g., "my stomach is rotting away") or both. Patients presenting with initial episodes of psychotic depressions are typically over the age of 40; patients with schizoaffective disorder are often younger.

Patients with **bipolar type** must be distinguished from patients in the psychotic phase of bipolar disorder (see Chapter 19). In patients with schizoaffective disorder, the disturbance in thinking is more typical of schizophrenia (e.g., blocking, illogical thinking, overinclusive thinking) rather than of mania (e.g., pressure to keep talking, racing thoughts). For patients with bipolar disorder in an excited psychotic episode to have an element of humor in their verbal productions is also typical. By contrast, patients with schizoaffective disorder are more likely to seem bizarre, and patients with schizophrenia, disorganized type, (sometimes older and more chronically ill) are more likely to appear silly and inappropriate. Patients with schizoaffective disorder usually have an episodic course with a good prognosis for a particular episode.

That patients with schizoaffective disorder were often classified as atypical or as having early forms of schizophrenia or bipolar disorder is understandable. K. Leonhard, who would have classified many of these patients as having cycloid psychoses, noted that their episodic course could eventually become chronic, with only partial remission from episodes once the illness pattern was well established. He considered these patients to have an independent endogenous psychosis that was neither schizophrenia nor bipolar disorder. Another alternative would be to see these disorders as reflecting a genetic mixing of bipolar disorder and schizophrenia. Careful observation of such patients suggests they are an extremely heterogeneous group; their family history patterns reveal more relatives with major depressive disorder and bipolar disorder and somewhat more relatives with schizophrenia and schizoaffective disorder than do those of control subjects. They also are likely to have first-degree relatives with alcoholism.

C. **Schizophreniform Disorder**

When G. Langfeldt introduced this term in 1939, it referred to acute reactive psychotic decompensations in previously well-functioning (i.e., normal) persons. Currently (i.e., in DSM-IV), this diagnosis is used for patients who appear to be having a more attenuated form of schizophrenia in terms of both duration and degree of disturbance in behavior and functioning. Rather than lasting for at least 6 months, the prodromal, active, and residual psychopathology in schizophreniform disorder lasts more than 3 months but less than 6 months with no severe impairment of functioning. Three modifiers are recommended.

1. **Provisional**. This term is used when schizophreniform disorder appears to be the appropriate diagnosis, but the patient is still ill (i.e., not enough time has elapsed since onset to assess whether recovery will take place before 6 months have passed). For patients who do not improve after 6 months, changing the diagnosis to schizophrenia is appropriate.

2. **With good prognostic features**. At least two of the following should be present:

   a. The time between any evidence of disturbed behavior and functioning and marked psychotic symptomatology is no more than 1 month (i.e., a relatively **more rapid onset** and **a short prodromal phase**).

   b. At the height of the psychotic decompensation, symptoms of **confusion or perplexity should be apparent**.

   c. Premorbid job or school and social role functioning should not be significantly compromised.

   d. Affect should not be flat or blunted.

3. **Without good prognostic features**.

D. **Brief Psychotic Disorder**

In the DSM-IV, this term is used for patients whose psychotic picture lasts for longer than 24 hours but for less than 1 month. The symptom pattern seen in these patients should be precipitated by an intensely distressing experience and should be followed by complete recovery of functioning to premorbid levels. As was noted earlier, the term **provisional** can be used as a modifier. The psychotic features should not be secondary to a medical condition or substance or medication use nor should they be part of a mood disorder or schizophrenia. One of four features (delusions, hallucinations, disorganized speech, and grossly disorganized or catatonic behavior) must be present, and this must not solely reflect a culture-bound behavior.

E. **Symptoms of Depression in Schizophrenia**

In addition to patients who have schizoaffective disorder, depressive type, other schizophrenic patients may show depression or depression-like symptoms at various times in the course of their disease. These symptoms may reflect the negative symptoms of schizophrenia. However, they may represent other conditions or manifestations of depression, broadly defined. The following subsections review selected considerations or conceptualizations that the author has found clinically useful, even though they are not incorporated into the DSM-IV or ICD-10.

1. **Depressive position**. Some patients appear to be in a depressive position or phase in their recovery from an acute episode of decompensation, as if they are demoralized about what has befallen them. Some appear to be grieving, whereas others appear to have shifted from paranoid thinking or delusions and distortions to depressive content (e.g., "They hate me" has become "I hate myself").

2. **Depression *per se***. Clinical experience clearly shows that schizophrenic patients are not immune to depression. For example, a schizophrenic

patient can experience and reveal a dysphoric mood or can move into an episode of major depressive disorder in connection with the loss of a significant person and yet not show further worsening of any preexisting schizophrenic symptoms. Antidepressant therapy added to the regimen of antipsychotic drugs may be of benefit to some of these patients. In other patients, depression may appear before the onset of psychotic symptoms in a first episode or during an exacerbation of symptoms in a patient who had been in remission. Although a few may benefit from antidepressants alone, more commonly these patients are likely to become more overtly psychotic when antidepressants are prescribed in the absence of antipsychotic agents.

3. **Neurasthenia**. These patients appear "stuck." They have often been chronically ill, or they have symptoms consistent with schizophrenia, residual type. They may seem depressed, without the will to reengage with active life outside an institutional or sheltered setting. Many seem demoralized (e.g., "Why bother! Nothing gets better"). In some patients, this may be an iatrogenic condition, a result of prolonged hospitalization or inadequate rehabilitation and socialization. In others, it may result when a well-meaning therapist tries to get the patient to do what the therapist wants for the patient rather than what the patient wants for himself or herself. The literature also contains a speculation that neurasthenia is a phase some patients must pass through as part of their reintegration process.

4. **Overmedicated patients**. Some schizophrenic patients who appear retarded and depressed may simply be overmedicated, especially those receiving **conventional antipsychotic agents (CAPs)**. Dosage reduction should produce an amelioration of their psychomotor retarded-depressed presentation.

5. **Akinetic parkinsonism**. Some patients may have neuroleptic-induced akinetic parkinsonism, especially those using CAPs, which presents to the observer as depression and psychomotor retardation. A trial of an antiparkinsonian agent may identify this subgroup.

II. Etiology and Genetic Factors

Although an in depth discussion of the etiology and pathobiology of schizophrenia is beyond the scope of this chapter, certain observations compel comment and these are mentioned in the appropriate sections. Schizophrenia tends to aggregate in families; data from investigations of twins and of children born to schizophrenic mothers but placed for adoption at birth argue for a major genetic factor in the etiology of the illness for some patients. About 50% of monozygotic twin pairs are concordant for schizophrenia; this argues against a simple genetic explanation. Nevertheless, there is reason to suspect that certain individuals inherit a susceptibility to the expression of schizophrenic disorganization. In some people, this susceptibility may lead to an early expression of symptoms, as in the schizophrenias of childhood and adolescence. More typically, the symptoms appear during adolescence or early adult life, perhaps when the stresses of separation from family or the requirements for living autonomously expose a schizophrenic vulnerability. An individual who is so burdened may be unable to cope with the stresses and demands of everyday life or to bear the losses, disappointments, or defeats that usually are encountered.

At the present time, genetic studies implicate several genes that may be linked to vulnerability to schizophrenia. This diverse group includes chromosomes 1q, 6p, 6q, 8p, 10p, 15q, and 22q. The strongest and most replicated evidence involves the α7-nicotinic receptor subunit gene (CHRNA7) at the 15q13-14 locus.

III. Differentiating Schizophrenia from Other Conditions that May Produce Similar Symptoms

The diagnosis of schizophrenia must still be made in part by exclusion. Table 20.5 lists some conditions and illnesses that can present with psychotic symptoms. Because so many of the symptoms of schizophrenia may be manifestations of a variety of local or systemic processes that alter central nervous system function, a complete consideration of these possibilities is beyond the scope of this chapter.

TABLE 20.5. SOME CONDITIONS AND ILLNESSES THAT CAN MANIFEST SCHIZOPHRENIFORM SYMPTOMS

Toxic and deficiency states
Drug-induced psychoses, especially those induced by amphetamines, cocaine, lysergic acid diethylamide, digitalis, steroids, disulfiram
Alcoholic hallucinosis
Wernicke encephalopathy
Korsakoff psychosis
Bromism and other heavy metal intoxication
Pellagra and other vitamin deficiencies
Uremia and liver failure
Infections
Syphilis
Toxoplasmosis
Viral encephalitis
Brain abscess
Schistosomiasis
Neurologic disease
Seizure disorders
Primary and metastatic neoplasms
Early presenile and senile dementias
Postencephalitic states
Cardiovascular
Lowered cardiac output
Hypertensive encephalopathy
Endocrine disorders
Thyrotoxicosis
Myxedema
Adrenal hyperfunction
Genetic and metabolic disorders
Acute porphyria
Homocystinuria
Niemann-Pick disease
Electrolyte imbalances
Diabetes mellitus
Collagen-vascular diseases
Central nervous system lupus arteritis

Of primary importance in this differential diagnosis is a careful personal and family history and physical examination, together with the judicious use of the clinical laboratory. Any history of exposure to drugs or toxins, a family history of a genetic disease, or the presence of neurologic deficits or the stigmata of systemic disease may be particularly significant.

IV. Epidemiology and Pathobiology

The lifetime risk for schizophrenia is estimated at 0.8% to 1.9%. The current estimate is that schizophrenia is present in about 2 million persons in the United States. The prevalence among men and women is probably approximately equal. Recently, some investigators have suggested a slightly higher prevalence among men; other investigators have concluded that more women develop schizophrenia. The age at onset of the first psychotic decompensation is in the mid-20s for women and is about 5 years earlier for men. Most men with schizophrenia have revealed obvious evidence of the disease before the age of 30. For men who develop schizophrenia to have shown a pattern of unsocialized aggression during their early adolescent years is not uncommon.

The risk of schizophrenia is 40% to 50% for the offspring of two schizophrenic parents and about 5% for those with one schizophrenic parent. A significantly greater likelihood is seen of finding schizophrenia among the first-degree relatives of schizophrenic patients than among the third-degree relatives (i.e., first cousins). The latter have rates that approximate the rate in the general population. As one might expect, the prevalence rates in second-degree relatives (aunts, uncles) fall between the two. These estimates are complemented by findings from adoption studies of children, both with schizophrenia and without, that were conducted in Denmark in the 1970s and 1980s. Rates for schizophrenia were higher among the first-degree biologic relatives of the adoptees with schizophrenia than among the relatives of the control subjects, and no increase in the rate of schizophrenia was observed among the adoptees who had nonschizophrenic parents but who were adopted by families in which one parent was schizophrenic.

Given the diverse symptomatology seen in patients with schizophrenia, that imaging studies (e.g., magnetic resonance imaging, positron emission tomography, single photon emission computed tomography) do not reveal consistent neuroanatomic changes is not surprising. Some of the following findings, however, occur with reasonable frequency: enlarged ventricles, widened sulci, hypofrontality as reflected in lowered glucose utilization, volume reductions in the gray matter of the left temporal lobe, and atrophy of the cerebellar vermis. The thalamus and striatum may also show changes. The frontal lobe changes are consistent with the defect state or negative symptoms seen in schizophrenic patients, and one group of investigators recently suggested that reductions in the volume of the left posterior superior temporal gyrus correlate with the degree of disordered thinking. Similarly, reduced insular gray matter volume and cortical surface size correlate negatively with the severity of psychotic symptomatology. In a meaningful proportion of patients with schizophrenia, reduced blood flow has been found in four brain regions—cerebellar vermis, parahippocampal gyrus, nucleus accumbens, and insular cortex—the latter three of which are limbic structures. A reasonable conclusion from these varied findings is that alterations in the interactions among frontal and mesolimbic pathways and structures may be the basis for many of the symptoms of schizophrenia.

An intriguing finding from postmortem brain tissue of persons known to have had schizophrenia is down-regulation of the gene for Reelin (RELN), a high affinity ligand for integrin receptors that is synthesized by γ-aminobutyric acid (GABA)ergic frontal cortex neurons. RELN is known to bind to the dendrites and dendritic spines of pyramidal neurons. Down-regulation is consistent with the shortened dendrites and the lower dendritic spine expression densities in pyramidal neurons that are found in the postmortem tissue from some deceased schizophrenic patients. Because similar changes have been found in cortical tissue from deceased patients who had bipolar disorder but not in those with major depressive disorder without psychotic features, this finding is not specific to schizophrenia.

Other findings suggest a reduction of GABAergic activity that may result in increased limbic and prefrontal area dopaminergic activity. A possible cause of these observations could be the disinhibition of glutamatergic activity or the hypofunction of N-methyl-D-aspartate receptors on GABAergic interneurons. This concept is consistent with the occurrence of schizophrenic-like symptoms after subanesthetic doses of the noncompetitive dissociative anesthetic N-methyl-D-aspartate receptor antagonists, such as phencyclidine, ketamine, and MK-801. The role of excitatory amino acids and their interactions with GABAergic interneurons and dopaminergic neurons remains an incompletely explored yet potentially important area of study that also includes the termination of glutamatergic activity by astrocytes.

Changes in dopaminergic activity, if they are not causal, appear to be at least contributory to the manifest symptomatology of schizophrenia. Mesolimbic and mesocortical dopaminergic tracts arise in the ventral tegmental area of the A10 region and project to the limbic areas (i.e., amygdala, pyriform cortex, lateral septal nuclei, nucleus accumbens) and to the prefrontal and frontal cortex and septohippocampal regions, respectively. Dopamine 2 (D_2) and D_3 postsynaptic receptors along these pathways appear to be important mediators of behavior. All currently marketed antipsychotic agents are antagonists at these receptors. D_3 (limbic area) receptor antagonism shows a strong correlation with the average therapeutic dose or potency of CAPs. The **atypical antipsychotic agent (AAP) clozapine** (see section VI.B.6.h) has a high affinity for D_4 receptors.

A more specific understanding of the actions of antipsychotic agents on various dopamine receptors is difficult to achieve at the present time because of the complicated interplay of regional receptor differences and actions at both presynaptic and postsynaptic sites. In the striatum, for example, D_2 receptors inhibit acetylcholine release. On dopaminergic nerve terminals, these receptors also function as autoreceptors; their activation reduces the firing rates, synthesis, and release of dopamine. Experimental dopamine autoreceptor agonists stimulate supersensitive but not "normosensitive" postsynaptic receptors. In the substantia nigra, CAPs acting on both presynaptic and postsynaptic D_2 receptors inhibit neuronal firing. **Clozapine, olanzapine, quetiapine, ziprasidone,** and **risperidone** show a reduced likelihood of decreasing the firing of these same neurons. As a group, these agents are all called AAPs. Mesocortical D_2, D_3, and D_4 receptor antagonism appears to be particularly important to the alleviation of psychotic symptomatology. **Clozapine** use may, however, actually increase prefrontal dopaminergic activity. This could explain how **clozapine** is beneficial for negative symptoms that have been hypothesized to be related, at least in part, to decreased dopaminergic activity in this area. Data from experimental autoreceptor agonists suggest that they too may improve negative symptoms. However, data from **clozapine, olanzapine, quetiapine, ziprasidone,** and **risperidone** *in vitro* studies also argue for an important linkage to concomitant 5-hydroxytryptamine (5-HT)$_2$ receptor antagonism for at least some patients. Indeed, a positive ratio favoring 5-HT$_2$ over D_2 receptor binding is central to the definition of an AAP (Table 20.6; see also Table 20.10).

V. Course, Outcome, and Prognosis

One of the crucial elements in Kraepelin's distinctions between manic-depressive psychosis and dementia praecox arose from data generated by followup examination. Dementia praecox was seen as an illness from which recovery was not common. In the 1910 edition of his textbook, Kraepelin, although he did acknowledge recovery in some 13% of patients, cited many contemporary investigations that emphasized deterioration and lack of recovery.

Eugen Bleuler's concept of a group of schizophrenias suggested the possibility of a broad spectrum of courses, outcomes, and prognosis. However, E. Bleuler emphasized that, despite periods of arrest or reversal, the patients would probably never be totally free of schizophrenia. As was noted earlier, Langfeldt emphasized a dichotomization of diagnoses based on outcome. Narrowly defined (nuclear) schizophrenic patients were predicted to have poor outcomes at followup. Another subset of patients was seen to recover and was considered schizophreniform by virtue of both their recovery and the presence of certain features in their behaviors and histories (e.g., acute rather than insidious onset, good rather than poor premorbid functioning, depressive symptoms). Langfeldt, noting

---

TABLE 20.6. A WORKING AND EVOLVING DEFINITION OF "ATYPICALITY" FOR ANTIPSYCHOTIC AGENTS

Beneficial effects on both positive and negative symptoms in patients with schizophrenia

Low or absent likelihood of extrapyramidal motor system (EPS) unwanted effects at therapeutic concentrations in patients

5-Hydroxytryptamine (5-HT)-2 receptor antagonism stronger than dopamine-2 (D_2) receptor antagonism in *in vitro* models

D_4 receptor antagonism stronger than D_2 receptor antagonism in *in vitro* models[a]

[a]Using all four criteria, **clozapine** is the most atypical antipsychotic agent.

M. Sakel's observation that 88% of schizophrenic patients recovered, suggested that this was based on diagnostic error and that the patient population must have included many reaction types with a tendency to spontaneous recovery. Many other clinicians have restated this position. J. H. Stephens, for example, wrote that "apparent 'schizophrenia' with a good prognosis is not a mild form of schizophrenia, but is a different illness."

Course and outcome must be considered not only in terms of manifest psychopathology but also with regard to adjustment or performance criteria as reflected by working capacity, interpersonal relationships, autonomy, and self-regard. Outcome may best be viewed as a process rather than as a dimension measured at a fixed point in time. Manfred Bleuler, for example, using observations from a study of over 500 schizophrenic patients seen by 1941, outlined seven possible longitudinal patterns to describe the course and outcome of schizophrenia as follows:

1. Acute onset leading to chronic severe psychosis;
2. Insidious onset leading slowly to chronic severe psychosis;
3. Acute onset leading to chronic mild psychosis;
4. Insidious onset leading slowly to chronic mild psychosis;
5. Several acute episodes leading to chronic severe psychosis;
6. Several acute episodes leading to chronic mild psychosis;
7. One or several acute episodes leading to recovery.

The first four patterns show a rather continuous evolution; the latter three are phasic. Having followed the life experiences of this cohort of schizophrenic patients for 23 years, M. Bleuler concluded that these patterns subsumed the experiences of 90% of patients. Other patterns, however, are certainly possible (e.g., insidious onset leading to recovery, chronic psychosis followed by acute episodes).

M. Bleuler began to accumulate a new cohort of over 200 patients in 1942. Twenty-six years later, more than a decade after the introduction of effective antipsychotic agents, Bleuler wrote about his 23-year follow-up of these 200 patients and indicated that the pattern "acute psychosis leading to chronic severe psychosis" had almost disappeared. He further suggested that cases evolving to a mild chronic psychosis had increased, whereas those involving severe chronic psychoses had diminished. He cautioned, however, that although the "most malignant **acute** schizophrenias are under control now, the most **chronic** schizophrenias are not. The percentage of chronic onset leading slowly to chronic severe psychosis has remained nearly the same within the last 25 years ... A further finding is also disappointing: it was not possible to increase the percentage of recoveries much over one-third of all cases." The reader should remember that M. Bleuler's data and perspective antedate the use of **clozapine** and other AAPs.

O. H. Arnold, who wrote in the mid-1950s before the advent of effective antipsychotic agents, described a large cohort of 500 schizophrenic patients that he followed for 3 to 30 years. His results revealed the following: (a) a phasic course of illness leading to complete remission in 15.6%, (b) a phasic course that became shift-like (new acute symptomatology that was followed by partial recovery) in 4%, (c) a phasic course leading to deterioration in 0.4%, (d) a phasic course leading to deterioration punctuated by exacerbations of symptomatology in 3.4%, (e) a shift-like course with some residual pathology in 9.6%, (f) a shift-like course leading to deterioration in 3.6%, (g) a shift-like course leading to deterioration punctuated by exacerbation in 14%, (h) a gradual deterioration in 7.2%, (i) a gradual deterioration punctuated by exacerbation in 38%, and (j) mixed psychotic courses in 6.6%. The important theme in his findings was that only about 16% recovered, whereas 67% of patients had chronic or eventually deteriorating courses, an ominous prognosis for patients with schizophrenia who do not receive effective antipsychotic therapies.

Many authors have examined and reviewed historical and clinical features that may not be dependent on treatment, yet they do correlate with improvement in schizophrenia. Table 20.7 summarizes some of the predictor variables that appear in these reviews. From this literature, one appears to be able to predict more

TABLE 20.7. SOME PREDICTORS OF OUTCOME IN SCHIZOPHRENIA

Poorer Prognosis	Better Prognosis
Insidious onset	Acute onset
Withdrawn behavior	Depressive symptoms
Emotional blunting	Good premorbid social and work history
Little overt hostility	Verbal aggression
Excessive persecutory delusions and paranoia	Concern with guilt and death
Schizoid or asocial premorbid personality	Tension and anxiety
Hebephrenic clinical picture	Clear precipitating factors
Clear sensorium	Confusion
Family history of schizophrenia	No family history of schizophrenia
Unmarried	Married
Absence of any affective symptoms	Family history of affective disorders

readily those who are less likely to do well than those who are likely to have a hopeful outcome.

Even with effective agents, can an individual really get over schizophrenia? Is remission merely a phase of arrest or reversal, as E. Bleuler suggested? Does he or she remain predisposed to decompensations under certain conditions? One cannot be cured of diabetes, for example, even though, with proper treatment, the expression of, and morbidity from, the illness can often be greatly modified. An ulcer may heal, but a predisposition to hyperacidity or infection by *Helicobacter pylori* may remain. Schizophrenia is not merely a pattern of overt symptomatology; it also appears to be an underlying vulnerability. Even when substantial or complete improvement has been achieved (either with or without treatment), does the patient still warrant the diagnosis of schizophrenia **in remission**? Unfortunately, no resolution has yet been reached for this perplexing question.

VI. Selected Aspects of the Treatment of Schizophrenia

A. Hospitalization as a Therapy

In this era of cost containment and managed care, ambiguity is present about the place of hospitalization in treatment planning for patients with schizophrenia. Historically, extended periods of hospitalization were observed to have negative effects. J. K. Wing in Great Britain and E. Goffman in the United States thoroughly described the harmful and dehumanizing effects of institutionalization. At the present time, the pendulum appears to have swung too far in the opposite direction, and patients may spend too little time in the hospital to benefit from the positive effects of hospitalization. Many patients now have an increased number of all too brief hospitalizations; others are rarely or never hospitalized, and instead they join the ever-growing ranks of the homeless.

The onset of symptoms of schizophrenia is not by itself an indication for psychiatric hospitalization. When sufficient support exists in the community and patients' symptomatology does not constitute a threat to themselves or others, outpatient treatment should almost always be attempted. Keeping patients in community-based care may help to preserve their existing matrix of social supports. Studies of why patients are hospitalized suggest that many hospitalizations can be avoided when adequate family and community resources are available.

When patients are a threat to themselves or others, hospitalization is usually recommended, even in today's cost-conscious managed care environment. Suicidal and homicidal ideation and attempts are especially serious in schizophrenic patients (see Chapter 17). Psychotic patients often lack the impulse control or judgment to modify such feelings, especially when they are having command hallucinations. They also may become distressed by delusional beliefs, especially persecutory ideation. However, one characteristic of many schizophrenic patients is that they often do not appear to feel distressed by experiences that others would find upsetting.

Moreover, when patients are confused or so anxious that they cannot adequately care for themselves, hospitalization is indicated. Although the sensorium is usually clear in schizophrenia, confusion and frank disorientation occasionally may occur. In assessing a patient's capacity for self-care outside the hospital, assessing factors such as the patient's abilities to plan daily activities or to have a full night's sleep is important.

Occasionally, temporary hospitalization of the schizophrenic patient becomes necessary when those caring for the patient in the community are unable to do so or when interpersonal pressures on the patient become intolerable. Such occasions may include the illness of a parent or sibling or the birth of a child in the patient's family. The ability and willingness of a backup hospital to help to support a patient, and indirectly the family, may influence the acceptance of the chronically disturbed patient within the community. Table 20.8 summarizes some of the major indications for hospitalization.

When the clinical decision to hospitalize the patient has been reached, the reasons for such an action should be clear; they should be explained to the patient in an unambiguous way. Whenever possible, the patient's collaboration and participation should be obtained. Although some patients may be too disturbed to participate in such a decision, most will be able to respond in some positive way to the clinician's firm resolve that temporary hospitalization will be helpful. Once patients are hospitalized, some experience the relief from

TABLE 20.8. SOME PURPOSES OF HOSPITALIZATION

Protective-custodial
  Safeguarding the patient's life
  Safeguarding specific persons or the community from the patient's behavior
  Removing the patient from a noxious or pathologic or overstimulating environment until it can be modified
  Protecting a person's reputation may also be a consideration for admission in some self-pay settings
Diagnostic
  Closer observation
  Availability of specialized procedures (e.g., imaging techniques)
Therapeutic
  Motivation of the patient and family
    To accept and support therapy
    To make necessary life changes
  Pharmacotherapy
    Administration of medication schedules too complex to be carried out at home or schedules that require careful observation by trained staff
    Rapid initiation of potentially problematic or toxic medications
    Assurance that confused or uncooperative patients take the prescribed medication
  Social-familial (*note:* these goals are rarely possible with current health maintenance organization mandated lengths of stay and cost concerns)
    Social rehabilitation, group therapy and group living experiences, exposure to a therapeutic community, assumption of social responsibilities in hospital setting
    Relief of family tensions so that exploration of critical relationships and issues can proceed without emergence of family crises
  Special therapies not possible outside the hospital (e.g., electroconvulsive therapy)

From Detre TP, Jarecki HG. *Modern psychiatric treatment.* Philadelphia: Lippincott, 1971, with permission.

being in a place where they can feel relatively safe and can obtain help in controlling their impulses. The moratorium of, and distance from, upsetting experiences may also be beneficial. Because the modal duration of acute hospitalization under some managed care plans is 7 to 14 days, engaging acutely ill patients in any form of milieu therapy is rarely possible.

Patients with schizophrenia often decompensate in unhealthy settings that are too stressful or too stimulating or in which abusable substances are available. Hospitalization may interrupt, not perpetuate, or even reverse this experience. Ideally, it should help patients regain interpersonal stability, and it should enable them to receive positive concern and regard from others. Adequate space and clearly written ward policies about passes, visitors, smoking, and personal possessions must exist. Stimuli in the ward setting that could encourage violence or sexual activity (e.g., television) should be minimized. Violence occurring within the ward setting is more likely to come from intolerance of restrictions or as a result of provocation by others than to be due to command hallucinations. Interpretive or oblique communications can increase patients' anxieties, anger, and disorganization. Communication with regressed patients must be clear, unambiguous, and brief.

Difficult management problems, such as acts of violence, inappropriate sexual behavior, and the refusal of food or medications, commonly occur. Because such activities can injure patients and those around them, the clinician should act in a firm but nonpunitive way to prevent such behavior. When the patient's behavior cannot be modified or contained by interpersonal interventions, such as clear verbal confrontation and exhortation, or by temporary placement in a quiet area, the use of physical restraints or seclusion may be indicated (see Chapters 25 and 26). Ideally, this need will be obviated by the patient's favorable response to antipsychotic agents.

The patient's refusal of food or fluids should not be allowed to endanger his or her health. This concern should be explained to the patient and his or her family. Although the legal issues regarding involuntary care and patients' rights to refuse treatment are being addressed, the emergency use of intravenous fluids and assisted feeding should be instituted when necessary. Acutely regressed, suicidal, or homicidal patients should not remain untreated when treatment is clearly indicated. When patients refuse oral medications, intramuscular administration or even electroconvulsive therapy (see Chapter 24) should be considered. After a short period of time, patients usually accept oral medications. Firmness in dealing with acutely regressed patients must not preclude efforts to reach an empathic understanding of their feelings or of what they may fear or of what they are trying to express.

In the past, hospitalizing the acutely schizophrenic patient allowed the clinician a more complete opportunity for clinical evaluation and a more controlled setting for effectively titrating the patient's dosage of antipsychotic medication. Currently, dosage titration is continued into the outpatient phase of care; unfortunately, some patients continue on the higher than needed doses that were previously necessary during hospitalization.

Discharge from the hospital-based phase of treatment to outpatient follow-up or community-based aftercare should be carefully planned. Premature discharge or discharge without adequate efforts to ensure that the patient is entering an environment that can tolerate his or her current level of functioning and psychopathology may make successful discharge and continued rehabilitation difficult if not impossible. These considerations are particularly relevant for acute exacerbations in chronically ill patients and for those who may have become alienated from family and friends. Table 20.9 summarizes many of the factors to be considered when evaluating the discharge readiness of patients.

B. Pharmacotherapy

The efficacy of CAPs (sometimes called neuroleptics or major tranquilizers) in treating acute and chronic schizophrenic patients has been established by a vast number of adequately designed controlled studies conducted over the

TABLE 20.9. SOME FACTORS TO BE CONSIDERED DURING DISCHARGE PLANNING

Patient shows sufficient improvement in behaviors that necessitated hospitalization, functions in an acceptable manner, or no longer constitutes a danger to self or others.

Patient shows a reduction in behaviors that are incompatible with living in the community; this change seems likely to be sustainable outside the hospital.

Patient has received maximum benefits that this hospitalization can provide; no further improvement is anticipated at this time in this setting.

Symptoms appear to be in stable remission, and immediate relapse does not seem likely.

Patients assumes responsibility for own behavior.

Appropriate aftercare arrangements are available, including living arrangements, and in place; patient is able to continue in therapy on an outpatient basis.

Patient in good contact with reality and is capable of discussing own situation.

Patient has gained socialization skills and is able to relate better to others.

Personal hygiene skills are acceptable.

Patient is capable of performing meaningful work independently and has a reasonable chance of obtaining employment.

Patient has adequate economic resources or identifiable sources of support.

Person is capable of following prescribed medication regimen alone or with the help of others.

The patient is not involved in pending litigation or under court-ordered hospitalization.

The patient has a history of repeated elopements while hospitalized.

The patient requests discharge against medical advice.

Modified from Katz RC, Woolley FR. Criteria for releasing patients from psychiatric hospitals. *Hosp Commun Psychiatry* 1975;26:33–36, with permission.

past 45 years. These studies repeatedly demonstrate the usefulness of antipsychotic agents for reducing disordered thinking, anxiety, delusions, hallucinations, and other symptoms associated with schizophrenia. Marked improvement of negative symptoms, such as apathy or social withdrawal, is not always demonstrated in studies with CAPs. After the introduction of the AAP **clozapine**, the fact that improvement in both negative and positive symptoms was more possible than was previously expected became apparent.

1. **Selection and specificity**. Although claims are made for differential therapeutic effectiveness among antipsychotic agents, controlled replications do not consistently substantiate such differences. One exception to this is **clozapine** (see section VI.B.6.h), which may have differential efficacy in some treatment-resistant patients. The choice of a particular antipsychotic medication rests primarily on a consideration of its main and secondary pharmacologic properties, its side effects, and its toxicity, as well as the patient's and the clinician's past experience with the drug. Cost may also be a factor in some settings. Clinical experience might suggest that a given patient should respond better to one drug than to another; however, in the absence of prior exposure or pharmacogenetic data, drug selection is empirical. In choosing an antipsychotic medication, the clinician must anticipate the patient's probable overall reaction. For instance, an agitated or sleepless young adult patient could benefit from the soporific effects of **thioridazine**, whereas an elderly or dehydrated patient might be harmed by the hypotensive and anticholinergic effects of this agent.

A patient's past experience with a particular medication may partially determine the clinician's current choice. In addition to inquiring about a past history of adverse drug reactions, including allergies, the clinician should try to ascertain which drugs the patient believes were of benefit and which were poorly tolerated because of particular unwanted effects. This investigation will not only supply the clinician with needed clinical information, but it will also promote the patient's cooperation with, and participation in, the treatment process.

Finally, clinicians should consider their own observations about a particular drug. Because many antipsychotic medications, including five AAPs, remain on the market today, extensive experience with all of these is unlikely. The author recommends that the clinician select about eight representative drugs from the currently available pool of CAPs and AAPs and become familiar with their clinical effects, both wanted and unwanted. Table 20.10 lists some features of eight representative antipsychotic agents.

2. **Dosage adjustments**. When titrating the dosage of a particular antipsychotic medication, the stage of the patient's decompensation and his or her target symptoms, body size, weight, and known response to the drug or similar agents must be considered. Antipsychotic medications exert their therapeutic effects over a broad dosage range; particular patients who do not respond favorably to a drug at one dosage level may respond at a higher or lower dosage.

When beginning the use of antipsychotic medication for the first time, administration of a small test dose of the drug is sometimes desirable (i.e., 25 to 50 mg orally or 25 mg intramuscularly [i.m.] of **chlorpromazine**, or the equivalent dose of another antipsychotic drug). This is particularly relevant for low potency CAPs. Doing so will give the clinician an opportunity to observe the patient for the development of orthostatic hypotension or other idiosyncratic effects. If such reactions do not occur within 2 hours of the administration of such a test dose, the clinician may then begin titrating the drug dosage into an effective antipsychotic range.

TABLE 20.10. SOME PROPERTIES OF SELECTED ANTIPSYCHOTIC AGENTS

Agents	5-HT$_2$/D$_2$[a] (K$_D$s)	Dosage Range[b] in mg (maximum) K$_D$s	Oral Dose Equivalence[c] in mg
Conventional			
Chlorpromazine	14	30–800	100
Thioridazine	1.2	50–400 (800)	60–100
Haloperidol	0.11	6–15 (100)	1–5
Atypical			
Clozapine	81	12.5–450 (900)	60–100
Quetiapine	25	25–750 (800)	25–75
Olanzapine	13	5–10 (15)	2–5
Risperidone	25	2–8 (16)	1–3
Ziprasidone	21	20–100 (160)	3–7.5

[a]These estimates are reproduced with permission from Richelson E, Nelson A. *Eur J Pharmacol* 1984;103:197–204; Wander TJ, et al. *Eur J Pharmacol* 1987;143:279–282; Richelson E, Souder T. *Life Sci* 2000;68:29–39, with permission.
[b]See page *xiv*. These data are based on the author's clinical experience and awareness of the literature; lower dosages are generally required for the elderly and slow titration, when clinically appropriate, is desirable; maximum doses reflect either manufacturers' recommendations or the author's synthesis of safety literature.
[c]Oral dosage equivalence is at best an approximation because of variables, such as formulation dissolution characteristics (e.g., particle size, excipients, presystemic extraction, amounts of liquid consumed); also equating conventional to atypical agents is not always straightforward because of tolerability differences.
Abbreviations: D$_2$, dopamine; 5-HT, 5-hydroxytryptamine; K$_D$s, dissociation constant.

Table 20.10 lists the approximate relative potencies of eight antipsychotic agents when given orally. These are at best rough approximations. For example, they may apply during the acute treatment phase but not to maintenance therapy. The values that are given are more accurate in the lower dosage ranges. Relative potencies of various drugs at high dosage ranges and for parenteral routes have not been studied adequately. Therefore, establishing the proper therapeutic dosage for a specific patient is largely an empirical process. These and the other dosage recommendations that follow are meant simply as guidelines to the clinician as he or she adjusts the dosage of a particular antipsychotic medication to meet the needs of the specific patient.

The usual antipsychotic dosage range for acutely ill schizophrenic patients, for example, is 2 to 8 mg per day of **risperidone** or 5 to 15 mg per day of **haloperidol** or an equivalent amount of another drug. Lower doses in such patients are not consistently effective, and higher doses, even if they are adequately tolerated, usually do not produce enhanced therapeutic effects. Although containing a patient's agitated, destructive, or regressed behavior is important, "snowing" the patient with excessive doses of antipsychotic medication may only treat the staff's anxieties, not the patient's turmoil or distress. The clinician should remember that antipsychotic drugs often have a cumulative or time-dependent therapeutic effect. Such an effect usually begins within the first 48 hours of treatment, but it may take up to several weeks after beginning a drug. In the author's experience, this is particularly common with **olanzapine**; initial concomitant use of **risperidone** or **haloperidol** during the first 5 to 21 days of treatment may hasten or improve the patient's response. As a general rule, the author advises titration of dosage until an adequate therapeutic response is achieved or troublesome side effects are encountered.

3. **Rapid tranquilization and parenteral administration**. Some authors advocate **rapid tranquilization** for acutely agitated schizophrenic patients, particularly when extreme agitation is present. This may involve frequent i.m. dosing (every 1 to 4 hours) until improvement is observed. Rapid tranquilization primarily achieves a quieting effect or sedation. The initial benefits are usually observed within 30 minutes to 2 hours. No rapid antipsychotic effect *per se* is present, unless calming the patient reduces his or her psychotic terror and agitation. Improvement often occurs within a day; frequent dosing for longer than 2 days is rarely beneficial.

Although i.m. **haloperidol** is not sedating, it is still used worldwide for rapid tranquilization by many clinicians. Supplementation with a benzodiazepine, such as **lorazepam**, is common. **Droperidol**, another butyrophenone, is also used in some emergency departments for rapid tranquilization. Because of its association with cases of ventricular tachyarrhythmias, **droperidol** is no longer available in some countries; in the United States, its use is restricted to those for whom other treatments have failed and who have no know risk factors for QT interval prolongation. **Risperidone** also enjoys some popularity when rapid tranquilization is needed but only when an oral medication (tablet or oral solution) is suitable.

Both i.m. **olanzapine** and i.m. **ziprasidone** have recently received United States Food and Drug Administration (FDA) approval for the treatment of agitation. In submitted studies, i.m. **olanzapine** in doses of 2.5 to 10 mg was shown to be statistically superior to the placebo and to be comparable with **haloperidol** or **lorazepam** on a scale that assessed positive and negative symptoms. In trials with **ziprasidone**, patients with schizophrenia and schizoaffective disorder, as well as patients with bipolar disorder, were given injections of either 10 mg every 2 hours (up to a maximum of 40 mg in 24 hours) or 20 mg every 4 hours (up to a maximum of 80 mg in 24 hours) for their agitation, and rapid improvement was noted. Both i.m. preparations appear to be well tolerated. Bradycardia secondary to **olanzapine** occurred in about 8%. This may reflect the drug's antagonist actions at the α_1-adrenergic receptors. According to the manufacturer, bradycardia and some degree of postural hypotension occur more often in the nonagitated control patients and in those who have not been previously treated with an oral dose. With **ziprasidone**, a concern about cardiac side effects (i.e., QT interval prolongation) does exist. Manufacturer's data suggest that the mean change in QTc after administration of i.m. **ziprasidone** does not exceed the prolongation found with the oral formulation, which averaged approximately 10 ms longer than that seen with **risperidone**, **olanzapine**, **quetiapine**, or **haloperidol**; that increment was less than the average change with a 300 mg dosage of **thioridazine**.

These parenteral approaches to treating psychotic agitation emphasize the frequency of, or time interval, between dosage increments. Although these procedures may be of value to some patients, especially in emergency situations, many clinicians do not believe this approach has an acceptable benefit-to-risk ratio.

4. **Dosage schedules**. After picking an antipsychotic medication and titrating its dose, the clinician should carefully rationalize the patient's dosage schedule. After the first few days of treatment, intensive administration of medication four to five times a day is usually unnecessary. Antipsychotic agents usually are generally well tolerated in large single oral doses. Reducing the number of daily administrations, while making appropriate increases in the tablet or capsule strengths, to a single bedtime dose or to two doses a day saves nursing time and costs, and it lessens the inconvenience to the patient and the cost per milligram of the medication. Furthermore, patient discomfort from many side effects is minimized by single bedtime doses, because the patient is asleep during the time of maximal anticholinergic or orthostatic hypotensive effects; this will not be beneficial unless the patient is sedated.

5. **Maintenance and discontinuation of treatment**. For first-episode patients, experience and published studies suggest that maintenance pharmacotherapy supplemented by psychosocial treatments, particularly family interventions when they are appropriate, is the best way to reduce relapse rates. Once the acute psychotic symptoms are controlled and the patient's condition has stabilized (usually 2 to 12 weeks), the daily dosage of medication may be slightly reduced over a period of weeks, but it should be kept at a full antipsychotic dose (usually about 100 to 400 mg per day [range, 100 to 600 mg per day] in **chlorpromazine** equivalents). Maintenance therapy is effective in more than 50% of patients. Benzodiazepines are sometimes used to reduce any exacerbations of symptomatology during maintenance treatment.

Drug-free intervals of 1 to 3 consecutive days a week (e.g., during weekends) are advocated by some clinicians to reduce the total amount of drug ingested by the patient, and these may be accomplished in many patients without ill effects. *At this time, drug-free periods do not appear to be needed with AAP use.* In contexts where CAP use is involved, whether this "holiday" approach alters the likelihood of serious side effects, such as tardive dyskinesias (TDs), from CAPs remains unclear.

Other than relapse or the emergence of serious unwanted effects, no clear guidelines exist for dictating the discontinuation or the switching of antipsychotic medications. Indeed, with AAPs, indefinite maintenance seems to be warranted. Discontinuation of maintenance medications in chronic ambulatory schizophrenic patients usually leads to relapse. Some clinicians still advocate a trial with no medication for patients who have attained a complete remission for about 6 months or for those who have been in chronic care settings and are being maintained on very low doses of medication. The clinician must remember that these agents leave the body slowly; therefore, drug-related relapse may not occur until weeks or months after discontinuation. One possible approach to trial discontinuation in chronically schizophrenic patients is to decrease the maintenance dosage by about 30%. If no deterioration is seen in 6 to 8 weeks, further decreases of 30% can be attempted at similar intervals. When a patient's aftercare program provides for reasonably frequent visits, the clinician should be able to see whether a patient's clinical status is beginning to deteriorate. In most instances, the medication can be reinstituted or the dosage can be increased before frank relapse occurs.

Many patients in aftercare status do not follow their prescribed treatment regimens. They may purchase or pick up their pills but then not swallow them. This may even happen when the pills are handed directly to the patient. Some data with CAPs suggest that a small number of very chronic patients require at least 2 years of antipsychotic drug treatment before changes are seen and that these changes are sometimes limited to more integrated behavior in a sheltered and structured living situation. What significant changes for which chronically ill patients can be accomplished in these expected outcomes with the use of **clozapine** or other AAPs has not yet been fully established.

Controlled studies generally show the benefits of the continuous use of antipsychotic agents to both chronic and acute schizophrenic patients. Depot medications may be necessary and appropriate for facilitating this in some patients.

6. **General comments and specific considerations**
   a. **Oral dosage forms** are usually effective. Time-release or sustained-action forms should not be necessary because of the long half-lives of these compounds. **Liquid forms** may be necessary for some patients, but they significantly increase the cost per milligram of most drugs.
   b. The use of **more than one antipsychotic agent** at a time is seldom indicated. Little evidence exists to suggest that combining drugs is more useful than raising the dose of one drug or switching to another drug. One exception may be the initial use of **haloperidol** or **risperidone** during the early weeks of exposure to **olanzapine**. (*Note:* Rather than combining agents, some clinicians prefer to use a loading dose approach with **olanzapine**, instead of following the usual strategy of gradual incremental dosing.)
   c. **Long-acting (depot forms) antipsychotic agents** may be indicated for patients who are unreliable medication takers. Estimates are that significant problems with adherence—not taking one's medication in the amount or frequency prescribed or missing days rather than merely skipping occasional doses—occur in 20% to 50% of chronically ill schizophrenic patients. Some studies suggest that most schizophrenic patients who stop their medications will relapse within 12 months. Several conventional agents are available in a variety of long-acting formulations as follows: **fluphenazine enanthate** (usually effective for 10 to 14 days), **fluphenazine decanoate** (usually effective for 14 to 21 days), and **haloperidol decanoate** (usually effective for 26 to 30 days). Dosage conversion is generally based on the assumption that 5 mg per day of oral **fluphenazine** equals 25 mg of either **fluphenazine enanthate** or **fluphenazine decanoate** given every 10 to 14 or 14 to 21 days, respectively; 5 mg per day of oral **haloperidol** is replaced by **haloperidol decanoate** given monthly (50 to 75 mg). Individual adjustment of dosage to meet a specific patient's needs is essential, and the lowest possible dose should be given. Customary maintenance doses of these depot

agents are 5 to 50 mg every 3 weeks for **fluphenazine decanoate**, 5 to 75 mg every 2 weeks for **fluphenazine enanthate**, and 50 to 150 mg every 4 weeks for **haloperidol decanoate**. A slightly increased incidence of neuroleptic malignant syndrome (see Chapter 3) and TD may be associated with the use of these depot forms. Some estimates suggest that the use of depot preparations can reduce relapse rates among chronically ill patients by up to about 45%.

   Risperidone is also available as a long-acting injectable microsphere formulation for i.m. use that is given every 2 weeks (25 to 75 mg). The microspheres are made from a biodegradable polymer. The side effects associated with its use are considerably milder than those seen in patients taking conventional depot antipsychotic agents; they consist mainly of headache, agitation, drowsiness, and increased anxiety.

d. **Drug interactions** are discussed in Chapter 29. Particularly noteworthy are the pharmacodynamic interactions involving other drugs with anticholinergic effects (e.g., **thioridazine** plus **amitriptyline**); **carbamazepine**'s ability to induce the metabolism of antipsychotic agents, such as **haloperidol**; and the increased clearance of **quetiapine** by **thioridazine** (putatively through induction of cytochrome P-450 [CYP] 3A4).

e. The use of **electroconvulsive therapy** for schizophrenic patients is discussed in Chapter 24.

f. The use of **antidepressants** in schizophrenic patients is briefly discussed in section I.E.2.

g. **Lithium** and **mood-stabilizing anticonvulsants**, when added to antipsychotic agents, may be beneficial in some schizoaffective patients of the excited type who do not respond adequately to the antipsychotic agents alone. (*Note:* The use of **lithium** for patients without a bipolar disorder diagnosis is not currently approved by the FDA.) In many instances, these patients actually may have an atypical bipolar disorder; subsequent episodes sometimes clarify the diagnosis. The dosage of **lithium** should be monitored and kept as low as possible. Some reports in the literature suggest a lowered threshold to neurotoxicity from **lithium** when it is combined with antipsychotic agents such as **haloperidol**. A few patients who have developed neurotoxicity while taking the combination of **lithium** and an antipsychotic agent were in seclusion rooms on extremely hot days or they had concomitant febrile illnesses. The importance of these factors for the appearance of neurotoxicity is not known (see Chapter 19).

h. **Clozapine** is a dibenzodiazepine derivative, and it is the first marketed agent in the United States to be considered an AAP. It is an effective treatment for both positive and negative symptoms in schizophrenic patients; its FDA approval is limited to refractory schizophrenia. About 50% to 60% of the 5% to 25% of patients with schizophrenia who do not respond to a CAP and perhaps half of the 5% to 20% who are intolerant to these agents because of the untreatable extrapyramidal side effects show noticeable improvement on **clozapine**. Moreover, **clozapine** provides an additional 20% benefit in the treatment of chronically ill schizophrenic patients. Although its current FDA approval is for use in refractory or treatment-resistant schizophrenic patients, it also appears to be beneficial in other schizophrenic patients and for psychoses secondary to L-**dopa** or **bromocriptine** (i.e., in patients treated for Parkinson disease). Its mechanism of action is not fully clarified, but it is an antagonist at D_4, D_3, D_2, and D_1 receptors and at 5-HT_{2A} and 5-HT_{2C} receptors. Its affinity for limbic D_2 receptors is three times greater than that for striatal D_2 receptors. In contrast to other CAP-type D_2 antagonists, it produces only transient elevations in plasma prolactin concentrations (secondary to its capacity to increase briefly dopamine turnover in tuberoinfundibular neurons). Other antipsychotic agents known to produce an increase in dopamine turnover are **thioridazine** and **quetiapine**; however, **thioridazine** produces a somewhat more sustained increase in prolactin levels.

Clozapine's half-life is about 8 hours, and its time to peak plasma concentration is about 2.5 hours. Up to 6 months may be required for **clozapine** to reach its full effectiveness. Plasma levels can be used to guide dosage; preliminary observations suggest that optimal levels may be in the range of 375 to 450 ng per mL. The manufacturer recommends divided dosing, and the dosage interval typically is twice a day.

Clozapine causes sedation, orthostatic hypotension, and hypersalivation (sialorrhea). Its most dangerous toxic effect, which occurs in about 1% to 2% of exposed patients, is agranulocytosis; the risk may be higher in Eastern European (Ashkenazi) Jews, elderly women, and people born in Finland. **Clozapine** has a low risk for causing TD, although a few cases have been reported in patients previously taking other CAPs. Other AAPs also are less likely than CAPs to put patients at risk for TD. Seizures are more common at doses greater than 600 mg per day. Weight gain and increased insulin resistance can occur.

i. **Risperidone** was the second AAP to be approved. Its approval is for the treatment of psychosis. A member of the benzisoxazole class, it binds with high affinity as an antagonist at both the 5-HT$_2$ and D_2 receptors (its D_2 affinity is 100 times greater than its D_1 affinity). Some authorities have been reluctant to classify **risperidone** as an AAP because, at higher doses, extrapyramidal side effects are not uncommon.

Risperidone is rapidly absorbed orally, and it reaches peak plasma concentrations after about 1 hour. Its elimination half-life together with its active metabolite 9-hydroxy**risperidone** is about 1 day. **Risperidone** is a CYP 2D6 substrate. Its modal effective dosage range is 4 to 8 mg per day, but a few studies have shown efficacy within the range of 2 to 16 mg per day. The manufacturer recommends once or twice daily dosing. Mild drowsiness, as well as tiredness and weakness, is not uncommon. As has been noted, some postural hypotension and extrapyramidal effects, particularly akathisia, have been observed, particularly in the higher dosage range. These effects are consistent with its profile of activity at various central nervous system receptors; in addition to its 5-HT$_2$ and D_2 effects, it shows H_1 antagonism and transient α_1-adrenergic antagonism. **Risperidone** raises prolactin levels in a pattern that is more similar to CAPs than to other AAPs.

j. **Quetiapine**, a dibenzothiazepine, is an orally administered AAP that is approved for the treatment of psychosis. As a CYP 3A4 substrate, it is affected by both CYP 3A4 inhibitors and inducers (see Chapter 29). Its half-life is 6 hours, and peak concentrations are reached in 1.5 hours. The manufacturer recommends that dosing occur on a twice or three times a day schedule. **Quetiapine** has predictable sedating properties and minimal anticholinergic activity, and some clinicians consider it to be particularly useful for elderly patients. One caution regarding this latter use is **quetiapine's** potential to cause orthostatic hypotension. Although periodic eye examinations are formally recommended, this precaution derives mainly from animal, rather than human, toxicity data.

k. **Olanzapine** is a thienobenzodiazepine AAP that is approved for the treatment of psychosis. A partial substrate for CYP 1A2, its clearance is subject to both inhibition and induction (e.g., from aromatic hydrocarbons in cigarette smoke) by agents affecting this pathway (see Chapter 29). Weight gain and increased insulin resistance are drawbacks to this effective and widely accepted AAP. Some data suggest that both **olanzapine** and **clozapine** are inverse agonists at 5-HT_{2C} receptors; this may be linked to the tendency of both of these agents to be associated with weight gain. Sedation and anticholinergic effects are moderate. After the oral administration of a single dose, **olanzapine** reaches peak concentrations after 6 hours. Its half-life ranges from 21 to 54 hours. The manufacturer recommends once daily dosing. A unique orally disintegrating tablet formulation is also available; this can be useful for selected patients, particularly those with swallowing difficulties.

   l. **Ziprasidone** is the most recently marketed AAP. The capsule formulation is approved for schizophrenia. Although it is an antagonist at both dopamine and serotonin postsynaptic receptors, **ziprasidone** also affects additional binding sites, including histamine (H_1) receptor antagonism and the blockade of presynaptic transporters for serotonin and norepinephrine. Unlike other antipsychotic agents, it is an agonist at α_1-adrenergic receptors. **Ziprasidone** has a half-life of 7 hours, and peak concentrations are reached 6 to 8 hours after a single oral dose. Twice daily dosing is recommended by the manufacturer. It is a CYP 3A4 substrate, but its major pathway is via aldehyde oxidase, which renders it less likely to be involved in pharmacokinetic drug interactions (i.e., no clinically used inhibitors or inducers of aldehyde oxidase are known). Only modest changes (30% to 40%) in **ziprasidone's** area under the plasma concentration curve are found when CYP 3A4 inducers or inhibitors are coingested. Product information warns of QTc interval prolongation; in perspective, though, use of this agent may convey a risk comparable with that of many other antipsychotic agents and may have less risk than that from **thioridazine, mesoridazine,** or **droperidol**.

   m. **Aripiprazole** is an AAP developed in Japan and marketed in Mexico that is now available in the United States. It has a unique binding profile because it accomplishes its postsynaptic D_2 effects not as a competitive receptor antagonist but as a partial agonist instead. It is also a partial agonist at the 5-HT_{1A} receptors and an antagonist at the 5-HT_{2A} receptors. The advantages and disadvantages of this drug are not yet fully understood. However, improved tolerability has been seen in "switching" studies. The improvements noted to date depend on the comparator drug (e.g., variable weight loss when given after **olanzapine,** lowered prolactin levels after **risperidone,** less extrapyramidal side effects [e.g., akathisia] compared with **haloperidol**). The typical daily dose is 30 mg per day.

7. **Additional comments on side effects**. Side effects and toxic reactions of antipsychotic drugs are varied; they potentially are extremely serious. They include neurologic and hepatic effects, hormonal alterations, weight gain, increased insulin resistance, blood dyscrasias, and pigmentary retinopathy (*note:* to avoid pigmentary retinopathy, an upper limit of 800 mg is placed on **thioridazine** dosage by the manufacturer). A full discussion of all possible reactions is beyond the scope of this chapter; nevertheless, prescribing clinicians must be thoroughly familiar with these reactions before using antipsychotic agents. Some side effects occur with sufficient frequency to merit brief review here (Table 20.11). *Even though some schizophrenic patients may not fully comprehend discussions of potential side effects from these agents, discussing side effects with the patient and with any family members whenever this is possible is important.*

   a. **Nonspecific sedation**. Agitation, hyperactivity, and disordered sleep are common manifestations of schizophrenia. Because antipsychotic

TABLE 20.11. PATTERNS OF SIDE EFFECTS OF ANTIPSYCHOTIC AGENTS DURING ACUTE TREATMENT[a]

Antipsychotic Agent	Anticholinergic (Muscarinic)	Extrapyramidal (Dopamine)	Hypotensive (Norepinephrine/ Adrenergic)	Sedative (Histamine)
Chlorpromazine	++	++	++[b]	++++
Fluphenazine	+	++++	+	+
Perphenazine	+	++++	+	++
Trifluoperazine	+	++++	+	+
Mesoridazine	++	+	++	++++
Thioridazine	+++	+	++	++++
Chlorprothixene	++	++	++	+++
Thiothixene	+	+++	+	+
Haloperidol	+	++++	+	+
Molindone	+	+	+	++
Loxapine	++	++	++	++
Pimozide	+	++	++	+
Clozapine	+++[c]	++	++	+++
Risperidone	+++	++[d]	+	+[e]
Olanzapine	++	+	+	+++
Quetiapine	+	+	++	++
Ziprasidone	+	+	+	++

+, slight; ++, mild; +++, moderate; ++++, strong.
[a] These estimates of the frequencies of selected side effects are based on the author's assessment of the use of these agents during the acute phase of treatment. Patterns may change during longer-term use (e.g., sedative effects usually are reduced).
[b] Intramuscular administration enhances orthostatic (postural) hypotension.
[c] Hypersalivation, particularly at night, is not uncommon.
[d] More likely at higher doses (e.g., >6 mg/d).
[e] Risperidone can be more sedating in youth.

agents ameliorate the contribution of any thought disorder responsible for such manifestations, any drug of this type can have a calming effect and can improve sleep in a psychotic patient. In nonpsychotic persons, antipsychotic agents produce variable nonspecific sedation that depends on the particular drug and the patient's sensitivity to it. Both CAPs and AAPs with histamine (H_1) receptor antagonist properties and, to a slightly lesser extent, piperidine phenothiazines and **ziprasidone** have sedative effects. Other CAPs and AAPs are less sedating. When sedation is the only unwanted effect of an otherwise effective agent, bedtime use or dosage reduction should be attempted before switching to another agent.

The spectrum of effects produced by antipsychotic agents may also be influenced by variables such as the underlying disease for which the agent is being given. A person taking **haloperidol** to relieve nausea and vomiting may experience little or no sedation, whereas the same dose may have a calming or even soporific effect when given to an agitated and sleepless schizophrenic patient.

b. **Adrenergic antagonism.** α_1-Adrenergic receptor antagonist properties of antipsychotic agents approximately parallel their nonspecific sedative effects. Aliphatic phenothiazines, thioxanthenes, and dibenzodiazepines are potent α_1-antagonists; piperazine derivatives, butyrophenones, dihydroindolones, and benzisoxazoles are weak antagonists. Dibenzoxazepines appear to be intermediate. Orthostatic (postural) hypotension is the most important consequence of this property; this effect must be considered, especially when **chlorpromazine**, **chlorprothixene**, **thioridazine**, or **clozapine** is prescribed. An increased risk may also be seen with **quetiapine**. In some instances, drug-induced hypotension has been serious or fatal, but exactly how frequently such events occur has not been established. As was noted earlier, taking the patient's blood pressure in supine and standing positions both before and after a test dose is recommended, particularly in the elderly. Patients who experience mild postural changes should be advised to get up slowly. Nighttime use of pressure (TEDS) stockings may also be beneficial.

A serious episode of orthostatic hypotension should not be treated with **epinephrine**, which is an agonist at both α-adrenergic and β-adrenergic receptors. β-Agonists are contraindicated. **Norepinephrine** and **phenylephrine** are the agents of choice. Serious hypotension and shock must be treated as a medical emergency (see Chapter 3).

A second consequence of α_1-adrenergic antagonism is inhibition of ejaculation. For reasons that are not completely clear, this troublesome side effect is most commonly reported with the piperidine phenothiazine CAPs, **thioridazine**, and **mesoridazine**.

c. **Extrapyramidal symptoms**. CAPs can induce a variety of involuntary motor movements. They are also seen more frequently with high doses of **risperidone** than with lower doses or with other AAPs. Antagonism at dopamine-2 (D_2) receptors in the basal ganglia is the postulated cause of these drug-related extrapyramidal movement disorders. Extrapyramidal effects appear to be correlated with the location and degree of D_2-receptor occupancy by antipsychotic agents (typically greater than 75% to 80%).

   (1) **Acute dystonic reactions**. These are the most troublesome of the extrapyramidal symptoms. These acute spasms of nuchal, truncal, buccal, or oculomotor muscle groups can be frightening or disabling; they typically occur within 10 to 14 days after the initiation of treatment. Because AAPs are currently the most commonly prescribed agents, many clinicians will never see a patient with an acute dystonia. When they do occur, dystonic reactions most frequently are induced by piperazine derivatives (e.g., **trifluoperazine**) or **haloperidol** or with initial high doses of **risperidone**. Acute dystonias can occur in young, otherwise healthy persons, particularly in younger men, after even a single dose of one of these drugs. **Prochlorperazine** is most often implicated in dystonic reactions in children (usually following accidental ingestions). Acute dystonic reactions may require parenteral treatment. **Benztropine** (0.5 to 2 mg) or **diphenhydramine** (25 to 50 mg) given intravenously or i.m. can provide a dramatic reversal of such reactions. For most patients with acute dystonic reactions who need to remain on the same antipsychotic medication, adding oral **benztropine** for the next 10 to 14 days protects them through their period of vulnerability. Treatment for longer than 6 weeks is almost never necessary.

   (2) **Akathisia and drug-induced parkinsonism**. More chronic, insidiously developing extrapyramidal symptoms can occur with any CAP. Occurrence is much less frequent with AAPs. These troublesome symptoms include the syndrome of motor restlessness or **akathisia** and the triad of akinesia, rigidity, and resting tremor resembling **parkinsonism** (often associated with increased salivation). Middle-aged and elderly chronic schizophrenic patients taking CAPs for weeks or months seem to be the most susceptible to drug-induced akathisia or parkinsonism.

Akathisia, which occurs in about 20% of persons receiving CAPs, is experienced subjectively as anxiety, emotional "disease," or inner tension and objectively as frequent pacing, foot shifting or rocking, or leg swinging while sitting. It can feel like a mobile internal anxiety that rushes from the abdomen into the chest. Reasonably predictable relief can be provided by β-adrenergic receptor antagonists (often called β-blockers). Lipophilic β-adrenergic receptor antagonists, such as **propranolol** (20 to 80 mg per day), may be more effective than the more hydrophilic ones (e.g., **nadolol, atenolol**). Anticholinergic antiparkinson agents or benzodiazepines, such as **lorazepam** (0.5 to 2 mg per day), may also provide mild benefit for some patients.

Drug-induced parkinsonism occurs in about 40% of patients treated chronically with CAPs; this can be ameliorated by antiparkinsonian drugs such as **benztropine** or **trihexyphenidyl** in oral doses of 2 to 8 mg per day. Oral antiparkinsonian drugs (Table 20.12) are effective in most patients when they are given once or twice a day. They do not compromise the efficacy of antipsychotic agents. Some authorities suggest that antiparkinsonian drugs should not be given prophylactically; instead, they should be administered only when the extrapyramidal reactions appear. Once therapy is started, it should not be continued indefinitely.

(3) **TD** (Table 20.13) appears in an undetermined percentage of patients who have received long-term treatment with CAPs; it is seen only rarely with AAPs. Signs of TD, however, may also appear in patients who have never received these drugs. The signs of TD may appear with dosage reduction or discontinuation or when another CAP is introduced at lower dosage equivalents. If an agent with D_2 antagonism is introduced at doses that block a sufficient number of receptors, the TD signs may disappear. This can be an effective treatment strategy (i.e., when a CAP is replaced by an AAP and the AAP is then tapered, some patients may no longer have TD). In the author's experience, this latter approach is quite different from the masking of TD that can occur when higher doses of a CAP are prescribed.

In some patients, these signs appear to be related to the patient's development of tolerance to a particular dosage level. Current hypotheses to explain TD generally assume that the condition results from rebound supersensitivity to dopamine in basal ganglion areas that have been subjected to prolonged antagonism at dopamine receptors. An interaction among the

TABLE 20.12. SOME ANTIPARKINSONIAN DRUGS IN CURRENT USE

Generic Name	Trade Name
Tropine derivatives	
Benztropine	Cogentin
Piperidine compounds	
Biperiden	Akineton
Procyclidine	Kemadrin
Trihexyphenidyl	Artane, Pipanol, Tremin
Ethanolamine antihistamines	
Diphenhydramine	Benadryl
Orphenadrine	Disipal

TABLE 20.13. PROMINENT FEATURES OF TARDIVE DYSKINESIAS

Lingual-facial hyperkinesias
  Chewing movements
  Smacking and licking of the lips
  Sucking movements
  Tongue movements within the oral cavity
  Tongue protrusion
  Tongue tremor with mouth open
  Myokemic movements (worm-like movement on the surface of the tongue)
  Blinking
  Grotesque grimaces and spastic facial distortions
Neck and trunk movements
  Spasmodic torticollis
  Retrocollis
  Torsion movements of the trunk
  Axial hyperkinesia (hip-rocking)
Choreoathetoid movements of the extremities

dopaminergic, serotonergic, and cholinergic systems is likely involved. Antiparkinsonian drugs are most often of no benefit; their use may exacerbate the symptoms of TD.

When a patient's clinical condition requires the continued use of antipsychotic agents, both the clinician and the patient must weigh the benefit derived from this against any adverse implications of their continued use. Patients who develop TD are at higher risk for clinical relapse.

d. **Cardiac toxicity**. Possible cardiotoxic effects, including prolongation of the QT interval, by antipsychotic agents also evoke concern. Reports of sudden unexplained deaths among previously healthy patients taking these drugs suggest that some antipsychotic agents may have the potential to precipitate fatal ventricular tachyarrhythmias, such as *torsade de pointes*. In general, caution should be exercised in any patient whose baseline electrocardiogram reveals a QTc interval of greater than 450 ms. Antipsychotic agents should be discontinued when a QTc interval of more than 450 ms occurs. **Thioridazine, mesoridazine**, and **droperidol** carry "black box" warnings about dose-dependent QTc interval prolongation based on accumulated clinical experience or clinical study data (see page **xiv**). The reader should note that drug interactions that reduce the clearance of any of these agents could enhance this risk. As was noted earlier, a concern exists about QTc interval prolongation from **ziprasidone**. Manufacturer's data suggest that the mean changes in the QTc interval after both oral and i.m. **ziprasidone** are comparable with, and that they do not exceed an average prolongation of approximately 10 ms longer than that seen with, **risperidone, olanzapine, quetiapine**, or **haloperidol**. These mean changes are also less than the average increment observed after a 300 mg dose of **thioridazine**.

Thioridazine and **mesoridazine** can also produce electrocardiographic changes resembling hypokalemia; these are almost always modifiable with small amounts of **potassium**. Because these latter changes are usually benign, adding **potassium** supplements is not generally advised. However, true hypokalemia could contribute to life-threatening arrhythmias in patients with prolonged QT intervals secondary to the use of antipsychotic agents.

     e. Cholinergic (muscarinic) receptor antagonism. Many antipsychotic agents have clinically important anticholinergic effects. Manifestations usually are limited to mild dryness of the mouth or tachycardia. In some people, these drugs can exacerbate untreated glaucoma or can precipitate urinary retention or intestinal obstruction. Antipsychotic agents can potentiate toxicity due to other medications with anticholinergic properties, and they should never be used to treat delirium or hyperpyrexia due to muscarinic receptor antagonists. Anticholinergic effects are particularly prominent with **thioridazine** and **clozapine**.

     f. Hepatic disturbances. Hepatic disturbances have been reported with most antipsychotic agents. The incidence of drug-induced jaundice appears to have diminished since the 1950s. **Chlorpromazine** has been more frequently implicated than other agents. Most cases develop during the third and fourth weeks of treatment. The clinical picture and time of onset suggest a hypersensitivity reaction; obstructive jaundice, fever, and eosinophilia are typical. Although some clinical experience suggests that cross-tolerance is rare and that some patients can even be placed back on the same drug without a recurrence, conservative treatment should include switching to another class of antipsychotic drugs (e.g., from a CAP to an AAP), preferably after a drug-free interval.

     g. Leukopenia and agranulocytosis. These rarely occur. Most cases occurring secondary to drugs other than **clozapine** typically appear during the interval between the end of the first month and the beginning of the fourth month. Elderly debilitated women appear to be at the greatest risk. However, careful clinical investigation should be made for any patient who develops pharyngitis or unexplained fevers. Immediate discontinuation of the offending drug and the use of antibiotics may be indicated. **Clozapine** causes agranulocytosis in about 1% to 2% of exposed patients, and regular monitoring of white blood cells is essential. When the white blood cell counts drop below 3×10^{12} per L, discontinuation of **clozapine** is essential. Other AAPs may be an alternative for those patients who cannot tolerate **clozapine**.

C. Psychotherapies

    Barring the unforeseen development of new techniques, Freud discouraged psychotherapeutic work with schizophrenics because he believed that their withdrawal of libido from the object world prevented the formation of a transference, a step he saw as essential to psychotherapy. Subsequent therapists modified this view. P. Federn, one of Freud's pupils, reformulated the therapeutic task as helping patients reestablish faulty ego boundaries. Other specific approaches were developed by M. Klein, M. Schehaye, J. Rosen, H. S. Sullivan, F. Fromm-Reichmann, G. Bychowsky, H. Searles, and many others. Understandably, well-designed studies of various psychotherapies for schizophrenic patients have been rare. A limited number have been conducted in both chronic and acute patients to assess the relative benefits of pharmacotherapies and individual or group psychotherapies. Comparisons among them are difficult because they lack consistency across a variety of important dimensions, including study design, stage of illness, type and frequency of psychotherapy, therapists' training, drugs and dosages used, and outcome measures.

    Despite this, stating some important conclusions is warranted—there are probably no acute or chronic schizophrenic patients who can be treated successfully by individual psychotherapy alone. From a public health point of view, the most useful single therapeutic intervention is antipsychotic medication, which is both the least costly and the most effective way to reduce schizophrenic symptomatology. However, a more preferable approach is a cogently designed multimodality treatment program that provides current pharmacotherapies and psychoeducation, reality-based ego-supportive psychotherapy, appropriate living situations, rehabilitation strategies (i.e., social and job skills training), family therapy, and ample community-based support systems.

For those who have the time and support to carry out such a program, an overview of one approach the author has found useful is presented here. In the first phase (usually hospital based), the focus is on providing the essentials of a trusting relationship, in which the therapist offers "lend-lease" ego strength, and on helping the patient to understand more about schizophrenia and to cope with regularly encountered reality-based issues. Establishing such a stable, trusting relationship is not an easy task for schizophrenic patients; their feelings of fear, indifference, distrust, worthlessness, and hostility may predominate. In beginning such a relationship, the therapist must find a way to establish affective contact with the patient before any understanding of the patient's concerns and feelings is likely to emerge. Because schizophrenic patients often do not communicate how they feel directly, the clinician must place importance on paying close attention to their nonverbal communications, including facial expression, posture, and activity. Furthermore, remembering that words can take on peculiar and concrete meanings for them is of great importance; the therapist must speak in simple, direct, and unambiguous terms. Clinicians must demonstrate constancy in their commitment to patients, together with an ability to share some aspect of their own human responses to the patient in an open constructive way.

During these acute stages, one should avoid making interpretations concerning the emotional conflicts that may have been temporally associated with the patient's decompensation into psychosis. Instead, the emphasis should be placed on gathering information about the patient's recent circumstances and any relevant past history. When this information cannot be obtained from the patient and permission is given by the patient, the patient's relatives or friends should be contacted. One goal of collecting such information is an understanding of any factors that may have contributed to the patient's later vulnerability to schizophrenia or of any events associated with the onset of decompensation. The clinician also needs to learn about the areas of healthy personal and occupational functioning available to the patient. These initial contacts should be brief; 15-minute to 20-minute sessions are often appropriate. Excessive closeness is invariably harmful.

In taking this history, the clinician not only demonstrates a concrete interest in the patient and the facts of his or her life, but he or she also observes the patient's characteristic avoidances of unpleasant feelings and experiences. Such observations of the patient's patterns of denial, distortion, and projection may later allow the therapist to help the patient understand the areas of his or her life that have been the most troublesome.

Bringing the issue of medication into the therapeutic work and exploring patients' feelings about taking medicine or any administrative issues are crucial so that they can be considered in planning treatment. The clinician should also help the patient to understand what is happening on the ward or in other therapeutic or living situations; clarifications about practical matters (e.g., ward policies) may also be beneficial.

As the acuteness of the psychotic process abates and the process of reintegration begins, many patients develop neurasthenic, hypochondriacal, obsessive-compulsive, or depressive symptoms. Suicide may become a serious risk at this time. During this time, the patient may also repeatedly challenge the therapist's interest in continuing the therapeutic relationship. Appointments are often missed by the patient, and both the patient and the therapist may begin to believe that the focus of the therapy has become obscure. From time to time, however, patients are able to use the therapeutic relationship at this stage to integrate some of the experiences and sources of lowered self-esteem that may have stressed them before their decompensation.

Coming to an empathic understanding with the patient of any specific stresses that may have contributed to the onset of the psychosis may also help the patient to anticipate future difficulties. The timing of this phase of the therapeutic work is crucial, and it is usually dependent on the clinician's experience and intuition and the patient's motivation and ability to go into such matters. Whenever possible, the clinician should demonstrate and encourage negotiation and compromise.

In advocating this approach, the author assumes that a schizophrenic patient's predisposition to disorganized thinking under stress has led to difficulties in adapting to and resolving problematic situations. This obviously affects the patient's self-image and experiential learning. The clinician tries to help the patient see what may evoke distortions of reality (e.g., not being able to "stand" feelings of loss, loneliness, helplessness, or rage), what consequences these distortions may have, or even how to limit their consequences. For example, not all patients are terrified by their auditory hallucinations. Some patients can learn to distract themselves from their voices by listening to music, exercising, or meditating. Some can even learn to ignore their voices. Others may learn to listen selectively and then to tell their negative voices that they have no time for them or that they will not listen to them. Still others set time limits for their voices (e.g., "I allow them to speak to me only from 9 p.m. to 10 p.m."). The clinician can try to help the patient increase his or her tolerance of uncertainty and ambiguity in interpersonal relationships. Evaluation of family interactions may provide useful information for therapeutic work, particularly when this reveals a pattern of highly expressed emotion in the family. Some patients are significantly helped by ongoing conjoint work with other family members that aims to lower the intensity of their interactions.

D. Rehabilitation and Psychosocial Therapies During Aftercare

Rehabilitation refers to the process of helping patients develop or relearn those personal, interpersonal, or job skills that could make them more self-reliant and productive members of the community. This process may be a major source of increased self-esteem because it should provide the patient with feelings of increased self-control, competence, and mastery. A patient's premorbid level of adolescent or adult functioning is one of the better indices of eventual ability to resume a more independent life. Those patients who are married or who had a successful vocational adjustment before their illness are more likely to achieve a successful adjustment. A given patient's probability of returning to community life often depends on the availability of adequate social supports.

Psychosocial therapies encourage rehabilitation and improved interpersonal relationships. Techniques such as major role therapy emphasize coping with personal and environmental factors that may contribute to relapse, and they try to determine what rates and types of activities lead to improvement rather than regression for each patient. For example, working on improving eye contact or on reducing any awkward or inappropriate gestures or facial expressions may be helpful. That a number of clinical studies have demonstrated that settings (e.g., families, groups, programs) that are too high in both positive and negative expressed emotions can be stressful for many chronically ill patients should not be surprising. Expectations should be appropriate to the current state of the patient and not to notions of what the patient should be accomplishing based on prior history (e.g., education, family background, prior work). Aftercare efforts that integrate medications, rehabilitation opportunities, and appropriate psychosocial therapies with family education and support, 24-hour crisis intervention teams, and varying community-based living arrangements have the highest likelihood of maintaining patients outside of hospitals and of improving their quality of life.

VII. The National Alliance for the Mentally Ill

National Alliance for the Mentally Ill (NAMI) is a critically important lay organization that provides support and education to families and patients and advocacy for improved and comprehensive services and research. NAMI's national telephone number is (800) 950-NAMI; more than 1,000 local chapters exist.

VIII. Treatment Algorithms

Algorithms for treatment of schizophrenia can be found in Appendix VII.

ADDITIONAL READING

Andreasen NC. Negative symptoms in schizophrenia: definition and reliability. *Arch Gen Psychiatry* 1982;39:784–788.

Arnold OH. *Schizophrener Prozess und Schizophrene Symptomgesetze.* Vienna: Maudrich, 1955.

Benkert O, Grunder G, Wetzel H. Dopamine autoreceptor agonists in the treatment of schizophrenia and major depression. *Pharmacopsychiatria* 1992;25:254–260.

Bleuler M. A 23-year longitudinal study of 208 schizophrenics and impressions in regard to the nature of schizophrenia. In: Rosenthal D, Kety S, eds. *Transmission of schizophrenia.* Oxford: Pergamon, 1968:3–12.

Carpenter WT Jr, Buchanan RW, Kirkpatrick B, et al. Diazepam treatment of early signs of exacerbation in schizophrenia. *Am J Psychiatry* 1999;156:299–303.

Chouinard G, Jones B, Remington G, et al. A Canadian multicenter placebo-controlled study of fixed doses of risperidone and haloperidol in the treatment of chronic schizophrenic patients. *J Clin Psychopharmacol* 1993;13:25–40.

Crespo-Facorro B, Kim JJ, Andreasen NC, et al. Insular cortex abnormalities in schizophrenia. *Schizophr Res* 2000;46:34–43.

Crespo-Facorro B, Paradiso S, Andreasen NC, et al. Neural mechanisms of anhedonia in schizophrenia. *JAMA* 2001;286:427–435.

Currier GW, Simpson GM. Risperidone liquid concentrate versus intramuscular haloperidol and intramuscular lorazepam for treatment of psychotic agitation. *J Clin Psychiatry* 2001;62:153–157.

Daniel DG, Potkin SG, Reeves KR, et al. Intramuscular (IM) ziprasidone 20 mg is effective in reducing acute agitation associated with psychosis: a double-blind, randomized trial. *Psychopharmacology* 2001;155:128–134.

de Leon J, Peralta V, Cuesta MJ. Negative symptoms and emotional blunting in schizophrenia. *J Clin Psychiatry* 1993;3:103–108.

Fenton WW. Evolving perspectives on individual psychotherapy for schizophrenia. *Schizophr Bull* 2000;26:47–72.

Freedman R, Leonard S, Gault JM, et al. Linkage disequilibrium for schizophrenia at the chromosome 15q13-14 locus of the α7-nicotinic acetylcholine receptor subunit gene (CHRNA7). *Am J Med Genet* 2001;105:20–22.

Glazer WM, Kane JM. Depot neuroleptic therapy: an underutilized treatment option. *J Clin Psychiatry* 1992;53:426–433.

Gottesman II. *Schizophrenia genesis.* New York: Freeman, 1991.

Grinspoon L, Ewalt JR, Shader RI. *Schizophrenia: pharmacotherapy and psychotherapy.* Baltimore: Williams & Wilkins, 1972.

Guidotti A, Auta J, Davis J, et al. Reelin and GAD67 expression is decreased in postmortem brain of schizophrenia and bipolar disorder patients. *Arch Gen Psychiatry* 2000;57:1061–1069.

Hogarty GE. Prevention of relapse in chronic schizophrenic patients. *J Clin Psychiatry* 1993;3:18S–23S.

Hogarty GE, Greenwald D, Ulrich RF, et al. Three-year trials of personal psychotherapy among schizophrenic patients living with or independent of family. II. Effects on adjustment of patients. *Am J Psychiatry* 1997;154:1514–1524.

Hogarty GE, Kornblith SJ, Greenwald D, et al. Three-year trials of personal psychotherapy among schizophrenic patients living with or independent of family. I. Description of study effects and relapse rates. *Am J Psychiatry* 1997;154:1504–1513.

Janicak PG, Keck PE Jr, Davis JM, et al. A double-blind, randomized prospective evaluation of the efficacy of risperidone versus haloperidol in the treatment of schizoaffective disorder. *J Clin Psychopharmacol* 2001;21:360–368.

Kane JM. Dosage strategies with long-acting injectable neuroleptics, including haloperidol decanoate. *J Clin Psychopharmacol* 1986;6:20S–23S.

Kay SR. *Positive and negative syndromes in schizophrenia.* New York: Brunner-Mazel, 1991.

Kerr IB, Taylor D. Acute disturbed or violent behavior: principles of treatment. *J Psychopharmacol* 1999;11:271–277.

Liberman RP, Evans CC. Behavioral rehabilitation for chronic mental patients. *J Clin Psychopharmacol* 1985;5:8S–14S.

Lieberman JA. Prediction of outcome in first-episode schizophrenia. *J Clin Psychiatry* 1993;3:13S–17S.

Marder SR. Depot neuroleptics: side effects and safety. *J Clin Psychopharmacol* 1986;6:24S–29S.

Melle I, Friis F, Hauff E, et al. Patients with schizophrenia after the acute ward: seven years' service utilization and clinical course. *Nordic J Psychiatry* 2000;54:47–54.

Meltzer HY, ed. *Novel antipsychotic drugs.* New York: Raven, 1992.

Nordström AL, Farde L, Wiesel FA, et al. Central D_2-dopamine receptor occupancy in relation to antipsychotic drug effects: a double-blind PET study of schizophrenic patients. *Biol Psychiatry* 1993;33:227–235.

Shader RI, DiMascio A, eds. *Psychotropic drug side effects.* Baltimore: Williams & Wilkins, 1970.

Stein LI. A system approach to reducing relapse in schizophrenia. *J Clin Psychiatry* 1993;3:7S–12S.

Stephens JH. Long-term course and prognosis in schizophrenia. *Semin Psychiatry* 1970;2:464–485.

Task Force Report. *Tardive dyskinesia.* Washington, D.C.: American Psychiatric Association, 1992.

Tran PV, Dellva MA, Tollefson GD, et al. Oral olanzapine versus oral haloperidol in maintenance treatment of schizophrenia and related psychoses. *Br J Psychiatry* 1998;172:499–505.

Tsuang MT, Stone WS, Faraone SV. Schizophrenia: a review of genetic studies. *Harvard Rev Psychiatry* 1999;7:185–207.

Tupin JP. Focal neuroleptization: an approach to optimal dosing for initial and continuing therapy. *J Clin Psychopharmacol* 1985;5:15S–21S.

Waddington JL. Schizophrenia: developmental neuroscience and pathobiology. *Lancet* 1993;341:531–538.

Wright JC, Ellison ZR, Sharma T, et al. Mapping grey matter changes in schizophrenia. *Schizophr Res* 1999;35:1–14.

21. APPROACHES TO THE PSYCHOPHARMACOLOGIC TREATMENT OF CHILDREN AND YOUTH

Jessica R. Oesterheld
Richard I. Shader
Dean X. Parmelee
Aradhana Bela Sood

The initial psychiatric evaluation of youth is often more complex and time-consuming than is the evaluation of adults. The following three sources of information must be tapped: parents (e.g., reason for referral, child's current and past functioning, child's past developmental and medical history, family functioning, and psychiatric history), teachers (e.g., child's cognitive functioning, learning style, symptoms present in school, and peer relations), and the youth (e.g., current and past symptoms and concerns, responses to important life events, and world view). Younger children may reveal information about themselves through their play and drawings. Most clinicians who evaluate children use a variety of standardized rating scales during the assessment process.

Parents and teachers may disagree on their views of the child because of bias or because children may behave differently in different settings (e.g., mild oppositional behavior may be evident only at home; bullying other children may be evident only on the playground). The clinician-evaluator must integrate all data and must place the information into a developmental, familial, cultural, and gender perspective to generate a differential diagnosis and to initiate a comprehensive treatment plan.

A modest research base for informing the development of psychologic and pharmacologic treatment plans for youth has hobbled clinicians. Because the United States Food and Drug Administration (FDA) and the National Institutes of Health have required or supported more research in pediatric psychopharmacology since 1995, a meaningful increase has occurred in studies and publications in this field. This has included the establishment of multicenter Research Units for Pediatric Psychopharmacology, which have begun to tackle questions about the efficacy of medications in youth for conditions such as anxiety disorders that have long been answered in adults. Disorders of childhood, such as Tourette disorder and attention deficit hyperactivity disorder (ADHD), are considered separately in Chapters 7 and 22. In this chapter, schizophrenia; autism; and disorders of conduct, mood, and anxiety are reviewed. Only issues of diagnosis and treatment specific to youth are included; the reader is referred to the appropriate general chapters for a more in-depth presentation of each disorder.

I. Major Depressive Disorder

Major depressive disorder (MDD) is a common psychiatric condition in youth that has been shown to be increasing in prevalence in each generation since the 1940s and that is developing in successively younger individuals (a cohort effect). Several decades ago, the diagnosis of MDD in youth was controversial because psychoanalytic theory precluded the possibility of the development of depression until the "superego" was formed. Although accurate diagnosis requires that the criteria of the *Diagnostic and Statistical Manual of Mental Disorders*, 4th edition (DSM-IV), are met (see Chapter 18), important, recognizable, developmentally based differences are evident in the presentation of depression symptoms in children and teenagers. Children are more likely to have concomitant anxiety (phobias, separation anxiety), somatic complaints (headaches and stomachaches), auditory hallucinations, irritability, frustration, temper tantrums, and behavioral problems. Adolescents show more irritability, sleep and appetite disturbances (e.g., hypersomnia and hyperphagia), delusions, and suicidal ideation and attempts. Recent research suggests that MDD may be chronic, familial, and recurrent. Childhood depression often persists into adulthood, and it is frequently compounded by comorbid bereavement (see Chapter 16), substance abuse, or anxiety or disruptive behavior disorders. Early identification, treatment, and diligent follow-up help to prevent the poor psychosocial and academic outcomes such as academic failure, teenage pregnancy, eating and substance abuse disorders, and attempted or completed suicide, that often result from this disorder.

Suicide prevention (see Chapter 17) is the highest goal for assessing and treating any child or adolescent with depression. Population studies suggest MDD prevalence rates of 0.4% to 2.5% for depression in children and 4% to 8% for adolescents. The lifetime prevalence rate of MDD for adolescents is about 15%, which is similar to the estimated adult prevalence rate of about 17%. The comparable figures for **dysthymic disorder** (DD) are 0.6% to 1.7% for children and 1.6% to 8% for adolescents. Although MDD in childhood occurs equally in boys and girls, adolescent girls over age 14 are affected at almost twice the rate of adolescent boys. This trend persists through the reproductive years, suggesting that hormonal and other developmental factors appearing during puberty may have an important etiologic role in this disorder.

In youth, a typical untreated episode lasts between 7 and 9 months. Relapse is common, and recurrence rates may be as high as 50% after 1 to 2 years and 70% after 5 years. Chronicity is evident in only 10% of first-episode cases. Youth with chronic depression have an earlier onset, a greater number and severity of prior episodes, poor compliance, psychosocial adversity, parental psychiatric illness, and adverse life events. For the diagnosis of DD, the child or adolescent must have had a 1-year period of dysphoric mood, wherein the signs and symptoms are quite similar to those of MDD but are fewer and less severe. Recent evidence shows that DD may have a chronic course and that it commonly acts as a "gateway" to the development of MDD. The clinician should remember that not all youth who show symptoms of depression develop a mood disorder.

Children and teens with MDD commonly have comorbid diagnoses (e.g., DD, anxiety disorders, substance abuse, disruptive behaviors, somatoform disorders, and personality traits), and the presence of comorbidity impacts the risk for recurrent depression, the duration of an episode, suicidal behaviors, poor psychosocial and/or academic function, and the benefits from treatment interventions. For example, youth with "double depression" (MDD plus DD) tend to have longer and more severe depressive episodes, increased suicidality, and poorer overall functioning. These youth are often significantly more impaired socially and less competent than their peers with either MDD or DD alone. Youth with co-occurring anxiety and MDD may also have poor outcomes.

A. Diagnosis, Etiology, and Assessment

Depression in a child or adolescent is the result of a confluence of biologic and environmental factors. Numerous twin and adoption studies have demonstrated that genetic factors account for at least 50% of the variance in the transmission of mood disorders for the adult population, and genetic studies have further indicated that environmental factors play a significant role in the onset, duration, and course of depression. Family aggregation studies have suggested that children of depressed parents are much more likely to have a lifetime episode of MDD, and the first-degree relatives of children with depression have lifetime prevalence rates of depression that range from 20% to 46%. Children appear to be highly sensitive to environmental events in both the development and the maintenance of depressive symptoms (e.g., children's depressive symptoms may relent when hospitalized for a short stay). Environmental factors that may predate the onset of signs and symptoms of a depressive disorder in a child or adolescent include adverse life events, such as loss or separation of a parent or other caregiver, the loss of a romantic relationship, change in peer group and/or school because of a family move, parental discord, and psychiatric illness in one or both parents. Studies suggest that depressed children may have cognitive styles that differ from nondepressed children in that they see the world more negatively. Many depressed children believe that they have less control over their lives, and they lack the social skills that seem to protect nondepressed children.

The most effective approach for the treatment of a child or adolescent who is depressed begins with a comprehensive assessment (Table 21.1). The clinical interview is the starting point for the evaluation of any child or adolescent with a possible depressive disorder. A careful assessment can reduce tension in the family; improve the bond between parents and child; reduce the risk of suicidal behaviors; and create a working alliance with the physician, which is necessary for treatment compliance. The parents and others who are important in the child's life serve as sources of information about changes in the child's mood and behavior. Although a careful detailed history from the parents is vital, the frequency of parents' lack of awareness of their children's suicidal thoughts or actions, hallucinations, delusions, or substance abuse is surprising. Children must therefore be afforded the opportunity to speak privately and must be given enough time to enable the clinician to explore the circumstances surrounding, and the progression of, mood and affect changes. Developmentally sensitive questioning about symptoms is essential. A series of pictures of different facial expressions may be used to initiate a conversation about feelings with younger children as follows:

What feeling does this face show?
After the identification of happy, sad, scared, angry, ask "Do you ever feel happy?"
When do you feel happy?
Do you ever feel sad?
When do you feel sad?

At times, clinicians may use a "mood thermometer," a ranking from 0 to 10 that indicates sad to increasingly happier faces.

If 0 is "I wish I were dead" and 10 is "I am feeling really, really happy," what number are you right now?
What is the highest number you ever feel?
When do you feel that way?
What is the lowest number you ever feel?
When did you feel that way?
Have you ever felt like a 0?

Children may prefer to interact with play or drawing materials as a way of displacing their feelings, or they may simply be more comfortable talking with an adult if they are allowed to engage in familiar activities such as drawing. Clinicians should be alert to any anhedonic quality and themes of death and destruction in the play of a depressed child. Several clinician and self-administered rating scales can be helpful in screening for depressive symptoms.

Medical conditions may first present with signs and symptoms of depression in children and adolescents, and they must be considered when evaluating for depression (e.g., hepatitis, influenza, infectious mononucleosis, acquired immunodeficiency syndrome, Cushing disease, hypothyroidism,

TABLE 21.1. ASSESSMENT OF YOUTHS WITH DEPRESSIVE SYMPTOMS

Clinical interviews of patient and caregivers, both separately and together
Family history of psychiatric illnesses
Identification of comorbid conditions, especially substance use
Review of medical conditions that may present with depression in this age group
Determination of suicide risk, "cleaning house" of possible weapons, setting a contract, if possible (see Chapter 17)
Use of rating scales (Children's Depression Inventory, Beck Depression Inventory, Reynold's Adolescent Depression Scale)

hyperparathyroidism, lupus erythematosus, porphyria, and uremia). Of importance is the recognition that youth with certain conditions may be prone to the development of mood disorders (e.g., diabetes mellitus, seizure disorders, velocardiofacial syndrome, physical abuse, anxiety disorders, eating disorders, substance abuse, conduct disorders [CDs]).

B. Treatment

1. **Psychoeducational approaches.** As outcome studies of schizophrenia and depression in adults have shown (see Chapters 18 and 20), patients and families benefit from learning about their illnesses. Children and adolescents and their families are often relieved to learn that they have a "treatable" or "understandable" illness. Furthermore, in describing the illness, the clinician can build rapport, enlist compliance with the treatment recommendations, and encourage patience with a prolonged treatment process. When the parents themselves suffer from depressive disorders, the appropriate referral should be initiated.

2. **Psychotherapy.** This approach has benefit for depressed children or adolescents who have mild or moderate forms of depression (some evidence for efficacy is also seen in severe depression). Individual and group cognitive-behavior therapy (CBT), interpersonal therapy, and psychodynamic psychotherapy have all shown benefit when tailored to the specific needs of the child or adolescent and his or her family. Dialectic behavioral therapy may be useful for teens with suicidal behaviors. The use of one or more of these psychotherapeutic approaches is important for more severely depressed children or adolescents and for those whose family backgrounds and situations (e.g., psychiatric and/or drug-dependent illness in parents, contentious divorce) place them at greater risk for chronic depression and suicidal behaviors.

3. **Pharmacotherapy.** Medication is not usually first-line treatment, except in certain contexts (e.g., unwillingness to participate in psychotherapy, a previously adequate but ineffective psychotherapeutic trial, a high suicidal risk, the presence of severe or psychotic symptoms). In contrast to adults, a limited number of double-blind, placebo-controlled studies demonstrate the efficacy of selective serotonin reuptake inhibitors (SSRIs) in the treatment of depression in children and adolescents. **Fluoxetine** is approved for use in youth 7 years of age and older. No similar studies of **bupropion, venlafaxine, mirtazapine,** or **nefazodone** nor of augmentation strategies have been conducted for treatment-resistant depression in youth. Tricyclic antidepressants (TCAs) are rarely used as an initial treatment in these age groups because no proven benefit over a placebo has been found in many drug trials. TCAs may have untoward side effects, especially cardiovascular ones; they may be lethal in overdose.

A few pharmacokinetic studies of youth have been completed, but dosing of the SSRIs in children is generally initiated in lower doses than in those seen with adolescents and adults because weight-corrected plasma levels in children are generally higher than they are in teens or adults. A typical regimen would be to initiate **fluoxetine** (5 to 10 mg per day orally) and to increase the dose up to 20 mg as tolerated after 2 to 3 weeks once evidence of at least minimal clinical improvement is seen (Table 21.2). Antidepressant dosing regimens of adolescents are similar to those for adults.

As in adults, adverse effects have been reported with all the SSRIs (see Chapter 18). Slight decreases in growth have been observed in youth on **fluoxetine.** Compared with adults, an increased rate of akathisia and behavioral activation may occur when these drugs (especially with higher doses of **fluoxetine**) are initiated in youth. (*Note:* Activation is *not* diagnostic of bipolar vulnerability.) Because some have suggested that as many as one-fourth of youth with depression develop manic symptoms, clinicians should be alert to frank manic symptoms that emerge later in the course of treatment after the depressive symptoms have relented.

TABLE 21.2. DOSING OF SELECTIVE SEROTONIN REUPTAKE INHIBITORS IN YOUTH

Drug	Usual dosage range (mg) in children less than 12 years of age
Citalopram	10–20
Fluvoxamine	25–200
Fluoxetine	5–20
Paroxetine	5–20
Sertraline	25–150

An increasing number of reports have been made of childhood central serotonin syndrome, which is now known as toxic serotonin syndrome (e.g., altered consciousness, hyperreflexia, myoclonus), after the initiation or a dosage increase of SSRIs or with the addition of other proserotonergic drugs (e.g., **clomipramine [CMI]**, **lithium**, and **meperidine**) (see also Chapters 3 and 29). After successful treatment with SSRIs (or other antidepressants), some youth who have been socially withdrawn or apathetic begin to demonstrate new-onset oppositional behavior. Amotivational syndrome, epistaxis, and easy bruising are rarely reported. Sexual symptoms should be investigated sensitively. Clinicians should obtain a careful drug history of all prescription drugs, over-the-counter medications, herbals and dietary supplements, and illicit drugs because all the newer antidepressants are cytochrome P-450 substrates and most inhibit P-450 cytochromes to varying degrees. Clinicians must be cognizant of possible drug interactions when SSRIs are combined with psychotropic or nonpsychotropic agents. For example, if **fluvoxamine** was added to **CMI**, a child could develop profound sedation secondary to an increased concentration of CMI. If **fluvoxamine** was then abruptly discontinued, the child could develop a flu-like syndrome from the abruptly reduced concentrations of CMI. Similar discontinuation symptoms may also occur when SSRIs are abruptly withdrawn, and they may be more common with **paroxetine** and **fluvoxamine**, but all SSRIs except **fluoxetine** should be gradually tapered.

If only some improvement is seen after administering the agent at full doses for 2 to 3 weeks, the clinician may augment the agent with **lithium** or **buspirone**. When no clinical improvement is seen or intolerable side effects have developed in 4 to 6 weeks, switching to another SSRI is common. Moving to a TCA (see Chapter 18), **venlafaxine**, **nefazodone**, **bupropion**, or **mirtazapine** may be indicated if the child or adolescent either fails to respond well to separate trials of two SSRIs or has a particularly adverse response to these agents. See Table 21.3 for dosing recommendations for these non-SSRI antidepressants.

TABLE 21.3. USUAL DOSING OF SELECTED ANTIDEPRESSANTS IN YOUTHS

Drug	Usual dosage range in children less than 12 years of age
Bupropion IR	3–6 mg/kg/d in t.i.d. dosing (no higher than 150 mg in a single dose)
Bupropion SR	150–300 mg/d in b.i.d. dosing
Mirtazapine	7.5–30 mg/d q.d.
Nefazodone	50–300 mg/d in b.i.d. dosing
Venlafaxine	1–3 mg/kg/d in b.i.d. or t.i.d. dosing

Abbreviations: b.i.d., twice a day; q.d., every day; t.i.d., three times a day.

Children or adolescents who do not substantially improve with any of these recommendations can be treated as if they were treatment-resistant adults (see Chapter 18). **Electroconvulsive therapy** (see Chapter 24) can and should be used in those youth who do not respond to a well-considered set of medication trials or whose level of sustained suicidal intent precludes the protracted time required for medication treatments. (*Note:* State laws rarely permit the administration of electroconvulsive therapy to children younger than the age of 14.) When psychotic features accompany MDD in a child or adolescent, adding one of the newer atypical antipsychotic medications to the antidepressant regimen can be considered (with careful attention to possible drug interactions). Unless the family support situation is particularly strong, inpatient hospitalization is likely indicated for the psychotically depressed child or adolescent.

A child or adolescent undergoing medication treatment for MDD should be seen weekly by the physician or another licensed and qualified clinician until clear signs of improvement are observed. The systematic use of one of the depression rating scales provides some objective information for the treating clinician, as well as for the patient and family. Once clinical improvement occurs (and the family "feels better" about the child), continuation of medication is recommended for at least 6 to 12 months. Visits to the treating clinician do not need to be as frequent unless ongoing psychotherapy with the child or family is being provided on a weekly basis. Because longitudinal studies show that MDD or DD starting in childhood or adolescence often persists into young adulthood (or recurs if it remits), plans should be made for regular follow-up visits for several years.

II. Bipolar Disorder

As in adults, youth who develop bipolar disorder (BD) can present initially with either depression or classic signs of mania, and one estimate is that 70% of individuals with teen-onset BD have an initial presentation of MDD. About one-third of prepubertal-onset children with depression and one-fifth of teenaged-onset depressives will develop mania. The mean onset of manic symptoms after MDD in the latter group is 4 years, and it occurs after two to four depressive episodes. Although prediction of a BD outcome in children with prepubertal-onset depression is correlated with parental and grandparental BD disease, only 12% to 15% of the offspring of parents with BD are diagnosed with BD, even in parents with early-onset BD or childhood ADHD.

Rarely children and more commonly those in their mid to late teens with BD present initially with hypomanic or full-blown manic symptoms. In community samples of teens, 6% to 13% have manic symptoms; however, when impairment and severity criteria are applied, less than 1% meet BD criteria. Youth with adolescent-onset BD have a prolonged course of mixed episodes and rapid cycling; psychotic features; an increased risk of suicide; comorbid substance abuse; and anxiety disorders, including panic disorder (PD), more often than do individuals with adult-onset BD. They may have other significant comorbid diagnoses, such as ADHD, CD, panic disorder, and Tourette disorder. The stability of a BD diagnosis of teen-onset BD has been shown through young adulthood, but the group of teens with *some* manic symptoms does *not* later develop BD.

Although individuals with teen-onset classic BD (especially those with comorbid childhood ADHD) are difficult to treat and they have high rates of relapse, no controversy is seen about their existence as a diagnostic entity. However, considerable controversy exists about whether the diagnosis of BD should be applied to a group of prepubertal children with chronic and non-episodic disabling behaviors and emotions that have many similarities to adolescent and adult BD. In the early 1990s, clinician-investigators began to describe a group of children who were extremely troubled and unresponsive to treatment. The hallmark of these children was their labile and irritable moods, which were termed "affective storms," that often occurred in combination with symptoms of impulsivity, hyperactivity, and distractibility. Hence, differentiating them from children with severe ADHD was difficult.

However, the serious "mood" instability, provocative irritability, and occasional belligerence and aggression that began as early as the age of 2 suggested a more serious disorder than ADHD. Family studies of relatives note an elevated risk for BD and depression among relatives when the proband child had BD type and ADHD symptoms but not when the proband had ADHD symptoms alone. This suggests that children who present with both ADHD and BD symptoms are a distinct subset from those with ADHD alone. Although these children did not meet DSM-IV criteria for BD, clinician-investigators began to refer to this group of children as bipolar and to treat them with mood stabilizers.

Currently, some investigators who are supported by the National Institute of Mental Health (NIMH) are using the diagnosis BD, not otherwise specified (NOS), for these children. Studies are being conducted over time to determine whether these children progress into cyclothymia or "true" BD diagnostic categories or, as often happens to teens with *some* manic symptoms, the evolution into a BD diagnosis does not take place (see Additional Reading).

A. Diagnosis and Etiology

Unfortunately, the term BD in children and teens has become a fad diagnosis for psychiatrists, pediatricians, and family practitioners. This is because of recent attention devoted to this diagnosis by a variety of media and lay publications, as well as the pressures of practicing in an environment controlled by managed care, which requires a biologically based diagnosis to make a payment. Many children with ADHD or CD are inappropriately diagnosed as BD. Diagnosis must be based on supporting data and not on the previous clinical diagnosis or even the hospitalization diagnoses of BD because of the inaccuracy and overdiagnosis of this condition.

Diagnostic instruments provide a standard format for assessing and quantifying mood-related symptoms (e.g., the Young Mania Rating Scale). However, clinical experience, a knowledge of development, and an understanding of the differences from and similarities to the other severe forms of psychopathology in childhood create the strongest basis for making an accurate diagnosis. Clinicians must search for comorbid ADHD, CD, anxiety disorders, and substance abuse. The latter is commonly found in teens with BD, but the clinician must also distinguish the symptoms of true BD from the "highs and crashes" of **amphetamine** use or from hallucinations caused by hallucinogens. Distinguishing the hallucinations of schizophrenia from those of BD is particularly difficult because the classic display of mood-congruent hallucinations (e.g., "I hear voices telling me that I am a bad person") is not always present. The presence of affective disorders in multiple generations of relatives is suggestive of a diagnosis of BD rather than of schizophrenia; for many youth, only long-term follow-up clarifies the diagnosis. Clinicians must be vigilant to hints of suicidality in youth with BD and must act to prevent its occurrence (see Chapter 17).

B. Treatment

1. **Psychoeducational approaches**. Families of youth with BD need education and psychologic support over time. Patients and parents must learn about the cyclical nature of this disorder, and they should be encouraged to create and maintain a **life chart**. This practice helps define precipitating stressors, as well as the outcome of specific therapeutic interventions. Appropriate residential placement can be a powerful remedial treatment, especially in youth with chaotic home environments that perpetuate their cyclic illness. Appropriate educational placements allow these youth to maximize their academic potential. Educating teachers and guidance counselors about the needs of youth with this disorder can facilitate a more positive attitude toward these youth, rather than viewing them merely as "that problem child."

2. **Psychotherapy**. **CBT** for children with BD is one of the preferred modalities of psychotherapy. A protocol has been formulated for the use of CBT with youth with BD (see Additional Reading) that helps them

learn to better manage the thoughts and behaviors that accentuate negative feelings and actions. Short-term, focused, insight-oriented psychotherapy may be useful for the management of poor medication compliance, especially among adolescents.

3. **Pharmacotherapy**. Developing a firm alliance and continuity of care with these youth and their families is crucial because the disorder usually persists through adulthood. Medication nonadherence is often the biggest obstacle to a youth's stability; a recent research study showed a 31% noncompliance rate. Regularly scheduled visits are necessary, and frequency should be increased during stressful times (e.g., parental discord, drug and/or alcohol experimentation, transition to a new school). Comorbid conditions should be vigorously treated.

The first multisite placebo-controlled study comparing **lithium, valproate**, and **carbamazepine** (CBZ) in these youth is underway. Several years are likely to pass before firm conclusions can be made about which drug is best for BD.

a. **Lithium** has FDA approval for the treatment of mania in children older than 12 years of age. It is the first line of treatment for classic mania, or it may be used as an add-on in valproate–treatment-resistant or CBZ–treatment-resistant mixed mania or rapid cycling. One double-blind, placebo-controlled study of adolescent-onset BD and concomitant substance abuse and of children with MDD with markers for future BD (i.e., delusions, TCA-induced mania, psychomotor retardation, family member with BD) reported an efficacy response of 43% to 46%.

Weight-based dosing should be considered when initiating treatment (see Additional Reading). Trough blood levels, complete blood count, thyroid-stimulating hormone, creatinine, calcium, and phosphorous need to be tested before treatment and at regular intervals; a pretreatment and follow-up urinalysis are also indicated. The treating clinician must monitor **lithium** trough blood levels and must remain vigilant for symptoms and signs of **lithium** toxicity; children may require higher dosing to obtain **lithium** blood levels within a therapeutic range because of their increased glomerular filtration rate and total body water. Younger children and those with **pervasive developmental disorder** (PDD) may be more sensitive to the side effects of weight gain, nausea, vomiting, tremor, and urinary frequency. Because nocturnal enuresis may develop and since this may be particularly embarrassing for children, using a once a day dosing regimen in the morning may be useful. (*Note:* The clinician should remember that, when shifting from three times a day to once a day **lithium** dosing, the once a day dose should be reduced to about two-thirds of the total three times a day dosing to obtain comparable trough **lithium** levels.) When nausea or vomiting is a prominent side effect, longer-acting preparations may be used. The following are key considerations when using **lithium**:

- Serum level of 0.8 to 1.2 mEq per L.
- Onset of action: 7 to 14 days, full benefit at 6 to 8 weeks.
- Side effects: nausea, diarrhea, tremor, enuresis, fatigue, ataxia, leukocytosis, malaise, acne, and weight gain.
- Other adverse effects: renal abnormalities, generally polyuria and polydipsia; electrocardiographic changes; and rare hypothyroidism; a subgroup of children may develop cognitive impairment at normal **lithium** levels.
- Importance of stable families to ensure medication adherence and to monitor levels.
- Importance of long-term maintenance because those who discontinue it have higher relapse rates in clinical trials.

b. **Divalproate (DVP)** is the current treatment of choice for mixed-episode presentations or rapid cycling. After liver function tests, complete blood count, and platelet count have been obtained, a loading dose of 7.5 mg per kg per day is tolerated by most youth. Alternatively, an initial oral dose of 250 mg twice a day can be gradually titrated upward. The following are key considerations when using **DVP**:

- Serum level target of 50 to 125 mg per mL.
- Onset of action: 4 to 10 days, full benefit at 6 to 8 weeks.
- Side effects: nausea, vomiting, sedation, weight gain, transient hair loss, tremor, and transient elevation of liver function tests.
- Other adverse effects: hepatotoxicity more likely in children under age 2 years treated with other anticonvulsants (*note:* findings from children with seizure disorders); high concentration of ammonia, blood dyscrasias, alopecia, and menstrual changes; rare cases of pancreatitis, benign hypothrombocytopenia, and decreased prothrombin times.
- In children with seizures receiving **DVP**, **polycystic ovary syndrome** (i.e., obesity, hyperinsulinemia, lipid abnormalities, and hyperandrogenism) is uncommon, but this may occur in those who start **DVP** as peripubertal girls.

c. **Carbamazepine** is an alternative treatment for BD in youth. It may be added to either **lithium** or **DVP** in treatment-resistant cases. Clinicians should be cautious with the latter combination because **CBZ** may induce glucuronidation and **DVP** inhibits the formation of **CBZ**-10,11-epoxide (a metabolite that is active but is not routinely measured). No loading dose strategies are available, but treatment can be initiated with 100 mg per day; therapeutic levels are reached by adding 100 to 200 mg weekly. The usual dose is 10 to 20 mg per kg per day twice a day or three times a day, but blood levels need to be checked because **CBZ** induces CYP 3A4 and reduces its own blood levels. Induction occurs within the first 2 weeks after a dose increase. Pretreatment complete blood count and platelet count and periodic blood should be drawn for both therapeutic levels and for a hematologic profile. The following are key considerations when using **CBZ**:

- Usual target dose of 200 to 600 mg per day for children; 400 to 1,200 mg per day for teens.
- Serum level of 5 to 10 mg per mL.
- Onset of action: 7 to 14 days, full benefit at 6 to 8 weeks.
- Side effects: drowsiness, loss of coordination, vertigo.
- Other adverse effects: leukopenia, aplastic anemia, thrombocytopenia, rashes, and drug–drug interactions via induction.
- In girls with seizures but without obesity, polycystic ovary syndrome rarely develops.

d. **Other anticonvulsants** with case reports of effectiveness for BD in youth include **lamotrigine** and **topiramate**. Children with seizures treated with **lamotrigine** have a higher incidence of rash than do adults, as well as a higher incidence of developing Stevens-Johnson syndrome or toxic epidermal necrolysis (1% versus 0.3%). These syndromes may be associated with a rapid titration of dosage and the concomitant usage of **DVP** in children with seizure disorders. A single case of cognitive impairment in a child with BD who was treated with **topiramate** has been reported, and a significant percentage of children with seizures who are treated with this drug have concentration and behavioral problems (14%). Concomitant usage of **lamotrigine** may be a predisposing factor. Weight loss in these children was reported to occur only in the first 12 to 18 months of treatment. These drugs need further study in the pediatric population before they can be recommended for routine usage, particularly because of problems such as confusion and memory impairment. Metabolic acidosis has been described in children with convulsive disorders.

   e. **Atypical antipsychotic agents (AAPs)** frequently need to be added to a mood stabilizer. These agents are useful in reducing aggression and the perceptual inaccuracies seen in these youth (see section IV). Clinical experience suggests that some AAPs may also have mood-stabilizing properties.

   f. **Psychostimulants** should not be added until the mood disorder is treated and fully stabilized. This is important because many children with BD may also have ADHD.

   g. Evidence suggests that **antidepressants**, such as SSRIs, improve the depressive episodes of BD, but, as in adults, SSRIs and TCAs may be associated with higher risks of mood destabilization. SSRI-treated children with BD may be at higher risk for induction of a manic switch and acceleration of an underlying BD illness than are teens who receive SSRIs. For treatment of BD depression, see Chapter 19.

   h. **Electroconvulsive therapy** may be considered in situations of acute suicidality and life-threatening mania.

III. Conduct Disorder

CD behaviors violate either the basic rights of others or societal rules. In addition, they should not be solely a response to a negative family or social context. These youth must be distinguished from those with **oppositional defiant disorder** (ODD) who have a recurrent pattern of behavior towards authority figures that is negative, defiant, disobedient, and hostile and that persists for 6 months. In less severe forms of ODD, youth may demonstrate these behaviors only at home (Table 21.4).

Accounting for up to one-half of clinical referrals to child psychiatry treatment services for both boys and girls, CD is the most common diagnosis seen in youth psychiatric clinics. It is often a pervasive, complex, and disabling chronic disorder that acts as a "gateway" to **antisocial personality disorder** in adulthood. The term "juvenile delinquent" describes youth who have become involved with police and the courts, and it may represent some youth with the most severe CD symptoms. No single path to antisocial personality disorder exists. Many children with CD do not have preexisting ODD. A small subset of children with ADHD and ODD will develop CD, but less than 50% of these youth will go on to antisocial personality disorder in adulthood. Additionally, the co-occurrence of anxiety or mood disorders and substance abuse may complicate CD and may predispose these individuals to later antisocial personality disorder. Parents of these youth can have significant psychologic impairments (e.g., psychiatric disorders, marital strife) and social disadvantages that may significantly impact the development, persistence, and treatment of this disorder in their children.

Scant information about girls with CD is found. Because aggression is not a necessary criterion for CD (Table 21.4), the symptoms of CD in girls may be quite different from those of boys. Girls may be less overtly aggressive and more likely to violate rules or to engage in deceitfulness or theft. The fact that girls have a different presentation of CD symptoms may influence the prevalence figures for CD (under the age of 18 years, 2% to 9% of females and 6% to 16% of males meet criteria for CD). However, the risk of developing antisocial personality disorder for girls with CD appears to be equal to that of boys, and these girls are at risk for early pregnancy with antisocial partners and for developing sexually transmitted diseases and significant medical problems. When compared with boys with CD, girls also have higher rates of **posttraumatic stress disorder** (PTSD), depression, and suicidality.

The following two types of CD have been described: **childhood onset** and **adolescent onset** (Table 21.5). Although this distinction may have heuristic value, it may not predict the outcome of an individual youth.

TABLE 21.4. DIAGNOSTIC CRITERIA FOR CONDUCT DISORDER

Three criteria must have been met in the past 12 months and one criterion in the last 6 months:

Aggression to people or animals (e.g., bullies or fights, demonstrates cruelty, forces sexuality)

Destruction of property (e.g., intentional setting of fires, vandalism)

Deceitfulness or theft (e.g., shoplifting, breaking into homes or cars)

Serious violation of societal rules (e.g., truancy, running away before the age of 13 years)

From the American Psychiatric Association. *Diagnostic and statistical manual of mental disorders,* 4th ed. Text revision. Washington, D.C.: American Psychiatric Association, 2000, with permission.

A. Diagnosis and Etiology

CD is a heterogeneous and complex disorder involving genetic, biologic, and environmental correlates. That as much as 50% of the variance for the development of CD may be genetic has been postulated. Some risk correlates in children that lead to CD include a "difficult" temperament; high novelty-seeking behaviors; chronic medical illness, especially that involving the central nervous system; co-occurring ADHD, especially with aggression, peer rejection, comorbid anxiety, depression, and substance abuse; and academic underachievement. Familial risk factors include parental antisocial personality disorder and substance abuse, exposure of children to parental discord, and inconsistent and harsh parental punishment. Low socioeconomic status and inner city residence are also associated with higher rates of CD. Physiologic correlates of youth with CD and aggressivity include "under-arousal" demonstrated by a low resting heart rate and low hypothalamic--pituitary–adrenal axis activity (decreased morning cortisol level or a restricted low range or salivary cortisol). Studies showing these correlates have not always controlled for comorbid conditions, especially depression or PTSD.

The purpose of the evaluation (e.g., forensic or treatment) and the role of the evaluator must be clarified by the clinician. If the psychiatric evaluation will be made available to the juvenile justice system, the clinician should tell the youth and the family before the start of the evaluation.

TABLE 21.5. CHARACTERISTICS OF CHILDHOOD-ONSET AND ADOLESCENT-ONSET CONDUCT DISORDER (ONSET AFTER 10 YR OF AGE)

Childhood onset (onset at or before 10 yr of age)
Usually boys
Usually meet the criteria for ODD before CD
Usually have concomitant ADHD
Family history of antisocial personality disorder and substance abuse
Comorbid substance abuse diagnosis that begins in adolescence
Poor prognosis

Adolescent Onset
History of normal functioning before the onset of the disorder
Occurs as frequently in girls as in boys
May have a concomitant mood disorder, early sexual activity, **alcohol** and **marijuana** abuse
May have a relatively "good prognosis"

Abbreviations: ADHD, attention deficit hyperactivity disorder; CD, conduct disorder; ODD, oppositional defiant disorder.
From the American Psychiatric Association. *Diagnostic and statistical manual of mental disorders,* 4th ed. Text revision. Washington, D.C.: American Psychiatric Association, 2000, with permission.

Although interviews of parents or other caretakers, teachers, or juvenile justice workers is essential for making a diagnosis of CD, the clinician should be aware that parents may minimize their children's problems. When the clinician's attitude conveys "I hear you have a tough reputation," the youth may volunteer a wealth of data, especially about covert acts unknown to the caretakers. The mental status examination is not useful in diagnosing CD, but a thorough and developmentally sensitive mental status examination is essential for assessing co-occurring mood disorders, anxiety disorders, ADHD, substance abuse, or PTSD. Youth with depression co-occurring with CD may have less severity of depressive symptoms, fewer anxiety symptoms, less guilt, and more self-injurious behaviors than do youth with MDD alone. Clinicians should be alert to any suggestion of neglect, abuse, traumatic brain injury, and seizure disorder; misperceptions that approach paranoia; or symptoms suggestive of mania. The clinician may use the parent or teacher-rated delinquency subscales of the Child Behavior Checklist or the Oregon Adolescent Depression Project Conduct Disorder Screener. Rating scales that may be clinically useful for aggressivity include the Overt Aggression Scale, the Children's Aggression Scale–Parent Version, and the Brown-Goodwin Assessment for Lifetime History of Aggression. Other scales should also be employed to evaluate comorbid conditions. Laboratory paradigms that assess cheating, stealing, and property destruction, such as the Temptation Provocation Tasks, have research utility only because they do not assess actual behaviors. Cognitive and educational assessments are essential to evaluate cognitive ability and learning disabilities, (e.g., reading disabilities in boys). Because youth with CD may be socially disadvantaged, undiagnosed medical conditions should be sought. A thorough neurologic evaluation should be completed. Substance abuse history and screening and a sexual history should be obtained. Parental psychopathology, marital discord, and parenting style should be evaluated.

B. Treatment

The ideal treatment plan is a multimodal one that addresses the educational, medical, psychosocial, and psychiatric needs of the youth and his or her family; however, because most evaluations are completed only when juvenile justice is threatened or involved, this ideal is rarely achieved.

1. **Psychoeducational approaches**. Parents of youth with CD and those with children at risk for the development of CD should receive detailed information about the risk correlates and treatment of CD.

2. **Psychotherapy**. Three treatments are well documented to be effective in youth (mostly documented in boys) and their families with ODD and CD.

   a. **Parent management training**. Although many treatment variants exist, general characteristics of these therapies include enhancing the quality of the parent–child relationship, establishing consistent rules, and fostering positive rewards and negotiation. Consequently, parental consistency is increased, harsh punishment is reduced, and parent–youth communication is improved. Dropout rates of 40% to 60% are common; these are associated with parental psychopathology and the parental perception of the difficulty and relevance of the therapy. Pretreatment parental psychoeducation, cultural sensitivity, and an understanding of "resistance" are crucial to improve compliance.

   b. **Youth cognitive problem-solving skills training** (for youth at least 10 years of age). By learning to assess and seek prosocial solutions to interpersonal problems, a child may correct negative attributions and may reduce impulsive antisocial choices.

   c. **Multisystemic therapy**. By using a home-based intensive model with many therapy modalities within the family, school, and community (e.g., parent management training, youth cognitive problem-solving skills training, marital therapy, contingency management), families can improve cohesion, consistency, and nurturance; and youth can improve their investment in education and in relationships with peers with prosocial behaviors. No evidence indicates that jail tours or "boot camps" will prevent or ameliorate CD symptoms without psychologic interventions.

3. **Pharmacotherapy**. No specific pharmacologic treatment exists for CD. The basis for pharmacotherapy is the treatment of comorbid disorders that may be related to the cause of the disruptive behavior (e.g., affective disorders, ADHD [*note:* psychostimulants have been shown to reduce aggression], anxiety disorder, PTSD, psychotic disorders, seizure disorder, traumatic brain injury). When aggression is a major problem in a youth with CD and the behavior does not respond to the psychologic therapies listed above or if the use of medication to treat a comorbid disorder has not improved aggressivity, the use of medication to treat aggressivity is warranted. "Affective aggressivity" associated with reactive impulsivity and lack of planning may be more responsive to psychotropic intervention than are "planful or proactive" aggression or "covert" aggression, such as lying and stealing. Although psychotropics are commonly used to treat aggression in this population, just a few placebo-controlled studies support the use of **lithium**, **valproate**, and **risperidone**. (*Note:* Nondrug factors may also contribute to reductions in aggressive behaviors in hospitalized youth.)

   a. **Antipsychotic agents** (see section IV). Although only **risperidone** has been shown to be effective in aggressivity in teens with CD, in practice all AAPs can be used with youth. In childhood-onset CD, youth may have paranoid thinking that is not well defined or significant enough to warrant a diagnosis of a thought disorder, but these youth may improve with AAPs. The clinician must collaborate with the family and the youth to decide if the benefit from the use of these agents outweighs the side effects that make them problematic (e.g., weight gain, prolactinemia) and to use the lowest amount of medication that results in a clinical effect (e.g., **risperidone**, 0.25 to 2 mg twice daily). Meticulous evaluation for extrapyramidal syndrome effects should be conducted when using **risperidone** or **olanzapine** because both, at some threshold dose, may "shift" to produce the side-effect profiles seen with CAPs, as well as an increased likelihood of the development of extrapyramidal syndrome and tardive dyskinesia.

   b. **Mood-stabilizing anticonvulsants and lithium**.

      (1) **Lithium** (see section II.B.3.a).

      (2) **Anticonvulsants** (see section II.B.3.b–d). **CBZ** has not been shown to be effective in children with CD and aggression. With **sodium valproate**, the least amount that will result in clinical effectiveness should be used. Blood levels are useful in monitoring compliance and preventing toxicity.

      (3) **Other agents**. A variety of other agents has been shown to have efficacy in youth with aggression and developmental disabilities in open studies, including β-adrenergic receptor antagonists, **buspirone**, α_2-adrenergic receptor agonists, and **trazodone**.

IV. **Schizophrenia**

   Investigators in the early 20th century, such as Kraeplin and de Sanctis, described schizophrenia occurring in childhood and adolescence as identical to that of adulthood. In the last mid-century, the term was expanded to include *all* severe childhood disorders. The term was further confused with autism after Kanner first described that syndrome in 1943. It was only after the studies of Kolvin and Rutter in the late 1960s and early 1970s that autism and schizophrenia in youth were differentiated. Now, the DSM-IV diagnostic criteria for schizophrenia in childhood and adolescence are identical to those of adult schizophrenia, except, in childhood, the definition of dysfunction is expanded to include "failure to achieve expected levels . . . of development." Similar to adults with schizophrenia, youth with schizophrenia have deficits of smooth pursuit eye movements; deficits in attentional and working memory tasks and autonomic responsivity; and neuroimaging abnormalities, including time-limited increases in ventricular size and decreases in frontal, parietal, and temporal gray matter.

The following two forms of schizophrenia in youth have been distinguished: childhood onset schizophrenia (COS), with onset occurring in youth less than 12 years of age, and early onset schizophrenia (EOS), with onset occurring in youth less than 18 years of age. Outcome studies of COS and EOS generally show stability of this diagnosis over time and a course that is indistinguishable from adult onset schizophrenia. Poor long-term outcomes for these youth have been demonstrated. (*Note:* Many of these are older studies, and youth had not received atypical antipsychotic agents and intensive treatment.) Unlike adults with schizophrenia, youth with schizophrenia show decreased intellectual functioning that continues after the onset of psychotic symptoms; this is related to hippocampal volume decreases that develop in the early stages of psychosis and that result in reduced information acquisition abilities. Schizophrenia in youth presents unique problems of diagnosis and treatment; this section focuses on these aspects only.

A. Diagnosis and Etiology

1. **Childhood onset schizophrenia**. Hallucinations in latency-age children must be distinguished from normal childhood experiences of imaginary friends, belief in monsters or angels, hypnogogic or hypnopompic illusions, and other developmentally based phenomena. True hallucinations (usually auditory) are believed by the child to be "outside his head" and are either commenting, conversing, or commanding.

   Clinicians are often misled by the presence of childhood hallucinations because they may *not* be symptomatic of schizophrenia but rather they may be related to major depression, PTSD, psychosocial deprivation, or cultural beliefs. Asking parents whether the family believes in spirits or ghosts is important. The diagnosis of COS is sometimes made in children with hallucinations and speech and language deficits or PDDs who superficially may appear to meet the schizophrenic criteria of "disorganized speech." Because of these factors and its extreme rarity (estimated to be 1 in 10,000), COS may be overdiagnosed by inexperienced clinicians.

   Patients with adult onset schizophrenia often have histories of abnormal language and motor development, low intelligence, or poor social development, but individuals who develop COS have even higher rates of these neurodevelopmental impairments. They may also have transient symptoms of PDD that precede the insidious development of frank psychotic symptoms (e.g., hand flapping, echolalia). Studies of offspring of schizophrenic parents support the presence of prodromal neurobehavioral deficits, especially in boys. Barbara Fish termed these traits "pandysmaturation"; they may be markers of schizophrenic vulnerability. Most children with developmental delays will not develop COS. In most studies of youth with COS, boys predominate. Auditory hallucinations are as common as delusions, and both symptoms have a less complex content than those of adults. A family history of schizophrenia (usually with an early onset), avoidant personality disorder, or schizotypal disorder and physiologic evidence suggestive of increased genetic risk from both parents may be present.

   In the NIMH study of COS, a subgroup of children who had been referred as "schizophrenic" by community psychiatrists were identified as having "multidimensionally impaired syndrome" and, later, as "psychotic disorder, NOS" (Table 21.6).

   Children with psychotic disorder, NOS, share the neurodevelopmental, neuropsychologic, and neuroimaging abnormalities of youth with COS. Both groups of children have a higher incidence of sex chromosome abnormalities and chromosome 22q11 deletions (velocardiofacial syndrome).

TABLE 21.6. CRITERIA FOR DIAGNOSIS OF MULTIDIMENSIONALLY IMPAIRED SYNDROME (MDIS) OR PSYCHOTIC DISORDER, NOT OTHERWISE SPECIFIED (PD-NOS)

Early onset of severe disturbance in boys
Hallucinatory experiences that do not meet criteria for schizophrenia (e.g., brief hallucinations or distorted perceptions)
Affective storms
Poor social skills
Excessive age-inappropriate fantasy or magical thinking (e.g., an 11-year-old who checks under sewer plates [covers] for Ninja Turtles)
Borderline intelligence (by IQ testing)
Comorbid ADHD

Abbreviations: ADHD, attention deficit hyperactivity disorder; IQ, intelligence quotient.
From Kumra S. Wiggs E, Bedwell J, et al. Neuropsychological deficits in pediatric patients with childhood-onset schizophrenia and psychotic disorder not otherwise specified. *Schizophrenia Res* 2000;42:135–144, with permission.

That some of the children with psychotic disorder, NOS, fall within the category of schizophrenia spectrum disorder has been hypothesized, but longer term studies are necessary to establish this connection.

2. **Early onset schizophrenia**. The clinical presentation of EOS is similar to that of adult onset schizophrenia. Symptoms may start at puberty, but they are more common after 15 years of age. As with adults, a first episode of psychosis in youth requires a thorough and complete psychiatric history from parents and other important adults, a thorough medical and neurologic assessment (see Chapter 20), and a meticulous mental status examination (see Chapter 2). Interviewing children for psychotic symptoms can be extremely challenging; children may need to be interviewed several times before the clinician is able to distinguish "true" hallucinations. Clinicians can begin this inquiry with the following questions:

Do you believe in spirits or ghosts or monsters?
Have you ever had any imaginary friends?
At night, most children see clothes or toys and think that they are something else. Has that happened to you?
Do you have any trouble with your ears or your eyes?
Have you seen or heard things and wondered if they were real?

The developmental history should be reviewed, both to assess premorbid functioning and to document the existence of neurodevelopmental disabilities and symptoms suggestive of PDDs (see section VI). Review of collateral information (e.g., previous school records, intelligence quotient testing, speech and language evaluations) can corroborate parental information. Youth with dysmorphologic features or mental retardation should be reviewed for chromosomal syndromes (e.g., fragile X, velocardiofacial syndrome). Because psychotic manic symptoms may be indistinguishable from those of schizophrenia and a history of affective disorders can be present in some families of youth with schizophrenia, long-term follow-up is essential to clarify the diagnosis. The differential diagnosis of youth with suspected schizophrenia should include BD, drug intoxications (drug usage occurs in about 50% of teens with schizophrenia, and it may be associated with first psychotic episode), MDD with psychosis, complex partial seizures, side effects of other medications, and other organic causes of hallucinations and personality changes (e.g., delirium, central nervous system lesions, neurodegenerative disorders).

When appropriate or in preparation for a medication intervention, laboratory, neurologic, and neuroimaging studies should be conducted to rule out other diagnoses. Neuropsychologic testing may be used to assess cognitive deficits and to improve treatment planning. Clinicians should be cognizant that anxiety symptoms, social withdrawal, and antisocial behavior may accompany psychotic symptoms.

Although the clinician is under pressure from managed care for rapid treatment, when possible, he or she should observe a youth over time before medication is initiated. The clinician should have an open mind about rediagnosis and drug-free reevaluations, because even the most rigorous of the diagnostic processes of the NIMH resulted in an almost 25% rediagnosis of youth with schizophrenia during a 4-week drug-free interval.

B. Treatment

1. **Psychoeducational approaches**. Informing the patient and family about the nature of schizophrenia and the value of medication compliance is vital. Although computer-based information programs are untested in teens, it may be particularly suited to this population. Substance-abuse educational interventions should be provided. Appropriate psychiatric, educational, and vocational placements should be sought with an eye toward maximizing future independent living.

2. **Psychotherapy**. Although few treatment studies of youth with schizophrenia have been conducted, clinicians can "borrow" treatment strategies from adults with schizophrenia, including family therapy, social skills training, and CBT.

3. **Pharmacotherapy**. A few studies of conventional antipsychotic agents (CAPs) and a small group of short-term studies of AAPs, mostly open trials and case reports, show efficacy in this condition. Most pediatric clinicians use only atypical antipsychotics. Schizophrenia can be a phasic illness, and the pharmacotherapy should be appropriate to the stage. When using antipsychotic medication, the therapeutic effect must be weighed against the potential side effects in each phase of the illness. With short hospitalizations and pressure from managed care, clinicians may give larger than necessary dosing of antipsychotic agents through the acute phase, and outpatient clinicians may be reluctant to reduce dosing during recuperative or residual phases.

   Clinicians must have a flexible stance toward the long-term usage of antipsychotic agents in youth. The development of a strong alliance with youth and their families is crucial because decisions about medications involve negotiations over years. Many youth will discontinue treatment without warning, especially when clinicians are insensitive about issues of their autonomy. A planned trial of medication tapering with mutual observation for "early warning signs" of symptom return may be suggested as a preemptive strategy.

   Youth with COS and EOS may have an increased or unique side-effect burden compared with that of adults (see individual medications below). Using the smallest effective doses and observing carefully for side effects is crucial. Latency children have both therapeutic effects and side effects at lower antipsychotic plasma levels than do teens or adults. Cognitive and/or behavioral syndromes in youth on antipsychotic agents are common. Typical symptoms include cognitive blunting (apart from that induced by the disease itself), behavioral problems, avolitional difficulties, dysphoria, separation anxiety, and school refusal. Youth may also be at special risk for parkinsonian bradykinesia, acute dystonias, withdrawal and treatment-emergent dyskinesias, cognitive or behavioral symptoms, and lethality from **neuroleptic malignant syndrome** (see section IV.B.3.a.(7)). Because of the reduced incidence of some of these side effects with AAPs, more recently trained clinicians who have not worked with CAPs may overlook the development of important side effects in youth. That some of these symptoms may have a diurnal variation must also be recalled, and clinicians should observe patients at different times of day.

a. Extrapyramidal syndrome in youth

   (1) Acute dystonia. Boys from the ages of 13 to 19 years with previous cocaine use and those with prior episodes of acute dystonia are at special risk. High potency CAPs (e.g., **haloperidol**) are more likely to precipitate acute dystonia, although this can occur with all antipsychotic agents, including but rarely **clozapine**. To reduce the incidence of acute dystonia, low initial dosing and slow upward titration of the antipsychotic agent are helpful, as is prophylaxis with a low-dose anticholinergic medication (e.g., **benztropine**, 0.5 to 1 mg three times a day, for 14 days in high-risk groups). When acute dystonia develops and the antipsychotic agent is discontinued, anticholinergic medication should continue for 4 to 5 days because of the extended duration of action of most antipsychotic agents and the possibility of renewed acute dystonia.

   (2) Parkinsonian symptoms. These may occur in about one-third of children receiving CAPs. Some prepubertal males may have atypical symptoms, and parkinsonism may be more common in older children with affective illness. Because these symptoms also may be associated with higher plasma concentrations of some AAPs, the clinician should be particularly vigilant in youth on combinations of other drugs and AAPs associated with cytochrome P-450 (CYP)–based drug interactions (e.g., **fluoxetine** and **risperidone**, **ciprofloxacin** and **olanzapine**).

   (3) Akathisia. Akathisia may be less common in youth receiving antipsychotic agents compared with adults.

   (4) Withdrawal dyskinesias. These appear as the tardive dyskinesia-like symptoms associated with lowering the dose or stopping an antipsychotic agent, and they may be present in 20% to 30% of children on CAPs. The symptoms are usually transient, but this should be monitored carefully.

   (5) Treatment-emergent dyskinesias. These dyskinesias may occur in 12% to 15% of children on CAPs.

   (6) Tardive dyskinesia. The true incidence of tardive dyskinesia in children is not known, but two studies of youth receiving CAPs revealed the presence of tardive dyskinesia in 3 of 17 children and in 2 of 40 teens (with 5 of 40 having some symptoms).

   (7) Neuroleptic malignant syndrome. In youth, neuroleptic malignant syndrome may not be associated with a higher incidence of affective disorders, but it may have a higher incidence of fatal outcomes.

b. Atypical antipsychotic agents in youth. A careful physical examination and medical history should be completed before starting youth on these agents. Particular attention should be directed to a history of abnormalities in liver and renal function. See Tables 21.7 to 21.9 for issues related to specific AAPs.

Data exist for psychosis in children treated with **clozapine**. Because the FDA encourages clinicians to reserve **clozapine** for treatment-resistant schizophrenia, no dosing recommendations are provided here. Despite some good clinical responses, youth with treatment-resistant schizophrenia may not tolerate this medication because of seizures, neutropenia, sedation, drooling, tachycardia, transient increases in liver function tests, weight gain, significant risk for hyperglycemia, and akathisia. Other side effects may include hypotension, development of arrhythmias, and fever. As yet, no published trials covering the use of **ziprasidone** in youth with psychoses are available.

TABLE 21.7. INFORMATION FOR PRESCRIBING RISPERIDONE FOR YOUTH

Pretreatment AIMS, liver function tests, fasting lipid profile and blood glucose, weight, and height; monitor these parameters

Common side effect of sedation and weight gain, especially in males

In association with weight gain, hepatitis rarely develops; this resolves with drug discontinuation

Children may be more sensitive to EPS (especially those with developmental disabilities) at lower doses

Potential for hyperprolactinemia because youth have increased D_2 receptors in the tuberoinfundibular system

Clinicians must inquire about sexual symptoms

There may be a vulnerable subgroup of children who have potential for hypertriglyceridemia

Target dosing range for youth: 0.25–3 mg/d in b.i.d. dosing

Shifts to CAP at high dosing

Abbreviations: AIMS, abnormal involuntary movement scale; b.i.d., twice a day; CAP, conventional antipsychotic agent; D_2, dopamine-2 receptor; EPS, extrapyramidal syndrome.

V. Anxiety Disorders

Throughout the lifespan, some amount of anxiety is normative; it provides the impetus for change. In childhood, anxiety may emerge at developmental transitions, such as stranger anxiety at 8 to 10 months of age; separation anxieties during the toddler years; various fears of the dark, bodily injury or integrity, or death during latency; and social fears during adolescence. Childhood fears are extremely common. For example, nighttime fears are present in 75% of children from the ages of 4 to 12 years. Parents may be unaware of or may minimize childhood anxieties. Clinicians must distinguish developmentally adaptive or transient fears from those that are excessive and that interfere with development.

Diagnosis and treatment of children with anxiety disorders can be challenging. Assessment of children can be difficult because children under the ages of 8 to 9 years may lack the cognitive and language skills to describe their internal states to parents and clinicians. Rarely does a child meet criteria for a single DSM-IV anxiety diagnosis; 75% of these children have coexistent psychiatric conditions, usually depression. Gender, family, and culture can shape the clinical presentation. Anxiety disorders in youth are both a source of distress and impairment for children, and, untreated, they may be the gateway to lifelong symptoms of anxiety and depression. Although separation anxiety disorder and

TABLE 21.8. INFORMATION FOR PRESCRIBING OLANZAPINE FOR YOUTH

Pretreatment screening of pulse, liver function tests, fasting lipid profile and blood glucose, height, weight, and AIMS; monitor same parameters

Children may have increased sedation (may be only initial), significant weight gain, and akathisia

Teens with EOS may have increased appetite, constipation, nausea, headache, sleepiness, concentration difficulties, tachycardia and transient elevations of SGPT, increased levels of prolactin and triglycerides

Clinicians must inquire about sexual symptoms

May not be very effective in treatment-resistant EOS

Target dosing range for youth: 2.5–10 mg/d

Shifts to CAP at higher dosing

Abbreviations: AIMS, abnormal involuntary movement scale; CAP, conventional antipsychotic agent; EOS, early onset schizophrenia; SGPT, serum glutamic-pyruvic transaminase.

TABLE 21.9. INFORMATION FOR PRESCRIBING QUETIAPINE IN YOUTH

In teens with psychosis, increased symptoms of sedation, postural tachycardia starting at 150 mg/d, initial insomnia only at low dosage and weight gain may be present.
In teens, target dosing range is 100–400 mg b.i.d.
In children with autism, the drug may not be effective; and it may cause increased sedation, behavioral activation and weight gain at 100–450 mg/d.

Abbreviation: b.i.d., twice a day.

selective mutism are the only anxiety disorders in the "Disorders Usually First Diagnosed in Childhood" section of the DSM-IV, other anxiety disorders commonly begin in childhood or adolescence. In general, the diagnostic criteria for generalized anxiety disorder (GAD), obsessive-compulsive disorder (OCD), PD, social phobias, and specific phobias are the same as those for adults (see Chapter 14), except for developmental considerations. Children may not recognize that the fear is "excessive or unreasonable"; the anxiety may be demonstrated by "crying, tantrums, freezing, or clinging." Other childhood modifications of DSM-IV anxiety diagnoses include the following: in social phobia, children have attained "age-appropriate social relationships" to exclude children with PDD, and their anxiety is also evident in peer relationships; and in GAD, only one symptom is required, not three.

A. General Issues of Diagnosis of Anxiety in Youth

Rarely do parents bring children for the evaluation of "anxiety" but rather for anxiety avoidant or oppositional behaviors (e.g., children with separation anxiety disorder may not want to go to school, children with social phobias will not speak to peers in school). Only infrequently do children volunteer that they have subjective anxiety or fearfulness to parents or clinicians because they may not have attained the cognitive development to recognize their feelings as excessive or unusual. Children may only be aware of physical symptoms (e.g., headache, "butterflies in the stomach"). Clinicians must interview parents and other adults to appreciate the degree of impairment in the child that is caused by the symptoms and must question the child to

TABLE 21.10. CHILDREN AND THE DIAGNOSTIC AND STATISTICAL MANUAL OF MENTAL DISORDERS, 4TH EDITION, POSTTRAUMATIC STRESS DISORDER CRITERIA

Follows a traumatic event: Children may not have feelings or show behavioral changes at the time of the event.
Reexperiencing the trauma criteria: Flashbacks may be uncommon—children may show repetitive play that links to the event and that does not relieve the anxiety; they may exhibit reenactments of the trauma; dreams may show nonspecific features; recollections of the trauma may be partial, skewed, or condensed.
Avoidance: Children must have the cognitive ability to link the traumatic event to their attempts to avoid it; instead of anhedonia, they may show loss of developmental skills (e.g., bedwetting) or the development of new fears; instead of detachment, they may show a restricted range of affect; many have a sense of "foreshortened or altered future" with beliefs in "omens" that, had they recognized them, they might have prevented the trauma.
Arousal: Arousal is usually present.

From the American Psychiatric Association. *Diagnostic and statistical manual of mental disorders,* 4th ed. Text revision. Washington, D.C.: American Psychiatric Association, 2000, with permission.

assess the extent and pervasiveness of his or her distress. Using interview techniques appropriate to the cultural and cognitive abilities of a child as follows is important:

"If a T. Rex came in this room, how would you feel?"
"Some kids feel [whatever their word] in their body or their head."
"How would you know when you are [their word]?"
"Does your heart go 'bunka-bunka' or do you have trouble breathing or something else?"
When a symptom is elicited, ask "When do you feel that way?" "When you are in bed at night?"
"When you speak in front of class?"
"What do you think about when you are lying in your bed at night?"
"Are you a worrier?"

Using self-report scales that children can complete or that parents or clinicians can read to them, such as the Multidimensional Anxiety Scale for Children and the Screen for Child Anxiety-Related Emotional Disorders-Revised, can be helpful. When parents have asked the questions of the child, rechecking of any endorsed symptoms by the clinician is crucial because children may not have understood the question. Clinician-driven rating scales, such as the Pediatric Anxiety Rating Scale, can provide a comprehensive diagnostic mini-interview.

B. General Issues of Treatment of Anxiety Disorders in Youth

Psychoeducation and CBT remain cornerstones of treatment in these conditions. Until recently, little research support existed for the use of pharmacotherapy in these conditions, although clinicians frequently used SSRIs or TCAs. The recent multicenter study of **fluvoxamine** in the treatment of social phobia, separation anxiety disorder, and GAD in children and teens and a double-blind study of **sertraline** in GAD have provided support for the pharmacotherapy of these conditions in youth

C. Separation Anxiety Disorder

School phobia is a general term that describes the clinical situation in which a youth avoids school. Children do not want to attend school for many reasons. These include the wish to avoid particular aspects of school or psychiatric symptoms that make attending difficult for them. Separation anxiety disorder is the most common psychiatric disorder causing school avoidance in prepubertal children. The cardinal feature of separation anxiety disorder is excessive anxiety engendered by separation from major attachment figures or the home environment that occurs for at least 4 weeks. Traits of separation anxiety disorder may continue to adulthood, but they are generally overshadowed by other psychiatric disorders, especially GAD, MDD, and PD. Indeed, separation anxiety disorder is a marker for the possible early onset of PD, and parental histories of PD or depression may be present.

  1. Treatment. Separation anxiety disorder can be a psychiatric emergency in childhood, and it should be treated vigorously.

   a. Psychoeducational approaches. Parents need to have a clear understanding of the manifestations and treatment of this disorder. Clinicians must address parental collusion with children with separation anxiety disorder; this may include an inability to set clear expectations for school attendance.

   b. Psychotherapy. Cognitive techniques can help a child learn to tolerate anxiety better. Behavioral plans or clear rules for school absences, scheduled phone calls, or beeper messages to parents each day from school are useful. Parents with psychiatric disorders, including anxiety disorders, should be offered treatment.

   c. Pharmacotherapy. Although **imipramine** was used for many years as the primary medication treatment for separation anxiety disorder, SSRIs are now the first-line treatment (see section I.B.3).

D. Shyness and Social Phobia (see Chapter 14)

Shyness is a trait with strong, but not immutable, continuity from childhood to adulthood. Behavioral inhibition is a research construct involving shyness; withdrawal avoidance; and fear of unfamiliar situations, objects, and people that can be shown to be present in a subgroup of children from the earliest months of infancy. This trait has only moderate stability over time; good parenting can change the outcome. Long-term follow-up reveals that some children with stable behavioral inhibition are at risk to develop social phobia (social anxiety disorder) in their teens. As in adults, the core symptoms for youth are blushing, trembling, palpitations, and sweating. For children, "butterflies in the stomach" may be experienced when speaking, writing, or eating at school or parties. The associated concern or fear of being scrutinized or evaluated by others may be lacking in young children.

The typical onset of symptoms of social phobia occurs in the mid-teens, with a higher prevalence in females. Of the two types of social phobia, the generalized form has an earlier onset than the specific form. The latter is most commonly a particular performance anxiety or fear of speaking. For youth with social phobia to seek treatment is highly uncommon; for them to resist treatment is quite common.

1. **Generalized type social phobia.** Children with early onset generalized social phobia (less than 12 years of age) are apt to develop depression and substance abuse in their teen years, and they less often report fearful cognitions. Comorbidity is usual—10% have GAD, 10% have ADHD, 10% have specific phobias (injections, high places), and 8% have **selective mutism**. These children are lonely and generally fearful, with poor social skills. They are dysphoric but not depressed. As they grow older, they may develop depression and suicidality. Most youth with later onset generalized social phobia also have comorbid conditions, including other anxiety disorders, depression, and substance abuse. Both groups may have behavioral problems that arise out of their anticipation of their poor performance in social situations, and they may develop school difficulties and chronic symptoms of social phobia. Two groups that have increased rates of social phobia are first-degree relatives of children with autism and girls with fragile X syndrome.

2. **Specific type social phobia.** This is more commonly associated with a traumatic event, and it usually develops in the late teens. Clinicians must distinguish these children from those with selective mutism. The latter fail to speak in certain social situations before the age of 5 years, and the syndrome usually comes to clinical attention when they fail to speak in school. It is more common in girls and in children with developmental delays, other anxiety disorders, encopresis, and enuresis. Whether this rare syndrome should be considered a subtype of social phobia or a separate anxiety disorder is not clear.

3. **Treatment.** In addition to psychoeducation and CBT, youth with social phobia benefit from individual or group therapies that promote improved social skills and assertiveness. Particular value may be found in providing interventions in a school-based setting where graded exposures can be supplied. Similar strategies may be useful for children with selective mutism when family, teachers, and treaters have a firm expectation of speech and offer positive rewards for speech as well. Concomitant treatment with SSRIs is useful for youth who do not respond to these interventions and for youth with coexisting depression because they have a more malignant outcome than do those without depression.

E. Panic Disorder (see Chapter 14)

Although panic attacks are uncommon in school-aged children, they may be present in 15% of teens. However, less than 1% of teens meet criteria for PD, and the onset peaks in the mid-teen years. Prevalence of early onset PD may be higher in the children of parents with early onset PD, regardless of the presence of associated depression. Clinicians should be aware of the following characteristics of PD in youth. Children with PD more commonly present with somatic symptoms (e.g., palpitations, shortness of breath, nausea, and sweating). Cognitive symptoms, fears of dying or going crazy, depersonalization, or derealization develop more commonly during adolescence. In the mid-teens, PD is often comorbid with GAD, agoraphobia, and other phobias; depression, which can be present before or after the onset of PD; and suicidal ideation or attempts.

1. **Psychoeducational approaches**. Families and youth must understand how mislabeling the usual physiologic sensations of fear, panic, and the "fear of fear" can lead to these anxiety symptoms.

2. **Psychotherapy**. CBT is the treatment of choice for all phases of PD—anticipatory anxiety, panic attacks, and avoidance. Learning self-monitoring and cognitive restructuring techniques can be crucial in a successful treatment.

3. **Pharmacotherapy**. Treatment of youth onset PD can be initiated with SSRIs (see section I.B.3) and ancillary high-potency benzodiazapines. Clinicians should be cautious about increasing dosages rapidly (as a way to avoid worsening of PD) with SSRIs and with benzodiazepines, as is the case with adults. **Clonazepam** with an initial dose of 0.25 mg twice a day can be useful in initiating treatment for PD while SSRIs are started and gradually titrated upward. Clinicians should be cautious with SSRIs that may increase the concentrations of benzodiazepines due to CYP interactions (e.g., **fluvoxamine** may increase **alprazolam** levels by up to 100%). After symptom relief is obtained, benzodiazepines may be tapered, if possible. TCAs are effective, but they are a second-line treatment because of their increased side-effect burden (see Chapter 18).

F. Specific Phobias

Specific phobias are more common in school-aged children (about 17%) than in teens (about 3%). Animal and natural environment phobias are the most common subtypes. More girls than boys receive the diagnosis of a specific phobia. Children rarely realize that their anxiety is excessive because they lack the cognitive abilities to assess their response compared with others. One-third of adolescents with specific phobias also have depressive and somatoform disorders. Although these teens may be significantly impaired, they rarely come to clinical attention. *In vivo* exposure is the best-studied intervention.

G. Generalized Anxiety Disorder (see Chapter 14)

Limited research data are available about GAD in youth. GAD is present in 3% to 4% of children and in 3.6% to 7.3% of teens. GAD symptoms in youth are believed to be similar to those in adults, but they may not be perceived as "excessive" by children. The focus of anxieties is success in school, sports, social, and child-related activities. Anxiety symptoms in children may result in an increased need for reassurance from parents. Teens more frequently resort to brooding. Once the diagnosis is made, almost one-half of youth with GAD continue to have the diagnosis more than 2 years later. As in adults, comorbid anxiety disorders, especially social anxiety disorder or PD, and depression are frequently present, and these predict more serious impairment.

1. **Diagnosis**. Medical conditions (e.g., hyperthyroidism, pheochromocytoma) should be excluded by physical examination and appropriate laboratory testing. A higher incidence of GAD and MDD has been found in youth with insulin-dependent diabetes mellitus.

2. **Treatment**. Education about the illness and parental support are necessary. CBT, including the recognition of anxiety and attendant cognitions and the development of coping treatment strategies (e.g., relaxation techniques), can be especially helpful. **Fluvoxamine** and **sertraline** have the best research support for efficacy in youth, and treatment with **buspirone** is supported by open studies. **Buspirone** may be used in three times a day dosing, up to 45 mg per day for children and 60 mg per day for teens. A single study supports the exclusion

of youth with BD from **buspirone** treatment because of an increase in agitation and aggressivity. TCAs and benzodiazepines remain options for treatment-resistant cases. Although **paroxetine and venlafaxine** are FDA approved for GAD in adults, insufficient experience with these exists to recommend their use in youth at this time.

H. Obsessive-Compulsive Disorder (see Chapter 6)

During preschool years, children may insist on sameness or symmetry, and latency-age children may develop rituals (e.g., avoiding cracks in sidewalks) or collecting behaviors (e.g., sorting baseball cards or spending hours dressing dolls). These normal developmental activities must be distinguished from the obsessions and compulsions characteristic of OCD (e.g., fear of dirt or contamination, fear of the death of a loved one or a terrible event, and washing or checking behaviors).

1. Diagnosis. About half of the children with OCD will continue to be affected in adulthood, but some characteristics of childhood onset OCD distinguish this condition from OCD in adults. Although OCD has been documented in very young children, it most typically develops at 12 to 14 years of age. For clinicians to discern prior "microepisodes" of OCD symptoms or a waxing and waning course that is exacerbated by stressful events is often possible. Clinicians may use psychologic instruments, such as the Children's Leyton Inventory, the medication-sensitive Children's Yale-Brown Obsessive-Compulsive Scale, or the NIMH Obsessive-Compulsive Scale, to assist in diagnosing OCD in children. Most often, these children fit the "poor insight" type of OCD, according to DSM-IV criteria, because they may not recognize their activity or thought as "senseless" and they may not experience or link a fearful thought with a compulsion.

The attributions of some children with OCD may seem bizarre to adults (e.g., contamination from "monster drool"), and they may incorrectly raise questions as to psychotic processes in less experienced clinicians. Unlike other anxiety disorders in childhood, boys can have a more severe or an earlier onset of symptoms of OCD, and they outnumber girls by 2 to 3 to 1 in prevalence of the disorder. Most children with OCD have other comorbid diagnoses, including depressive disorders, other anxiety disorders, motor tics, and learning disabilities. The child may hide his or her symptoms from the family for several months. Parents may inadvertently collude with their children by tacitly encouraging the carrying out of rituals in an attempt to avoid family conflict, or their own symptoms of anxiety may reinforce the child's attitudes toward his or her symptoms.

Because an association may exist between group A β-hemolytic streptococcal infections and the acute development of OCD, clinicians should document this association when it is present (this is termed PANDAS[1], see Chapter 7). Increases in the levels of antistreptococcal (ASO) titers and the nonhuman lymphocyte antigen DR-positive cell marker (D8/17) *may* be nonspecific markers of susceptibility to PANDAS. If documented by a positive throat culture, the vigorous treatment of future streptococcal pharyngitis should occur, but immunomodulatory treatments with plasmapheresis or intravenous immunoglobulin remain investigatory.

2. Treatment. Therapy for this disorder in childhood may be challenging.

a. Psychoeducational approaches. Using these approaches with youth and family members is essential because this condition may be lifelong. Recognition and early identification of subsequent episodes is one goal, as is the disengagement of parental collusions with the child's rituals.

b. Psychotherapy. CBT techniques adapted for children, especially exposure and response prevention, habit reversal, and behavioral

---

[1]PANDAS is the acronym for pediatric autoimmune neuropsychiatric disorders associated with streptococcal infection.

rewards, are extremely useful. The addition of a CBT family component may be helpful.

c. **Pharmacotherapy**. As in adults, SSRIs are the first-line medication for treatment. Although CMI is one of a few pharmacologic treatments with sound research support in children, most clinicians reserve it for treatment-resistant cases because of its side-effect burden (e.g., decreased seizure threshold, QTc interval prolongation on electrocardiogram). Clinicians should initiate treatment with either drug class at a low dosage because rapid titration can worsen the OCD symptoms. Clinicians should wait a full 10 to 12 weeks before trying a second SSRI because obsessive-compulsive symptoms diminish slowly.

Resistant cases can be treated with the addition of **CMI** at 25 mg per day to **fluvoxamine** because this combination preserves the higher CMI to desmethyl-CMI ratio best. Trough blood levels of CMI and desmethyl-CMI should be obtained after 3 weeks when the metabolite reaches steady state concentrations. Electrocardiograms should be obtained before and after treatment with CMI. The clinician can also try adding an AAP to any SSRI as long as he or she is mindful of possible drug interactions between these classes. If drug treatment is discontinued, this should be as a slow taper to prevent triggering a relapse. Regretfully, although a significant proportion of children's OCD symptoms may respond to treatment, these children may still meet the criteria for this disorder, even after pharmacotherapy.

I. Posttraumatic Stress Disorder

Youth are the victims of sexual and physical abuse, motor vehicle accidents, natural disasters, medical procedures, gang warfare, or other traumatic events. They may witness parental discord, and they see an estimated 10% of parental murders, rapes, and suicides. Of this potential pool of victims and witnesses, only about one-third of youth will develop symptoms that meet the full criteria of acute stress disorder or PTSD (see Chapters 14 and 27). Although the following are not absolutely related to the type, severity, or frequency of the traumatic event, possible risk factors for developing PTSD after a single event include the severity of the trauma and the distress of parents or caretakers. In community samples, 3% to 6% of school children have PTSD, whereas 12% to 36% of urban teens are affected.

1. **Diagnosis**. The DSM-IV criteria for PTSD best fit adults who have experienced a single traumatic event. Teens are more likely to meet these criteria than are younger children. Table 21.10 highlights the differences of children's symptoms when compared with DSM-IV criteria. Many children who are either very young or who are victims of chronic physical or sexual abuse will meet only some of the criteria for PTSD. Especially, they may fail to meet the "avoidance" criteria.

Many clinicians fail to ask youth about symptoms of PTSD because of a belief that children are too young to understand what they have seen or because of a wish to protect them. Psychiatric assessment of youth should always include questions about "What bad things have happened to you?" or "Have you ever been hurt or ever seen anyone get hurt?" A sensitive face to face interview must be conducted to assess PTSD symptoms. Details or clarifications may be elicited after the children have been allowed to tell their whole story. When particular PTSD symptoms have not been volunteered, the clinician should inquire about them. Estimates of both frequency and intensity should be elicited.

Because children often recall traumatic events just before they go to sleep, the clinician can ask children what they think about at night. The interview should include questions about the child's ideas of how he or she could have stopped the event and any ideas about the future. Because childhood PTSD is highly comorbid, questions about new fears, grief, and depression should be included. Watching the child's play may be crucial to recognize posttraumatic play (i.e., joyless and relentless repetition of the trauma with little disguise, such as when a child who witnessed his father drop his baby brother from a window repeatedly pretends during play that small figures are being dropped from heights and rescued by Superman). Clinicians should ask teens about coexistent depression, dissociative features, self-abuse, and substance abuse. If adults have also been involved in the trauma, they should also be interviewed if this is appropriate. The following inventories can be useful: the Children's PTSD Inventory delineates acute and chronic PTSD, and the Children's Impact of Traumatic Events Scale, revised, may be especially useful for sexually abused children. Children who fail to meet PTSD criteria but who are significantly impaired should nevertheless be considered for treatment.

2. **Treatment of single-event traumas**
   a. **Psychoeducational approaches**. Providing parents, guardians, teachers, and youth with an understanding of the nature and treatment of PTSD is essential, particularly with regard to educating caretakers to recognize and manage their children's everyday PTSD symptoms.
   b. **Psychotherapy**. CBT interventions are the cornerstone of treatment. Identifying specific reminders of the trauma is crucial, and these are coupled with teaching techniques that reduce anxiety and promote a sense of mastery. Techniques of hierarchical imaginal exposure to reduce anxiety and exploration of cognitive attributions of the cause of the trauma and of how the future will be changed by the trauma can be helpful.
   c. **Pharmacotherapy**. A few pharmacologic studies support the use of α_2-adrenergic receptor agonists (e.g., 0.05 to 0.3 mg per day of **clonidine** or 1 to 3 mg of **guanfacine**) or β-adrenergic receptor antagonists (e.g., **propanolol**, 2 mg per kg per day) to help children's symptoms of hyperarousal, agitation, or sleep disturbance. Other psychotropic agents (e.g., **trazodone**, TCAs, **mirtazapine**) may be used as hypnotics. Because SSRIs or **nefazodone** have been shown to be effective in adults with PTSD, the clinician may borrow these findings as evidence to justify the use of these drugs in children. Although para-hallucinatory experiences may occur in youth with PTSD, atypical antipsychotics should be reserved for those with coexistent psychosis or serious aggression or self-injurious behaviors. Comorbid conditions should be diagnosed and appropriately treated.

3. **Treatment of multiple-event PTSD** is more complex. Children may have long periods (e.g., months to years) of "numbing" symptoms that alternate with periods of "reexperiencing" symptoms. Children often have increased PTSD symptoms at times of the year when they were significantly abused, when they disclose their abuse, during legal processes, or in response to subtle cues (e.g., seeing a man who looks like their abuser, seeing a kitchen floor similar to that where parents fought). "Pulsed" therapies that either close down symptoms or open them up need to be used judiciously over the long-term course of this condition. Pharmacotherapy needs to be targeted to specific symptoms, and it should be withdrawn when symptoms relent.

VI. **Pervasive Developmental Disorders**

PDDs develop in early childhood; they are characterized by significant deviations in social interactive, language, and communicative skills. Additionally, children with these syndromes may have restrictions in interests or activities, and they may demonstrate repetitive behaviors. The use of the term "pervasive" is controversial because many children with one of these disorders have areas of normal functioning or areas of highly developed "islets of abilities." However, the term is used because it does differentiate PDDs from one of the "specific" developmental disorders (e.g., expressive/receptive language disorder, reading disorder). The five PDD subtypes are autistic disorder (AD), PDD-NOS, Asperger disorder, Rett disorder, and childhood disintegration disorder. The latter two are extremely rare and so are only briefly described. Although the spectrum of ADs shares common characteristics, these disorders may not share a common etiology.

A. Autistic Disorder

AD has attracted much scientific investigation since its first naming in the mid-20th century. Over the past 50 years, much has been learned about its natural history. The medical community is better at diagnosing it, and it also has some evolving ideas about its cause(s), and some modest headway is being made in its treatment. Prevention remains a mystery.

Before 1988, the prevalence of AD was 4 to 5 cases per 10,000, but recent surveys have increased that number severalfold. When children with the presence of some symptoms or "atypical" presentation are included (i.e., PDD-NOS), the figure rises to 26 to 60 cases per 10,000. Although this term can be interpreted in several ways (see Cohen and Volkmar in Additional Reading), PDD-NOS is best understood as a lesser form of AD—a condition in which a definite diagnosis of AD cannot be made because not all the sign and symptom criteria are met. Children with PDD-NOS may be less impaired than those with AD. The diagnostic process and treatment options are identical, however.

In AD, boys are more commonly affected than girls by a ratio of almost 5 to 1, but affected girls may be more seriously impaired than boys. Mental retardation is present in most individuals (75% to 80%) who receive an AD diagnosis. AD occurs with the same frequency in families of all socioeconomic levels, and a family that has one autistic child carries a small increased risk (4% to 5%) of having a second child with AD.

1. **Diagnosis and etiology**. The etiology of AD is likely heterogeneous, but little question remains that AD is genetic. Studies of twins demonstrate concordance rates of more than 50% in identical twins and a less than 3% concordance rate in nonidentical twins. Although the rate of mental retardation is not higher among nonautistic siblings of children with autism, both parents and siblings of children with AD are more likely to have social and cognitive deficits (e.g., awkward expressions and odd verbal interactions) than are the family members of nonautistic children. About 10% of children with AD also have tuberous sclerosis, neurofibromatosis, Angelman syndrome, intrauterine rubella infection, fragile X syndrome, Möbius syndrome, and fetal valproate or thalidomide syndrome. Visual and hearing impairments occur at a higher rate in these children than they do in the general population. Retinopathy of prematurity is overrepresented in children with AD. Currently, evidence exists of an association between AD and chromosomes 7q, 13q, and 15q and perhaps with the serotonin transporter gene. An association is also found between unfavorable events during pregnancy and delivery in children with AD, but no evidence indicates that any particular "difficulty" during a mother's pregnancy or in the perinatal period leads to the onset of AD. Furthermore, *none* of the currently used childhood immunizations has been found to cause the disorder.

Neuroimaging technology holds great promise for delineating the anatomic and metabolic abnormalities present in AD. Although studies of the brains of autistic individuals are relatively few in number, these do show evidence of abnormalities in limbic or cerebellar areas. More than 10% of individuals with AD have macrocephaly, especially in the occipital and parietal areas. Numerous neurochemical and neuroendocrine studies have been inconclusive, except for the discovery of hyperserotoninemia in as many as 30% of individuals with AD.

The diagnosis of AD should be considered when significant deviations in a child's development are seen in the following areas:

- Social relatedness: demonstrates little or no interest in either caregivers or peers; avoids eye contact with them; does not seek or give emotional or physical affection.

- Communication and play: demonstrates delayed or absent speech or nonverbal communications to express needs and wants; may have extremely idiosyncratic, repetitive, stereotypic speech; fails to respond to the communication of others, both verbal and nonverbal; does not use imaginative or "make-believe" play or engage in play with others or even with stuffed animals.
- Restricted interests and activities: engages in repetitive stereotyped behaviors (e.g., twirling a small piece of string in front of his or her face, spinning, toe walking) or becomes extremely upset with any change in routine.

Often the child with symptoms of AD who is under 3 years of age avoids eye contact and does not point to objects (e.g., toys, pets). "Pretend play" and communicative speech are not present. These children may not develop ritualistic, repetitive, stereotypic, and rigid behaviors until in their later preschool years. In the past, these children were often not diagnosed with AD until their school years. Because physicians, other professionals, and parents "waited" for more normal development to occur (i.e., "he will grow out of it"), opportunities were missed to provide early intervention services that could possibly have changed the long-term outcome.

As always, the process of assessment begins with the clinical history, the interview with the parents and child, and a careful observation of behaviors among the child, parent, and physician. Characteristically, these children will lack functional and imaginative play and will favor spinning or twisting toys. The medical history must consider the genetic disorders already noted, and the other possible disorders of the PDDs need to be systematically excluded. About 30% of children with AD develop a seizure disorder (usually peaks in early childhood and at puberty), compounding their disability. The Childhood Autism Rating Scale and, in 18-month-olds, the Checklist for Autism in Toddlers may be used as screening tools. The Autistic Diagnostic Interview-Revised and the Autism Diagnostic Observation Schedule-Generic are the most reliable and validated diagnostic instruments for the diagnosis of AD and PDD-NOS, although they do not differentiate specific PDDs particularly well.

2. **Treatment**. The approach to children with autism must concentrate on the interrelated goals of improving communication, cognition, and social development.

   a. **Psychoeducational approaches**. Every few months, reports are seen in the media of "cures" of AD with the use of some medication, hormone (e.g., secretin), special diet, megavitamin, allergy treatment, or some other "new" technique (e.g., facilitated communication). To date, none of those touted treatments or approaches has been found to make any sustained difference in the behaviors of these children. The clinician must play an active role in educating parents about the need for evidence that something new works and must help parents not to fall prey to false hope engendered by the publicity generated by the many charlatans who delight in the headlines of a cure for AD. Clinicians can realistically tell parents that their child's social interactions may improve over time with appropriate services. Clinicians need to help families select the validated interventions that best fit their child's needs. Parents can find information, support, and assistance from other parents through their state branch of the Autism Society of America (*http://www.autism-society.org/*).

   b. **Psychotherapy and education**. Many useful approaches involve behavioral therapy or structured intensive education. Heflin and Simpson provide an excellent summary of approaches that may be recommended to parents (see Additional Reading). The earliest intervention was the Treatment and Education of Autistic and Related

Communication Handicapped Children program. This is a package of interventions for individuals with AD using visual cues, schedules, and workstations to promote skill acquisition. More recently, a specialized behavioral modification approach entitled discrete trial format training (Lovaas training), a method of applied behavioral analysis, has been found to be beneficial. Applied behavioral analysis is a one to one intervention, and parents and teachers and even peers can be trained in the techniques. Target behaviors (e.g., making eye contact, stopping self-stimulatory rituals, using words) can be enhanced by positive reinforcement or reduced by the absence of reinforcement or consequences. An essential element of Lovaas training is the constant evaluation of the child's performance to measure his or her progress. Other interventions that are more naturalistic (e.g., peer-initiated social interactions) may generalize better than one to one interventions do. A recent focus on developing techniques to target initiation of speech and nonverbal referential cues and then to "fade" them out systematically may improve outcomes. Other techniques may be used with older verbal children (e.g., increasing verbal responses through self-monitoring techniques, improving verbal interactions with scripted videotaped conversations or social stories, improving understanding of the affect of others through social skills groups). For children who are nonverbal, augmentative and alternative communication systems may be used (e.g., sign language, Picture Exchange Communication System, computer systems).

c. **Pharmacotherapy**. Although evaluating children with AD and PDD-NOS is sometimes challenging, clinicians must evaluate these children thoroughly. Psychiatric conditions (e.g., mood disorders, anxiety disorders) can develop, and treating these disorders with the same medications used in non-AD children is appropriate. However, because some children with AD or PDD-NOS may not communicate well, for the clinician to use one of the rating scales based on observation by parents and teachers to evaluate the medication effects objectively (e.g., Aberrant Behavior Checklist) is important.

No specific pharmacologic treatments exist for AD. Behaviors that interfere with the acquisition of language and social skills and that fail to respond to behavioral techniques may be helped by psychotropic agents. Repetitive behaviors, aggression, hyperactivity, and self-injurious behaviors are the most common reasons for psychiatric consultation. In the past, low dosage **haloperidol** was well documented to reduce social withdrawal, repetitive behaviors, hyperactivity, and aggression in about 50% of children with AD. However, its side effects (e.g., sedation and subtle cognitive changes) interfered with learning, and more than one-third of the children developed withdrawal dyskinesias. Sixty percent of adults with AD show improvement in aggressivity, repetitive behaviors, and emotional lability with low dose **risperidone**. A controlled study by the Research Units for Pediatric Psychopharmacology Autism Network of the effectiveness and tolerability of **risperidone** in children with AD has shown efficacy for self-injurious behavior and aggression. AAPs may be used to improve the symptoms listed above (e.g., start with 0.25 to 0.5 mg per day of **risperidone** or others; see section IV.B.3).

Fluvoxamine has been shown to be effective in ameliorating repetitive thoughts and/or behaviors, maladaptive behaviors, and aggression in about half of treated adults with AD. However, children with AD who were treated with the same drug failed to improve, and many developed behavioral activation or insomnia. Other SSRIs have not been sufficiently studied.

For the symptoms of hyperactivity often seen in children with AD, psychostimulants have been tried with some success. Because psychostimulants are known to worsen stereotypic movements in non-AD children sometimes, inventorying carefully and videotaping existing stereotypic movements before treatment are wise. Clinicians should also be alert for the side effects of dysphoria and aggression in these children. **Clonidine** may also be useful in selected cases (see Chapter 22). The symptom of inattention has not been well studied in this population.

B. Asperger Syndrome

Children with this disorder have social deficits but normal cognitive functioning and a history of normal language development. Their social deficits may include impaired nonverbal behaviors (e.g., eye contact, facial expressions, body postures, and gestures) and an inability to "read" social cues in others. Despite normal language development, they also have impaired speech (e.g., poor prosody and modulation of volume) and hyperverbosity about special areas of interest (e.g., clouds, clocks, a particular WWE wrestler). These interests may shift every few years. They have been dubbed "little professors" because of these traits. As a result, although they desperately want friends, they often fail to develop good peer relationships. Because they often have motor skill difficulties, they are clumsy and they have an awkward gait. They may be quite intelligent, and some individuals show high verbal intelligence and deficits in performance intelligence that are suggestive of a nonverbal learning disability. Exact epidemiologic figures for this disorder are lacking, but this condition is believed to be less common than is AD. Data about comorbidity of Asperger syndrome with other psychiatric conditions is just emerging: As many as 20% of these youth have OCD, ADHD, or MDD (seen especially in the teen years when they become aware of their deficits), and a percentage of children with Asperger syndrome also have Tourette disorder.

Treatment of children with Asperger syndrome should follow the principles used with children with AD, focusing on social awareness and social skills development. Psychopharmacologic interventions should be used to address specific comorbidities.

C. Rett Disorder

This very rare condition (1 in 10,000 to 15,000) continues to be included in the psychiatry nomenclature although almost all of its manifestations, except for autistic features, fall in the neurologic realm. Girls develop normally through their first 5 months. Then, their head circumference decelerates and their acquired hand skills are lost; later, stereotyped hand movements develop and social and communication skills atrophy. Classic Rett disorder is persistent and progressive. Occasionally, a girl with Rett disorder may have some modest developmental and social interaction gains in later childhood or adolescence; however, the deficits in communication and motor difficulties persist through life (e.g., by the third decade, as many as 80% will be nonambulatory). Usually, this condition is sporadic, but it is occasionally familial. Recently, mutations in the X-linked gene that codes methyl-CpG-binding protein-2 (MeCP2) have been identified in some children with Rett disorder. This protein is a "transcriptional silencer" that affects the normal development of other genes, including those regulating many neurotransmitters. In affected families, a broad range of phenotypes is present, extending from mildly learning disabled girls to those with the classic progressive encephalopathy. Although Rett disorder was believed to be present solely in girls because males had only a single affected gene, boys with the variants of this genetic abnormality and severe mental retardation have been identified.

D. Childhood Disintegration Disorder

Formerly called Heller syndrome, this extremely rare condition has a poor prognosis. It has two key features. First, during the first 2 years of life, normal verbal and nonverbal communication and social development are seen. Second, between the ages of 2 and 10 years, a loss of language, adaptive behavior, bowel and/or bladder control, and play or motor skills occurs. The condition is seen more frequently in boys than in girls, and the syndrome is often accompanied by a seizure disorder. Very limited improvement is seen with age. Although any evidence of brain damage or a neurologic disease has yet to be found, cognitive abilities decline into the severe or profound range of mental retardation. Its presentation and course are similar to that of dementia in adult life, including the development of stereotypical behaviors and unusual responses to the environment. Commonly, affected children require long-term residential care. In rare instances, the child with childhood disintegration disorder regains some self-care skills. Making a definitive diagnosis is difficult because childhood disintegration disorder is a diagnosis of exclusion.

ADDITIONAL READING

American Academy of Child and Adolescent Psychiatry. Practice parameters for the assessment and treatment of children and adolescents with depressive disorders. *J Am Acad Child Adolesc Psychiatry* 1998;37:63S–83S.

Anonymous. Fluvoxamine for the treatment of anxiety disorders in children and adolescents. *N Engl J Med* 2001;344:1279–1285.

Anonymous. National Institute of Mental Health research roundtable on prepubertal bipolar disorder. *J Am Acad Child Adolesc Psychiatry* 2001;40:871–878.

Basco MR, Rush AJ. *Cognitive-behavioral therapy for bipolar disorder.* New York: Guilford Press, 1996.

Biederman J, Faraone SV, Chu MP, et al. Further evidence of a bidirectional overlap between juvenile mania and conduct disorder in children. *J Am Acad Child Adolesc Psychiatry* 1999;38:468–476.

Birmaher B, Ryan ND, Williamson DE, et al. Childhood and adolescent depression: a review of the past 10 years. Part I. *J Am Acad Child Adolesc Psychiatry* 1996;35:1427–1439.

Bryden KE, Carrey NJ, Kutcher SP. Update and recommendations for the use of antipsychotics in early-onset psychoses. *J Child Adolesc Psychopharmacol* 2001; 11:113–130.

Cohen DJ, Volkmar FR, eds. *Handbook of autism and pervasive developmental disorders,* 2nd ed. New York: John Wiley & Sons, 1997.

Findling RL, McNamara NK, Branicky LA, et al. A double-blind pilot study of risperidone in the treatment of conduct disorder. *J Am Acad Child Adolesc Psychiatry* 2000;39:509–516.

Fombonne E, Simmons H, Ford T, et al. Prevalence of pervasive developmental disorders in the British nationwide survey of child mental health. *J Am Acad Child Adolesc Psychiatry* 2001;40:820–827.

Geller B, Cooper TB, Sun K, et al. Double-blind and placebo-controlled study of lithium for adolescent bipolar disorders with secondary substance dependency. *J Am Acad Child Adolesc Psychiatry* 1998;37:171–178.

Goodwin R, Gould MS, Blanco C, et al. Prescription of psychotropic medications to youth in office-based practice. *Psych Serv* 2001;52:1081–1087.

Greenhill LL, Pine D, March J, et al. Assessment issues in treatment research of pediatric anxiety disorders: what is working, what is not working, what is missing, and what needs improvement. *Psychopharmacol Bull* 1998;34:155–164.

Grothe DR, Calis KA, Jacobsen L. Olanzapine pharmacokinetics in pediatric and adolescent inpatients with childhood-onset schizophrenia. *J Clin Psychopharmacol* 2000;20:220–225.

Heflin LJ, Simpson RL. Interventions for children and youth with autism. *Focus Autism Other Dev Disab* 1998;13:194–211.

Keenan K, Loeber R, Green S. Conduct disorder in girls: a review of the literature. *Clin Child Fam Psychol Rev* 1999;2:3–19.

Kumra S, Jacobsen LK, Lenane M, et al. Childhood-onset schizophrenia: an open-label study of olanzapine in adolescents. *J Am Acad Child Adolesc Psychiatry* 1998;37:377–385.

Kumra S, Wiggs E, Bedwell J, et al. Neuropsychological deficits in pediatric patients with childhood-onset schizophrenia and psychotic disorder not otherwise specified. *Schizophrenia Res* 2000;42:135–144.

Lambert EW, Wahler RG, Andrade AR, et al. Looking for the disorder in conduct disorder. *J Abnorm Psychol* 2001;110:110–123.

Leonard HL, Swedo SE. Pediatric autoimmune neuropsychiatric disorders associated with streptococcal infection (PANDAS). *Int J Neuropsychopharmacol* 2001;4:191–198.

Lewinsohn PM, Klein DN, Seeley JR. Bipolar disorder during adolescence and young adulthood in a community sample. *Bipolar Disord* 2000;2:281–293.

Lombroso PJ. Genetics of childhood disorders. XIV. A gene for Rett syndrome: news flash. *J Am Acad Child Adolesc Psychiatry* 2000;39:671–674.

Lovaas OI, Smith T. A comprehensive behavioral theory of autistic children: paradigm for research and treatment. *J Behav Ther Exp Psychiatry* 1989;20:17–29.

Malone RP, Delaney MA, Luebbert JF, et al. A double-blind placebo-controlled study of lithium in hospitalized aggressive children and adolescents with conduct disorder. *Arch Gen Psychiatry* 2000;57:649–654.

March JS, Parker JD, Sullivan K, et al. The Multidimensional Anxiety Scale for Children (MASC): factor structure, reliability, and validity. *J Am Acad Child Adolesc Psychiatry* 1997;36:554–565.

Martin A, Koenig K, Scahill L, et al. Open-label quetiapine in the treatment of children and adolescents with autistic disorder. *J Child Adolesc Psychopharmacol* 1999;9:99–107.

Martin A, Landau J, Leebens P, et al. Risperidone-associated weight gain in children and adolescents: a retrospective chart review. *J Child Adolesc Psychopharmacol* 2000;10:259–268.

McConville BJ, Arvanitis LA, Thyrum PT, et al. Pharmacokinetics, tolerability, and clinical effectiveness of quetiapine fumarate: an open-label trial in adolescents with psychotic disorders. *J Clin Psychiatry* 2000;61:252–260.

McCracken JT, McGough J, Shah B, et al. Risperidone in children with autism and serious behavioral problems. *N Engl J Med* 2002;347:314–321.

McDougle CJ, Scahill L, McCracken JT, et al. Research Units on Pediatric Psychopharmacology (RUPP) Autism Network. Background and rationale for an initial controlled study of risperidone. *Child Adolesc Psychiatr Clin North Am* 2000;9:201–224.

Monga S, Birmaher B, Chiappetta L, et al. Screen for Child Anxiety-Related Emotional Disorders (SCARED): convergent and divergent validity. *Depress Anxiety* 2000;12:85–91.

Myers K, Winters NC. Ten-year review of rating scales. I. Overview of scale functioning, psychometric properties, and selection. *J Am Acad Child Adolesc Psychiatry* 2002;41:114–122.

Nguyen M, Murphy T. Olanzapine and hypertriglyceridemia. *J Am Acad Child Adolesc Psychiatry* 2001;40:133.

Potenza MN, Holmes JP, Kanes SJ, et al. Olanzapine treatment of children, adolescents, and adults with pervasive developmental disorders: an open-label pilot study. *J Clin Psychopharmacol* 1999;19:37–44.

Wagner KD. Generalized anxiety disorder in children and adolescents. *Psychiatr Clin North Am* 2001;24:139–153.

Walkup J, Labellarte, M. Complications of SSRI treatment. *J Child Adolesc Psychopharmacol* 2001;11:1–4.

Weller EB, Weller RA, Fristad MA. Lithium dosage guide for prepubertal children: a preliminary report. *J Am Acad Child Psychiatry* 1986;25:92–95.

Wilens T, Biederman J, Millstein BA, et al. Risk for substance use disorders in youth with child- and adolescent-onset bipolar disorder. *J Am Acad Child Adolesc Psychiatry* 1999;38:680–685.

Woolfenden SR, Williams K, Peat J. Family and parenting interventions in children and adolescents with conduct disorder and delinquency aged 10–17. *Cochrane Database Syst Rev* 2001;2:CD003015.

22. DIAGNOSIS AND TREATMENT OF ATTENTION DEFICIT HYPERACTIVITY DISORDER IN YOUTH AND ADULTS

Jessica R. Oesterheld
Richard I. Shader
Paul H. Wender

Attention deficit hyperactivity disorder (ADHD) is the current designation for a group of disorders previously known as minimal brain dysfunction, hyperkinesis, the hyperactive child syndrome, minimal brain damage, and minimal cerebral injury, as well as others. The recognition of ADHD has its roots in pediatric practice, and attribution is usually given to the British pediatrician, George Still, who was made an honorary member of the American Academy of Pediatrics. In 1975, Paul Wender recognized the connection between the dopamine agonist properties of the then available psychostimulants and their efficacy in ADHD. ADHD is among the most common disturbances of behavior seen in the pediatric age group, and it is likely to persist into adulthood. The core symptoms of inattention, hyperactivity, and impulsivity can lead to significant disturbances in family and peer relationships, as well as in school or work.

Treatment of ADHD with psychostimulants was first described in 1937. During subsequent years, countless placebo-controlled trials have established their short-term efficacy. Since 1990, psychostimulant usage has increased fourfold to fivefold in the United States. Critics have written that ADHD is overly diagnosed and have claimed that these symptoms in children are a function of ineffective parents or teachers. Others have asserted that prescribing psychostimulants is unnecessary, addictive, and dangerous. In response, the Drug Enforcement Administration and the National Institutes of Health have undertaken an evaluation of the current scientific data on ADHD. The American Medical Association and the McMaster University Evidence-Based Practice Center in Canada have conducted extensive literature reviews. All sources have affirmed that the diagnosis of ADHD can be made accurately and that treatment with psychostimulants is effective in the short run. Data from the National Institute of Mental Health Multimodal Treatment of Children with ADHD trial have corroborated these findings. Some studies have shown that, although some geographic areas in this country have excess diagnoses of ADHD, it continues to go unrecognized in others.

Recognition of this syndrome in adults and children is important because effective therapy is available and comparatively inexpensive, and the benefit-to-risk ratio is extremely favorable. The American Academy of Child and Adolescent Psychiatry and the American Academy of Pediatrics have developed practice guidelines. The reader is referred to their publications for further information (see Additional Reading).

I. **Attention Deficit Hyperactivity Disorder in Youth**
   A. **General Commentary and Principal Clinical Features**
      Criteria for the diagnosis of ADHD have evolved over the years. The *Diagnostic and Statistical Manual of Mental Disorders,* 4th edition (DSM-IV), recognizes the following three subtypes of ADHD: predominantly inattentive, predominantly hyperactive-impulsive, and combined types (Table 22.1).

      The DSM-IV requires that the symptoms of ADHD be present before 7 years of age, but this requirement is viewed as arbitrary by numerous clinicians. When the onset is quite early (usually with symptoms of aggression or extreme hyperactivity), the conservative approach is to institute behavioral interventions and to defer the diagnosis of ADHD until the persistence of symptoms is established. Often, waiting until the child has entered school may be reasonable. This avoids making an incorrect diagnosis in a child who may be age-appropriately hyperactive or in one who is undergoing a transient form of disturbance in concentration and activity (e.g., as a direct reaction to parental strife or divorce). If symptoms are severe and unremitting, a full

TABLE 22.1. DIAGNOSTIC FEATURES OF ATTENTION DEFICIT HYPERACTIVITY DISORDER IN CHILDREN AND ADOLESCENTS[a]

Symptoms and behaviors characteristic of ADHD must (a) appear before the age of 7 years; (b) must be apparent in at least two contexts (e.g., school, play, home, work); (c) must not appear just during a psychotic disturbance or as a manifestation of an anxiety, mood, dissociative, or personality disorder; and (d) must produce significant clinical distress or impairment of functioning. Either **inattention** or **hyperactivity-impulsivity** or both must be present and must be developmentally inconsistent.

Inattention (*at least six of the following and present for at least 6 months*):
Failure to pay proper attention to detail, makes careless mistakes
Difficulty sustaining attention
Does not seem to be listening
Poor follow-through, failure to finish tasks
Poor organizational skills
Avoids or expresses dislike for tasks requiring sustained mental effort
Loses or misplaces items necessary for completion of activities or tasks
Distractible, often by extraneous stimuli
Forgetfulness

Hyperactivity-impulsivity (*at least six of the following and present for at least 6 months*):

Hyperactivity	Impulsivity
Fidgets, squirms	Blurts out answers before questions are completed
Gets up or leaves before it is appropriate	
Runs about, climbs excessively when it is inappropriate to do so (for adolescents, subjective restlessness or feelings of restlessness)	Has difficulty waiting in line or taking turns
	Interrupts others or intrudes
Has difficulty being quiet while playing or engaging in leisure activities	
Seems to be "on the go," revved up, as if "driven by a motor"	
Talks excessively	

[a] Criteria from the *Diagnostic and Statistical Manual of Mental Disorders,* 4th edition.
Abbreviation: *ADHD,* attention deficit hyperactivity disorder.
From the American Psychiatric Association. *Diagnostic and statistical manual of mental disorders,* 4th ed. Text revision. Washington, D.C.: American Psychiatric Association, 2000, with permission.

assessment and the development of a multimodal treatment plan are indicated. Part of this plan should include a medication trial to assess response.

Referrals for the evaluation and treatment of ADHD are usually made when schoolwork or home tasks require a greater degree of self-initiated or self-motivated behaviors or more continuous involvement than the child can sustain—at school entry; in elementary, junior high, or high school; in college; or even professional school. The following sections highlight certain important clinical and behavioral aspects of ADHD.

1. **Problems with attention**. These include (a) difficulty sustaining attention as shown by an inability to complete tasks once initiated or by a disorganized approach to carrying out tasks; (b) impairment in maintaining focused or selective attention (i.e., a short attention span); (c) frequent forgetting of demands or requests; (d) high levels of distractibility, impaired alertness, or excessive arousal (these children appear fidgety, restless, and often flit from one activity to another); or (e) worsening of

attentional processes in unstructured situations or when the tasks at hand require independent functioning and performance. Teachers and parents alike report that the child has difficulty with "stick-to-it-iveness" both in play patterns and in schoolwork. Some children are even unable to sit through a favorite half-hour television program.

Children with predominantly **inattentive form of ADHD** may represent the most common subtype of ADHD in community samples. Although boys with inattentive ADHD still predominate, the incidence of girls in this subgroup may be higher than it is in other subtypes. These children may be less aggressive and less oppositional than children with the combined form, and they usually present as lethargic and socially passive ("couch potatoes"). Consequently, they may be less disliked by their peers than are children with the combined forms of ADHD. These youth may have a later onset of symptoms and a later age of referral than their counterparts with the combined form of ADHD. Whether they have higher rates of learning or anxiety disorders is not clear. Barkley (1990) asserted that the inattention in these children is related to focused or selective attentional processing deficits that are qualitatively different from the deficits in persistence and distractibility in youth with the combined type.

2. **Impulsivity**. Impulsive behavior may be manifested as (a) sloppy school work despite a reasonable effort to perform adequately; (b) frequent speaking out of turn in class or making noises; (c) frequent interruption of, or intrusion into, other children's activities or conversations; (d) difficulty waiting for one's turn in games or in group situations; or (e) frequent fighting with other children, indicating low frustration tolerance rather than calculated intention—trouble seems to "bump into them." Patterns of impulsive behaviors may change as a function of age. In toddler and preschool years, the condition may manifest as a tendency to aggression; once the child is in elementary school, it may be rushing off to pursue his or her own interests, irrespective of those of the teacher. The child usually has marked difficulty tolerating delays. In preteen and adolescent years, impulsivity may be manifested as talking excessively in class or becoming "the class clown."

3. **Hyperactivity**. Hyperactivity *per se* is neither pathognomonic of ADHD nor is it necessarily present in ADHD. Some children with ADHD are actually hypoactive (see the inattentive form of ADHD above). When hyperactivity is present during preschool and early school years, the child may incessantly, haphazardly, or impulsively run, climb, or crawl. During middle childhood or adolescence, a marked inability to sit still, up and down activity, and fidgeting are characteristic. Hyperactivity often diminishes with age, and it may actually disappear in most children, although an inner sense of restlessness and other signs of ADHD may persist. These activities differ from age norms in both quality and quantity.

4. **Additional features**. Many clinicians believe the following signs and symptoms are seen with increased frequency in children with ADHD.

   a. **Coordination deficits**. About half of ADHD children show some form of incoordination. These may be in the area of fine motor coordination, with children showing difficulty in learning to tie their shoelaces, cutting with scissors, and coloring and later with handwriting. These difficulties may also be in the area of balance; the child may have difficulty learning to roller skate or to ride a two-wheeled bicycle. Finally, difficulties may be present in the area of hand–eye coordination; the child may be inept in sports, particularly those requiring throwing, catching, or hitting balls.

   b. **Emotional behavior**. Many ADHD children show age-inappropriate characteristics of younger children, including affective lability (moodiness), a short temper (or "short fuse"), and a low frustration tolerance. Their parents often describe them as being "too emotional" or as having "mood swings."

c. **Interpersonal behavior**. Children with ADHD typically show abnormalities in interpersonal behavior with their peers or with adults. The child with ADHD may appear outgoing and extroverted. Friendships may be pursued, but they are easily lost due to immaturity, bossiness, or domineering behavior. Because of unpopularity or a need to dominate, the child with ADHD may choose to associate with younger children or peers who are more compliant.

In relationships with adults, youth with ADHD are frequently refractory to the usual social reinforcers; they seem as if they are insensitive to the consequences of their behavior. Parents and teachers report that discipline or punishment appears to be ineffective in curbing undesirable behaviors. Similarly, positive reinforcers (e.g., praise, extra attention) may not be effective in strengthening desired responses; the child may need more than the typical amount of reinforcement or may perform less well with intermittent levels of reinforcement. A lack of responsiveness to discipline together with impulsivity, which is sometimes interpreted by parents and teachers as willful, is often the basis for referral for psychiatric or pediatric intervention. ADHD should always be considered in the child who is globally described as having "behavior problems."

d. **Learning problems**. An appreciable proportion of ADHD children shows impaired learning in school despite normal intelligence quotients. In fact, academic underachievement with variability of output in school is almost a hallmark of the syndrome. Poor achievement may be a product of decreased attentiveness or "stick-to-it-iveness," low frustration tolerance, or specific learning disorders that are frequently seen in association with ADHD. Because routine psychologic examination often does not include the evaluation of educational performance, such an evaluation should always be made in an underachieving child with ADHD.

B. Co-occurring Disorders

Between one-half and two-thirds of youth with ADHD have comorbid conditions, and therefore clinicians must seek out the presence of co-occurring disorders. Common among these are oppositional defiant disorder, conduct disorder, anxiety disorders, and depressive disorders.

Clinical presentation, prognosis, and treatment are affected by comorbidity. For example, both boys and girls with conduct disorder or oppositional defiant disorder and ADHD have a poorer prognosis and a significantly higher risk for psychopathology, drug or alcohol abuse, and school failure. Both groups should be treated with behavioral interventions in addition to medication to optimize the outcome. Children with comorbid anxiety disorder and ADHD may respond equally well to behavioral treatments or psychostimulants. A comprehensive treatment plan that includes comorbidities is essential for effective care.

Discrimination must be made between symptoms of **demoralization** secondary to academic or social failure and clinical **depression**. School evaluation and remediation of ADHD symptoms should precede pharmacotherapy for co-occurring depression or anxiety. The finding by Biederman et al. that 11% to 21% of children with ADHD have bipolar affective disorder is not universally accepted. They described children who were angry, active, and difficult to manage, and they did not require the presence of mania with grandiosity or euphoria, depression with vegetative changes, or periods of euthymia. Some clinicians believe that their finding is a consequence of overlapping symptoms in the criteria for ADHD and bipolar disorder rather than representing true comorbidity.

C. Prevalence and Prognosis

ADHD is more common in boys than in girls. Depending on the population studied (e.g., community, school, or clinical samples) and the diagnostic criteria and methods used, the male-to-female ratio varies from 3 to 1 to 9 to 1. These same issues apply to estimates of the overall prevalence of ADHD. A reasonable prevalence estimate for planning for the needs of children and their families and school systems is between 3% and 6% in elementary and high school. Approximately two-thirds of children who have demonstrable ADHD during their elementary school years will continue to manifest symptoms of ADHD into their teenage years. Prominent among these are problems with substance abuse and community adjustment

Follow-up and retrospective studies suggest that motor hyperactivity frequently decreases before adolescence, although other problems may persist. As was noted above, ADHD occurring with a concomitant conduct disorder may be the forerunner of a number of important adult problems, especially adult antisocial personality disorder. From epidemiologic studies, ADHD without comorbidity appears to predispose individuals to early cigarette usage, substance abuse, and alcoholism; the presence of these additional behaviors may obscure the diagnosis of ADHD and may cause it to be undetected in adulthood. Untreated, ADHD is a frequent cause of school dropout, motor vehicle accidents and injuries, and trouble with the law.

D. Gender Differences

Girls with ADHD may be less impulsive than are boys with ADHD, although they may be more impaired socially. Female teens with ADHD have more distress, anxiety, and depression than do their male counterparts.

E. Etiology

Historically, ADHD was usually thought to be secondary to intrauterine or postnatal brain damage; many early cases were recognized in children with postencephalitic behavioral dysfunction after the World War I influenza pandemic. Because the influenza virus affects dopaminergic neurons in adults and after von Economo had observed that brain lesions in children involved dopaminergic neurons, Wender (1971), linking the effectiveness of **amphetamines** to these findings, proposed the "**dopamine hypothesis**" for ADHD. Current evidence indicates that most cases of ADHD are genetically determined. A higher concordance for the disorder is seen among monozygotic twins than among dizygotic twins. A disproportionate number of parents of ADHD children show problems such as alcoholism, antisocial personality disorder, and mood disorders. Twenty percent to 30% of parents of both boys and girls with ADHD had or have ADHD themselves. Evidence that ADHD and major depression share a genetic vulnerability and that ADHD with conduct disorder may be a genetic subtype is beginning to accumulate. By contrast, parents who adopt children with ADHD do not have a higher incidence of these disorders. Whether ADHD is a discrete heritable disorder or is at the high end of a continuum of heritable behavioral traits is moot. Candidate genes within the dopamine system have been investigated. For example, two copies of the 10-repeat allele of the dopamine transporter gene *DAT1* on chromosome 5 and the 120-base pair repeat in the 5′ untranslated region of the dopamine receptor *D4* gene on chromosome 11 appear to be associated with a poor response to **methylphenidate**. The seven-repeat allele of the dopamine receptor *D4* gene on chromosome 11 appears to be linked to a positive response to **methylphenidate** (within the monoamine oxidase system, the DXS7 locus). Positive associations of these genes and ADHD have been both replicated and refuted in studies, and therefore their association with ADHD awaits clarification. Transgenic mice without *DAT1* are calmed by **methylphenidate**, whereas wild-type mice are activated by this agent.

Food allergies and increased sugar intake have been asserted to cause ADHD; appropriate controlled trials have not supported these claims. Fetal alcohol syndrome, fragile X syndrome, Asperger syndrome, very low birth weight, and lead poisoning are associated with a higher prevalence of ADHD. **Socioeconomic factors** influence both tolerance for the symptoms of ADHD and the likelihood of their detection, but neither poverty nor poor parenting can cause ADHD.

F. Diagnosis

1. **History and current level of functioning**. The diagnosis of ADHD is best made based on a detailed psychologic and behavioral history together with a careful description of the child's current level of functioning and an age-appropriate mental status examination. Adequate history-taking requires not only a survey of the kinds of target symptoms already reviewed here—and which are presented in DSM-IV—but also a thorough developmental history. The creation of a timetable or sequence of the appearance of symptoms in relation to family interactions and behaviors at home, school functioning, and peer interactions may also be useful. Open-ended interviews in this situation can often elicit a history of signs and symptoms of ADHD. If these are uninformative, a structured inquiry covering development and the common areas of psychologic malfunctioning should be completed. Informants should include all those who have observed the child, including parents; parent surrogates; and, after permission is obtained from guardians, teachers. Careful inquiry about family history should also be made, including the presence of alcoholism or drug abuse, tic disorders, or ADHD. *ADHD is a syndrome*; not all signs and symptoms need to occur in a single patient. Avoiding the use of one's own observation of the child as the sole determinant of an ADHD diagnosis is crucial because, with one to one adult attention, children with ADHD can sometimes function quite well. Use of the standardized instruments described below after discussions with the child's parents and teachers is essential. In addition, careful inquiry must be made about drugs of abuse, over-the-counter products, herbal preparations, and prescribed drugs because symptoms similar to ADHD can be seen with antipsychotics, bronchodilators, chronic marijuana usage, and others.

2. **Standardized inventories** for which normative data are available may be useful for assessing the response to treatment. Among the most frequently used are the Connors Global Index for Parent and Teachers; the Swanson, Nolan, and Pelham questionnaire; the Attention Deficit Disorders Evaluation scales; the Child Behavior Checklist; and the Behavioral Assessment System for Children. Impairment should be evident in two domains, but a lack of concordance is sometimes seen between raters. Obtaining additional information from teachers about a child's school functioning or a classroom observation sometimes clarifies discrepancies. Computerized performance testing does not reliably discriminate children with ADHD from control subjects, but it may be used adjunctively when reliable information from two or more settings is not available. A careful mental status examination of the child, including his or her perceptions of his or her problems and strengths and his or her attitudes about medicine, should be obtained.

3. **School information and psychologic testing**. No psychologic tests are diagnostic. When possible, the school nurse or physician should also be contacted and interviewed. As was noted, many children with ADHD have academic underachievement as a direct result of the behavioral abnormalities or as a consequence of coexistent learning disorders. The underachieving child with suspected ADHD must receive cognitive testing (e.g., Wechsler Intelligence Scale for Children, third edition [WISC-III]) and standardized achievement testing to assess the presence of learning disorders and to obtain a profile of intellectual abilities and vulnerabilities.

4. **Neurologic examination**. Schools frequently request a neurologic examination to determine if the child is neurologically impaired and therefore if he or she is eligible for special placement. The electroencephalogram has no diagnostic utility, and it does not need to be obtained unless a history of seizure disorder is entertained separately. As for any child or adolescent with a psychiatric disorder, every child suspected of having ADHD should have a concurrent pediatric or medical examination.

5. **Assessing environmental components**. Separating the relative contributions of a presumptive biologic abnormality from a familial or social problem in the etiology of a child's difficulties may be challenging. Because children with ADHD often have parents with ADHD, problems in the home do not rule out ADHD. Familial strife may reflect biologic abnormalities in the parents and may actually strengthen the diagnosis rather than indicate that psychologic forces are producing the ADHD syndrome in the child. Obviously, parental pathology may aggravate the problems of a child with ADHD, even though this does not cause the disorder. Diagnosing the child may be impossible until family pathology is reduced or eliminated. Establishing whether the family is able to monitor medication usage is also crucial because psychostimulants can be misused or abused by the patient or family members.

Based on history and psychologic test performance measures, the physician may suspect the syndrome. Even with a comprehensive diagnostic workup, uncertainty may remain. In such instances, the physician should discuss this uncertainty with the parent(s) (or guardian[s]) and the child and should schedule a reevaluation for a later date.

G. Management and Treatment

1. **Education of the family and child**. An essential component of the management and treatment of ADHD is explaining the problem to the child's parents and, with proper modifications appropriate to his or her developmental level, to the child. Many parents of youth with ADHD are confused, guilty, and angry, believing that their child's problems reflect their inadequacies as parents. Blame of the other parent and guilt can often be produced or aggravated by contact with a therapist or teacher or family member who attributes the child's psychopathology to parental pathology. Most often, parents do not know how to handle the child, they frequently disagree, and they are highly liable to blame each other. Parents should be helped to distinguish the child's symptoms that may or may not respond to medication from those that are generated or aggravated by their management of the child. Parents should be given a good understanding of which problems will **not** be ameliorated by improved psychologic management, such as attention deficits, and of those that **may** be benefitted, such as noncompliance or disobedience. The advantages of parent education in ADHD are demystification, adjustment of expectations, and acquisition of more effective management techniques. As part of the education of the family, aspects of childrearing should be introduced and discussed, including both general techniques, as well as more specific approaches, such as contingency and behavioral management techniques. Some parents will not allow physicians to prescribe psychostimulants or other medications to their children with ADHD. When parents eschew medication, they should be urged to leave the option open if behavioral treatments are insufficient. Organizations such as Children and Adults with Attention Deficit Disorder (CHADD; *http://www.chadd.org/*) and the National Attention Deficit Disorder Association (*http://www.add.org/*) can provide helpful information. CHADD support groups can be found in many areas of the country; they provide perspective and support to parents caring for children with ADHD and to adults who struggle with ADHD.

2. **School placement**. When educational problems exist, proper educational placement is essential. As has been noted, many children with ADHD perform badly in school because of their inattentiveness and lack of "stick-to-itiveness," which are characteristics of the syndrome, whether or not they also have associated learning disorders. Medications may improve important symptoms of ADHD, but they do not improve specific learning disorders. No technique of parental management or pharmacotherapy can succeed unless the child is given an academic placement consistent with his or her needs. This may require special

classes when learning disabilities are present or catch-up classes if the child is of adequate intelligence and has no learning disabilities but has fallen behind in school. Seating the child where the teacher makes the most eye contact allows better supervision and attentional cueing. Working closely with school personnel is essential to optimize the educational environment (e.g., the use of paraprofessionals, resource room, behavioral management strategies that stress positive rewards for appropriate classroom behavior, decreasing distractions). Unfortunately, many desirable educational placements are harder to obtain as economic and political factors shift resources away from the educational system. Clinicians should encourage parents and guardians to be active and effective advocates for the best educational placements for their children.

3. **Medications**. Some important principles govern the use of medication with children in general and in children with ADHD in particular. Boys and girls respond equally well to psychostimulants. Most youth are not able to describe or they do not experience a subjective difference when taking medication. A frank discussion of this fact with the youth should precede treatment.

The clinician should titrate the medication against specific behaviors, so appropriate monitoring requires reports from parents and teachers. Standardized rating instruments are useful because they can be used to quantify the type and degree of behavioral improvement, and review of these forms or discussion with the teacher before medication adjustment is invaluable. Psychostimulants help approximately 70% to 80% of ADHD children; however, their beneficial effects, although they are at times dramatic, are symptomatic only. Medication may have to be continued for years to control the child's and, later, the adolescent's and adult's signs, symptoms, and behaviors. The fact that medications are not curative, however, should not be interpreted as denigrating their value to the individual with ADHD. By suppressing the symptoms of ADHD, children will be more likely to grow both intellectually and socially.

As children approach middle school age, they may resist using medication, particularly if they are oppositional at school. This can happen in those who have responded extremely well and even in the child who acknowledges benefits from taking medication. Because this may stem from many factors (e.g., adolescent denial of problems, a reluctance to be stigmatized as ill, a need for increased autonomy), clinicians should anticipate this possibility and should discuss the children's feelings about medication with them during elementary school. This may help to strengthen the clinician's alliance with the child.

By remaining flexible and inventive, clinicians can encourage appropriate medication usage through positive rewards and planned discontinuations. Trial periods without medication or of placebo substitution (where ethically and legally sanctioned) with a systematic review of changes in rating scale assessments provide objective evidence of whether continued use of medication is warranted and necessary.

Clinicians need to discuss whether medication will be given only during the school week or on weekends and vacations as well with parents or guardians. In instances in which the child with ADHD has difficulty with peers and parents as well as school problems, medication helps the child by improving his or her ability to work and play with others. To the extent that the child's self-esteem is benefitted by good interaction with others, treatment outside the school setting can be expected to provide further benefit. If the child obtains a good response from medication, trial discontinuations at intervals should be used to determine if medication is still useful. One policy is to offer such medication "holidays" during psychologically less demanding times (e.g., during the summer vacation) and, when they are successful, to resume medication use when school begins again. Clinical experience suggests that having a child start the school year with medication and later carrying out a trial off the medication is better.

Assessing the adequacy of psychostimulants to monitor behavior while the medication is affecting the child is particularly important. If psychostimulants are given as they typically are in the morning and at noon and the parent sees the child in the afternoon after the medication has worn off, he or she may inaccurately deem them ineffective. In some schools, local regulations prevent children from receiving medications during the school day. This has made the availability of longer acting alternatives particularly important. Attention to all these aspects of treatment involves considerable clinician time and requires a strong alliance that is fostered by regular and unhurried appointments with the child and family.

    a. Psychostimulants. When psychostimulant medications are maximally effective, they frequently reverse many of the psychologic abnormalities that have been described and promote psychologic growth to an extent not seen before the drugs were administered. Many children will demonstrate a longer attention span, an increased tolerance of frustration, greater emotional stability, and increased sensitivity to the requests of peers and parents. The current psychostimulant medications used are the amphetamines (***d*-amphetamine, Adderall**), **methylphenidate**, and **pemoline** (Table 22.2).[1]

    Methylphenidate and **d-methylphenidate** (also called **Focalin** or ***d-threo*methylphenidate**) are available in an immediate release (IR) formulation (lasting 2.5 to 4 hours) and in the following six longer acting preparations: **Ritalin-LA**, **Ritalin-SR**, **Methylin ER**, **Metadate-ER**, and **Metadate-CD**, which are 8-hour preparations; and **Concerta**, a 12-hour osmotically controlled-release formulation.

    Ritalin-SR is available only in a 20 mg dosage. Some clinicians and research groups report that this particular wax matrix preparation, which has a slower onset of action compared with IR preparations, is actually not longer acting than IR formulations, and they believe it is effective for only 4 to 6 hours. Some also suggest that it also may be more vulnerable to tolerance development than are the IR preparations; similar suggestions have been made about Metadate-ER and Methylin-ER. Some suggest that Ritalin-SR tablets can be divided into halves; note that this is contrary to product labeling.

    Limited data exist for all the longer acting forms of **methylphenidate**. The authors have had clinical experiences that suggest that the **Concerta** formulation can adequately substitute for the three times a day dosing of the IR preparations and that it lasts at least 8 hours. Concerta is generally well tolerated. When dosages are increased, additional side effects may develop. In some children, a dysphoria develops toward the end of the expected duration of effect; this dysphoria may be lessened by adding 2.5 to 5 mg of an **IR** formulation about an hour before the dysphoria is expected to occur.

    Manufacturers' product labeling specifically recommends that **methylphenidate** should not be used for children under the age of 6 years, even though at least six studies support its efficacy and safety in these younger children.

    ***d*-Amphetamine** (lasting 4 to 6 hours), **Dexedrine spansules** (lasting about 6 to 8 hours), **Adderall** (a mixed salt lasting about 5 hours), and **Adderall-XR** (lasting 6 to 8 hours) have a longer duration of action than does **IR methylphenidate**, and they may

---

[1]Although **methamphetamine** is still available in a 5 mg oral dosage form, its use is not recommended because of the abuse potential of **methamphetamine**.

TABLE 22.2. CURRENTLY AVAILABLE ORAL PSYCHOSTIMULANTS APPROVED FOR ATTENTION DEFICIT HYPERACTIVITY DISORDER[a]

Agent (estimated duration in hours)[b]	Initial Dose	Usual Maximum Dose[b]
Immediate-release (IR) methylphenidate (2.5–4)[c] (many names) d-*threo*methylphenidate (2.5–4)[d]	2.5–5 mg in a.m. or b.i.d. or t.i.d.	60 mg/d[b]
Extended-release methylphenidate		
Ritalin-LA (8)[e]	20 mg in a.m.	60 mg/d
Ritalin-SR (4–6, 8 [see text])[f]	20 mg in a.m.	60 mg/d
Metadate-ER (8)[g]	10 mg in a.m.	60 mg/d
Metadate-CD (8)[h]	20 mg in a.m.	60 mg/d
Methylin-ER (8)[i]	10 mg in a.m.	60 mg/d
Concerta (10–12)[j]	18 mg in a.m.	72 mg/d
Immediate-release d-amphetamine Dexedrine (3.5–6)[k] d,dl-amphetamine Adderall (5)[l]	2.5–5 mg in a.m. or b.i.d.	40 mg/d
Sustained-release d-amphetamine Dexedrine spansules (5–8)[m]	5 mg in a.m.	40 mg/d
d,dl-amphetamine Adderall-XR (6–8)[n]	10 mg in a.m.	40 mg/d
Pemoline Cylert (5–10)[o]	18.75 mg in a.m.	112.5 mg/d

Abbreviations: b.i.d., twice daily; t.i.d., three times a day.
[a] Currently, these psychostimulants are classified as class II with the exception of pemoline, which is class IV.
[b] These estimates of the duration of effect reflect the authors' clinical experience and may differ from the product's labeling. Usual maximums are sometimes exceeded because of factors such as age, weight, or tolerance development. The usual range for methylphenidate in youth is 30–40 mg/d, but a few require up to 70 mg/d.
[c] Currently available as 5 mg, 10 mg, and 20 mg tablets; this formulation can be opened and the beads can be placed into soft foods such as applesauce.
[d] Currently available as 2.5 mg, 5 mg, and 10 mg tablets.
[e] Currently available as 20, 30, and 40 mg capsules.
[f] Currently available as 20 mg sustained-release (wax matrix) tablets.
[g] Currently available as 10 mg and 20 mg extended-release tablets.
[h] Currently available as a 20 mg (biphasic delivery) tablet.
[i] Currently available in the following two tablet strengths: 10 and 20 mg.
[j] Currently available in the following four extended-release (osmotic) capsule strengths: 18, 27, 36, and 54 mg.
[k] Currently available as 5 mg tablets (contain tartrazine).
[l] Currently available in the following seven tablet strengths (each at 1 : 1 : 1 : 1 ratio of dextroamphetamine saccharate, dextroamphetamine sulphate, amphetamine aspartate, and amphetamine sulphate): 5, 7.5, 10, 12.5, 15, 20, and 30 mg.
[m] Currently available in three sustained-release capsules as follows: 5, 10, and 15 mg (contain tartrazine).
[n] Currently available as 10 mg, 20 mg, and 30 mg capsules.
[o] Currently available as 18.75 mg, 37.5 mg, and 75 mg tablets; also as a 37.5 mg chewable tablet.

reduce the total number of daily doses. Dexedrine spansules have a slightly later onset of action than that of **d-amphetamine**; these two formulations may be given together in the morning to enhance efficacy. **Adderall** has a similar duration of action to that of **d-amphetamine**; the XR formulation may be used for once a day dosing.

For *d*-amphetamine, the product labeling recommendation is for usage in children ages 3 or over. A few clinical trials support this statement.

Overall, **methylphenidate** and the **amphetamines** appear to be about equally effective, and most physicians start with one and switch to the other when the child's response is not optimal. Although the overall percentage response may be the same for both, about one-third of children will do better on one class than they do on the other.

Longer acting preparations (e.g., **Methylin-ER**, **Metadate-ER**, **Metadate-CD**[2], **Concerta**, **Dexedrine spansules**, and **Adderall-XR**) may facilitate once daily dosing, thus avoiding the need to depend on a mid–school-day dose administered either by the school nurse, a teacher, or the child (sometimes, an older sibling). Some school-aged children are highly sensitive to being identified as "different" from their peers, and they may refuse to take the medication during school hours.

Pemoline has fallen into disfavor because of its linkage to hepatic failure and death. Although it is still marketed in the United States, its product information contains a "black-boxed" warning indicating these concerns. (*Note:* **Pemoline** is no longer marketed in some countries [e.g., Canada, the United Kingdom].) Currently, **pemoline** is usually considered only if the youth or family has a history of drug abuse or when **methylphenidate**, **amphetamines**, and other options have been ineffective. In the past, some physicians prescribed **pemoline** because it is scheduled in Class IV rather than in Class II; it may be prescribed and renewed for 6 months, rather than having to be prescribed every month. As was noted above, a major concern with **pemoline** is that a very small percentage of individuals can develop evidence of hepatitis that ranges in severity from asymptomatic increases of serum aminotransferases to acute hepatic failure and even death. Written informed consent outlining these risks and other options for treatment should be obtained before **pemoline** is prescribed. Obtaining pretreatment liver function tests to establish a baseline is also crucial. That some cases of **pemoline**-induced hepatic failure developed after many years of apparently safe use and in the presence of previously normal liver function tests should be emphasized. How often on-treatment liver function tests should be obtained is debatable; some clinicians recommend every 2 weeks, and others advocate informing parents or guardians about the signs and symptoms of hepatic dysfunction and obtaining laboratory tests every 6 months. **Pemoline** also has the potential to cause insomnia, and it may be the psychostimulant with the highest likelihood of causing choreiform movements and tics. Contrary to previous belief, its onset of action is rapid and dose related. Although the usual recommendation is to dose it once daily, many youth require a second dose in the afternoon.

Atomoxetine is a recently introduced treatment for ADHD. It appears to be a selective inhibitor of the norepinephrine transporter. Because, to date, data do not suggest that it causes euphoria or withdrawal, **atomoxetine** is not classified as a controlled drug. **Atomoxetine** is metabolized by cytochrome P-450 (CYP) 2D6. Patients who are poor metabolizers of CYP 2D6 and those who are being treated concurrently or those who have recently been treated with potent 2D6 inhibitors (e.g., **paroxetine**, **fluoxetine**) will usually have increased plasma concentrations of **atomoxetine** (increases of up to fivefold). As with other psychostimulants, **atomoxetine** should not be taken with

[2]This formulation consists of immediate and extended release beads. The clinician should keep in mind that these capsules can be opened and placed into soft foods to facilitate ingestion. However, removing some beads and diverting them for other, possibly inappropriate, uses is also possible.

MAOIs, and it is not recommended for us in patients with narrow angle glaucoma. **Atomoxetine** can modestly affect weight gain, blood pressure, and heart rate; these parameters should be monitored. Less than 2 percent of patients experience orthostatic hypotension. Common side effects include GI symptoms, fatigue, dizziness, mydriasis, and mood swings. For youth who are at least 6 years of age and less than 70 kg in body weight, this agent should be initiated at 0.5 mg per kg per day and then should be gradually increased to 1.2 mg per kg per day, either as single or twice daily dosing. Total daily dosing should not exceed 100 mg (or 1.4 mg per kg per day). For youth above 70 kg in body weight, 40 mg per day is the initial dose. The dosage can typically be increased to 80 mg per day. The manufacturer suggests that **atomoxetine** can be discontinued without tapering (*note:* the authors recommend tapering whenever possible until more clinical experience has confirmed this advice from the manufacturer). This agent is available in 10, 18, 25, 40, and 60 mg capsules.

A number of other medications have been used in the treatment of ADHD uncomplicated by comorbid conditions when psychostimulants are ineffective or as "add-ons" to psychostimulants in the presence of comorbid conditions or with incomplete or partial response. These include a variety of antidepressants, such as the less sedating tricyclic antidepressants (TCAs) **bupropion** and **venlafaxine**. Of the TCAs, only **desipramine** has proven efficacy in ADHD, yet many clinicians avoid its use because of the reports of seven deaths of children treated with this agent; some prescribe **imipramine** or **nortriptyline** instead. Unlike in depression, the response of ADHD to treatment with TCAs may occur rapidly, but whether their positive effects are sustained beyond a few months is still debated. Those claiming a continued response argue that TCAs must be dosed at maximum dosing of 5 mg per kg per day to be effective in younger children; because many clinicians are reluctant to use such high doses, TCA use is not common. Many clinicians find that these agents treat the inattention symptomology less adequately. Providing parents with a balanced informed consent discussion about the TCAs and doing a careful pretreatment workup are important (Table 22.3).

Latency children may have a profile of side effects on TCAs that differs from those in adults, including dysphoria, irritability, or aggression; weight loss; increased heart rate; and increased blood pressure (especially diastolic). Although youth appear to be less sensitive than adults to the peripheral anticholinergic side effects, they may be more sensitive to the central anticholinergic symptoms (e.g., confusion, sedation).

Starting dosing at night is useful for minimizing daytime sedation and treating comorbid insomnia. The dose should be gradually titrated upward as clinical effectiveness is assessed. Latency children should be dosed based on weight. Three to 5 mg per kg per day

TABLE 22.3. PRETREATMENT WORKUP FOR TRICYCLIC ANTIDEPRESSANTS

Careful inquiry into patient and family cardiac history, including any history of early or sudden death in first-degree relatives
Complete blood count with differential, blood urea nitrogen, creatinine, liver function tests
Electrocardiogram
Pulse rate
Standing and supine blood pressure readings to assess the presence of postural (orthostatic) changes

TABLE 22.4. CARDIOVASCULAR PARAMETERS AND TRICYCLIC ANTIDEPRESSANTS

Consultation with a pediatric cardiologist and concomitant reduction of dosage or discontinuation of the TCA is indicated when any one of the following circumstances prevails

Age (yr)	Resting Heart Rate (beats/min)	Resting Blood Pressure in mm Hg (sec)	PR Interval (sec)	QTc Interval (sec)
≤10	≥110	≥140/90 or ≥135/85 for more than half the time for 3 weeks	≥0.18	≥0.5
>10	≥100	≥150/95 or ≥140/85 for more than half the time for 3 weeks	≥0.20	≥0.5

Abbreviation: TCA, tricyclic antidepressant.
From Kye C, Ryan N. Pharmacologic treatment of child and adolescent depression. *Child and Adolesc Psych Clin North Am* 1995;4:261–281, with permission.

is a typical target dose range for **imipramine**, with 5 mg per kg per day as the highest dose. For **nortriptyline**, 3 mg per kg per day is the highest dose because of its potency. Because of possible cardiac effects from **imipramine** or other TCAs, a pretreatment electrocardiogram should be obtained, with follow-up electrocardiograms at 3 mg per kg per day and again at the highest dose. Resting blood pressure and pulse should also be obtained (Table 22.4).

Although the response to treatment has not been shown to correlate with specific blood levels, at least one blood level should be obtained at low dosing to ensure that the child is *not* a poor metabolizer of CYP 2D6 substrates (see Chapter 29). Because of the potentially serious consequences of overdose, clinicians should emphasize to parents the importance of protecting other children, especially toddler siblings, from accidental ingestion.

Bupropion has limited research support for efficacy in ADHD, and many clinicians find that it has only mild treatment effects; some clinicians try it because it is scheduled in Class V. **Bupropion** was voluntarily removed from the United States market in 1986 because of an increased incidence of seizures in bulimic patients, but it was then reentered in 1989. Before treatment is instituted, a history of eating disorders and seizures should be ruled out. Its IR formulation is dosed in a range of 3 to 6 mg per kg per day, divided into three doses, because of **bupropion's** short half-life. Any single dose should be below 150 mg because higher doses have been associated with an increased risk for seizures (4 in 1,000 in adults). The **SR** formulation may be dosed twice daily, and it has a lower risk for seizures. The generally accepted maximum daily IR dose for children is 300 mg, and for teens, 450 mg. (*Note:* The maximum dose for **bupropion-SR** is 400 mg per day.) Amelioration of symptoms of ADHD may begin as early as the third day. Side effects are generally mild, and they include rash, appetite increases, nausea, stomachache, minimal weight loss, blood pressure fluctuations, agitation, aggravation of tics, and, more seriously, cognitive distortions and delirium. The onset of rash may signify a serious allergic reaction, similar to an autoimmune "serum sickness" profile, and it thus

necessitates discontinuation of the medication. Adding psychostimulants on to **bupropion** may be necessary to improve its effectiveness. Increased **valproic acid** levels have been found with
coadministration; these are likely related to competition for glucuronide formation.

The use of α_2-adrenergic agonists has research support; both
clonidine and **guanfacine** are commonly used to treat children
with ADHD, particularly those with impulsivity and hyperactivity,
comorbid tic disorders, aggressivity, or stimulant sleep problems.
Because **clonidine** affects many receptors (it is sometimes referred
to as a "dirty drug"), it can cause more sedation, more hypertensive
rebound after sudden discontinuation, and more hyperglycemia than
does **guanfacine**. The pretreatment workup for both should include
an inquiry about abnormal heart rhythms, and early sudden death
of relatives and the exclusion of Raynaud disease and diabetes mellitus. An electrocardiogram should be conducted if it is indicated,
and baseline blood pressure and pulse should be recorded as well.
Dosing is titrated against behavioral effects. **Clonidine** dosing is
calculated at 5 to 8 μg per kg per day in three to four times daily
scheduling. A single dose is begun at night. Sedation typically is immediate, but maximum behavioral effectiveness may occur gradually over 2 or 3 months. Although the elimination half-life of
clonidine is prolonged, the "behavioral half-life" may be only 3 to
6 hours. Commonly, sedation, dry mouth, and dizziness may be experienced early in treatment. Later, nighttime awakening, nightmares, and night terrors can occur. Depression may appear in about
5% of children, particularly those with a history of depression.
Parents should be aware of the potential for the serious consequences of overdose. Many parents complain of "see-saw" effectiveness, and a **clonidine patch** is useful in youth who do not have skin
reactions to it because the blood levels of the drug are sustained over
the day. Some protection against skin rash is provided by spraying
the skin area to which the patch will be applied with a nasal steroid
spray (e.g., beclomethazone). Although recommendation is made for
weekly patching in the drug insert, many children have better results with 5-day patching with a 2-day overlap of a second patch.
TCAs and **trazodone** inactivate the presser effects of **clonidine**
and possibly its behavioral effects. Some protection against skin rash
is provided by spraying the skin area to which the patch will be applied with a nasal steroid spray (e.g., beclomethazone). Although the
deaths of four children on **methylphenidate** and **clonidine** were
reported, further evaluation has not implicated the combination.
Guanfacine use is increasing in acceptance; it is dosed in a range
from 1.5 to 4 mg per day, often twice daily. When shifting from **clonidine** to **guanfacine**, the clinician should "cross-taper" these drugs
to prevent withdrawal reactions.

b. **Administration**. **The general procedure of administration** is
to begin any of these drugs at a low dose and then to increase the
dose until the point of maximum therapeutic benefit is reached or
some unpleasant side effect develops. That clinicians use a side-
effect scale (e.g., Barkley Side Effect Questionnaire) before and after
treatment is recommended to help track psychostimulant side effects. Although psychostimulants may minimally increase pulse and
blood pressure, monitoring is not necessary unless the patient has a
history of a preexisting arrhythmia or hypertension. These changes
are least likely with **pemoline**. The long-term consequences of these
cardiovascular effects are believed to be benign.

Common side effects of the psychostimulants include appetite
loss, irritability, stomachaches, headaches, and insomnia. Some par-

ents express concern about the possible effects of stimulant medication on growth during these critical years. New studies suggest that adult height and weight are unaffected by **methylphenidate**, except for a small number of individuals with side effects of nausea and vomiting. Weight and height should be monitored at least every 6 months to track growth. Tics, stereotypes, and tremors can appear *de novo* or they can worsen, but some individuals with preexisting tics will experience little or no change in their severity. Previously, the presence of tics was accepted to be a contraindication to stimulant use, but now many clinicians will use psychostimulants (sometimes covering the tics prophylactically with an anti-tic medication; see Chapter 7) in this population. **Amphetamines** may be more likely to produce compulsive behaviors, whereas **methylphenidate** may induce more perseverative behaviors and movement disorders. Rarely, hallucinations (usually of insects crawling) may develop in children with a prior history of hallucinations. Physical dependence to these drugs usually does not occur in childhood, and, in general, tolerance does not occur. Occasionally, tolerance will develop to one of the psychostimulants, and the usual practice then is to switch to a drug of another class. Clinicians should carefully explain all this information to parents or guardians in an informed consent discussion before initiating treatment.

IR methylphenidate is usually administered in two or three daily doses, in the morning, at noon, and possibly after school. Although some physicians, especially pediatricians, dose **methylphenidate** by weight (from 0.3 to 0.6 mg per kg per day), little empirical support is seen for this strategy. However, in children weighing less than 25 kg, more than 35 mg per day is associated with increased side effects. The **amphetamines** are about twice as potent on a per milligram basis as **methylphenidate**. The spacing of doses for either class of IR drug is purely empirical and is usually every 2.5 to 6 hours. Children with difficulties that are confined to school may require dosing once or twice each day; children with severe difficulties both at home and in school may require three or more doses per day. In children, appropriate "bunching" of dosing of agents with a short (2 to 3 hours) duration of effect is crucial in maximizing effectiveness, but the need for more frequent dosing may not be evident unless the clinician speaks directly to the teacher. Less experienced clinicians may be reluctant to increase individual doses above 5 to 10 mg, but dosing should be increased in a stepwise fashion to maximum levels until the agent is effective or side effects become evident. If medication is given too late in the day, some youth experience sleep difficulties; others show improved sleep and behavior with an early evening dose. If 60 mg is set as a somewhat arbitrary maximum daily dose, obviously some portion of the day will remain "uncovered" in children with severe difficulties. Discussion of these dosage issues with guardians and youth is essential in order to individualize regimens that optimize academic and social development. Although oral psychostimulants taken in usual therapeutic doses are not addictive, without a doubt, children or parents can abuse or misuse psychostimulants by taking them in high doses or by snorting or injecting them. Clinicians must evaluate the parents' and school personnel's ability to monitor for misuse of these medications.

4. **Specific psychologic therapies for the child and the family**. Efficacy has been demonstrated in training parents and teachers in contingency management techniques (e.g., time-out, token or point reward systems, response cost). Psychoanalytic psychotherapy and cognitive-behavioral treatments have not been shown to be effective in the treatment of children with ADHD. However, without a doubt, the reduction of family tensions and the structuring of a child's environment are fre-

quently of benefit. Because children with ADHD often have parents with ADHD, a parent's psychiatric pathology sometimes prevents him or her from modifying his or her behavior toward the child. Parental guidance or psychopharmacologic or psychotherapeutic treatment may help to alter the unwanted parental behavior(s). In children with ADHD whose problems have received attention only after they have suffered the accumulative psychologic effects of the syndrome for some years, psychotherapy may potentially be of benefit.

II. Attention Deficit Hyperactivity Disorder in Adults

At present, a growing body of research and other information about ADHD in adults exists. Although a decrement in ADHD symptomology often occurs over time, the evidence for the persistence of ADHD from childhood into adulthood is clear from a number of studies. In the outcome study of Weiss et al. (1985) of the 15-year course of children with ADHD, 30% to 40% of individuals had no significant symptoms, 10% had severe problems (usually drug abuse or antisocial behaviors), and 50% to 60% had moderate symptoms in their work or interpersonal domains. Factors that moderated these adult outcomes included female gender, low aggressivity, no learning disability, no parental pathology, high socioeconomic status, and high intelligence quotient. Increased symptoms of ADHD may emerge as life situations change. For example, a man may function well as an outdoor worker but then may become disorganized and inefficient when he is promoted to management. A housewife whose family tolerated her "relaxed style" may return to college and become overwhelmed by her own lack of organization. In general, adults with ADHD can be expected to have more job impairments, troubled relationships, parenting difficulties, and automobile accidents when compared with non-ADHD adults. The incidence of women and men diagnosed with ADHD in adulthood is roughly equal; the general assumption is that women were "missed" in childhood because of their lack of impulsivity or because of cultural bias.

Adults who present for psychiatric evaluation often come with diagnosis "in hand" after their child has been diagnosed with ADHD or after they have been "diagnosed" by a spouse or friend. Because the DSM-IV requires that symptoms of ADHD must be present before the age of 7 years, the likelihood of an accurate diagnosis is increased when adults remember a trial of **methylphenidate** as a child or when they recall efforts by their teachers to keep them quiet.

Adults with ADHD have been shown to describe accurately their childhood symptoms. Consistent with their history of childhood psychopathology, adult women describe more dissatisfaction with their childhood relationships, and they endorse a poorer self-concept than do men with ADHD. Comorbidity may be even more common in adults than in children; estimates of comorbidity are setting dependent (e.g., in a prison setting, the co-occurrence of ADHD with antisocial personality disorder will be extremely high). Clinicians in many instances can also rely on the available parents of adult patients to ascertain childhood ADHD symptoms, to complete retrospective ADHD scales, or to supply any report cards they may have saved. Current adult ADHD symptomology is sometimes reported most accurately by those who live with or work with the adult patient rather than by the adult patient *per se.*

The studies of Weiss et al. (1985) and Mannuzza et al. (1998) established that certain behaviors of children with ADHD could persist into adulthood. Another group (Wender et al.) subsequently developed two scales to assess these childhood symptoms retrospectively. The Parents Rating Scale is based on the Connors 10-item hyperactivity index, and the Wender Utah Rating Scale is a 61-item questionnaire on which the index adult rates his or her own recalled symptoms from childhood. DSM-IV criteria for ADHD are based on behaviors (signs) in contrast to symptoms. Another diagnostic scale is the Connors Adult Attention Rating Scale; it has good statistical properties and it is recommended by many experts. The Connors Adult Attention Rating Scale comes in two formats—observer and self-reports. Both contain 66 items and, within these, are items reflecting the DSM-IV criteria. Some items seem quite straightforward (e.g., "I don't finish things I start," "I am restless or overactive"); other items seem more appropriate for youth (e.g., "I have trouble waiting in line or taking turns with others," "I blurt things out"); and others may not be interpreted consistently (e.g., "I step on people's toes without meaning to")—it is the intention of the scale's creators that this is taken figuratively rather than literally. Another useful scale is the 18-item ADHD Behavior Checklist for Adults with its two nine-item subscales, one for inattention and the other for hyperactivity and/or impulsivity (Murphy and Barkley, 1996).

The Wender group developed criteria to delineate a group of adults who were likely to benefit from psychostimulant treatment; these criteria focus both on signs and symptoms. In addition to meeting two behavioral criteria (signs) for combined-type ADHD in childhood (i.e., attentional problems and hyperactivity), these adults must currently have at least two of the following five symptoms, which can be remembered by the following mnemonic **TIMID**: (a) hot **T**emper, (b) **I**mpulsivity, (c) **M**ood lability, (d) **I**ntolerance for stress, and (e) **D**isorganization. A structured interview, the Targeted Attention Deficit Disorder Scale, elicits data on all seven of these dimensions—the two behavioral and the five just listed.

Methylphenidate, *d*-**amphetamine**, and **pemoline** have all shown efficacy in adults selected by these criteria. Some adults with comorbid anxiety who are treated with **Adderall** may have an increase in anxiety. Clinical observations suggest that, in addition to symptom reduction, improvements in vocational or educational performance and in relationships with spouse or partner, children, or extended family are seen (e.g., rather than getting fired, they get promoted; rather than failing in school, they graduate; rather than divorce, their marriages improve). Specifically, a reduction in the number and intensity of outbursts of temper (rages); an increased ability to cope with stress; increased attention and decreased distractibility; decreased motor restlessness, if present; and improved executive functioning will be seen.

Attentional deficits may present as problems of "executive functioning" (e.g., trouble organizing tasks, persisting in tasks, or managing affect during tasks). Adults with ADHD show a treatment response to psychostimulants that is similar to that seen in children and adolescents with ADHD (i.e., they do not have the euphoric response to treatment-range doses of psychostimulants that is seen in many non-ADHD adolescents and adults). Similarly, they do not become tolerant to the beneficial effects of psychostimulants.

Dosing of **IR methylphenidate** to 1 to 2 mg per kg per day or of equivalent **amphetamines** is typical in adults. The duration of action of **IR methylphenidate** is about 2 to 3 hours in adults; *d*-**amphetamine's** duration of action is about 3.5 to 4.5 hours. A typical dosing regimen for **IR methylphenidate** could be 10 to 15 mg every 2.5 to 3 hours or about five to six times per day. *d*-**Amphetamine** is usually given as 7.5 to 15 mg every 4 hours or three to four times per day. When Dexedrine spansules are given to adults, some clinicians add to these 5 to 7.5 mg of *d*-**amphetamine**. More experience is needed with the newer long-acting formulations of **methylphenidate** to clarify their durations of effect. Because of their characteristic disorganization, some adults with ADHD use multiple-alarm wrist watches to alert them to take their medications as prescribed.

Unlike children, adults generally feel subjectively better when the psychostimulants are effective, and they often describe feeling "calm and collected and able to think about one thing at a time," "being centered," "being less impulsive," or "getting things done." Adults with ADHD have an increased rate of automobile accidents, and psychostimulants have been shown to improve simulated driving. For these reasons, some appropriately selected adults may benefit from the use of medication while driving, especially during "boring" long-distance driving. Of theoretical concern is the possibility that ADHD adults and some adolescents could obtain euphoric effects from larger doses of psychostimulants or that they would be more likely than children to divert them to others for illicit use. Many clinicians, therefore, are disinclined to use amphetamines and **methylphenidate** in older adolescents and adults, to the disadvantage of such patients.

Although less well studied, many agents that have shown at least some efficacy in children with ADHD can be administered to adults in usual adult doses. Positive results have been found in small to moderate sample size, double-blind, placebo-controlled trials with **guanfacine, desipramine, bupropion**, and **atomoxetine**. Monotherapy is the ideal, but combined pharmacotherapy is often necessary. Many adults with ADHD do not find traditional psychotherapies useful. Rather, an approach emphasizing specific organizational skill acquisition and "coaching" individually or in groups can be helpful. Couples therapy can be useful as the adult with treated ADHD renegotiates couple and parental roles.

III. **Online Clinical Practice Guidelines**
   The American Academy of Pediatrics has an online version of their 2001 ADHD treatment guidelines, *Treatment of the School-Aged Child With Attention-Deficit/Hyperactivity Disorder*. The online version includes a PDF file called AAP Parent Pages. This file is a useful handout for parent or patient education. It can be found at *http://www.aap.org/policy/s0120.html*.

ADDITIONAL READING

American Academy of Child and Adolescent Psychiatry. Practice parameters for the assessment and treatment of children, adolescents and adults with attention-deficit hyperactivity disorder. *J Am Acad Child Adolesc Psychiatry* 1997;36:85S–121S.

Barickman LL, Perry PJ, Allen AJ, et al. Bupropion versus methylphenidate in the treatment of attention-deficit hyperactivity disorder. *J Am Acad Child Adolesc Psychiatry* 1995;34:649–657.

Barkley RA. *Attention-deficit hyperactivity disorder: a handbook for diagnosis and treatment.* New York: Guilford Press, 1990.

Barkley RA. *A clinical workbook: attention-deficit hyperactivity disorder.* New York: Guilford Press, 1998.

Barkley RA, Murphy KR. *Attention-deficit hyperactivity disorder,* 2nd ed. New York: Guilford Press, 1998.

Conners C, Erhardt D, Epstein J, et al. Self-ratings of ADHD symptoms in adults. I. Factor structure and normative data. *J Attention Dis* 1999;3:141–152.

Conners C, Erhardt D, Sparrow E, et al. *The Conners Adult ADHD Rating Scale (CAARS).* Toronto: Multi-Health Systems, 1998.

Faraone SV, Biederman J, Mennin D, et al. A prospective four-year follow-up study of children at risk for ADHD: psychiatric, neuropsychological, and psychosocial outcome. *J Am Acad Child Adolesc Psychiatry* 1996;35:1449–1459.

Findling RL, Short EJ, Manos MJ. Developmental aspects of psychostimulant treatment in children and adolescents with attention-deficit/hyperactivity disorder. *J Am Acad Child Adolesc Psychiatry* 2001;40:1441–1447.

Goldman LS, Genel M, Bezman RJ, et al. Diagnosis and treatment of attention-deficit/hyperactivity disorder in children and adolescents. Council on Scientific Affairs, American Medical Association. *JAMA* 1998;279:1100–1107.

Greenhill LL, Osman BB, eds. *Ritalin theory and practice,* 2nd ed. Larchmont, NY: MA Liebert, 2000.

Hechtman L. Families of children with attention deficit hyperactivity disorder: a review. *Can J Psychiatry* 1996;41:350–360.

Hechtman L, Weiss G. Controlled prospective fifteen year follow-up of hyperactives as adults: non-medical drug and alcohol use and anti-social behaviour. *Can J Psychiatry* 1986;31:557–567.

James RS, Sharp WS, Bastain TM, et al. Double-blind, placebo-controlled study of single-dose amphetamine formulations in ADHD. *J Am Acad Child Adolesc Psychiatry* 2001;40:1268–1276.

Mannuzza S, Klein RG, Bessler A, et al. Adult psychiatric status of hyperactive boys grown up. *Am J Psychiatry* 1998;155:493–498.

McCann BS, Scheele L, Ward N, et al. Discriminant validity of the Wender Utah rating scale for attention-deficit/hyperactivity disorder in adults. *J Neuropsych Clin Neurosci* 2000;12:240–245.

Michelson D, Faries D, Wernicke J, et. al. Atomoxetine in the treatment of children and adolescents with attention deficit/hyperactivity disorder: a randomized, placebo-controlled, dose-response study. *Pediatrics* 2001;108:e83.

Murphy K, Barkley RA. Attention deficit hyperactivity disorder adults: comorbidities and adaptive impairments. *Compr Psychiatry* 1996;37:393–401.

Murphy K, Barkley RA. Updated adult norms for the ADHD behavior checklist for adults. *ADHD Rep* 1996;4:12–13.

Nadeau K. *A comprehensive guide to attention deficit disorder in adults.* New York: Brunner-Mazel, 1995.

Schachar R, Taylor E, Wieselberg M, et al. Changes in family function and relationships in children who respond to methylphenidate. *J Am Acad Child Adolesc Psychiatry* 1987;26:728–732.

Shader RI, Harmatz JS, Oesterheld JR, et al. Population pharmacokinetics of methylphenidate in children with attention-deficit hyperactivity disorder. *J Clin Pharmacol* 1999;39:775–785.

Spencer T, Biederman J, Wilens T, et al. Effectiveness and tolerance of tomoxetine in adults with attention deficit hyperactivity disorder. *Am J Psychiatry* 1998;155:693–695.

Spencer T, Wilens T, Biederman J, et al. A double-blind, crossover comparison of methylphenidate and placebo in adults with childhood-onset attention-deficit hyperactivity disorder. *Arch Gen Psychiatry* 1995;52:434–443.

Swanson J, Lerner M, March J, et al. Assessment and intervention for attention-deficit/hyperactivity disorder in the schools: lessons from the MTA study. *Pediatr Clin North Am* 1999;46:993–1009.

Taylor FB, Russo J. Comparing guanfacine and dextroamphetamine for the treatment of adult attention-deficit/hyperactivity disorder. *J Clin Psychopharmacol* 2001;21:223–228.

Weiss G, Hechtman L, Milroy T, et al. Psychiatric status of hyperactives as adults: a controlled prospective 15-year follow-up of 63 hyperactive children. *J Am Acad Child Psychiatry* 1985;24:211–220.

Weiss M, Hechtman-Trokenberg L, Weiss G. *ADHD in adulthood: a guide to current theory, diagnosis, and treatment.* Baltimore: Johns Hopkins University Press, 1999.

Wender PH. A possible monoaminergic basis for minimal brain dysfunction. *Psychopharmacol Bull* 1975;11:36.

Wender PH. Attention-deficit hyperactivity disorder in adults. *Psychiatr Clin North Am* 1998;21:761–774.

Wender PH. *ADHD: attention-deficit hyperactivity disorder in children and adults.* New York: Oxford University Press, 2000.

Wilens TE, Biederman J, Spencer TJ, et al. Pharmacotherapy of adult attention deficit/hyperactivity disorder: a review. *J Clin Psychopharmacol* 1995;15:270–281.

23. MEDICAL USES OF HYPNOSIS

Richard I. Shader
Claire M. Frederick
Stephen G. Pauker

The understanding of **hypnosis** has come a long way since 1794 when a special commission of the French Academy (including Benjamin Franklin, Lavoiser, and Guillotine) dismissed Anton Mesmer's work with the rather ironic charge that it was merely "imagination." Some believe that the first description of hypnosis occurred in *Genesis 2:21–22,* which says that "God caused a deep sleep to fall upon Adam, and while he slept God took one of his ribs. . . ." Hypnosis can be thought of as a state of intense focal concentration with diminished peripheral awareness that is usually coupled with a high degree of relaxation. It is part of the continuum of normal attention, and it is composed of heightened absorption in perceptions, the dissociation of mental states from one another, heightened suggestibility, and diminished critical judgment.

The use of hypnosis as a therapeutic tool has been sanctioned by the American Medical Association since 1958. Recognizing the value of hypnosis, the American Medical Association has recommended that medical students should be trained in hypnosis; only rarely is this recommendation implemented. When hypnosis is appropriately applied, it can facilitate diagnostic and therapeutic procedures in clinical medicine. Even though the field of hypnosis has been a focus of much research and many therapeutically helpful developments, a great deal of misinformation and prejudice about it still remains.

I. **Suggestion**
   Clinicians cannot help but use suggestion; at issue is whether it is used knowingly for patient benefit or inadvertently in ways that may cause harm. When a clinician asks a patient, "How is your pain today?", he or she is indirectly suggesting that the patient still has pain. A more helpful suggestion might be, "I wonder whether you're more comfortable today." The kind of **indirect suggestion** illustrated here can be quite effective. Suggestions are even more effective when they are connected to strong emotions. Patients' expectations about the future clearly play a part in shaping the future and in how they perceive it. "It is not simply mind over matter, but it is clear that mind matters" (Spiegel, 1999).

II. **The Trance State**
   The trance state is an altered, but natural, state of consciousness. Hypnotizable people can enter this state in a matter of seconds, and good hypnotic subjects (*note:* when hypnosis is used for medical purposes, the word subject is interchangeable with the word patient) often slip in and out of trance states without realizing it (see sections III and IV). One common kind of trance experience is being totally absorbed in reading a book or magazine or in watching a movie or television to the extent that one is unaware of peripheral distractions. This intense concentration on a focal issue permits subjects to "ignore" or modify their perception of unwanted stimuli, such as noise or pain. Moreover, suspending critical judgment or focusing selectively on alternative feelings or behaviors is possible. During a trance, many different subjective phenomena may be experienced, depending on variables such as the expectations of the patient, the suggestions of the therapist, and the depth of the trance (Table 23.1).

   Typically, a person in a hypnotic trance wants to comply and cooperate with the suggestions offered by the therapist who induces the trance. When subjects profoundly object to suggestions, they are unlikely to comply. When obtaining consent for the medical use of hypnosis, reassuring patients that, while in the trance state, they will not involuntarily reveal any secrets, lose consciousness, or have weakened will power is important. On the other hand, during a trance

TABLE 23.1. SOME TRANCE (HYPNOTIC) PHENOMENA

Catalepsy
Amnesia
Dissociation
Analgesia and anesthesia
Hyperesthesia
Ideosensory activity
Somnambulism
Hallucinations
Hyperamnesia
Age regression
Ideomotor activity
Age progression
Time distortion
Depersonalization
Induced dreams
Relaxation

patients may occasionally recall deeply repressed material about which they were consciously unaware and with which they may still be unable to deal or process. During the trance, these recollections are communicated to the therapist. In such situations, the therapist may sometimes suggest that, upon alerting, the patient "will remember those things that are safe and useful but will remember to forget material that is not, until it is safe to do so."

Currently, contemporary research techniques are being applied to clarify the processes and changes in physiology underlying trance states. One recent study, for example, revealed increased cerebral blood flow occipitally and increased delta wave activity as measured by the electroencephalogram. In time, that the biology of trance states will be more fully understood seems probable.

III. The Trance Induction

All hypnosis is, in reality, self-hypnosis, whereby the subject allows himself or herself to slip into a mode of intense concentration. The therapist can systematically teach a patient how to use this capacity, while stressing from the beginning that nothing will be "projected" or forced onto the patient. An atmosphere of repose, free of coercion, that enables the therapist and patient to choose a focus of fixed concentration is extremely important. The particular ritual or technique of trance induction (Table 23.2) is less important than is the patient's conviction of its efficacy and of the need for therapeutic relief. In fact, some of the benefits of positive suggestion can be obtained without inducing formal trance. Clinicians can sometimes use suggestion *en passant* during other clinical activities, such as the physical examination or the performance of minor procedures. Rather than engaging in random conversation with the patient at these times, the clinician may choose to use **waking suggestions** to make the patient more comfortable, to improve adherence, to diminish anxiety, to facilitate healing, and to shape behavior. When a formal trance is used, providing the patient with the demonstration and recall of some manifestation of trance is useful for ratifying its existence (e.g., temporary *glove anesthesia* or some *posthypnotic suggestion*) (Table 23.3).

IV. Diagnostic Uses

Because people vary in their ability to go into a hypnotic trance, a growing body of experience now exists that recommends a systematic assessment of this trance capacity as a way of providing useful diagnostic information quickly. The trance experiences of comparatively healthy persons seem clearly distinguishable from those of persons with severe personality disorders, schizophrenia, or nonpsychogenic amnesic or pain syndromes (e.g., toxic states, head trauma). Patients with these more severe problems can enter the trance state only errat-

TABLE 23.2. A SAMPLE PROTOCOL FOR HYPNOSIS

- Assess the patient and establish rapport.
- Orient the patient and dispel any misconceptions.
- Create a positive expectancy about the hypnotic experience.
- Develop therapeutic goals and plans.
- Fix the patient's attention using an induction technique.
- Deepen the level of trance using suggestions and trance phenomena.
- Accomplish the planned therapeutic strategy; note the patient's responses; and modify the plan, using what patient says and does.
- Ratify the trance state, giving the patient a signal that something special has happened.
- When posthypnotic suggestions are indicated, introduce them.
- Make ego-strengthening suggestions about the future.
- Remove or time limit any unwanted suggestions or phenomena elicited during induction.
- Realert the patient.

TABLE 23.3. DEPTH OF TRANCE—POTENTIALLY OBSERVABLE PHENOMENA

Light trance (hypnoidal state)
Slower, deeper breathing
Progressive feelings of lethargy
Observable relaxation
Inhibition of voluntary movements
Eyelid catalepsy
Limb catalepsy
Medium trance
Glove anesthesia
Partial posthypnotic anesthesia
Partial amnesia
Partial age regression
Some degree of time distortion
Positive mental imagery
Ability to have dream-like experiences
External noises can be heard yet ignored
Deep trance (somnambulism)
Full age regression (revivification)
Positive and negative hallucinations
Extensive anesthesia
Posthypnotic anesthesia
Spontaneous amnesia
Responds to suggestions for amnesia
Eyes-open trance
Decrease in spontaneous mental activity
Highly responsive to posthypnotic suggestion
Perceptual distortion and body dissociation
Circumoral pallor > 1 cm
Plenary trance (stuporous state)
Timelessness
Lack of awareness of physical body
Loss of one's ordinary identity
Potential to be anyone or anything
Feeling at one with the universe
Marked decreases in respiratory and pulse rates
Cessation of spontaneous mental activity
Lack of awareness of the external world except for the therapist

ically, and they have difficulty maintaining the continuous concentration that is required. For example, hypnosis may assist in the difficult differential diagnosis of a dissociative disorder from other, possibly psychotic, conditions. The response to trance induction may be expected to differ strikingly in these two clinical situations. The hypnotizability of patients with dissociative disorders (see Chapter 4), posttraumatic stress disorders (see Chapters 14 and 27), and some eating disorders (e.g., bulimia nervosa) (see Chapter 8 and Esplen et al., 1998) is higher than normal, whereas that of patients with schizophrenia is quite low. Although hypnosis has yet to be studied adequately in toxic and other medical conditions, difficulties similar to those experienced with schizophrenic patients may reasonably be expected.

One brief (10-minute) assessment of trance capacity (Table 23.4) that may be incorporated as part of the clinical induction procedure is known as the hypnotic induction profile (Spiegel and Spiegel, 1978). It is usually carried out when evaluating patients for treatment with hypnosis or when hypnosis is used to assist in differential diagnosis. A series of behavioral instructions can be given after a brief hypnotic induction. The therapist suggests that a subject's hand will remain light and in an upright position. The patient shows hypnotizability by the degree to which he or she acts in accordance with this instruction and to which he or she experiences reversible alterations in sensation and motor control in the hand. Other good hypnotizability scales that have been adapted for clinical use are also available (e.g., Hilgard and Hilgard, 1975). However, many clinical

TABLE 23.4. SOME ILLUSTRATIVE ELEMENTS ADAPTED AND MODIFIED FROM THE HYPNOTIC INDUCTION PROFILE

Phase	Action	Instruction to Patient[a] and Observation
Pre-induction	Up gaze	Say: "Look upward toward your eyebrows and up to the top of your head." Evaluate: how much sclera is visible between the iris and the lower lid, as well as the extent to which the iris is hidden by the upper lid.
Induction	Eye-roll sign	Say: "Continue to look upward, close your eyes slowly. Good. Close, close, close." Evaluate: scleral exposure and iris coverage by upper lid.
	Arm levitation	Say: "Imagine a floating feeling, right down through the chair. Concentrate on your arm and hand. Notice the movement sensations that develop in your fingers, causing the hand to feel buoyant. Let your hand be a balloon." Evaluate: the extent to which the patient's arm slowly rises.
Post-induction	Cut-off	Having previously suggested arm levitation and that the feeling of dissociation of the arm will disappear with a nonverbal cue (typically a touch of the elbow), provide the cue, saying "Now note this." Evaluate the extent to which the patient reports a change in sensation after the cue is provided.

[a] Note that the maneuvers of the hypnotic induction profile (HIP) produce a light trance in suggestible patients. Any suggestions made should be removed or nullified before completing the evaluation. From Spiegel H, Spiegel D. *Trance and treatment: clinical uses of hypnosis.* New York: Basic Books, 1978, with permission. There are many procedures for trance induction. These selected items are illustrative of one approach. The interested reader should consult the original text for the complete approach to the use and scoring of the HIP.

reports suggest little difference in therapeutic outcomes from hypnosis based on the hypnotizability of the patient.

The therapist should be alert to at least two sources of artifact in this assessment. If the patient feels coerced or untrusting, the response may be below the individual's real capacity. In addition to this problem of motivation, when a patient is medicated, that sedative-hypnotics and antipsychotic agents, and possibly other classes of agents, would interfere with trance capacity is probable. Enough patients have sufficient trance capacity to make hypnosis a clinically useful tool, even if their hypnotic induction profile score is only modest. For this reason, many clinicians do not formally assess suggestibility or hypnotizability. Instead, they presume that the patient has an adequate capacity for trance and simply proceed. This is particularly important when hypnosis and suggestion are used as an adjunct to other medical therapies. For example, if the patient is about to undergo a procedure (e.g., catheterization, endoscopy, lumbar puncture, or even the suturing of a laceration), performing the hypnotic induction profile before deciding to use suggestion to mitigate the patient's discomfort would be inappropriate. Suggestion or even formal trance should be used in such circumstances as a matter of course.

Approximately 10% of the population are refractory to or uncooperative about hypnosis. Of the remaining 90%, about one-third are capable of light trance, one-third of moderate trance, and one-third are highly responsive (Hammond, 1998). Children tend to use trance more easily than do adults, with peak responsivity between the ages of 8 and 12 years. Experienced pediatricians skilled in hypnosis report the ability to induce trance in infants, even newborns, using nonverbal techniques (S. Pauker, *personal communication*, 2000).

V. Therapeutic Applications

Many psychiatric inpatients may be incapable of sustained trance experiences. In general medical settings and in outpatient treatment, however, hypnosis can augment a variety of therapeutic strategies; the higher that the patient's hypnotizability is, the more likely a positive outcome will be. The clinician must remember, however, that a patient's hypnotizability *per se* does not make hypnosis an effective treatment for that person. Other important factors include motivation to change, the presence of secondary gain, and the transference and/or alliance with the therapist (see Chapter 1).

A. Pain

Hypnosis can be remarkably effective in controlling pain, whether of psychogenic or nonpsychogenic origin. In the last century, Esdaile reported better than 80% surgical anesthesia with hypnosis. Esdaile's series of 3,000 patients also showed a 10-fold decline in operative mortality, from 50% to 5%, that presumably resulted from avoiding the effects of shock. Although hypnosis has been used successfully as the sole anesthesia in major surgery, very few medical indications are found for performing major surgery with hypnosis as the sole anesthesia. Rather, hypnosis should be considered an adjunct that permits comfort with lower doses of anesthetic agents and that may speed recovery and diminish intraoperative blood loss, especially if those expectations are established preoperatively. Highly hypnotizable subjects often can achieve full anesthesia; persons with a lower responsiveness can learn to transform their perceptions or to divert their attention from the pain. Hypnosis may be underrecognized as a helpful technique in natural childbirth; it is also potentially useful for the relief of preoperative anxiety that will usually augment the postoperative pain. Furthermore, patients with postsurgical or trauma-induced pain, as well as some with chronic distress, may be taught to hypnotize themselves to cope with pain better. Remembering that opiates and sedative-hypnotics, by clouding the sensorium, interfere with hypnotic capacity is important.

Before any treatment approach is chosen, establishing an accurate diagnosis is essential. Hypnosis can be used in a number of ways to control pain. One could produce a state of tingling numbness, warmth or coolness, and reduced sensitivity in an unaffected area (e.g., the left hand in a right-handed person) and could then recreate these feelings in the affected area. This is a substitution strategy. The patient can also be told to imagine that a local anesthetic has been applied to the painful area, although care should be taken to determine that the patient is not allergic to local anesthetics, lest the suggestion induce an allergic reaction, a rare complication of such suggestions. Another variation could shift or displace attention from the affected area to a neutral or unaffected area (e.g., from the lower back to the left hand). These strategies can be combined. In addition, use of repeated sessions to reduce the perceived magnitude of the pain decrementally at each successive session is often reasonable.

These examples illustrate one of the main elements in the control of pain by hypnosis, perceptual filtering. Another element is induced physical relaxation. The patient is taught to concentrate on a metaphor that connotes muscle relaxation, such as floating. This can often produce relaxation in the painful area and can thereby reduce pain signals. Among the strategies that can be useful in managing pain, suggestion can be used to alter the intensity of the sensation and its quality and duration, which refers to the ability of trance and posthypnotic suggestion to produce time distortion. When patients have difficulty decreasing the discomfort (a less jarring word than "pain"), a useful approach can be to have the patient *increase* the severity of the pain. Once this has been accomplished, patients can be guided to the realization that they do have the ability to affect their own pain. At that point, the realization that they can, if they so desire, "take the hurt out of their discomfort" is a small step for them. Ewin (1983) noted that happiness and joy often override painful situations. In treating patients with acute thermal burns, he has found the suggestion that patients visit their "laughing place" to be useful.

Because chronic pain syndromes are so often accompanied by demoralization or depression, the treatment of pain must always be undertaken in a context that addresses the broader needs and problems of the patient (see Chapters 18 and 28). Even then, however, showing patients that they have some control over their discomfort can be liberating, and it can increase their coping capacity. To help patients manage chronic pain, therapists often use the trance to show the patient how to alter the severity or quality of the sensation and they use time distortion to modify its frequency or duration. A useful metaphor can be to ask the patient to scan their bodies and minds to locate the switch or rheostat that controls their sensation in that area and then to turn it to change its volume or tone.

B. Medical and Surgical Procedures

Hypnosis is a powerful adjunct for patients undergoing a variety of procedures. The relaxation and dissociation it provides decrease anxiety and discomfort. Its influence on the autonomic nervous system can produce selective vasoconstriction and can thereby diminish intraoperative bleeding. Hypnosis, even if it is introduced only in the preanesthetic induction setting, can establish positive expectations about surgical outcomes and can speed recovery. A recent controlled study demonstrated that formal hypnosis can diminish the procedure and recovery time (Lang et al., 2000). Pediatricians may find that providing their healthy young patients with a "magic spot," which the patient controls and can apply as needed (e.g., for immunizations, for suturing lacerations), to be useful.

C. Medical Conditions

Hypnosis has been applied, with mixed success, to a broad variety of medical conditions. Unfortunately, the results remain mostly anecdotal, with few well-controlled trials in the literature. Nonetheless, because the risks of hypnosis are quite low (barring inadequate diagnostic evaluation and masking of important symptoms), clinicians may find the use of suggestion and hypnosis to be beneficial in many different settings (Pinnell and Covino, 2000). Among the conditions reported to respond to hypnosis are irritable bowel syndrome, asthma, migraine, warts, and psoriasis. (*Note:* Each of these is an episodic condition in which exacerbations can be produced by stress.)

D. Psychosomatic Illnesses

Some medical conditions with large affective and stress-related components, such as asthma, can be susceptible to intervention with hypnosis. The technique is similar to that used for anxiety; it consists of teaching the patient to master his or her somatic responses in the face of an atopic or emotional stress to prevent further decompensation.

E. Anxiety

Patients with recurring anxiety can be helped to interrupt the "snowballing" effect of their somatic and psychologic tension. In such situations, hypnosis can be used to disconnect the somatic symptoms from the subjective psychologic distress. Patients are taught to use self-hypnosis. In one self-hypnosis exercise, for example, the patients imagine themselves relaxed and floating in a comfortable chair while picturing their concerns on an imaginary split movie screen. On one half of the screen are seen the anxieties and problems; on the other half are the patient's own internal resources—stabilizing relationships, achievements, and abilities.

Patients with **panic attacks** can be helped with hypnosis in several ways. One is the use of relaxation and the split screen technique. Patients are instructed to picture a feared situation on one side of the screen and a means of coping with it, or other psychologic resources, on the other, all the while maintaining the feeling of floating. The screen may also be used to estimate the real risk and to diffuse the confusion between probability and possibility that affects many patients with panic attacks or phobias. The enhanced control over the physical response that is obtained through hypnosis can help anxious and phobic patients master their physical symptoms instead of feeling frightened by them. This technique enhances relaxation and promotes a sense of mastery. The initial stimuli remain, but the helplessness and immobilization are contained. The success of this particular technique is compromised when the anxious patient is unable to bind or contain the anxiety long enough to permit focused concentration. Self-hypnosis works best for minimal to mild anxiety (see Chapter 14). Hypnosis can also be used for the identification of triggers for panic attacks and for desensitization to both the triggers and the panic experience itself. Hypnoanalytic work has the potential for uncovering and repairing unresolved conflicts that may be expressing themselves in panic attacks.

F. Simple Phobias

These respond well to behavior therapy, but they may also respond to hypnosis, which, in some instances, is less time consuming. Phobic patients can be taught to bring on a sense of relaxation and well-being using the technique described in section E. For example, patients with flying phobias are taught to use a self-hypnotic feeling of "floating with the plane," as if the plane were an extension of their own bodies. For all simple phobias, the patient and therapist work out a series of steps involving exposure to the feared object or situation coupled with a self-hypnotic state of relaxation. Again the goal is to contain the anxiety and to promote a sense of mastery (see Chapter 14).

Alternatively, some clinicians find that phobias, such as fear of flying, can be approached by asking patients to visualize a successful outcome in the future (e.g., walking off the plane at the planned destination) and slowly playing their mental tape or imagery backward until they can see the entire sequence (e.g., from leaving their home to arriving at their destination) as a series of successes. These same approaches can be helpful in patient who is extremely anxious about a procedure, such as surgery, or something they must accomplish, such as a performance or a sporting event.

G. Obsessions and Compulsions

A special case of anxiety control involves the alleviation of some of the distress and anxiety that either alters the threshold and produces an increased frequency of obsessive thoughts and compulsive actions (see Chapter 6) or results from attempts (or an inability) to resist them. The goal is to enhance the patient's sense of calmness and comfort, thereby raising the threshold for the emergence of these unwanted experiences; one approach involves using hypnosis to place time boundaries around them. Once the patient with a compulsion to clean has been hypnotized, for example, he or she is asked to imagine spending 1 hour a day thoroughly cleaning the bathroom. After several sessions, the patient would then be asked (while in the trance state) to describe the activities and feelings involved. Next, the therapist uses posthypnotic suggestion to give the patient the task of actually cleaning the bathroom in question within the 1-hour limit. If this goal is met, the patient is then helped to reduce the time (e.g., to 15 min per day).

Hypnosis can also be used to determine whether thoughts or contexts exist that lower the patient's threshold for the emergence of the obsessive thoughts and actions. For patients with more severe symptoms and distress (e.g., those meeting the criteria for obsessive-compulsive disorder) (see Chapter 6), hypnosis rarely works as a primary treatment. It can have value as an adjunctive therapy in further reducing an unwanted behavior (e.g., hair pulling) in a patient who has had a partial response to medication or behavior therapy.

Obsessive-compulsive symptoms can be thought of as existing on a spectrum ranging from the most biologically determined to the most psychologically determined. Many patients with obsessive-compulsive symptoms have dissociative difficulties as well (Frederick and McNeal, 1999). At times, hypnoanalytic work can help to resolve the psychopathologic underpinnings of obsessions and compulsions.

H. Dissociative Disorders and Conversion Symptoms

Although hypnosis is considered by many to be extremely helpful in working with patients who have dissociative disorders (see Chapter 4), the nature and treatment of these disorders has become a theoretical, forensic, and political battleground in recent times (Brown et al., 1997). Many patients with dissociative amnesia or fugue can be treated with simple hypnotic age regression. Highly hypnotizable people may be prone to conversion symptoms. They may be "willing" to give up or to eliminate these symptoms when the secondary loss has exceeded the gain. Hypnotic suggestion can be used to reduce, to exaggerate, or to transfer a symptom, thereby showing the patient how to enhance control over that symptom. This should be done in the context of a rehabilitation program that reinforces improvement and that does not interpret resistances. A nonhypnotizable patient is more likely to have hypochondriasis or a nonpsychogenic problem.

The diagnosis and treatment of trauma and dissociation is a rapidly developing field. The use of newer diagnostic tools has led many to believe that the incidence of serious dissociative disorders, such as dissociative identity disorder, is much higher than was previously believed. The diagnosis and treatment of dissociative identity disorder can be extremely complex. Although age regression and *abreaction* (recalling and reexperiencing or reliving suppressed or repressed events) of traumatic memory material can be used at times in the treatment of dissociative identity disorder and other serious dissociative conditions, emphasis has shifted to **phase-oriented treatment models**, in which the use of hypnosis for stabilization, ego strengthening, and mastery achieve prominence. Current standards of care require that hypnotically facilitated abreaction be conducted only in stabilized patients who have good ego strength and who have learned how to exercise mastery over trauma material. The therapist must always use extreme caution in avoiding any suggestion to patients that trauma or abuse has occurred.

When working with the patient, the therapist must be prepared to deal with emerging traumatic memory material, which may or may not be associated with accurate recall of actual traumatic events *per se,* and the traumatic transference and countertransference associated with childhood trauma or abuse. Training in trauma and dissociation is now considered to be necessary for those who treat posttraumatic and dissociative disorders, and additional advanced education in hypnosis is essential for those who wish to use it for treating these populations, especially for the victims of rape (see Chapter 27).

I. Habits

Hypnosis can facilitate a strategy of self-affirmation in dealing with difficult problems such as smoking. Self-hypnosis is a widely used aid to smoking cessation. It is used in the context of the cognitive restructuring of the urge to smoke, and it involves having the patient focus instead on a commitment to respect and protect his or her body. For example, the patient is instructed during the trance to repeat, "For my body, smoking is a poison; I need my body to live; I owe my body the respect and protection of not smoking; I am responsible for my body; I am a nonsmoker." Patients learn to stop smoking not by fighting the urge to smoke but rather by connecting this urge to broader interests in health and protection of the body. Some clinicians present the patient with a model in which smoking is seen as a conditioned response to external stimuli, such as situation-specific stress. Patients are then shown how to use hypnosis to extinguish that conditioned response by playing out in their trance how the presentation of the stimulus (stress) does not need to be followed by the evoked response. Hypnosis is used to illustrate to patients the way that they relate to their bodies and how their bodies are dependent on them. Hypnosis is likely to be most successful when it is incorporated into a total treatment plan that includes group therapy and possibly the use of **nicotine**-containing preparations (e.g., patches, gum) or the prodopaminergic agent **bupropion**.

Similar approaches are used to help some patients who overeat, especially those who overeat when they are anxious (see Chapter 8). Little success has been found for the use of hypnosis in the treatment of addiction to alcohol or other abusable substances. Hypnosis has also been applied to bruxism, nail biting, gagging, tongue thrusting, enuresis, and other habit disorders.

J. Spontaneous Hypnosis

A subgroup of patients may require training in how not to enter the trance mode. These extremely hypnotizable people are constantly being "entranced" by others, are working to please them, and are suspending their own critical judgment. Here the trance induction is used as a demonstration of how susceptible they are, and they are taught how to control their own tendency to slip into trance states. Spontaneous hypnosis can also be observed to occur in houses of worship and in the emergency departments of hospitals.

VI. Cautions and Contraindications

Hypnosis should never be attempted under threat or coercion. The therapist should explain briefly the nature of hypnosis and should emphasize that trance is a natural state into which all enter on a daily basis, that all hypnosis is really self-hypnosis, that the patient will remain aware of what is happening, and that he or she is free to break the trance state at any time. The purpose of the hypnotic intervention should be explained clearly, and the nature of the induction procedure should be briefly reviewed. The clinician must remember that hypnosis is only a technique, and clinicians should never attempt to do anything with hypnosis that they are not trained to do without hypnosis. Even with some of the patients noted in the next three subsections, hypnosis can sometimes be used successfully to ease the discomfort associated with specific interventions, such as dental phobias, preoperative preparation, or obstetric and gynecologic procedures.

A. Severe Depression

Many hypnotic techniques can help with the mitigation and resolution of depression. Hypnosis can be used to augment both psychodynamic and/or object relations-oriented psychotherapy and cognitive-behavioral approaches (Yapko, 1996; Frederick and McNeal, 1999). Hypnotically facilitated ego strengthening can be "of unparalleled value" with suicidal patients when conducted by therapists well trained in therapeutic hypnosis (Brown and Fromm, 1986; Frederick and McNeal, 1999). However, the inexperienced should approach depressed patients with extreme caution. Persons who are severely depressed and suicidal may have their hopes for a magical cure raised and then dashed by an attempt at a hypnotic induction. A patient could view an unsuccessful induction as one more failure in life, and, if he or she is suicidal already, this experience could be used as an excuse for a suicide attempt. *Careful assessment of level of depression, expectations, and suicidal tendencies is critical.*

B. Paranoid Thinking of Psychotic Proportion

At one time, hypnosis was thought to be contraindicated with psychotic and borderline patients because it activates archaic preoedipal transferences, thus producing a state of regression. Later work (Baker, 1981–1994; Frederick and McNeal, 1999; Murray-Jobsis, 1985–1991) showed that hypnosis can be a premier tool for developmental repair with such patients when it is used by those who are highly trained in this area. The regression is actually a "regression in the service of the ego," and hypnosis can be used with psychotic patients for relaxation and stabilization and as a significant medium for transitional experiences, boundary formation and strengthening, affect containment, impulse regulation, the correction of cognitive defects, and other aspects of developmental repair (Fromm and Nash, 1997; Frederick and McNeal, 1999). However, certain cautions must be exercised. A person who has developed a projective framework of thinking (see Chapter 4), for example, is not likely to appreciate the subtleties of hypnosis or self-hypnosis as distinct from mind control. He or she may attribute great powers to the therapist and may get quite angry at what seems to be a loss of control. This does not need to be the case, however, and paranoid persons may discover, to their surprise, that they achieve even greater control with hypnosis. *But care must be taken, and hypnosis with paranoid patients should not be approached by the inexperienced.* Most paranoid persons will make the therapist's decision to use hypnosis an unnecessary one by simply refusing to participate.

C. Patient With a History Suggestive of Abuse: Attempting to Use Hypnosis to Find Out "What Really Happened"

This issue often arises with patients who have a history suggestive of abuse. These patients are often problematic for the casual hypnotherapist, and the concerns noted in section V.H are important considerations, especially the realization that, although material accessed through hypnosis may bear some relationship to historical reality, it may also be untrue, distorted, or even symbolic of the patient's conflicts.

Recent clinical and legal cases have focused on the issue of patients coming to believe that certain events occurred when they in fact had not. The use of hypnosis when sexual abuse may be involved or suspected creates some legal exposure for the therapist. Many hypnotherapists require an informed consent from patients with whom they work.

D. Patients Who May Have to Testify in Court

In many jurisdictions, patients who have had hypnosis for the exploration of **memory material** or for any other reason whatsoever may be precluded from providing testimony in court. Hence, patients should be warned about those legal risks before any hypnotic encounter. *Generally, using hypnosis with patients who may have to testify in court is most unwise.*

VII. Comment

Many insurance companies will reimburse some portion of the charges for medical hypnosis when it is provided by a licensed clinician. However, referral to a well-trained clinician who uses hypnosis is not easily accomplished in some areas of the country. Because the practice of hypnosis is not regulated in many states, checking with a national organization may be advisable. The American Society of Clinical Hypnosis may be reached at 630-980-4740 (*http://www.ASCH.net*) and The Society for Clinical and Experimental Hypnosis can be contacted at 509-335-2097 (*http://www.hypnosis-research.org*).

ADDITIONAL READING

Baker EL. An hypnotherapeutic approach to enhance object relatedness in psychotic patients. *Int J Clin Exp Hypnosis* 1981;29:136–147.

Baker EL. Resistance in hypnotherapy of primitive states: its meaning and management. *Int J Clin Exp Hypnosis* 1983;31:82–89.

Baker EL. *The therapist as transitional object in intensive hypnotherapy*. Presented at the Annual Meeting of the American Society of Clinical Hypnosis, March 16, 1994, Philadelphia, Pennsylvania, 1994.

Baker EL. The use of hypnotic dreaming in the treatment of the borderline patient: some thoughts on resistance and transitional phenomena. *Int J Clin Exp Hypnosis* 1983;31:19–27.

Barabasz A, Barabasz M, Jensen S, et al. Cortical event-related potentials show the structure of hypnotic suggestions is crucial. *Int J Clin Exp Hypnosis* 1999;47:5–22.

Berkowitz B, Ross-Townsend A, Kohberger R. Hypnotic treatment of smoking: the single treatment method revisited. *Am J Psychiatry* 1979;136:83–85.

Braun BG, ed. *Treatment of multiple personality disorder*. Washington, D.C.: American Psychiatric Association, 1986.

Brown D, Fromm E. *Hypnotherapy and hypnoanalysis*. Hillsdale, NJ: Lawrence Erlbaum Associates, 1986.

Brown DP, Scheflin AW, Hammond, DC. *Memory, trauma, treatment, and the law*. New York: WW Norton, 1997.

Crasilneck HB, Hall JA. *Clinical hypnosis: principles and applications,* 2nd ed. New York: Grune & Stratton, 1985.

Esdaile J. *Hypnosis in medicine and surgery*. New York: Julian Press and the Institute for Research in Hypnosis, 1957.

Esplen MJ, Garfinkel PE, Olmstead M, et al. A randomized controlled trial of guided imagery in bulimia nervosa. *Psychol Med* 1998;28:1347–1357.

Ewin DM. Emergency room hypnosis for the burned patient. *Am J Clin Hypnosis* 1983;26:5–8.

Frederick C, McNeal S. *Inner strengths: contemporary psychotherapy and hypnosis for ego-strengthening*. Mahwah, NJ: Lawrence Erlbaum Associates, 1999.

Friedman H, Taub HA. The use of hypnosis and biofeedback procedures for essential hypertension. *Int J Clin Exp Hypnosis* 1977;25:335–347.

Fromm E, Nash M. *Psychoanalysis and hypnosis*. New York: International Universities Press, 1997.

Gilbertson AD, Kemp K. The use of hypnosis in treating anxiety states. *Psychiatr Med* 1992;10:13–20.

Gill MM, Brenman M. *Hypnosis and related states: psychoanalytic studies in regression*. New York: International Universities Press, 1959.

Graffin NF, Ray WJ, Lundy R. EEG concomitants of hypnosis and hypnotic susceptibility. *J Abnorm Psych* 1995;104:123–131.

Hammond DC. *Handbook of suggestions and metaphors*. New York: WW Norton, 1990.

Hammond DC. *Hypnotic induction and suggestion*. Chicago: American Society for Clinical Hypnosis Press, 1998.

Hammond DC, Garver RB, Mutter CB, et al. *Clinical hypnosis and memory: guidelines for clinicians and for forensic hypnosis*. Chicago: American Society for Clinical Hypnosis Press, 1995.

Hilgard ER. *Divided consciousness: multiple controls in human thought and action*. New York: Wiley, 1977.

Hilgard ER, Hilgard JR. *Hypnosis in the relief of pain*. Los Altos, CA: William Kaufmann, 1975.

Holroyd J. The uncertain relationship between hypnotizability and smoking treatment outcome. *Int J Clin Exp Hypnosis* 1991;39:93–102.

International Society for the Study of Dissociation. Guidelines for treating dissociative identity disorder (multiple personality disorder) in adults. *J Trauma Dissoc* 1997;1:117–134.

Kluft RP. The use of hypnosis with dissociative disorders. *Psychiatr Med* 1992;10:31–46.

Lang EV, Benotsch EG, Fick LJ, et al. Adjunctive non-pharmacological analgesia for invasive medical procedures: a randomized trial. *Lancet* 2000;355:1486–1490.

Levoie G, Sabourin M. Hypnosis and schizophrenia. In: Burrows GD, Dennerstein L, eds. *Handbook of hypnosis and psychosomatic medicine.* New York: Elsevier, 1980.

Lynn SJ, Rhue JW. *Casebook of clinical hypnosis.* Washington, D.C.: American Psychological Association, 1996.

Melzack R, Wall PD. Pain mechanisms: a new theory. *Science* 1965;150:971–979.

Miller ME, Bowers KS. Hypnotic analgesia and stress inoculation in the reduction of pain. *J Abnorm Psych* 1986;95:6–14.

Miller ME, Bowers KS. Hypnotic analgesia: dissociated experience or dissociated control? *J Abnorm Psych* 1993;102:29–38.

Mott T. Untoward effects associated with hypnosis. *Psychiatr Med* 1992;10:119–128.

Murray-Jobsis J. An exploratory study of hypnotic capacity of schizophrenic and borderline patients in a clinical setting. *Am J Clin Hypnosis* 1991;33:150–160.

Murray-Jobsis J. Ego building. In: Hammond DC, ed. *Handbook of hypnotic suggestions and metaphors.* New York: WW Norton, 1990:136–139.

Murray-Jobsis J. Exploring the schizophrenic experience with the use of hypnosis. *Am J Clin Hypnosis* 1985;29:34–42.

Murray-Jobsis J. Hypnosis with severely disturbed patients. In: Wester WC II, Smith AJ Jr, eds. *Clinical hypnosis: a multidisciplinary approach.* Philadelphia: Lippincott, 1984:368–404.

Murray-Jobsis J. Renurturing: forming positive sense of identity and bonding. In: Hammond DC, ed. *Handbook of hypnotic suggestions and metaphors.* New York: WW Norton, 1990:326–328.

Nash MR. The truth and the hype of hypnosis. *Sci Am* 2001;285:47–55.

Nash MR, Lynn SJ, Stanley S, et al. Hypnotic age regression and the importance of assessing interpersonally relevant affect. *Int J Clin Exp Hypnosis* 1985;33:224–235.

Olness K, Kohen DP. *Hypnosis and hypnotherapy with children,* 3rd ed. New York: Guilford, 1996.

Pettinati HM. Measuring hypnotizability in psychotic patients. *Int J Clin Exp Hypnosis* 1982;30:404–416.

Pettinati HM, Horne RL, Staats JM. Hypnotizability in patients with anorexia nervosa and bulimia. *Arch Gen Psychiatry* 1985;42:1014–1016.

Pinnell CM, Covino NA. Empirical findings on the use of hypnosis in medicine: a critical review. *Int J Clin Exp Hypnosis* 2000;48:170–194.

Rainville P, Hofbauer RK, Paus T, et al. Cerebral mechanisms of hypnotic induction and suggestion. *J Cogn Neurosci* 1999;11:110–115.

Spiegel D. Healing words: emotional expression and disease outcome. *JAMA* 1999;281:1328–1329.

Spiegel D. Hypnosis. In: Hales RE, Yudofsky SC, Talbott JA, eds. *American Psychiatric Press textbook of psychiatry.* Washington, D.C.: American Psychiatric Press, 1988.

Spiegel D. Uses and abuses of hypnosis. *Integr Psychiatry* 1989;6:211–222.

Spiegel D. The use of hypnosis in the treatment of PTSD. *Psychiatr Med* 1992;10:21–30.

Spiegel D, Hunt T, Dondershine HE. Dissociation and hypnotizability in posttraumatic stress disorder. *Am J Psychiatry* 1988;145:301–305.

Spiegel H. A single treatment method to stop smoking using ancillary self-hypnosis. *Arch Environ Health* 1970;20:736–742.

Spiegel H, Spiegel D. *Trance and treatment: clinical uses of hypnosis.* New York: Basic Books, 1978.

Torem M. Hypnosis in the treatment of depression. In: Wester WC, ed. *Clinical hypnosis: a case management approach.* Cincinnati, OH: Behavioral Science Center, 1987:288–301.

Wain HJ. Pain as a biopsychosocial entity and its significance for treatment with hypnosis. *Psychiatr Med* 1992;10:101–118.

Watkins JG. *The practice of clinical hypnosis.* Vol 1: Hypnotherapeutic techniques. New York: Irvington Publishers, 1987.

Whorwell PJ, Houghton LA, et al. Physiological effects of emotions: assessment via hypnosis. *Lancet* 1992;340:69–72.
Wickramasekera I, Pope AT, Kolm P. On the interaction of hypnotizability and negative affect in chronic pain: implications for the somatization of trauma. *J Nerv Ment Dis* 1996;184:628–635.
Yapko MD. A brief therapy approach in the use of hypnosis in treating depression. In: Lynn S, Kirsh I, Rhue J, eds. *Casebook of clinical hypnosis.* Washington, D.C.: American Psychological Association, 1996:75–79.

24. ELECTROCONVULSIVE THERAPY

Laura J. Fochtmann
Chester Pearlman
Richard I. Shader

Since its first use in 1938, **electroconvulsive therapy (ECT)** has been effective for several psychiatric disorders. The development of effective psychotropic medications in the 1950s reduced the need for ECT, and negative media portrayals influenced public perceptions of ECT. Patients were often fearful, and the availability of ECT decreased, particularly in the public sector. More recently, studies have led to technical improvements and an enhanced knowledge of risk-to-benefit considerations. Because few psychiatrists in the United States administer ECT, more than one psychiatrist is usually involved. In such cases, communication among them must be more frequent and more detailed than with the medical-surgical model. Psychiatrists who do not provide ECT also must understand the indications and procedures to make appropriate referrals.

This chapter reviews the clinical use of ECT. It covers indications and assessment of potential benefits and risks. An overview of ECT administration is provided. More detailed practice guidelines can be found in the reports of the American Psychiatric Association Committee on Electroconvulsive Therapy and the Royal College of Psychiatrists Special Committee on ECT (see Additional Reading).

I. **Indications**
   A. **General Factors**
      Patients who have failed adequate medication trials are the most appropriate candidates for ECT. A past response of patients or their biologic relatives to ECT also suggests that ECT will be efficacious. For this reason, some patients prefer ECT as a first-line treatment. ECT is also indicated as primary treatment for severe symptoms (extreme suicidality or inanition) where the risk of a failed drug trial would be unwise. In such patients, ECT usually produces more rapid improvement, particularly for vegetative symptoms. An advantage of ECT for the medically ill is that exposure is brief and that it is associated with careful monitoring and ready management of complications. For pregnant patients, ECT may be advantageous by avoiding the long-term use of potentially teratogenic medications.
   B. **Diagnostic Considerations**
      1. **Major depression**. ECT is the gold standard for treatment of depressive episodes both in major depressive or bipolar disorder. Greater efficacy of ECT has been shown in comparisons with tricyclics, monoamine oxidase inhibitors, and selective serotonin reuptake inhibitors. Response rates are 80% to 90%, although some evidence exists to indicate that failure of an adequate drug trial is associated with a lower response rate. Those with comorbid personality disorders tend to do less well, but older patients and those with psychomotor retardation respond better. ECT is also highly effective in patients with psychotic features. It is somewhat superior to, and is often better tolerated than, therapy with an antidepressant combined with an antipsychotic agent. In patients with dementia, depression often contributes to cognitive impairment and makes caregiving more difficult. When other treatments are unsuccessful, ECT can safely and effectively treat such depression. A somewhat increased risk of acute delirium or more persistent cognitive impairment may be present, but this risk can be minimized by the adjustment of treatment frequency or other parameters if indicated.
      2. **Mania**. ECT is the only antidepressant treatment that is also effective for mixed or manic episodes. In acute mania, ECT is generally reserved

for those who do not respond to the usual combinations of mood stabilizers (e.g., **lithium**, **valproic acid**), benzodiazepines (e.g., **clonazepam**), or antipsychotic agents (e.g., **olanzapine**). ECT is indicated as the primary treatment in severe excited states and for those who are unresponsive to medication or who have required frequent physical restraint during previous episodes. Comparison studies have shown equivalent or superior efficacy to that of **lithium** or antipsychotic agents. Before the advent of **lithium**, maintenance ECT was the standard treatment; it remains useful for patients who do not tolerate medications or who relapse in spite of them.

3. **Catatonia**. This syndrome involves symptoms such as mutism, severe hypokinesia, and dystonia (catalepsy or rigidity). It is much more common in mood disorders than it is in schizophrenia. Although the initial treatment is usually with a benzodiazepine (e.g., **lorazepam**), ECT is highly effective if symptom resolution is incomplete. Although benzodiazepine use is generally minimized during an ECT course to avoid possible interference with efficacy, it may augment the ECT response in some catatonics. In neuroleptic malignant syndrome, which shares many signs and symptoms with catatonia, some patients will respond better to ECT than to other treatments.

4. **Schizophrenia and related disorders**. Although schizophrenia, schizophreniform, and schizoaffective disorders are generally less responsive to ECT than are the mood disorders, ECT may also improve symptoms of these conditions. Hallucinations, delusions, and changes in mood show more improvement when ECT is given in combination with an antipsychotic agent. Patients with longer duration of illness, insidious onset, or premorbid paranoid or schizoid personality traits do less well. However, even with an extensive history of minimal response to antipsychotic agents, some improve with ECT.

5. **Other diagnoses**. For some medical conditions, ECT may benefit the syndrome itself. Presumably due to the dopaminergic effects of ECT, patients with Parkinson disease may show an increased benefit of antiparkinson drugs and improvements in rigidity or "on–off" periods. In intractable seizures, ECT has been beneficial by increasing the seizure threshold and stimulating the release of endogenous anticonvulsant substances involved in termination of seizure activity.

C. **Age-Related Considerations**

Age is not relevant in determining appropriateness for ECT. For those under 18 years of age, concurrence should be obtained from a consultant familiar with the treatment of children and adolescents (two should be obtained for those under 13 years of age). Because adult psychiatrists administer most ECT, this process ensures the consideration of the unique aspects of treatment of children and adolescents. As was discussed above, the elderly often tolerate ECT better than drugs.

D. **Considerations Relating to Medical Conditions**

1. **Pre-ECT medical and anesthetic evaluation**. This involves a complete medical history; a physical examination, including assessment of the teeth; laboratory screening tests, including a pregnancy test for women of childbearing age; electrocardiogram; and chest x-ray, as defined by local policies for brief procedures involving general anesthesia. Preanesthesia assessment by an anesthesiologist includes questions about adverse reactions to barbiturates and a personal or family history of abnormal responses to succinylcholine (e.g., prolonged apnea or malignant hyperthermia) and the assignment of American Society of Anesthesiologists (ASA) risk status according to the ASA system (Barash et al., 1991).

2. **Medical conditions associated with increased risk**. Although no absolute contraindications to ECT exist, some of the following conditions are associated with increased risk: severe or unstable cardiovascular

disorders, such as recent myocardial infarction, unstable angina, poorly compensated congestive heart failure, severe valvular heart disease, aneurysm, or vascular malformations, and recent gastrointestinal bleeding. In the central nervous system, a substantially increased risk is associated with increased intracranial pressure. Others with increased risk are those ranked as ASA status 4 (i.e., incapacitating illness that is a threat to life [heart failure, renal failure]) or ASA status 5 (i.e., a moribund patient not expected to survive 24 hours [ruptured aneurysm, head trauma with increasing intracranial pressure]). ECT is not done in ASA 5 patients.

E. **Technical and Pharmacologic Modifications to Optimize Benefit and to Minimize Risk**

1. **Medical comorbidities**. Table 24.1 lists suggested ways to minimize risks of specific conditions. Some standard medications, such as hypoglycemic agents and diuretics, should be held until after ECT, and the dosage of antiparkinson agents should also be decreased by 50%. Antihypertensive, antianginal, antiarrhythmic, and antireflux agents; bronchodilators; glaucoma medications; corticosteroids; and other medications that may reduce side effects should be given with a minimum amount of water before ECT.

2. **Modifications in psychotropic medications**. Antipsychotic agents and antidepressants can generally be continued during an ECT course. Some evidence of synergistic effects of antipsychotic agents in patients with schizophrenia does exist. The use of antidepressants is less clear. One report has been made of possible synergism, and no evidence of increased risk is seen. Concern among anesthesiologists regarding hypertensive reactions with monoamine oxidase inhibitors is based on the use of indirect sympathomimetic agents during emergency surgery and is not relevant to current practice. **Lithium** doses should be reduced or discontinued when feasible because of the increased potential for neurotoxicity. With unilateral electrode placement, benzodiazepines may interfere with the efficacy due to the necessity for greatly suprathreshold stimulation. For this electrode placement, agents without active metabolites should be used and no benzodiazepines should be given for 8 hours before ECT. In patients receiving anticonvulsants for seizure disorders or mood stabilization, bitemporal ECT is advised to avoid the necessity for greatly suprathreshold stimulation. Morning doses of these medications should be held before ECT, and sometimes the preceding evening doses should be held as well.

3. **Modifications in electrode placement and treatment frequency**. At comparable stimulus intensities, fewer cognitive effects occur with right unilateral ECT than with bitemporal ECT. However, unlike bitemporal placement, optimum benefit with unilateral ECT requires stimulation that is at least five to six times the threshold. Medications that increase the seizure threshold (e.g., benzodiazepines, barbiturates, anticonvulsants) are likely to diminish the efficacy of unilateral ECT. Although the seizure threshold is usually much lower with unilateral ECT, United States Food and Drug Administration restrictions on the energy output of ECT devices in the United States may make sufficient suprathreshold stimulation impossible. Several strategies have been used to minimize the cognitive side effects while maximizing response. One is to begin with right unilateral ECT with stimulus intensity significantly above the seizure threshold and to change to bitemporal placement if minimal response is seen after about 2 weeks. Another strategy is to begin with bitemporal ECT and to change to unilateral placement or twice weekly treatment if cognitive side effects become a problem. Other electrode placements are less studied, but these may provide comparable therapeutic efficacy to bitemporal placement with less impact on cognition. They include bifrontal positioning and a

TABLE 24.1. MEDICAL CONDITIONS AND ELECTROCONVULSIVE THERAPY MODIFICATIONS

Medical Condition	Suggested Modification
Addison disease or other steroid-dependent conditions	Additional steroid boluses may be needed at the time of electroconvulsive therapy (ECT)
Aneurysms	Use antihypertensive agents to blunt the surge in blood pressure that occurs with seizure induction
Asthma or chronic obstructive pulmonary disease	Pre-ECT bronchodilators and additional oxygenation may be required; discontinue theophylline or decrease dose to avoid prolonging seizures
Bone or joint disease	If severe, increase muscle relaxant dosage
Cardiac arrhythmias	Lidocaine interferes with seizure induction; bradycardia or asystole may require treatment with anticholinergic agents; tachycardias may require treatment with β-adrenergic receptor antagonists; in patients with pacemakers, cardiology consultants should comment on whether a change to a fixed firing rate is indicated; in patients with implanted defibrillators, cardiology consultants should comment on whether this function should be disabled during ECT
Central nervous system tumor or other mass lesion	Antihypertensive agents, steroids, diuretics, or hyperventilation can minimize the likelihood of increases in intracranial pressure
Diabetes mellitus	More frequent glucose monitoring may be needed; dosages of oral hypoglycemic agents or insulin may need to be adjusted
Esophageal reflux	H_2-receptor antagonists or sodium citrate can be given before ECT to minimize and neutralize stomach acids; metoclopramide can promote gastric emptying; cricoid pressure at the time of ECT may decrease aspiration risk; consider intubation for high-risk patients
Glaucoma	Prescribed antiglaucoma medications should be given before ECT
Hyperthyroidism	If clinically significant, give β-adrenergic receptor antagonists to decrease the risk of thyroid storm
Intracranial shunt	Ensure shunt patency before ECT
Ischemic cerebrovascular disease	Avoid induction of low blood pressure with ECT
Myasthenia gravis	Decrease the dose of succinylcholine
Parkinson disease	Decrease the dose of dopaminergic agonists, such as L-dopa, to minimize post-ECT delirium
Pheochromocytoma	Give medications to block α-adrenergic receptors, β-adrenergic receptors, and tyrosine hydroxylase synthesis
Porphyria	Use only nonbarbiturate anesthetics

(continued)

TABLE 24.1. MEDICAL CONDITIONS AND ELECTROCONVULSIVE THERAPY MODIFICATIONS *(Continued)*

Medical Condition	Suggested Modification
Pregnancy	Depends on the stage of pregnancy and recommendations of obstetrical consultants; modifications may include altered patient position with a wedge placed under the right hip at the time of ECT after 20 wk gestation, altered doses of anesthetic medications due to pharmacokinetic changes of pregnancy; to prevent and reduce risks of aspiration, minimize the use of anticholinergic agents, use antireflux agents and consider intubation near-term; ensure good oxygenation without hyperventilation; fetal monitoring, including fetal heart rate before and after ECT past 14–16 wk gestation and a 30-min to 60-min fetal heart rate strip (nonstress test with a tocometer) before and after ECT past 24 wk gestation
Seizure disorders	Optimal anticonvulsant dosages
Traumatic brain injury	Avoid placing stimulus electrodes directly over a skull defect
Upper motor neuron disease	Decrease doses of succinylcholine

Abbreviation: H_2, histamine-2.

right frontotemporal–left frontal electrode placement (see Additional Reading).

II. Electroconvulsive Therapy Procedures

A. Number and Frequency of Treatments

The number of treatments in an ECT course is determined by the patient's response. With major depressive episodes, the time course with ECT is similar to that with antidepressant drugs. Some show improvement after one or two ECT treatments, but full response usually requires 3 to 4 weeks. With schizoaffective disorder or schizophrenia, longer courses may improve the outcome. Regardless of diagnosis, however, benefit is unlikely if no response is seen after 4 weeks. In the United States, ECT is generally administered three times per week on nonconsecutive days. Twice weekly ECT is also effective, and it has fewer cognitive effects, especially with bitemporal placement.

B. Informed Consent

From a legal perspective, capacity to consent to a standard procedure like ECT is presumed. However, when the clinical evaluation of the patient suggests that this capacity may be impaired by cognitive deficits or psychotic beliefs, a formal assessment of capacity is warranted before obtaining informed consent. To have this capacity, a patient must show a clear understanding of the risks, benefits, and alternatives to the proposed treatment. For individuals lacking this capacity, individual state laws govern consent procedures. A typical method involves surrogate consent from a family member, legal guardian, or health care proxy, but judicial proceedings for court-ordered treatment may be required. In such instances, consideration should be given to opinions expressed by the patient when this capacity was not compromised by acute illness. The consent process for a patient or surrogate involves the rationale; a description of the procedure; a range of likely number of treatments; possible complications, including memory disturbance; activity restrictions during and after the ECT course; and the likely need for some form of continuation or maintenance treatment. For persons influenced by negative media imagery, consultation with other psychiatrists or educational videotapes may be helpful. If videotapes are used, the clinician should review them before giving them to the patient to ensure their appropriateness for that particular patient, as well as their current accuracy.

C. Treatment Environment

As a procedure involving general anesthesia, ECT is administered in an area with appropriate monitoring equipment and emergency medical support. When the ECT treatment area is distant from the psychiatric unit, familiar personnel and occasional preanesthetic medication may minimize patient anxiety.

D. Anesthetic Considerations

1. **General factors**. Throughout the procedure, monitoring should include electrocardiogram, serial blood pressures, and pulse oximetry. Ventilation with 100% oxygen should be delivered using positive pressure at a rate of at least 5 L per min with 15 to 20 breaths per min. Additional preanesthetic oxygenation is indicated for patients at risk of myocardial ischemia.

2. **Anticholinergic medications**. Though common in clinical ritual, such agents may increase the cardiovascular risk by inducing tachycardia and increased hypertension. Their appropriate use is restricted to documented bradyarrhythmias or to situations in which subconvulsive stimuli are used to determine the seizure threshold, especially in patients treated with β-adrenergic receptor antagonists. Rarely, anticholinergic medications are also indicated when the oral secretions are excessive.

3. **Anesthetic medications**. **Methohexital** (0.5 to 1 mg per kg intravenously [i.v.]) is generally used to induce ultrabrief general anesthesia for ECT. Some practitioners use **thiopental** (1.5 to 3.5 mg per kg i.v.). **Etomidate** (0.15 to 0.35 mg per kg i.v.) does not appear to impact the seizure threshold or duration, and it may be useful when adequate seizure induction is difficult. **Propofol** (0.75 to 1.5 mg per kg i.v.) is useful for patients with barbiturate allergies or conditions requiring minimal hypertensive reaction, but it requires bitemporal ECT because of its significant increase in seizure threshold. **Ketamine** (2 to 3 mg per kg i.v.) has also been used to enhance efficacy with unilateral ECT, but postictal delirium is a significant complication.

4. **Muscle relaxants**. Muscle relaxants are used to minimize motor convulsive activity and also to facilitate airway management. The usual muscle relaxant agent used for ECT is the depolarizing neuromuscular blocking agent **succinylcholine** (0.5 to 1 mg per kg i.v.). In patients particularly susceptible to fractures, more complete relaxation is required via the use of higher doses of **succinylcholine**. The rare patients who lack plasma cholinesterases are unable to metabolize **succinylcholine** rapidly; they are at risk of prolonged apnea. For these patients, nondepolarizing (competitive) neuromuscular blocking agents, such as **mivacurium** or **atracurium**, can be used because they have a prompt onset of action, they are not long acting[1], and they are nonenzymatically degraded at pH 7.4. **Succinylcholine** also causes transiently increased serum **potassium**. Patients at increased risk for **succinylcholine**-induced hyperkalemia (e.g. burns, muscle trauma, paraplegia, or other conditions involving neuromuscular degeneration) should be treated with a nondepolarizing agent. In all patients, muscle relaxation must be ensured before delivering the electrical stimulus. With **succinylcholine**, muscle relaxation is unlikely to be sufficient before fasciculations have stopped. Adequacy of relaxation may also be checked by lower extremity reflexes or the response to peripheral nerve stimulation. Muscle relaxation

---

[1]Although short-acting, atracurium has a longer duration of action than mivacurium; cholinergic reversal with neostigmine or edrophonium can be used to terminate its effects.

is never complete, however, and residual muscle activity produces carbon dioxide that may contribute to cardiac arrhythmias. Thus, adequate postictal ventilation is essential.

5. **Cardiovascular medications**. The initial parasympathetic activation with stimulus delivery and subsequent sympathetic activation with seizure induction are associated with alterations in heart rate and blood pressure. These changes are generally self-limited. Rarely, anticholinergic agents are needed acutely to treat asystole or bradyarrhythmias. More often, medications are used to attenuate tachycardia and hypertension. For example, in patients with cardiac disease, β-adrenergic receptor antagonists may be used to decrease tachycardia and cardiac workload. The most commonly used is **esmolol** (0.25 to 0.5 mg per kg), an ultra–short-acting β_1-selective adrenergic receptor antagonist, whose brevity allows use in conditions where β-adrenergic receptor antagonists are typically contraindicated. Short-acting antihypertensive agents may also be used to reduce the cardiac workload and to minimize the risk of increased intracranial pressure and intracranial bleeding. The most effective agents are calcium channel blockers, such as **nifedipine** (10 mg crushed and swallowed 0.5 hours before ECT) or **nicardipine** (1.25 to 5 mg i.v.). **Nitroglycerin** (as a paste, sublingual tablet, or sublingual spray) is less reliable, but it may facilitate coronary artery dilation. These agents are short acting, and they do not cause hypotension or orthostasis after recovery from ECT.

E. Seizure Elicitation

1. **Stimulus parameters**. The use of a constant current, brief, pulse stimulus is recommended because sine waveforms produce increased cognitive impairment with only rare reports of increased efficacy. Adjustments in stimulus intensity are most efficiently accomplished by altering the duration of the pulse train.

2. **Stimulus dosing**. Stimulus dosing with ECT resembles individualized dosing of psychotropic agents and aims to minimize adverse cognitive effects while still producing an effective response. Such procedures include formula-based dosing procedures and stimulus titration. With empirical stimulus titration, an initial dose is selected, generally based on age and gender, that would rarely be expected to elicit a generalized seizure. If no seizure occurs, the stimulus energy is increased, generally by about 50%, and another stimulus is given after a delay of at least 20 seconds. This upward titration continues until a generalized seizure occurs or until four or five stimulations have been unsuccessful. The empirically estimated threshold is taken to be the stimulus intensity at which a seizure occurred. At subsequent treatment sessions, stimulus energy is used that is 1.5 to 2.5 times the seizure threshold for bilateral ECT or 2.5 to 6 times the seizure threshold for unilateral ECT. Common formula-based strategies apply the observation that seizure thresholds vary with age—younger patients require lower stimulus intensities, whereas the elderly require much higher stimulus intensities to produce an adequate seizure. Thus, for bitemporal ECT, half of the patient's age as a percentage of maximum stimulus output is a good estimate of seizure threshold. More complex formula-based dosing strategies include variations in seizure threshold by gender and electrode positioning. Regardless of the method by which an initial stimulus dose is selected, adjustments in dosing are generally necessary during a series of ECT. For many patients, the seizure threshold may increase significantly, requiring a comparable increase in stimulus energy by the end of the treatment course.

3. **Stimulus administration**. For efficacy and safety, ensuring optimal contact between the skin and the electrode is important; this is produced by cleansing the underlying skin and applying conducting paste to the electrodes. To prevent injury to the teeth and tongue from contraction of

the masseter muscles induced by the stimulus, a flexible protective device is placed between the teeth before stimulus delivery and the chin is supported manually.

4. **Seizure monitoring**. The duration of the induced seizure may be monitored by electroencephalogram (EEG) or by convulsive movements. Although motor signs are usually clear, visualization can be ensured by placing a blood pressure cuff on a wrist or ankle and inflating it above the systolic pressure before the muscle relaxant is administered. When unilateral placement is used, the cuff is placed ipsilateral to the electrodes to be sure of seizure generalization. EEG monitoring is done with a frontomastoid lead placement. With unilateral ECT, the leads are placed contralateral to the electrodes to ensure generalized seizure induction. EEG monitoring is essential for detection of prolonged nonconvulsive seizure activity. Prolonged seizures (longer than 180 seconds by motor or EEG) are rare, and these require termination by an i.v. benzodiazepine or additional barbiturate anesthetic and oxygenation throughout the seizure activity. More often, delivery of the electrical stimulus induces only a brief seizure or none at all. For seizures lasting less than 15 seconds, a neuronal refractory period requires a delay of 45 to 90 seconds before restimulation with a stimulus intensity of 1.5 to 2 times that of the original. When no seizure activity is noted, the delay can be as short as 20 seconds, but restimulation is done with a similarly increased intensity.

When inducing an adequate seizure at a given treatment session is not possible, several factors should be considered. Hyperventilating the patient before seizure induction and ensuring adequate hydration are always helpful. In addition, reducing the anesthetic dose or using an anesthetic with less anticonvulsant effect may be possible. When feasible, the doses of benzodiazepines and other anticonvulsant medications should be decreased and held before ECT. If the benzodiazepine dosage cannot be reduced, the benzodiazepine receptor antagonist **flumazenil** may be given immediately before ECT to achieve an adequate seizure. Except as noted, no relation is observed between seizure duration and clinical outcome. Although the specific features of the EEG waveforms are a subject of ongoing research, whether these may predict efficacy is not clear.

III. Complications
A. Mortality
Despite the increasing use of ECT in patients with serious medical conditions, morbidity and mortality remain low. The report of the American Psychiatric Association Committee on ECT estimates mortality at 1 in 10,000 patients or 1 in 80,000 treatments, approximately the same as that associated with minor surgical procedures or with childbirth.

B. Cardiovascular Effects
Electrocardiogram changes after ECT include ST segment depression, T-wave inversion, premature ventricular contractions, and, rarely, ventricular tachyarrhythmias. They result from the sympathetic activation, and they are rarely associated with myocardial enzyme changes. A history of arrhythmia increases the risk of arrhythmia with ECT. Similarly, a history of myocardial ischemia increases the risk of morbidity due to ischemia with ECT. The modifications in treatment procedures discussed in section II.D.5 have mostly eliminated such complications.

C. Adverse Cognitive Effects
These show a great deal of individual variability. The most frequent are anterograde or retrograde amnesia. With anterograde amnesia, new information is forgotten more rapidly, whereas with retrograde amnesia, recall of autobiographical events and public information shows spotty deficits. Typically, the recall of public information is affected more than that of personal details, and recent events are affected more than distant ones.

Amnesia is most prominent during and immediately after a course of ECT, and it fades within a few weeks. Some patients report longer lasting difficulty with memory, and they may show inability to recall items remembered before ECT when tested 6 months later. Because no problem is seen with relearning, distinction from normal forgetting may be difficult. Patients with prominent white matter hyperintensities in the head of the caudate nucleus and prefrontal subcortex on magnetic resonance imaging (most parkinsonian patients) are at increased risk of more severe cognitive effects, including delirium (see Chapter 5). Cognitive effects are also more pronounced with sine wave stimulation, bitemporal brief pulse stimulation given thrice weekly, and possibly high stimulus doses relative to the seizure threshold. Modifications that minimize cognitive side effects include changing electrode placement and decreasing treatment frequency or stimulus intensity. Several nootropic agents have been given with ECT in the attempt to counteract such effects, but none has been shown clinical efficacy despite benefit in animal trials. In most patients, improvement in psychiatric symptoms with ECT leads to improved attention, concentration, and global cognitive performance. Thus, patients with persisting subjective memory complaints should be assessed for residual depression. Because ECT affects memory and cognition, many individuals have expressed concern about possible brain damage. ECT does produce increases in cerebral blood flow and metabolism and a transient increase in blood–brain barrier permeability, but extensive study with computed tomography, magnetic resonance imaging, and neuronal enzyme markers has shown no evidence of injury to brain tissue.

D. Other Adverse Effects
1. **Prolonged apnea.** Prolonged apnea is rare, and it results from the slow metabolism of **succinylcholine**. If adequate oxygenation is maintained, it usually resolves spontaneously without sequelae after 30 to 60 minutes.
2. **Postictal agitation.** Delirium and agitation upon awakening are rare but troublesome complications of ECT. Young men are most susceptible, but no relation to previous history or other treatment factors has been determined. Although this is usually managed supportively, physical restraint (see Chapter 26) may be necessary, and i.v. doses of a benzodiazepine may be useful.
3. **Headache.** Headache is common, occurring in up to 45% of patients. It generally responds to rest under dim lighting or to analgesics, such as **acetaminophen**; nonsteroidal antiinflammatory agents; or 5-hydroxytryptamine (5-HT)$_{1B/D}$ agonists, such as **sumatriptan**.
4. **Nausea or vomiting.** Nausea and vomiting may be associated with headaches, anesthesia, or recent changes in psychotropic medication dosages. These symptoms are usually well controlled with dopamine receptor antagonists, such as **prochlorperazine** or **metoclopramide**.
5. **Muscle aches.** This is a known complication of **succinylcholine**, and it is treated symptomatically with analgesics.
6. **Treatment-emergent mania.** All antidepressants may cause a switch to hypomania or mania, but only ECT can treat it. Thus, more ECT leads to mood stabilization. If continuation or maintenance ECT is not used, treatment with a mood-stabilizing agent is advisable.

IV. Ambulatory or Outpatient Electroconvulsive Therapy
With the increasingly restrictive criteria for inpatient psychiatric care, ECT is increasingly being provided in an outpatient setting. In such instances, the patient's symptoms must be safely manageable as an outpatient. Those with significant suicide risk, substantial psychotic or cognitive impairment, or a risk of serious medical complications should be treated as inpatients. Outpatients must be willing and able to comply with specific requirements during the ECT course. These include avoiding activities that could be influenced by the cognitive effects of ECT, complying with medication regimens, and abstaining from

oral intake for about 8 hours before each ECT. Outpatients must also be able to make reliable reports of changes in their medical condition or of the adverse effects of ECT or anesthesia. Except for stable outpatients receiving maintenance ECT, this requires at least one significant other or caregiver to ensure the patient's safety and compliance with the treatment plan and to transport the patient to and from treatment sessions. For a more detailed discussion, see the report by Fink et al. (1996).

V. **Continuation or Maintenance Electroconvulsive Therapy and Continuation Pharmacotherapy**

After a successful course of ECT, continuation therapy is advisable to reduce the risk of relapse. Although some may respond to a class of antidepressants that they have not already failed, many will fare best with maintenance ECT. The decision to use this approach is complicated by the unpredictable duration of spontaneous remission that is obscured by maintenance drug treatment guidelines. When ECT is used, treatments are given at intervals ranging from weekly to monthly, with treatment schedules adjusted to clinical response. As suggested by guidelines for drug treatment, the need to continue ECT is assessed at intervals that are based on the number of previous episodes, with patient preferences playing a major role in the decision to continue treatment. One recent study suggested that over 80% of responders to ECT who were treated with an oral placebo relapsed within 6 months after ECT if no additional treatment was given. In this study, **nortriptyline** combined with **lithium** was found to reduce the relapse rate to 39%. The use of **nortriptyline** alone led to a 60% relapse rate.

VI. **Possible Mechanisms of Action**

Although the mechanism of ECT is unknown, some data are suggestive. The anticonvulsant hypothesis is based on observations that the therapeutic outcome is correlated with the magnitude of increase in seizure threshold during the ECT course, especially with right unilateral stimulation. A relation to the increasing role of anticonvulsants in mood disorders may be present. The neuroendocrine hypothesis suggests that therapeutic benefits result from diencephalic stimulation and the consequent release of mood-regulating neuropeptides. With **electroconvulsive shock (ECS)**, the animal analogue of ECT, many neuropeptides (e.g., **thyrotropin-releasing hormone, somatostatin, β-endorphin, enkephalin, neurokinin A, neuropeptide Y, nerve growth factor, brain-derived neurotrophic factor**) show increased levels in discrete brain regions. The difficulty is determining which, if any, of these is responsible for benefits of ECT. A similar problem exists with neurochemical hypotheses of ECT. With a time course like clinical ECT, ECS increases brain levels of norepinephrine. Repeated ECS also increases cortical and amygdalar α_1-adrenergic receptors while decreasing the numbers of α_2- and β-adrenergic receptors in the cortex and hippocampus. Dopamine levels are also increased with repeated ECS, particularly in the striatum. Although dopamine D_2 receptor numbers are generally unchanged, altered dopaminergic responses are seen with repeated ECS, and these relate to the increased numbers of nigrostriatal dopamine D_1 receptors. ECS also leads to acute increases in brain serotonin, but basal serotonin levels remain unchanged. Cortical 5-HT$_2$ receptor numbers are increased after repeated ECS, but only in male rats. This contrasts with the down-regulation of 5-HT$_2$ receptors with antidepressant drugs. Repeated, but not single, ECS also affects other receptors, enzymes, and neuronal ion channels. Second messengers (e.g., cyclic adenosine monophosphate [AMP] and phosphatidyl inositol) and multiple transcriptional regulatory factors are also differentially modulated. Despite the limitations of animal models, these findings establish that electrically induced seizures produce a complex array of neurochemically specific changes that are localized to specific neuroanatomic regions. Consequently, they refute the idea that ECT acts as a "global reset button" for brain electrical activity. In addition, these results suggest that specific neurochemical alterations may relate to the specific effects of ECT. Future research will need to detail the mechanisms by which such neurochemical changes are translated into the therapeutic benefits of ECT.

VII. Useful Websites

Readers may wish to contact the following for more useful information: the National Institute of Mental Health (800-421-4211 or *http://www.nimh.nih.gov/*), the American Psychiatric Association APA Answer Center for Electroconvulsive Therapy (*http://www.psych.org/*), or the JAMA Patient Pages (see Patient Page Index for March 14, 2001; *http://www.jama.com/*).

ADDITIONAL READING

General References

Abrams R. *Electroconvulsive therapy,* 3rd ed. New York: Oxford University Press, 1997.

American Psychiatric Association Committee on Electroconvulsive Therapy. *The practice of electroconvulsive therapy: recommendations for treatment, training, and privileging,* 2nd ed. Washington, D.C.: American Psychiatric Association, 2001.

Beyer JL, Weiner RD, Glenn MD. *Electroconvulsive therapy: a programmed text,* 2nd ed. Washington, D.C.: American Psychiatric Press, 1998.

Kellner CH. *Handbook of ECT.* Washington, D.C.: American Psychiatric Press, 1997.

Royal College of Psychiatrists Special Committee on ECT. *The ECT handbook: the second report of the Royal College of Psychiatrists' Special Committee on ECT.* London: Royal College of Psychiatrists, 1995.

Specific References

Avramov MN, Stool LA, White PF, et al. Effects of nicardipine and labetalol on the acute hemodynamic response to electroconvulsive therapy. *J Clin Anesth* 1998;10: 394–400.

Bailine SH, Rifkin A, Kayne E, et al. Comparison of bifrontal and bitemporal ECT for major depression. *Am J Psychiatry* 2000;157:121–123.

Barash PL, Cullen BF, Stoelting RK. *Handbook of clinical anesthesia.* Philadelphia: J B Lippincott, 1991:4.

Beale MD, Kellner CH. Proposed titration schedule. *Convuls Ther* 1997;13:44.

Bloch Y, Levcovitch Y, Bloch AM, et al. Electroconvulsive therapy in adolescents: similarities to and differences from adults. *J Am Acad Child Adolesc Psychiatry* 2001;40:1332–1336.

Ende G, Braus DF, Walter S, et al. The hippocampus in patients treated with electroconvulsive therapy: a proton magnetic resonance spectroscopic imaging study. *Arch Gen Psychiatry* 2000;57:937–943.

Fall PA, Granerus AK. Maintenance ECT in Parkinson's disease. *J Neural Transm* 1999;106:737–741.

Fink M. Delirious mania. *Bipolar Disord* 1999;1:54–60.

Fink M, Abrams R, Bailine S, et al. Ambulatory electroconvulsive therapy: report of a task force of the Association for Convulsive Therapy. Association for Convulsive Therapy. *Convuls Ther* 1996;12:42–55.

Fochtmann LJ. Animal studies of electroconvulsive therapy: foundations for future research. *Psychopharmacol Bull* 1994;30:321–444.

Folk JW, Kellner CH, Beale MD, et al. Anesthesia for electroconvulsive therapy: a review. *J ECT* 2000;16:157–170.

Glass RM. Electroconvulsive therapy. *JAMA* 2001;285:1346–1362.

Krystal AD, Watts BV, Weiner RD, et al. The use of flumazenil in the anxious and benzodiazepine-dependent ECT patient. *J ECT* 1998;14:5–14.

Lisanby SH, Maddox JA, Prudic J, et al. The effects of electroconvulsive therapy on memory of autobiographical and public events. *Arch Gen Psychiatry* 2000;57: 581–592.

Manly DT, Oakley SP Jr, Bloch RM. Electroconvulsive therapy in old-old patients. *Am J Geriatr Psychiatry* 2000;8:232–236.

McCall WV, Reboussin DM, Weiner RD, et al. Titrated moderately suprathreshold vs fixed high-dose right unilateral electroconvulsive therapy: acute antidepressant and cognitive effects. *Arch Gen Psychiatry* 2000;57:438–444.

Petrides G, Divadeenam KM, Bush G, et al. Synergism of lorazepam and electroconvulsive therapy in the treatment of catatonia. *Biol Psychiatry* 1997;42:375–381.

Rabheru K, Persad E. A review of continuation and maintenance electroconvulsive therapy. *Can J Psychiatry* 1997;42:476–484.

Rao V, Lyketsos CG. The benefits and risks of ECT for patients with primary dementia who also suffer from depression. *Int J Geriatr Psychiatry* 2000;15:729–735.

Rasmussen KG, Jarvis MR, Zorumski CF. Ketamine anesthesia in electroconvulsive therapy. *Convuls Ther* 1996;12:217–223.

Sackeim HA. The anticonvulsant hypothesis of the mechanisms of action of ECT: current status. *J ECT* 1999;15:5–26.

Sackeim HA, Haskett RF, Mulsant BH, et al. Continuation pharmacotherapy in the prevention of relapse following electroconvulsive therapy. *JAMA* 2001;285:1299–1307.

Sackeim HA, Prudic J, Devanand DP, et al. A prospective, randomized, double-blind comparison of bilateral and right unilateral electroconvulsive therapy at different stimulus intensities. *Arch Gen Psychiatry* 2000;57:425–434.

Swartz CM. Asymmetric bilateral right frontotemporal left frontal stimulus electrode placement for electroconvulsive therapy. *Neuropsychobiology* 1994;29:174–178.

Tharyan P, Adams CE. Electroconvulsive therapy for schizophrenia. *Cochrane Database Syst Rev* 2002;2:CD000076.

Walter G, Rey JM, Mitchell PB. Practitioner review: electroconvulsive therapy in adolescents. *J Child Psychol Psychiatry* 1999;40:325–335.

Weiner RD, Coffey CE, Krystal AD. Electroconvulsive therapy in the medical and neurologic patient. In: Stoudemire A, Fogel BS, Greenberg D, eds. *Psychiatric care of the medical patient.* New York: Oxford University Press, 2000:419–428.

25. SECLUSION AS A TREATMENT MODALITY

Thomas G. Gutheil
Richard I. Shader

Limiting anyone's freedom is always a serious matter. Although sending a child to his or her room as a "time out" technique may be common and many children will learn from this type of control, some of these will always feel abandoned and rejected. Restricting the freedom of movement of any patient, particularly a psychiatric patient, is also a serious and almost always controversial decision that should never be taken lightly, even though considerable clinical experience suggests that restricting the amount of space and degree of stimulation available to carefully selected psychiatric patients can play a useful and safety-promoting role in their treatment, either as an adjunct or as an alternative to medication or other behavioral or somatic therapies.

Noting that the use of seclusion has decreased in recent years is important. Many factors are involved, including a changing medicolegal and social climate regarding its use, the availability of increasingly effective medications, a reduction in the number of hospital units with appropriately constructed spaces, and nursing staff changes that result in fewer personnel familiar with its use, as well as rotation practices that reduce the continuity of care. However, paralleling these factors is an increase in overcrowding on some units or admixtures of patients that may put dual diagnosis adolescents alongside frail elderly patients with dementia (situations that may promote the very circumstances that could benefit from the appropriate and judicious use of some forms of seclusion).

Most physicians will not need to prescribe seclusion, but, for those who must do so, this chapter outlines some important considerations. Varying degrees of restriction may be appropriate. The most minor form may be requesting that a patient remain in hospital clothing. More limiting forms include requesting that patients do not leave the ward, asking them to spend increased time in their own rooms, placing them in monitored confinement in a specified section of a ward, and instituting voluntary or forced confinement to a specially designed room (i.e., a "quiet" or seclusion room). The utility of these treatment strategies depends, in part, on careful and appropriate application and patient selection.

Jurisdictions vary in their criteria and requirements for seclusion, which are generally outlined in statutory law or administrative regulations. At the federal level, the Children's Health Act of 2000 (PL 106-310) established standards for the use of seclusion in all psychiatric facilities that receive federal monies (e.g., Medicare) and in nonmedical community-based facilities for children and youth. Interestingly, these standards are less rigorous than the prototypical set of criteria for the use of seclusion that is outlined at the end of this chapter. Because the use of seclusion continues to occasion forensic and clinical controversy, a brief discussion of the principal legal issues involved is also included.

I. Definition

Seclusion as part of a therapeutic regimen for an inpatient is placement alone in a room especially designed for this purpose. The definition of seclusion does not include the distinction of whether it is involuntary. Indeed, when seclusion is indicated and can be explained to and understood by patients, they should first be asked to comply voluntarily with the therapeutic strategy. Although the door may be unlocked, "seclusion" usually implies a door that is locked for specified periods of time. The length of time varies according to specific state statutes; a designated time interval is clinically desirable and is usually interposed (e.g., 10 to 20 minutes every 1 to 2 hours) during which the door is opened and appropriate staff–patient contact (called "breaking seclusion") is made for clinical observations, feeding, toileting, hygiene, and other medical care, as discussed below. These considerations should be articulated fully in hospital or departmental policies, regional guidelines, legislation, or some combination of these.

II. Basic Principles of Seclusion Room Design

The fundamental consideration in designing a seclusion room is to make it safe **for the patient** (i.e., free from sources of potential self-injury) and **from the patient** (i.e., sturdy enough to resist destructive abuse). Seamless construction, special paneling, industrial carpeting, or similar materials should be used. When possible, the simple device of high ceilings (out of the reach of the patient) permits the use of standard lighting fixtures and heating and cooling apertures. This type of construction, however, necessitates that patients do not have access to materials such as torn sheets or towels that can be used as ropes. Otherwise, fixtures must be recessed or designed to eliminate sources of danger to the patient such as jagged edges, glass, and electrical wiring. Adequate ventilation is essential; many patients have impaired or potentially impaired thermoregulation (e.g., excited or retarded catatonics, patients on antipsychotic agents with hypothalamic effects or peripheral α_1-adrenergic receptor antagonist properties). Because a padded room is still used for seclusion in some locales, the matter of control of the room's ambient temperature must be monitored and adjusted. Properly designed doors are also an essential feature; for example, doors should be designed to open out and to facilitate rapid entry and exit. Doors should have external hinge pins; safety-glass observation windows that permit a view of the entire room; and key locks, not knob locks. Placement near the nursing station is recommended, and an intercom or closed-circuit television monitoring system may be helpful.

III. Theory of Seclusion and Clinical Management of Space

Acutely psychotic or regressed patients may be particularly vulnerable to surprise and the unexpected. Many acutely disturbed patients startle easily, they are confused and terrified by their psychotic distortions, they are fearful of assault, or they are so hyperaroused that they cannot calm themselves or modulate their responses to stimuli in their immediate environment. All these factors can provoke extreme anxiety and distress. A specific and limited space in which to move around may temporarily promote a sense of safety and familiarity. Having a recently admitted patient move in a planned and graduated way from smaller to larger areas of the overall unit may be helpful. A step-wise expansion of territory permits patients to experience a gradual increase in the demands placed on them, to integrate stimuli, to deal with other people, and to master unfamiliar terrain and experiences. Increasing space offers more chances for exploration, interpersonal encounters, and responsibility for one's self-control. When a patient's capacity to integrate stimuli or to contain impulses is impaired or strained, a decrease in the available (external) space may prove therapeutically supportive and may enhance the patient's sense of control. Thus, being moved to a quiet corner, one wing of the ward, a lounge, or his or her own room may calm an agitated patient. Both the decreased stimulation and distance from others may be helpful, as this chapter details later. Patterns of space limitation may range all the way from having patients stay within the grounds of a large hospital complex to secluding them; actual seclusion represents one end point on the continuum of planned space allotment as a clinical treatment.

A. Mechanisms of Action

Seclusion likely operates through its effects on perception, interpersonal relatedness, and behavior.

   1. **Perception**. Seclusion decreases sensory input in all forms by producing an environment of relative sensory sameness or monotony. This sameness may be particularly helpful when the patient's clinical state or degree of regression has produced a heightened vulnerability to sensory bombardment and distortion; stimulus generalization or overstimulation; or an inability to integrate stimuli, whether from within the body or from without.

   2. **Interpersonal relatedness**. The effect of seclusion on interpersonal relatedness is to isolate or distance patients temporarily from persons in their perceptual field. The isolation is not total because other patients

and staff are visible and audible through the door and its observation window. Enough distance is provided, however, to minimize the patient's fears of others, whether from a loss of his or her sense of boundaries or feelings of fusion or from his or her experiences of staff and other patients as sources of persecution, threat, or attack.

3. **Behavior**. Compassionate seclusion can prevent out of control patients from harming themselves and others by removing their opportunity for violence and subsequent guilt or embarrassment. In addition, the bareness and absence of objects in the room and the ease with which the patient can be observed closely may reduce his or her self-destructive behavior.

B. Conditions for Which Seclusion May Be Useful

Seclusion is indicated as a treatment for clinical states in which the mechanisms mentioned earlier—sensory hyperesthesia, pathologic intensity or distortions in interpersonal relatedness, and pathologic excitement and behavioral dyscontrol—apply. These include (a) psychotic disorders (e.g., schizophrenia, especially with catatonic excitement, and bipolar disorder, especially with acute mania in all its forms), (b) acute paranoid reactions (e.g., delusional disorder) and extreme panic, (c) toxic conditions and withdrawal states (e.g., **amphetamines**, hallucinogens, and **phencyclidine** psychoses) and deliria of various origins (see section III.F for exceptions), (d) cognitive disorders (e.g., certain forms of dementia that produce difficulty in integration of stimuli, reality perception, or modulation of affects), (e) transient but severe situational disturbances (e.g., a host of circumstances that may evoke overwhelming panic, rage, or self-destructive or outwardly directed assaultiveness on either basis), and (f) acutely suicidal patients for whom seclusion offers temporary freedom from objects that may be put to self-destructive use. Infrequently, a patient may be placed in temporary seclusion solely for the protection of other patients, a use that always requires considerable thought and documentation.

C. When to Seclude a Patient

Seclusion should be instituted as (a) an elective (patient-requested) measure to provide calm, quiet time for reflection; (b) a planned measure to head off a developing crisis when the patient's typical pattern is known or can be anticipated; (c) an adjunct to other treatments, such as medication, particularly for the dangerously aggressive patient; or (d) an alternative when other interventions have not been effective. Though the clinical effects may be quite similar, legal statutes or mental health regulations tend to distinguish involuntary from voluntary seclusion. Involuntary seclusion is usually sanctioned by law in cases of emergency, which are defined in one state, for example, as "the occurrence of, or serious threat of, extreme violence, personal injury, or attempted suicide." In certain instances, such as toxic states, both secluding and restraining patients may be necessary and helpful.

D. How to Seclude a Patient

Seclusion should preferably be initiated only after the ordering physician has evaluated the patient and has discussed other treatment options with involved staff. In an emergency, if the physician cannot see the patient immediately, the ordering physician should see the patient no more than 1 hour after the order is carried out. The patient should be conveyed to the seclusion room in a manner that permits maximum safety for the patient, other patients, and staff. This method may involve merely a staff escort of one or more persons, or it may entail a five-person face-down carry, with one person to each limb and another holding the head and managing doors. When the patient is in seclusion, he or she should be searched, and potentially hazardous articles, such as pocketknives, matches, belts, and sharp objects, should be removed. If medically indicated, the appropriate medications should be administered, giving careful attention to the seclusion room context (e.g., hydration, thermoregulation). Secluded patients should be told that they are being placed in the room for their own protection (or for the protection of others when this is the indication), that they will be observed frequently and regularly and will be given time for necessities such as toileting and eating, and that they will be released when their self-control makes this possible. Such information may provide some reassurance against abandonment feelings.

E. Continuation of Seclusion

As an emergency situation, seclusion requires extremely careful monitoring. The patient must be observed at regular intervals. Seclusion must be "broken" regularly (e.g., 10 to 20 minutes out of every 1 to 2 hours) to allow for feeding; conversation (if it is not too stimulating to the patient); bathing; toileting (usually every 4 hours); medication; monitoring of vital signs; medical procedures; drawing of blood; and, most important, clinical assessment of the patient's condition to determine the need for continuing or terminating seclusion. In addition, patients should be checked through an observation window at designated intervals, usually every 15 minutes, but surveillance should occur more frequently or even constantly if it is required by a patient's clinical condition. Because staff may be in danger when seclusion is broken, adequate staffing patterns must be ensured. Staff must be alert to potential dangers, and they must be trained to deal with them.

F. Termination of Seclusion

Because no absolute clinical assessment criteria are available for determining when to terminate seclusion, the responsible physician must rely on his or her judgment and experience and on consultation with other treatment team members. The most important indicator for ending seclusion is a worsening of the patient's clinical state in response to seclusion. Though ill effects are relatively rare in practice, seclusion may communicate to the patient, despite reassurances, a sense of being unwanted, abandoned, or isolated that may vitiate its calming effect. Some patients (e.g., those with cognitive disorders or toxic deliria) may need the reassurance of having a familiar person close by. Their disorganization may derive in part from feelings of isolation or from sensory deprivation, and seclusion may worsen their agitation rather than help it, a phenomenon similar to that seen in some patients with "black patch" psychosis after cataract surgery or in some elderly patients who "sundown." On occasion, worsening may also result from inadequate or inappropriate concomitant pharmacotherapy or from staff whose fear of the patient prevents them from establishing reassuring contact. Unfortunately, no obvious way for predicting the outcome of seclusion is available, short of a brief trial.

Seclusion should be terminated as soon as it has produced its desired effects. In most instances, seclusion and the appropriate medication can calm a patient sufficiently to avert or arrest an emergency or an upsurge in symptoms. At that point, the patient should return to a larger environment. A common first step is to open the door with adequate numbers of staff in attendance and then to begin increasing the number and duration of forays out of the seclusion room. The return (a) should be discussed and negotiated with the patient to maintain or reestablish the treatment alliance; (b) should be graduated to allow the patient to acclimate to gradually increasing levels of stimulation, spatial expansion, and responsibility for self-control; (c) should be monitored to assess the need for additional treatment that might include a return to seclusion for additional periods; and (d) should include a debriefing of the patient to elicit his or her responses to the intervention and to answer any questions.

IV. Misuses of Seclusion

Seclusion is a valuable addition to the therapeutic armamentarium, but it is subject to misuse. PL 106-310 requires that seclusion should only be used to ensure the patient's safety. In the authors' opinion, seclusion is misused when it is used in the following ways:

1. As "punishment" for "bad" behavior (as a child is sent to his or her room).
2. As an aversive stimulus in the context of an involuntarily imposed behavior modification paradigm.

3. As an intervention for a patient who is obnoxious, pestering, irritating, insulting, or provocative when this behavior is voluntary and is not due, for example, to the intrusive, irritable clinical escalation that can occur in mania.

4. As an expression of milieu countertransference. Seclusion as a treatment is meant to benefit the patient and, indirectly, other patients, and it is not for the unconscious or conscious needs of staff. Protection from this contingency typically is achieved by peer assessment, consultation, supervision, and legal safeguards.

5. As a procedure unaccompanied by planned close observation and monitoring. This misuse of seclusion may represent clinical abandonment or neglect of the patient.

Seclusion should not be used as a substitute for staff attention; it must be prescribed in concert with attention.

V. Adverse or Unwanted Effects of Seclusion

Almost no lasting unwanted effects specific to seclusion are observed when it is appropriately prescribed and monitored. As was noted earlier, seclusion can temporarily worsen certain clinical states as a result of sensory deprivation, but, except for the transient grudges that sometimes develop over seclusion, this is not a serious problem. Self-injury is always possible, but patients who are not placed in seclusion may just as easily harm themselves. Improper use of seclusion or an improperly designed or monitored room can result in injuries, exhaustion states, dehydration, pneumonia, and death. Careful search procedures are essential to protect against hazards from objects taken into seclusion by patients or smuggled in by others.

In addition to physical and emotional dangers to patients, the use of seclusion can cause splitting or lack of cohesion among staff. Ample time must be given for staff to air their views and to review carefully the issues concerning a particular patient. Unresolved differences among staff can be communicated to patients and may potentially increase their turmoil. At times, providing other patients with an opportunity to voice their fears and other feelings about seclusion (e.g., in a ward community meeting) may also be helpful.

VI. Forensic Aspects of Seclusion

Forensic problems around seclusion rest on three interrelated factors.

A. Confusion Between the Proper Use and Abuse of Seclusion

If seclusion is used to approximate the solitary confinement of a prison, no therapeutic goal for the patient is served, and the patient is, in effect, imprisoned without due process. Attorneys not uncommonly view this abuse of seclusion as if it represents all uses of seclusion. Some accept the concept of seclusion as equivalent to a public health quarantine.

B. The View of Seclusion as Punitive, Without Therapeutic Effect or Clinical Justification

This view draws its force from the ignorance of many attorneys of clinical psychiatry, that perhaps is coupled with an antiillness bias from reading the works of certain authors such as Thomas Szasz, an author frequently represented in law school curricula.

C. A Clouded View of the Custodial Versus Treatment Role of Psychiatric Inpatient Care for Some Patients

Many attorneys contend that patients have the right to receive treatment and, increasingly, the right to refuse it, and yet the hospital is not free to discharge the treatment-refusing or uncooperative involuntary patient. No parallel exists to the disciplinary code of school systems, which permits detention in the principal's office or expulsion from school to prevent harm to others. Furthermore, physicians may feel compromised in their responsibility, ability, and freedom to treat when legal authorities see the behavior in question not as the result of illness but as freedom of expression by the patient.

Seclusion, in some instances, may represent the "least restrictive alternative" currently sought by some jurists because it usually permits brief placement in the seclusion room, followed by return to an open ward, instead of more restrictive alternatives such as transfer to a closed-door high-security facility. An exception would be an unremittingly assaultive patient who does not respond to short-term interventions. In such cases, transfer to a secure facility is often less restrictive, because such a patient's clinical condition might require long-term seclusion in the average inpatient setting, whereas in a secure facility with structured programs, trained personnel, and adequate physical design, the patient might be able to leave his or her room or walk around a courtyard. In addition, seclusion may be safer for some specific patients in both the short and long term than the two alternative approaches to the same symptoms—medication or electroconvulsive therapy (see Chapter 24)—a fact often overlooked by legal authorities.

Some clinicians believe that using **restraints** (see Chapter 26) is a less restrictive alternative than seclusion, in part because the restrained patient can have closer and more human contact. In the authors' clinical experience, the feeling of being physically restrained is more troubling to some patients than is seclusion. The use of restraints carries its own hazards, such as aspiration and exhaustion. The main indications for restraints are probably limited to awakening from a delirium, constant self-destructive acts, or potential injury to staff during necessary clinical activities such as taking vital signs (see Chapter 26).

As this chapter was being put into its final form (2002), the Health Care Financing Administration promulgated an "Interim Final Rule" (HCFA-3018-IFC) on seclusion and restraint. This rule contains stronger provisions than the Children's Health Act; it permits seclusion or restraint **only** under emergency conditions and when other interventions have failed to be effective. As the reader can imagine, the proposed rule is being vigorously debated. Among the arguments against the rule is that, given current staffing and funding levels and the composition of many patient cohorts, its adoption could force the closure of some clinical settings.

VII. A Prototypical Set of Principles for Clinicians

The following factors or principles are offered as guidelines to the therapeutic use of seclusion.

1. All personnel working with patients in seclusion must receive careful orientation about the medical, legal, and ethical issues involved before they are assigned to patient care duties.

2. Patients should always be asked to enter seclusion voluntarily before they are involuntarily secluded.

3. As soon as possible, a responsible member of the patient's family, if one can be found, should be told of the symptoms requiring seclusion. Any questions should be answered to permit families to exercise their right to seek treatment elsewhere (at present, many families view seclusion only in negative terms). On the other hand, confidentiality and right to privacy issues must also be considered.

4. The decision to seclude should be documented by a clearly written order on the physician's order sheet. This order may be signed by the ordering physician, and it should include both the date and the time. The ordering physician should preferably see the patient before seclusion is initiated or within 1 hour if he or she cannot be immediately present.

5. The option of telephone orders should only be considered rarely. Telephone orders should be used only in extreme emergencies, and they should be countersigned in person by the ordering physician within a specified time interval (e.g., 30 minutes or long enough to permit the physician time to evaluate the patient's condition before signing). No more than 1 hour should be acceptable for this delay. An American Psychiatric Association Task Force report (see Additional Reading) recommends that the patient be seen within 1 hour of entering seclusion but allows up to 3 hours to adjust for physician availability.

6. Whenever possible, the need to seclude should be anticipated and discussed with the patient and staff as part of a total treatment program. The conditions

and symptoms to be treated by seclusion should be documented clearly in the patient's treatment plan. This point is controversial because many hospitals and some jurisdictions believe that standing orders for "as needed" seclusion are always improper.

7. While in formal seclusion, the patient should be seen by a physician at least two to three times per 8-hour shift.

8. A single seclusion order should have a defined duration of applicability (e.g., a maximum of 8 hours). The physician making the assessment must then write new orders with documentation of the patient's condition and including reasons for continuation.

9. A physician must evaluate the patient to end seclusion and to assess the consequences of seclusion and its termination.

10. Progress notes should document all incidents of seclusion; their positive and unwanted consequences; and the reason(s) for seclusion, including a description of the target symptoms and behaviors.

11. Any patient who requires two or more seclusion episodes in a week should be reviewed formally (e.g., at a team or ward conference) by the responsible physician; at least one other physician, preferably a physician from another service who is knowledgeable about the benefits and risks of seclusion; and the nursing service. This discussion should include review of alternative treatment, including transfer to another ward or facility. Many hospitals require that patients in continuous seclusion be evaluated by the hospital's chief medical officer (or his or her designee) after 72 hours and before further seclusion orders can be written.

12. Hospital seclusion must be subjected to regular review by the medical staff, utilization review personnel, quality assurance staff, other standard-setting groups within the hospital, and relevant external bodies.

13. Any death during seclusion or within 24 hours after the termination of seclusion must be reported to the appropriate agencies.

ADDITIONAL READING

Binder RL. The use of seclusion on an inpatient crisis intervention unit. *Hosp Commun Psychiatry* 1979;30:266–269.

Binder RL, McCoy SM. A study of patients' attitudes toward placement in seclusion. *Hosp Commun Psychiatry* 1983;34:1052–1054.

Chamberlin J. An ex-patient's response to Soliday. *J Nerv Ment Dis* 1985;173:288–289.

Convertino K, Pinto RP, Fiester AR. Use of inpatient seclusion at a community mental health center. *Hosp Commun Psychiatry* 1980;31:848–850.

Curie CG. Use of restraints, seclusion, and exclusion in state mental hospitals. *Pennsylvania Department of Public Welfare, Mental Health, and Substance Abuse Services Bulletin.* OMHSAS-99-01. Harrisburg, PA: Pennsylvania Department of Public Welfare, Mental Health, and Substance Abuse Services, 1999.

Curran WJ. Law-medicine notes. The management of psychiatric patients: courts, patients' representatives, and the refusal of treatment. *N Engl J Med* 1980;302:1297–1299.

Department of Health and Human Services, Health Care Financing Administration. Medicare and Medicaid Programs: hospital conditions of participation: patients' rights: Interim Final Rule. 42 CFR 482. *Federal Register* 1999;64:36069–36089.

Fitzgerald RG, Long I. Seclusion in the treatment and management of severely disturbed manic and depressed patients. *Perspect Psychiatr Care* 1973;11:59–64.

Guirguis EG. Management of disturbed patients: an alternative to the use of mechanical restraints. *J Clin Psychiatry* 1978;39:295–303.

Gutheil TG. Observations on the theoretical bases for seclusion of the psychiatric inpatient. *Am J Psychiatry* 1978;135:325–328.

Gutheil TG. Restraint versus treatment: seclusion as discussed in the Boston state hospital case. *Am J Psychiatry* 1980;137:718–719.

Hammill K, McEvoy JP, Koral H, et al. Hospitalized schizophrenic patient views about seclusion. *J Clin Psychiatry* 1989;50:174–177.

Jensen K. Comments on Dr. Stanley M. Soliday's "A comparison of patient and staff attitudes toward seclusion." *J Nerv Ment Dis* 1985;173:290–291.

Mallya AR, Roos PD, Roebuck-Colgan K. Restraint, seclusion, and clozapine. *J Clin Psychiatry* 1992;53:395–397.

Mattson MR, Sacks MH. Seclusion: uses and complications. *Am J Psychiatry* 1978;135: 1210–1213.

Ng B, Kumar S, Ranclaud M, et al. Ward crowding and incidents of violence on an acute psychiatric inpatient unit. *Psychiatr Serv* 2001;52:521–525.

Oldham JM, Russakoff LM, Prusnofsky L. Seclusion: patterns and milieu. *J Nerv Ment Dis* 1983;171:645–650.

Plutchik R, Karasu TB, Conte HR, et al. Toward a rationale for the seclusion process. *J Nerv Ment Dis* 1978;166:571–579.

Ramchandani D, Akhtar S, Helfrich J. Seclusion of psychiatric inpatients. *Int J Soc Psychiatry* 1981;27:225–231.

Schwab PJ, Lahmeyer CB. The uses of seclusion on a general hospital psychiatric unit. *J Clin Psychiatry* 1979;40:228–231.

Soliday SM. A comparison of patient and staff attitudes toward seclusion. *J Nerv Ment Dis* 1985;173:282–286.

Soloff PH, Gutheil TG, Wexler DB. Seclusion and restraint in 1985: a review and update. *Hosp Commun Psychiatry* 1985;36:652–657.

Soloff PH, Turner SM. Patterns of seclusion: a prospective study. *J Nerv Ment Dis* 1981;169:37–44.

Steel E. *Seclusion and restraint practices: a review and analysis.* Alexandria, VA: National Mental Health Association, 1999.

Tardiff K, ed. *The psychiatric uses of seclusion and restraint.* Task Force Report No. 22. Washington, D.C.: American Psychiatric Press, 1984.

Tardiff K. *Concise guide to assessment & management of violent patients.* Washington, D.C.: American Psychiatric Press, 1989.

Wadeson H, Carpenter WT. Impact of the seclusion room experience. *J Nerv Ment Dis* 1976;163:318–328.

Wells DA. Use of seclusion on a university hospital psychiatric floor. *Arch Gen Psychiatry* 1972;26:410–413.

Whaley MS, Ramirez LF. The use of seclusion rooms and physical restraints in the treatment of psychiatric patients. *J Psychiatr Nurs Ment Health Serv* 1980;18:13–16.

26. USE OF PHYSICAL RESTRAINTS AS AN EMERGENCY TREATMENT

Thomas G. Gutheil
Richard I. Shader

The use of physical restraints is perhaps the most controversial treatment method described in this text. Because it can be both protective and life saving for patients and staff, this chapter provides a brief discussion of physical restraint in the following four most common forms: the geriatric chair, the Posey belt, plastic handcuffs, and four-point restraints (wrist and ankle bracelets). All forms of physical restraint require constant monitoring and consideration of a patient's physical needs and status. Adequate numbers of staff are essential both for patient monitoring and for safe placement of patients in restraints. As with the use of seclusion (see Chapter 25), restraints should not be ordered by a physician when other safe and effective methods of temporary control are available that have not been used (see also section IV.C). A persuasive clinical argument involving safety to the patient, other patients, or staff must be documented each time a decision is made to use restraints. Most jurisdictions have laws governing the use of restraints in hospitals, nursing homes, and other settings. Some believe that the movement toward more restrictive laws was prompted by perceptions that restraints were not being used primarily for the benefit of patients (see also section VI.C in Chapter 25 for information about proposed interim rules from the Health Care Financing Administration).

I. Geriatric Chair

The geriatric chair is used most often with demented elderly patients. It is a broad-based chair (rarely, a wheeled chair) that is fitted with a lap desk secured to its arms. The chair prevents the confused, agitated, and disoriented patient from wandering around or off the ward or intruding on other patients, either to their detriment or so as to provoke an aggressive reprisal or response.

A. Advantages

The advantages of this method are that the patient sits in a comfortable position; most activities of the hands such as occupational therapy, eating, writing, and taking medication are possible; and the device is generally safe for the occupant as long as the chair cannot be tipped over. In addition, ongoing staff contact can be readily maintained.

B. Possible Hazards

1. **Contact hazards**
   a. Skin abrasion.
   b. Abdominal compression.
   c. Chair sores.
   d. Impairment of circulation, including (in rare instances) venous stasis, thrombosis, or embolism. These complications are the result of problems with the use of the chair, including a failure to adjust the chair to the patient, faulty chair design, insufficient supervision, or inadequate hygienic monitoring of the patient.
2. **Treatment hazards**
   a. Deliberate avoidance and neglect of the patient after placement in the chair, leading to failures of feeding, toileting, and interpersonal contact.
   b. Sensory deprivation, leading to agitation.
   c. The creation of a false sense of security; the patient is supposedly "all right" and is no longer in need of nursing staff attention.
3. **Other hazards**. Severe increases in agitation resulting in injury from the chair itself or by its tipping over.

II. Posey Belt

A Posey belt is a broad canvas, leather, or web belt that is secured around the patient's waist and fastened to the bed frame or chair. Used with side rails in a bed, it may help to keep a wandering demented patient in the bed when rest is required by the patient's medical condition. This method may also be used when specially designed geriatric chairs are not available. The hazards are circulation impairment; abdominal compression; abrasion; and, if the patient tries to slide out of the belt, strangulation, a hazard that severely limits the value of the Posey belt.

III. Plastic Handcuffs

A patient who, because of dangerous assaultiveness or terror, is judged incapable of being evacuated from an area or a building for clinical or administrative purposes (e.g., fires, fire drills, or emergency evacuations) can be temporarily restrained by plastic handcuffs. These plastic cuffs resemble metal handcuffs, but they are made of noninjurious plastic, often with additional padding. The cuffs facilitate ambulation and add a degree of safety for other patients being evacuated. After the emergency or drill is over, the cuffs should be removed immediately.

IV. Four-Point Restraint

Four-point restraint usually consists of foam-padded leather wrist and ankle bracelets attached securely to the frame of a hospital bed or to a specialized bed frame that is sometimes secured to the floor. Sufficient slack should be left in the placement of the restraints to permit needed positional changes, especially side to side movement and toileting. The use of this method of restraint is an intensive and specialized medical procedure that requires specific training and careful monitoring and supervision.

A. Indications

In general, restraints are considered when a patient's loss of control is of dangerous proportion, and little or no response is seen with medication, temporary isolation or seclusion (see Chapter 25), or verbal intervention. Under certain circumstances, patients with toxic psychoses, such as those induced by **phencyclidine or lysergic acid diethylamide (LSD)**, that promote violence toward the self or others may be protected and treated in restraints until the offending agent is metabolized or is countered by an effective antidote. Deliria, especially delirium tremens or other drug-withdrawal deliria, also may be so treated, especially if the patient must be briefly left unattended. A patient ill enough to be restrained should in no instance be left unattended for more than 10 to 15 minutes; some jurisdictions require that the patient never be left unattended.

Severe paranoid and manic states may require emergency restraint when other methods, such as seclusion or medication, have been ineffective or have not yet had time to work. Agitated depressions involving severe unremitting self-injury (e.g., self-mutilation, eye enucleation, self-strangulation) may mandate the use of restraints to keep the patient safe until emergency electroconvulsive therapy can be initiated or medications have taken effect. In addition, violent patients with comorbid medical disease in a combination that prohibits other treatment measures may need restraints to allow time for safe medical treatment or nursing care. **Although the following is controversial, some clinicians advocate restraints instead of medication in psychotic women who are pregnant, believing that the temporary use of restraints gives time needed for the consideration of the risks of medication exposure during pregnancy**. In any patient, the clinical benefits of restraints must exceed or outweigh the risks, both psychologic and physical.

B. How Do Restraints Help?

Restraints are thought to act through direct physical control of the patient's ability to harm the self or others. In addition to preserving life and bodily safety, restraints communicate to patients who may fear loss of control that they do not need to rely only on their own fragile internal controls. Some clinicians believe that the inherently calming effect of this message is a likely factor in the efficacy of restraint. In certain clinical states, a period in restraints may be the only time an acutely agitated patient can relax.

Physical restraint also allows disturbed patients a period of safe interpersonal contact. Medication, other treatments, and diagnostic procedures may be achieved in an atmosphere of safety for the patient and staff; the patient obtains crucial human contact without fearing the effect of his or her own impulses.

A third mechanism is the induction of a state of relative sensory sameness, which is advantageous, as with seclusion, in aiding patients prone to sensory overload and stimulus generalization. This latter mechanism is especially relevant when a patient requires physical restraints while in the seclusion room.

C. Contraindications

Restraints should not be used (a) when other effective treatment measures are available; (b) as a replacement for staff attention; (c) except for brief emergency situations for the habitually violent, those with impulse disorders or explosive personalities, or very angry nonpsychotic patients (these patients should receive other types of treatment or, when appropriate, legal or administrative controls); or (d) in place of transfer to a secure facility when this is indicated and is possible.

D. Technique

Restraints should be used only by physicians, nursing staff, or treatment teams familiar with and trained and practiced in their use. All staff must be thoroughly oriented to the theory of restraints and should be comfortable with their use, especially because a positive nonpunitive attitude, when communicated to the patient, should reassure him or her about being controllable. Annual retraining is strongly recommended. **For pregnant patients whose level of dyscontrol requires restraints, placing the patient on her left side or using a pillow to raise the right hip to avoid aortocaval compression has been recommended** (see Additional Reading). In general, patients should be restrained in a supine position; some authorities further suggest elevation of the head of the bed to decrease the likelihood of aspiration.

The patient should be offered restraints on a voluntary basis whenever possible. The possible future use of restraints and a review of alternative aids to control should also be discussed. A request for restraint that is initiated by a patient should almost always be honored. All patients in restraint should be told as clearly as possible that this is occurring for their own protection or the protection of others; that they will be carefully observed and followed closely; and that, when their control returns, they will be released promptly. Once the patient is in restraints, he or she must be viewed as being under intensive care and requiring more observation, not less. Attention to feeding, toileting, vital signs, concurrent medical conditions, the careful use of medications, and body position changes must be regular and systematic. At the same time, the staff must continue to assess the beneficial effects of restraint and whether the patient's self-control has been reestablished.

Recent guidelines from the American Academy of Child and Adolescent Psychiatry (see Additional Reading) largely track the recommendations provided in this chapter and emphasize the alertness to any potential for airway obstruction and avoidance of this as a possibility.

E. Hazards and Risks

These are mostly short term, and they include abrasion or injury from the straps, cuffs, or bed; asphyxiation or aspiration from vomiting or while feeding; and bladder and bowel disturbances secondary to position. **In pregnant patients, compression of venous return through the inferior vena cava must be avoided**. With prolonged use, restraints may cause bed sores, muscle atrophy, bone demineralization, and other metabolic disturbances. Attention to exercise and metabolic needs is essential. Psychologic hazards are posed particularly for the types of patients described in section IV.C, who may regress when placed in restraints, and for those with cognitive disorders (e.g., dementias) for whom excessive sensory deprivation could worsen their mental state.

Limited data are available on the rates of accidental deaths attributable to the use of restraints. One recent survey examined 1,403 incidents of restraints use in a 150-bed county psychiatric facility over a 5-year period, with the following two findings. First, in keeping with national trends, annual use rates fell steadily from 9.2 per 1,000 patient days in 1994 to 1.5 per 1,000 patient days in 1999 for an average rate over the 5 years of 4.6 per 1,000 patient days. Second, more importantly, no deaths were attributable to the use of restraints.

F. Termination

The decision to terminate restraint is as critical, and requires as much clinical care, as the decision to initiate it. As with the termination of seclusion (see Chapter 25), restraints must be removed in a graduated stepwise manner that has been negotiated with patients as part of an ongoing assessment of their clinical state. The staff must be ready to resume restraints at a certain stage after release to allow the patient to acclimate; nevertheless, an inconsistent, impulsive, nongraduated, or non-negotiated "on-again, off-again" approach should be studiously avoided.

G. Forensic Issues

These are similar to those with seclusion (see Chapter 25). Some authorities suggest that when a voluntary patient must be restrained involuntarily, involuntary commitment proceedings should be initiated immediately. The use of physical restraint is a sensitive and controversial subject. It is a source of potential distress to patients, families, and staff, so its use must be the subject of active review and discussion. To ensure high standards of practice, each episode of restraint must be the subject of careful internal review and documentation of indications and response; the review itself must be documented.

ADDITIONAL READING

Bursten B. Using mechanical restraints on acutely disturbed psychiatric patients. *Hosp Commun Psychiatry* 1975;26:757–759.

Carmel H, Hunter M. Compliance with training in managing assaultive behavior and injuries from inpatient violence. *Hosp Commun Psychiatry* 1990;41:558–560.

Department of Health and Human Services, Health Care Financing Administration. Medicare and Medicaid Programs: hospital conditions of participation: patients' rights: Interim Final Rule. 42 CFR 482 *Federal Register* 1999;64:36069–36089.

Fisher WA. Restraint and seclusion: a review of the literature. *Am J Psychiatry* 1994;151:1584–1591.

Guirguis EF, Durost HB. The role of mechanical restraints in the management of disturbed behavior. *Can Psychiatr Assoc J* 1978;23:209–218.

Hay D, Cromwell R. Reducing the use of full-leather restraints on an acute adult inpatient ward. *Hosp Commun Psychiatry* 1980;31:198–200.

Mallya AR, Roos PD, Roebuck-Colgan K. Restraint, seclusion, clozapine. *J Clin Psychiatry* 1992;53:395–397.

Masters KJ, Bellonci C, Bernet W, et al. Practice parameter for the prevention and management of aggressive behavior in child and adolescent psychiatric institutions with special reference to seclusion and restraint. *J Am Acad Child Adolesc Psychiatry* 2002;41:4S–25S.

Miller WH, Resnick MP. Restraining the violent pregnant patient. *Am J Psychiatry* 1991;148:269.

Pinninti NR, Rissmiller D. Incidence of restraint-related deaths. *Psychiatr Serv* 2001;52:975.

Raskin VD, Dresner N, Miller LN. Risks of restraints versus psychotropic medication for pregnancy. *Am J Psychiatry* 1991;148:1760–1761.

Rosen H, DiGiacomo JN. The role of physical restraint in the treatment of psychiatric illness. *J Clin Psychiatry* 1978;39:228–232.

Soloff PH. Behavioral precipitants of restraint in the modern milieu. *Compr Psychiatry* 1978;19:179–184.

Tardiff K, ed. *The psychiatric uses of seclusion and restraint.* Task Force Report No. 22. Washington, D.C.: American Psychiatric Press, 1984.

Tardiff K. *Concise guide to assessment & management of violent patients.* Washington, D.C.: American Psychiatric Press, 1989.

27. RAPE AND SEXUAL ASSAULT

Janet E. Osterman
Jane E. Barbiasz
Richard I. Shader

Rape is an act of sexual violence perpetrated by one person against another. Rape should not be delimited to the common stereotype of a male stranger attacking a woman. Rape may occur in diverse situations and across the life span; children and the elderly are not spared. In the United States, where rape has an estimated prevalence of 9% to 13% for women and 0.7% to 5% for men, strangers account for only 22% of rapes. Boyfriends or domestic partners commit 19% of rapes, and another 38% are perpetrated by other family members.

Whether the event consists of the attack of an unknown male against a woman, the sexual subjugation of a woman by invading troops in a war zone, the molestation of a child by a pedophile or parent, the unwilling "use" of a weaker inmate by a stronger inmate in a prison setting, or the exploitation of a person subdued by alcohol or sedatives during a date, the central themes of rape are exploitation, domination, intimidation, humiliation, and force.

From a legal perspective, **rape** is defined as sexual intercourse perpetrated against the victim's will and consent or as sexual intercourse with a person who is unable to give consent due to age or mental impairment. **Sexual assault** is the term used for other forms of nonconsensual sexual activity, such as forced fellatio or forced anal penetration. Recently, **date** or **acquaintance rape** appears to have become more common; its true prevalence may be obscured or complicated by the use of amnesic drugs, such as the benzodiazepine **flunitrazepam** (Rohypnol) and the γ-aminobutyric acid agonist γ-**hydroxybutyrate**, which leave the victim without memory of the rape. How frequently these agents are used is unknown because their detection is obscured by rapid hepatic clearance and the lack of standard testing for γ-hydroxybutyrate.

Completed rape and sexual assault are common traumatic experiences. The National Comorbidity Survey found that 9.2% of women and 0.7% of men have been raped. The National Women's Study estimated that 12.7% or over 12 million adult women in the United States have experienced a completed rape and that an additional 14.3% or 13.5 million women have been sexually assaulted. For perspective, selected statistics from the National Victim Center for 1992 are listed in Table 27.1.

College student surveys found that 20% of women and 4% of men experienced forced sexual activity from a date or acquaintance. The 1994 Bureau of Justice's National Crime Victimization survey reported that 5% of adolescent rape victims were males.

According to the United States Department of Justice, a quarter of a million children are victims of sexual abuse each year. However, it is widely acknowledged that child rape and sexual assault are underreported and thus do not come to the attention of child protection services or other agencies. Child victims of rape or sexual assault often live with, are related to, or know the perpetrator. Up to 16% of American women are the victims of rape, attempted rape, or molestation before the age of 18. Limited data are available on the incidence of rape and childhood sexual abuse perpetrated against boys despite the recent media attention to victimization of boys by "trusted" members of the community.

I. Psychologic Sequelae of Rape and Sexual Assault
A. Consequences of Adult Rape and Sexual Assault

The psychologic sequelae of rape have been described in the literature since 1974 with the initial description of the "rape trauma syndrome" by Burgess and Holmstrom. The rape trauma syndrome is a two-phase reaction with an acute and a reorganization stage. The acute phase is characterized by disorganization, denial, and shock; the reorganization phase includes

TABLE 27.1. SELECTED STATISTICS FOR RAPE

The United States has the world's highest rape rate for countries that publish statistics—3 times higher than Germany, 13 times higher than the United Kingdom, and 20 times higher than Japan.

In the United States, 1.3 women are raped every minute; this translates into about 700,000 rapes per year.

One of three women in the United States will be sexually assaulted in her lifetime.

One of seven women will be raped by her husband.

Seventy-eight percent of rape victims know the perpetrator.

One of 12 male students responding to a survey had committed acts against women that met the legal definition of rape.

Seventy-five percent of male and 55% of female students involved in acquaintance rape had been drinking or using drugs.

Compared with nonvictims, rape victims are almost nine times more likely to attempt suicide.

From the National Center for Victims of Crime & Crime Victims Research and Treatment Center. *Rape in America: a report to the nation.* Arlington, VA: National Center for Victims of Crime, 1992.

nightmares, fear, and avoidance behaviors. The symptoms of the reorganization phase are now subsumed under the diagnosis **posttraumatic stress disorder (PTSD)**; the acute phase is most similar to the new *Diagnostic and Statistical Manual of Mental Disorders,* 4th edition, (DSM-IV) diagnosis of **acute stress disorder**.

1. **PTSD**, a clinical syndrome that may follow a traumatic event, such as rape and sexual assault, causes significant distress and morbidity. PTSD is characterized by the following three symptom clusters: reexperiencing of the traumatic event, avoidance of reminders of the traumatic event and emotional numbing, and hyperarousal symptoms. For example, a rape victim may experience intrusive thoughts of the rape, may suffer from nightmares of threat or rape, or may experience flashbacks of all or some portions of the rape experience. Avoidance of reminders of the rape are common, and these may include avoidance of the site of the rape or similar places, avoidance of sexual relations, or avoidance of people who are similar to the perpetrator. Rape victims may experience emotional numbing, such as a sense of being unable to have loving feelings, feeling detached from others, or having decreased interest. Difficulty falling asleep, being easily startled, irritability, and hypervigilance are common hyperarousal symptoms. Table 14.10 provides the formal diagnostic criteria for PTSD.

   Since the 1980 inclusion of PTSD in the diagnostic nomenclature in DSM, 3rd edition, the psychologic sequelae of rape and the incidence of rape-related and sexual assault-related PTSD have been frequently studied. The National Comorbidity Survey found that 49.5% of women and 65% of men who had been raped suffered PTSD. In the National Women's Study, 12.4% of the 12 million American women rape victims and 6.7% of the 13.5 million sexual assault victims developed chronic PTSD. Foa et al. reported that 90% to 95% of female rape victims suffered symptoms of PTSD in the first 2 weeks after a rape, with nearly 50% continuing to suffer from PTSD 3 months later. In other studies, Foa found that, of the 52.4% of women suffering PTSD 2 months after being raped, 47.1% continued to suffer PTSD at 9 months. Thus, PTSD after rape may not be self-remitting but can become chronic and debilitating.

2. **Acute stress disorder**, a recent addition to the diagnostic nomenclature, is characterized by dissociative reexperiencing, avoidance, and hyperarousal symptoms. Symptoms must begin between 2 days and 4 weeks after the index traumatic event. Dissociative experiences fre-

quently predominate; they may include derealization, depersonalization, being in a daze, numbing, and amnesia. Some preliminary studies suggest that the presence of acute stress disorder is predictive for the development of PTSD; many studies show that peritraumatic dissociation is a risk factor for PTSD.

3. **Anxiety and depression** are also common consequences of rape. Seventy-seven percent of rape victims reported significant fears in the year after a rape. One author reported that 41% of women suffered from depression 15 to 30 months after rape. Others have reported that the likelihood in women rape victims of suffering depression was related to the number of rapes, increasing from 46% after a single rape to 80% after two or more rapes. However, some studies report that the depressive response in the first year after the rape is no different than the frequency observed in control subjects.

4. **Dissociative reactions**, such as dissociative amnesia and depersonalization, may be both an acute and chronic consequence of rape.

5. **Suicidal ideation** has been estimated to occur in up to 50% of rape victims with reports of 3% in the first month, a figure that increases over time. A large random population survey found that 19% of rape victims reported a suicide attempt and that 44% reported suicidal ideation.

B. Consequences of Childhood Rape and Sexual Assault

Childhood rape and sexual assault frequently result in psychologic consequences both in childhood and in adulthood. PTSD in children is often characterized by repetitive play reenacting the trauma; thus, in the case of rape or sexual assault, children show repetitive sexual play behaviors. Recurrent dreams may be frightening, but without recognizable content. These behaviors must be differentiated from normal childhood sexual curiosity and other causes of nightmares or night terrors. Children who are subjected to sexual abuse may also exhibit somatic complaints, anxiety, and depression.

Adults with histories of childhood sexual abuse may meet the diagnostic criteria for PTSD, depressive disorders, borderline personality disorder, somatization disorder, and dissociative disorders. Childhood sexual abuse is one of the most common causes of adult PTSD, which afflicts 10% of the population. A survey of adult women found that 64% of those who had been raped as a child and 33% of those who were molested suffered from PTSD. Childhood sexual abuse is presumed by many to be a risk factor for the development of dissociative identity disorder (see Chapter 4). One study reported that 68% of a sample of 100 dissociative identity disorder patients suffered incest. In addition, childhood sexual assault is a significant risk factor for adult sexual victimization, with one study showing that 50% of adult rape victims reported childhood histories of sexual abuse.

A new concept, **disorders of extreme stress (DES)** or **complex PTSD**, has been proposed by van der Kolk, Herman, and others to define a posttraumatic clinical syndrome characterized by problems in self-regulation of affect and impulses; disordered interpersonal functioning; somatization; and alterations in attention or consciousness, perceptions of the perpetrator, self-perceptions, and meaning systems. These symptoms are currently described as associated features of PTSD in DSM-IV. Findings from the field trials for the DSM-IV found that adult survivors of childhood sexual abuse were about four times more likely to suffer from disorders of extreme stress. Adults who suffered both childhood sexual and physical abuse were about 14 times more likely to suffer from this symptom complex.

II. Emergency Treatment of Rape Victims

Rape is a psychologic crisis for the victim. The victim's family and friends may also suffer a psychologic crisis. Rape victims may present to the emergency room for treatment of physical or psychologic injuries, or they may be brought by the police for a forensic examination. In cases with **severe or life-threatening injuries**, the urgency of the patient's medical status will preclude early mental health interventions. However, for most rape victims, the need for medical treatment and forensic examination affords the emergency mental health clinician an opportunity to assess the patient's psychologic status, to provide early mental health interventions, and to address any family needs for clinical intervention. The mental health clinician is often part of a rape treatment team that addresses the physical, psychologic, and forensic needs of the patient, and he or she must be knowledgeable about all aspects of the emergency treatment of rape.

A. Psychologic Interventions

Recognizing that rape or sexual assault victims will likely be psychologically overwhelmed on arrival to the emergency department and that they will need interventions to diminish their distress is essential. Ideally, the patient will be immediately triaged to a private, quiet, supportive area within the emergency department. Family members or friends, with the patient's consent, should be contacted to provide additional support for the patient. If the patient is unwilling to contact family or friends, the clinician should explore the reasons with the patient because rape frequently induces issues of shame that may prevent the patient from making use of family and community support. Acknowledgment of this nearly universal response and a discussion of patients' needs for support may help patients include family or friends in their treatment. In addition, a sensitive exploration may help to determine if a family member or partner was the perpetrator. Upon the arrival of family or friends to the emergency department, the mental health clinician must assess their ability to provide support and must supply the interventions necessary to maximize their ability to give support.

A patient's initial presentation in the emergency department or to emergency personnel in the field almost always reflects persisting survival mode functioning. "Survival mode" functioning, as described by Chemtob, is characterized by specialized cognitive-affective mechanisms organized as "flight," "fight," and "freeze" behaviors. High levels of anxiety and avoidance are seen with persisting "flight" responses, patients with anger reflect persisting "fight" responses, whereas persisting "freeze" responses appear clinically as dissociation. The highly anxious ("flight") or angry ("fight") patient typically receives mental health interventions in the emergency department, whereas patients with dissociative or numbing ("freeze") reactions present as quiet and withdrawn and they may not elicit a similar level of emergency mental health intervention. Despite this presentation, patients with dissociative reactions are at high risk for developing PTSD and they need specialized interventions.

Persistence of survival mode functioning after rape may complicate both the forensic evaluation and the medical treatment. Helping the patient move from a survival mode response to psychologic safety will also promote cooperation and a willingness to consent to the medical and forensic examinations. Although the physical examination and the collection of evidence are essential in the treatment of a rape victim, the physical contact and the vaginal, rectal, or oral examinations may act as triggers that stimulate further survival mode functioning and behaviors. Addressing the patient's psychologic needs for safety before proceeding to these examinations is essential unless severe or life-threatening injuries require immediate treatment.

The emergency five-step approach to the emotionally traumatized person as described by Osterman and Chemtob is (a) to restore psychologic safety, (b) to provide information, (c) to correct erroneous attributions (often called "misattributions"), (d) to restore and support effective coping, and (e) to ensure social support. Table 27.2 summarizes the steps in emergency care of the rape or sexual assault victim.

Psychologic safety must be restored by helping patients recognize that the rape is over and that they are now safe in the hospital. For patients who present with dissociation, providing grounding strategies, such as having them touch the examination table or other medical equipment (e.g., a stethoscope), is often necessary. Once the patient reports a sense of safety and knowledge

TABLE 27.2. EMERGENCY INTERVENTIONS FOR THE MEDICALLY STABLE RAPE VICTIM

Stage 1: Psychologic interventions
Restore psychologic safety.
Provide information.
Clarify or correct any misattributions.
Restore and support effective coping.
Ensure social support.
Stage 2: Medical and forensic examinations
Use SANE Program or rape kit.
Stage 3: Psychologic reassessment
Assess for reactivation of symptoms.
Repeat stage 1 interventions, as needed.
Stage 4: Review aftercare plan

Abbreviation: SANE, Sexual Assault Nurse Examiner.

that the danger has passed, providing information will allow the patient to begin to develop a cognitive map for understanding what has happened.

Rape victims and sexually assaulted patients require **specialized information** concerning their current medical status. They also typically have concerns and fears about future health problems, including sexually transmitted diseases (STDs) and pregnancy. It is common for victims of rape to have concerns about human immunodeficiency virus (HIV) and acquired immunodeficiency syndrome. The patient may also have questions about the legal implications of this crime and may need information about the legal system and police involvement. She or he may have fears of reporting the crime or may need information or assistance about how to report the crime. The clinician should discuss the patient's concerns, acknowledging that the patient may not wish to press charges at this point but that the medical care providers will collect the evidence in the event she or he wishes to pursue charges at a later time.

Patient's concerns and needs for information provide an opportunity for a sensitive discussion of both the need for medical and forensic examinations and how these examinations will be conducted. The clinician must acknowledge the patient's fears about being touched and about having a vaginal or rectal examination. The mental health clinician should discuss that the examination might trigger a flashback or intrusive memory of the actual rape or sexual assault and should assure the patient that psychologic support will be given. The patient should be asked if she or he wishes to have a family member or friend present and should be informed about which members of the rape treatment team will be present during the examination. Informing the patient that he or she might have a reexperience of the trauma that is induced by the examination will prevent the patient from feeling as if she or he is "going crazy," when or if a flashback occurs. Assuring the patient that a family member or friend may be present and that the mental health clinician will assist in managing any reexperiencing symptoms will help the patient cope with the examinations.

Victims of rape and sexual assault typically have erroneous beliefs or "misattributions" and frequently blame themselves (e.g., "I should not have been out alone," "I should not have worn a skirt that was this short"). Helping patients recognize the catastrophic nature of such beliefs, correcting any cognitive errors, and exploring their experience more realistically should decrease their anxiety, guilt, and anger.

The clinician should work to **restore and support effective coping and to ensure social support**. Psychoeducation for the patient and his or her family and friends about normative responses to trauma and common symptoms after rape can help restore the patient's sense of psychologic competence and can allay fears, for the family and friends and the patient, that he or she is "crazy" or has "lost control." Families and friends should be assisted in developing strategies to provide necessary social support, and they must understand that their support is an essential component of the patient's ability to cope and recover. The mental health clinician should discuss potential problems with arousal, irritability, sleep, memory and recall, intrusive thoughts, nightmares, avoidance, and numbing. Validation of typical trauma responses by family and friends may decrease patients' shame or fears and allow them to accept support.

The impact of rape on intimacy and the potential for subsequent sexual touching to trigger a survival response should be discussed with the patient's sexual partner. This may help the partner understand that these responses are common after rape and that they are not a reflection on him or her, which may prevent the partner from responding to this perceived rejection with an angry statement that further increases the patient's transition to fight, flight, or dissociation. Patients should be encouraged to be active participants in their medical and mental health care and to help the clinician in assessing their coping skills and access to community resources.

A referral for crisis intervention should be made before the patient is discharged from the emergency service. When possible, patients should speak with the clinician they will see, and a firm appointment time should be set to maximize the likelihood of keeping the appointment. In addition, patients should be informed that they should return to the emergency service or the crisis center if they are having difficulties managing feelings, physical symptoms, or adjustment following the rape. In addition to the support from family and friends, referrals to appropriate community agencies, self-help groups, and outpatient mental health treatment are needed for ongoing social support. Some states provide financial support for mental health treatment following rape, and the patient should be informed about how to obtain such services.

B. Medical and Forensic Examinations

Many emergency services have initiated the use of the **Sexual Assault Nurse Examiner (SANE)** program that was developed in 1976 through a collaboration of nurses, physicians, hospital administrators, district attorneys, local police, and rape crisis advocates. A standardized approach, such as the SANE program, is necessary because medical care providers frequently do not have education and training in forensic issues, and thus they may be reluctant to testify in court. The SANE program aims to strengthen victims by advocating for them and by providing the necessary evidence in the event that a victim wishes to pursue criminal charges. That medical care providers are knowledgeable and skilled in meeting the medical and mental health needs of the patient and in evidence collection and handling is essential.

The primary goals of the SANE program are to assist the patient in returning to his or her pretrauma level of health, to involve him or her in medical decision making, and to collect forensic evidence that will withstand judicial scrutiny. The SANE program includes treatment for STDs, pregnancy prevention, and psychologic counseling. The SANE clinician is able to provide witness testimony for victims who elect to report the case and to involve the judicial system. *Clinicians must be trained in the specific protocols of the SANE program for their state, because variations exist in legal standards among states.*

If the SANE program is not used, the rape treatment team should be trained in the proper collection of evidence, as required by their state laws, and they should be familiar with the standard rape kit. Despite variations across jurisdictions, some protocols are standard across settings, and these are discussed. Although mental health clinicians may not perform the medical and forensic examination, they must be familiar with the procedures to assist fearful patients and to provide correct information.

For the medically stable patient who is able to **consent** to and to cooperate with evidence collection and whose rape or sexual assault occurred within the past 3 to 5 days, the nurse or physician can begin the medical and forensic examinations. The accepted time interval between the rape or sexual assault and evidence collection is determined by the state's legal standards. If these time standards are exceeded, only the medical examination is performed.

The patient's **history** must be obtained by a member of the rape treatment team. When a native language problem is present, a hospital interpreter is required because using a family member or friend both is inappropriate and is in violation of state evidence collection rules. The history will become part of the patient's legal statement if she or he wishes to seek legal recourse, and it must include the patient's account of the rape or sexual assault. The location of the assault, the number of assailants, and, if possible, the identity of the assailant(s) must be obtained. The clinician must document the patient's account of the rape, including what orifices were penetrated and with what and whether the rape or assault involved force, threats, or weapons. In addition, the patient's general medical information, including medical illnesses; past or present psychiatric disorders; allergies; and current pregnancy status and date of last menstrual period, if applicable, should be obtained and documented. A family history of psychiatric disorders is important, because this may be predictive of mental health sequelae following rape. Describing the examination and ascertaining if the patient understands the examination procedures are important.

When the patient arrives immediately after the rape or sexual assault, all of his or her clothing is collected; however, only the undergarments are collected if the patient's clothing was changed before admission. Some patients wish to change their clothing immediately upon admission to the emergency room. This request should be accommodated while ensuring the proper collection of evidence. It is recommended that the patient undress over a paper covering to maximize the collection of evidence. Ideally, only the patient should touch his or her clothing to prevent the contamination of the evidence, but medical personnel wearing gloves can provide assistance.

1. **The physical and forensic examinations**. These examinations include a general medical evaluation with attention to signs of physical trauma and the collection of legal evidence. The medical and forensic examinations may trigger **reexperiencing** symptoms in some patients. Speaking in a supportive manner to the patient and holding her or his hand throughout may help the patient recognize that she or he is not still "back there," alone and helpless. Such interventions may assist patients in recognizing that they are now safe, are in the hospital, and are undergoing a physical examination.

   Overwhelming trauma, such as rape, may result in amnesia for important aspects of the trauma, and therefore the patient may not be able to identify accurately which orifices were penetrated. A complete medical and forensic examination must include oral, anal, and vaginal examinations for trauma and sperm and seminal fluid collection. Evidence is obtained from fingernail scrapings; swabs of areas containing blood, saliva, or seminal fluid; and hair and fibers from the victim's body or clothing. The pubic area is combed for the collection of loose hair, and specimens of the patient's head and pubic hair are obtained for forensic comparison.

2. **Laboratory analyses**. Laboratory evidence includes blood for DNA screening and a saliva sample to determine the patient's secretor status. A urine specimen for a drug analysis is obtained, especially if the patient is suspected to have been drugged by the assailant. Ascertaining the patient's current hepatitis B status is common, whereas collection of cultures for STDs are obtained only when they are clinically relevant or are required by institutional protocols.

3. **Prophylaxis for STDs**. Prophylactic medical treatment of STDs varies with the treatment center's protocol. Most programs will administer prophylactic antibiotics for chlamydia, gonorrhea, trichomonas, and syphilis. When the victim does not know his or her hepatitis B status, the first dose of the vaccine is recommended, and the patient is given instructions regarding follow-up doses in 1 month and 6 months.

Prophylactic emergency treatment for **HIV** infection is currently being implemented in most settings. These protocols are likely to change and to undergo refinement as more is learned about this disease. Rape characteristics that are considered high risk for HIV exposure are stranger rape, multiple assailants, and vaginal or anal penetration with tearing. When a patient consents to prophylactic medications, she or he must know that strict adherence to the medication regime is crucial. Because the prophylactic protocols may change over time based on our current knowledge, consultation by the rape treatment team with their infectious diseases expert is essential.

4. **Prophylaxis for pregnancy**. Because estimates of risk of pregnancy resulting from rape range from 1% to 10%, female patients of childbearing age may be offered medications for prophylaxis. However, determining the patient's pregnancy status before administering pregnancy prophylaxis is essential. The patient should be informed that this treatment is 75% effective and that, if she does not menstruate within 21 days, she should have a repeat pregnancy test.

5. **Psychologic reassessment and interventions**. Once these examinations are completed, the mental health clinician should reassess the patient's status and should provide interventions for any psychologic symptoms that might have developed during the examination. After the examination, the mental health clinician should assess the patient for the reactivation of anxiety, anger, or dissociation and should provide interventions to ensure psychologic safety. The patient's coping status and his or her plans for follow-up treatments for both medical and mental health should be reviewed.

III. **Acute Mental Health Treatment**

Few studies of acute treatment of psychologic distress after rape are available to guide interventions for victims of recent rapes. Many rape crisis centers provide acute interventions based on the debriefing models of Mitchell and Bray, which were developed for disaster interventions. However, the efficacy of such interventions for rape victims has not been established. *In the authors' clinical experience, rape-focused groups in which patients are asked to provide details of the rape incident and their responses are not indicated as an initial intervention.* Experience suggests that this approach tends to be overwhelming to patients and that it provides multiple triggers for the reexperiencing of the assault when no skills have evolved as yet to manage the sequelae of this. In addition, patients may come to "redefine" their rape experience as even more traumatizing when they learn of other, more frightening outcomes. The authors recommend an individual treatment that incorporates psychoeducation about the effects of trauma and rape, provides psychologic support, and assists the patient with processing the rape.

Some researchers have suggested that a brief prevention program consisting of exposure, relaxation training, and cognitive restructuring prevents the development of PTSD. However, subsequent work by these same authors found that this approach held no advantage over supportive counseling or routine assessment.

IV. **Treatments for Posttraumatic Stress Disorder After Rape**

According to recently published treatment guidelines for PTSD, both exposure-based therapies and pharmacotherapy are efficacious for the treatment of PTSD. **Cognitive-behavior therapy (CBT)** receives the highest endorsement. The more recently developed **eye movement desensitization and reprocessing**

(EMDR) approach is also identified as an option. Recommended medications are selective serotonin reuptake inhibitors, **venlafaxine**, and **nefazodone**. Group therapy and psychodynamic psychotherapy, although both are widely used to treat PTSD, have not been systematically or adequately studied. All therapies for PTSD aim to reduce the patient's anxieties and fears, to assist the patient with mastering and integrating the memories of the traumatic event, and to return the patient to psychologic health. The development of a good working relationship and therapeutic alliance is essential to effective treatment. Involvement of selected family members or partners either in family or couples therapy or in periodic involvement in the patient's individual therapy may be beneficial to both the patient and the family.

A. **Cognitive-Behavior Therapeutic Approaches**

Early behavior theories conceptualized PTSD as a conditioned fear response and adapted treatments known to be effective for other anxiety disorders. Imaginal exposure or "flooding" was introduced in the early 1980s for the treatment of male veterans suffering from PTSD. According to behavior theory, exposure to the feared memories as seen in imaginal exposure relieves symptoms through habituation or extinction; the patient becomes less fearful of reminders of the trauma. Another variant, **anxiety management training**, was also adapted for the treatment of PTSD. This approach assists in overcoming fears through the development of anxiety management skills. **Stress inoculation therapy** (SIT), was formulated specifically for rape victims. SIT provides education and coping skills, including relaxation skills, breathing control, role playing, cognitive restructuring, thought stopping, and guided self-dialogue. Studies of SIT in the treatment of rape have demonstrated significant reductions in PTSD symptoms.

Emotional processing theory attributes any fear reduction to the correction of stimulus–stimulus and stimulus–response associations and erroneous attributions. In exposure therapy, the patient's fear is activated while corrective material that is incompatible with the fear structure is presented. The patient learns that being reminded of the rape while in a safe setting is not dangerous and that he or she can discriminate between remembering and "being there." The patient learns that anxiety and fear can be reduced and that having anxiety or other PTSD symptoms does not result in a loss of control.

1. **CBT** for PTSD after rape, as developed by Foa et al., uses imaginal (prolonged) exposure (PE) in a safe therapeutic setting. The patient is instructed to go back to the time of the rape, to relive the rape in his or her imagination, and, with eyes closed, to describe the rape as if it were presently occurring. The session may be taped, and the patient is given homework to repeat the exposure between sessions. The goal is to diminish the patient's distress rapidly through repeated exposure until the patient is able to recall the rape without becoming symptomatic.

    A limited number of studies comparing PE and SIT have found that both are effective for treating PTSD after rape. Patients treated with PE continue to improve after treatment, yet SIT-treated patients show no additional gains. Studies of combined PE–SIT, SIT, and PE find that all three treatments produce significant improvement in both PTSD and depressive symptoms, although anxiety and overall social adjustment are most helped by PE.

2. **Cognitive processing therapy** was developed by Resick and Schnicke for the treatment of rape victims with PTSD. Cognitive processing therapy combines exposure therapy, anxiety management training, and cognitive restructuring. Patients are asked to describe the rape in writing and to read the account as the means of exposure. The cognitive component addresses faulty thinking patterns and focuses on the following five core themes for rape victims: safety, trust, power, esteem, and intimacy. In one recent study comparing cognitive processing therapy, PE, and a waiting list control group, cognitive processing therapy and PE were found to be equally effective in decreasing symptoms of PTSD.

B. Eye Movement Desensitization and Reprocessing

Eye movement desensitization and reprocessing (EMDR) is a treatment program developed by Shapiro for the treatment of PTSD. *EMDR is indicated only when no likelihood of legal testimony exists as testimony following EMDR may not be admissable in some jurisdictions.* EMDR includes exposure to memories and images of a traumatic event, an assessment of the psychologic distress and self-beliefs relating to these images or memories ("negative cognition"), identification of a competing cognitive appraisal ("positive cognition"), and examination of the physiologic reactions to the recalled memory or images ("body scan"). Exposure to the traumatic image, body sensations, and negative cognition during rapid lateral eye movements is thought to assist the patient with processing the traumatic event and with modifying both cognitive and emotional responses. Progress toward these goals is measured by a decreased level of distress and an increased acceptance of the positive cognition. Some evidence supports the efficacy of EMDR in the treatment of PTSD.

C. Psychodynamic Psychotherapy

This therapy conceptualizes PTSD as a failure of integration of the traumatic experience into the patient's overall meaning structure that results in the continued intrusions of thoughts and subsequent avoidance. The aims of psychodynamic treatment are to assist patients in reframing of their cognitive appraisal of the experience to reduce fears and feelings of helplessness and to facilitate and support emotional processing. This is expected to promote integration of the trauma into enduring schemas about self and others. To date, no well-designed studies of either group or individual psychodynamic psychotherapies have been reported for the treatment of PTSD or rape.

D. Psychopharmacology

Only a limited number of pharmacologic studies of rape victims having PTSD have been published, and no studies of combined cognitive-behavioral approaches and pharmacotherapy are seen in the literature. Early pharmacologic drug trials for PTSD focusing on the use of monoamine oxidase inhibitors or tricyclic antidepressants yielded mixed results. More recent studies have used the selective serotonin reuptake inhibitors because of their greater tolerability and improved safety margins, and a few have shown benefit (e.g., **citalopram**, **fluoxetine**, **fluvoxamine**, **paroxetine**, **sertraline**). One anecdotal study of **sertraline** (mean dose, 150 mg per day) in rape victims reported that four of five women with chronic PTSD had a greater than 30% reduction in PTSD symptoms after a 12-week trial. In another 12-week open trial in 17 patients (2 had been raped as adults and 7 had been sexually abused as children [the remainder were victims of nonsexual assault]) of **paroxetine** (mean dose, 42.5 mg per day), some improvement was noted for intrusive thoughts, avoidance behaviors, and hyperarousal, as well as in associated symptoms of anxiety, depression, and dissociation. Studies of both **sertraline** and **fluoxetine** in mixed community populations, including sexual assault victims and victims of childhood sexual abuse, found efficacy for the arousal and avoidance and/or numbing symptom clusters but reported no change for the reexperiencing symptoms. Several other medications, including **nefazodone**, **valproate**, **carbamazepine**, **lithium**, **propranolol**, **trazodone**, **venlafaxine**, **mirtazapine**, **clonidine**, **alprazolam**, and **clonazepam**, have been investigated in open-label, small-sample studies of chronic PTSD, although none of these has been specifically studied in a population of rape victims. Except for the two benzodiazepines, all these agents have shown improvement in at least one aspect of PTSD. Given the degree of comorbid substance abuse in patients with PTSD, any use of benzodiazepines beyond a brief exposure could become problematic. In addition, some of the subjective sleep disturbance experienced by sexual assault victims may be the result of sleep-related movement or breathing disorders, and benzodiazepine use is not likely to be optimal for these causes of disturbed sleep.

Limited and preliminary studies suggest that both β-adrenergic receptor antagonists (e.g., **propranolol**) and α_2-adrenergic receptor agonists (e.g., **clonidine**) may have some beneficial effects, particularly with the arousal and reexperiencing symptoms of PTSD. Based on the observations of Raskind et al., the editor of this text (R.I.S.) has observed in uncontrolled clinical use that the α_1-adrenergic receptor antagonist **prazosin** (1 to 3 mg per day) reduces hyperarousal and related nightmares, flashbacks, anxiety, and dissociative behaviors in a few women with childhood sexual abuse histories and current adult PTSD.

Unfortunately, no double-blind studies have been conducted of drug treatments in the immediate aftermath of trauma. For patients with persisting anxiety who are not responsive to acute psychologic interventions, judicious and temporary use of a benzodiazepine may calm the patient sufficiently to allow his or her engagement in psychologic interventions.

V. Special Populations
A. Children

Children who have been raped are rarely brought to medical attention, unless they have suffered injuries requiring medical treatment. The care of children who have been raped, sexually assaulted, or sexually abused includes the same treatment as that discussed for adult rape victims but it must also include additional knowledge of pediatric growth and psychosocial development.

Emergency interventions for the child rape victim are complicated because the adult who brings the child for treatment is sometimes the perpetrator or she or he may have complex issues regarding her or his relationship to the perpetrator. The perpetrator may in fact be a person respected by the family, as has been seen in the publicized cases of the rape of children by clergy, coaches, teachers, and other trusted members of the community. Pedophiles typically "groom" their victims, and they may devote much time and energy to developing a trusting relationship with the family, child, and community to increase access to a child or children.

When child sexual abuse or rape is suspected, it is essential that a clinician speak to the child without the accompanying adult(s) being present. Interviewing the child alone may provide an opportunity for the child to identify the perpetrator and may allow medical care providers to assure the child that appropriate protective steps will be taken. Furthermore, the presence of an accompanying adult may be distracting to the child, and it may limit the adult's ability to act as a witness in legal proceedings.

Mandatory reporting to child protection services may be required if the rape or assault was perpetrated by a person responsible for the child's care or one who is in a position of authority or who has a significant relationship with the child (e.g., relative or someone living in the home) or if parental neglect is suspected. Child protection and police notification requirements vary across jurisdictions. Clinicians must be aware of the reporting regulations for their state.

Recognizing that the parent(s) or guardian(s) of this child typically present with posttraumatic responses, exhibiting anger, anxiety, or dissociation as previously described, is important. Support and psychoeducation as outlined in the five-step approach are indicated to maximize the parents' or guardians' functioning and ability to help care for their traumatized child. Common themes include a sense of failure as a parent, a sense of betrayal if the perpetrator was a trusted individual, and fears about the effects of the rape or sexual assault on the physical and emotional well-being of the child. The parent or guardian may be able to provide information about the suspected perpetrator, and he or she can give information about how he or she learned of the abuse, rape, or sexual assault.

The **pediatric physical and forensic examinations** follow many of the protocols of the adult examination, including collection of evidence and screening and prevention of STDs, HIV, and pregnancy, but they must provide additional psychologic support. When possible, the child should be examined in a pediatric area or a quiet area of the hospital with toys or coloring materials available. The interview is critical for obtaining evidence about the rape, assault, or abuse, and it should take place as soon as possible to avoid suspicion that the statements were influenced by others. The clinician must be sensitive to the child's readiness and ability to talk, his or her emotional and physical needs, and the time of the last suspected incident. If the last incident of abuse or rape occurred within 72 hours, the physical and forensic examinations must be carried out.

The initial task of the interviewer is to provide a safe and trusting environment and to explain to the child the purpose of the interview. Beginning with neutral questions about school, friends, and favorite activities and then moving to inquiries about what happened is best. The child should tell of his or her experience, and he or she may use anatomical dolls or drawings; however, the use of anatomical dolls is controversial, and the admissibility of information generated by using anatomical dolls varies from state to state. Dolls and drawings are useful to help define the child's language for body parts and to give details of what happened. All drawings should be labeled, dated, and signed by the child and entered into the medical record.

Consent laws vary across states, with some allowing only a parent or guardian to authorize the examination, unless the parent or guardian is the suspected offender. Other states allow police, social services, or the court to authorize the examination, and, in some states adolescents are able to consent for themselves. In addition, the child must agree (i.e., give consent) to the examination.

The physical and forensic examination is similar to the adult examination, with some modifications. In prepubertal girls, a speculum examination is indicated only if vaginal injuries are present, and, if required, it may be done under general anesthesia. Specimens can be collected using a sterile cotton swab. STD testing is performed when the suspected offender is known to have an STD or is at high risk for an STD, when the child has signs and symptoms of an STD, or if the community has a high prevalence of STDs. Treatment for STDs is considered if the offender is known to have an STD, when the child at risk for STDs is not likely to come for follow-up visits, if the assault was a single episode by a stranger, or when multiple assailants were involved. The American Academy of Pediatrics recommends that adolescents should be offered prophylaxis for syphilis, gonorrhea, and chlamydia, as well as for pregnancy.

Disclosure of sexual abuse or assault by a child requires significant **psychologic support**. As in the adult patient, survival mode functioning may be present, and the child will need to move to a place of psychologic safety. The child may feel both relief and fear with the disclosure, as well as regarding the ensuing disruption of family or community that may follow depending on the role of the perpetrator. Shame, guilt, anger, confusion, fear, betrayal, isolation, sadness, and fear of abandonment are common emotions. As in the adult patient, the medical examination may induce flashbacks with which the child has few psychologic resources for coping. The mental health clinician's role is to support the child's coping, to provide protection, and to allow the child to discuss his or her fears and concerns.

The **developmental phase** of the child, which is not necessarily the same as his or her chronologic age, must be understood and should be incorporated into the treatment strategies. Children younger than 2 years of age typically react to trauma with clinging; crying; or aggressive behaviors, such as biting. The 2-year-old to 6-year-old child may reenact the trauma repeatedly, may develop separation anxiety, or may show regressive behaviors. Six-year-old to 10-year-old children often develop multiple somatic complaints, loss of appetite, and sleep disturbances, as well as regressed behaviors. The preteen to early teen may exhibit anger, mood swings, withdrawal from family and friends, somatic complaints, or denial or repetition of the trauma. Adolescents may become critical of parents and authority figures; may withdraw from others; may have sleep and appetite disturbance; or may turn to risk-taking behaviors, drugs, or alcohol. Children and adolescents may develop PTSD, depression, and suicidality after a rape or sexual assault. A national survey of adult women survivors of childhood rape identified a threat to life, physical injury, testifying about rape, and multiple rape types as predictors of PTSD after rape.

The family must be informed of the pattern of responses and of the need for early mental health treatment to assist their child with coping with the trauma of rape or sexual assault. Because the needs of families after disclosure of sexual abuse or assault are complex, all families, in addition to the child, must be referred for mental health assessment and treatment. Contacting the family a few days after the disclosure to offer support and additional resources and information is recommended.

Psychotherapeutic approaches to the traumatized child often combine CBT, psychodynamic, and family-based interventions; exposure is typically seen as a necessary component. Few controlled studies for the treatment of childhood PTSD and still fewer after rape or sexual assault have been conducted. In a study of 90 sexually abused children, CBT for the child and the child–parent dyad reduced PTSD symptoms, depression, and externalizing behaviors in the children and increased parenting skills, as compared with community care. CBT limited to the parents improved parenting skills, but it did not improve symptoms in the child. Another study of 32 mother–daughter pairs after sexual abuse of the daughter found that both CBT and supportive psychotherapy decreased the child's PTSD symptoms, as well as both internalizing and externalizing behaviors. The mothers in the CBT group showed decreases in self-blame and in expectations of negative impact on the child. EMDR has not been studied in children who have been raped or sexually assaulted; however, a controlled study of EMDR for the treatment of children with PTSD after natural disasters demonstrated significant improvement in PTSD symptoms, anxiety, and depression. No controlled studies of pharmacologic treatments of childhood PTSD have been conducted.

B. Disabled Persons

Few studies exist about rape of physically or mentally disabled persons, whether mentally retarded or psychotic persons. However, this population is an especially vulnerable group because the disabled person may be incapable of preventing rape or fearful of reporting a sexual assault, especially if the perpetrator is a caretaker. Mentally disabled persons have additional barriers in communicating about abuse because they may not be able to describe or articulate their experience. As is the case in the treatment of children, the patient may be accompanied by the perpetrator who will present the "history" of injuries or assault. Interviewing the disabled patient alone is essential to allow him or her to identify the perpetrator. In some states, the treatment team is mandated to report abuse of disabled persons if the perpetrator is a caretaker or family member.

The approach to the **medical and forensic examination** is modified to accommodate the patient's mental status and functional age. The cognitively impaired or psychotic patient may not comprehend the need for the medical or forensic examination and thus may require additional support and education from the mental health clinician. The rape treatment team must proceed only with the cooperation of the patient, and it should continue to assess the patient's understanding of the examination and should provide education as needed. Psychotherapy interventions for rape sequelae must take into account the patient's functional age and mental functioning.

C. The Elderly

The true incidence of rape in elderly women is unknown; however, in 1995, the United States Department of Justice estimated that rape occurred in only 4 of 10,000 women over age 65 years. It is likely that elderly women underreport rape because of shame and social fears. The elderly rape victim typically is a woman who lives alone and who is raped at home, although elderly women may also suffer rape from an acquaintance or caregiver. In addition to the psychologic distress that may result from rape at any age, rape in this age group may increase feelings of vulnerability for both the victim and her family regarding common life-span issues, such as independence versus dependence. The elderly rape victim and family may need assistance in determining if this patient could or should live independently.

D. Domestic Violence and Rape

Domestic violence includes not only physical violence but also partner rape. An estimated 33% to 46% of women who have been physically abused by a partner have also been raped or sexually assaulted by the partner. A community study found that nearly 24% of the rape cases were committed by husbands. A 1996 study of domestic violence in gay relationships reported that 39% of men have been raped by their partners.

Domestic violence continues to be underreported and underrecognized in emergency settings because of multiple barriers, including the failure to ask about domestic violence or partner rape, staff perceptions that they are too busy to address such complex social issues, staff frustrations that victims will return to the abusing partner, or concerns about invading family privacy. Women often do not report spousal or partner rape as unwanted or coerced sexual acts, and, in the context of marriage, such acts are rarely defined by women as rape. Women and men presenting with injuries or suspected domestic violence should also be asked about coerced sexual acts and partner rape. When the patient does not wish to acknowledge the domestic violence or to receive services, safety planning or information about shelters should be provided.

E. Male Rape

Both adult and child male victims of rape and sexual assault, including forced anal intercourse, forced fellatio, and forced ejaculation, are underidentified and are poorly served by the current systems of care. No estimates are available of the numbers of male rapes in the community. In prison populations, the estimate is that 0.5% to 3% of inmates are raped. Studies estimate that 6% to 10% of people being treated in rape crisis centers are male, although the fact that male victims rarely seek treatment is frequently noted. Barriers include social beliefs that a man should be able to defend himself; the victim's fears that his sexual orientation will be questioned; the male ethic that men are self-reliant; and significant shame, guilt, and humiliation.

The **emergency treatment** of male victims of rape may be complicated by injuries, because men are more likely to have suffered greater physical harm, to have had multiple assaults and assailants, to be held longer in captivity, to be attacked by strangers, and to have had weapons displayed or used. Themes common to men that may need to be addressed in emergency interventions include issues surrounding masculinity and perceptions that the victim is "weak," fears raised by him about his own sexual identity or orientation, or worries that others will now question his sexual orientation. Several studies noted that a common clinical presentation in male rape victims is that of anger and hostility, although the other survival responses of anxiety and dissociation may also present.

Long-term themes have been reported to include sexual dysfunction and sexual identity or orientation confusion that is most pronounced if the victim was forced to ejaculate. Male victims of anal penetration may not be aware that penile pressure on the prostate may cause involuntary erections and even orgasms. The victim who does not understand the physiologic nature of this response may feel shame and confusion about his response. Currently, no treatment outcome studies of male rape victims are available; however, the PTSD literature may be used as a guide while bearing in mind themes and misattributions common to male victims. Further study is essential to increase the knowledge of male rape, its consequences, and treatments.

F. Date and Acquaintance Rape

This applies when the perpetrator is someone known to or someone who is dating the rape victim. Victims of date rape rarely report the rape to the authorities, and they frequently attribute the rape to their own poor judgment.

Estimates from college samples range from 13% for date and acquaintance rape to 68% for coerced sexual activity by a date or acquaintance. Use of drugs and alcohol by the victim or the perpetrator is highly correlated with coerced sexual activity. As was previously noted, unwitting victims may be given a "date rape drug," such as **flunitrazepam** or **γ-hydroxybutyrate**, leaving them without any memory of being raped.

G. Gang Rape or Rape by Multiple Perpetrators

This is estimated to occur in up to 2% of college samples and 26% of police samples. Gang rapes, because they involve multiple assailants and sexual assaults, lead to prolonged assault duration and thus to an increased risk of injury, STDs, and PTSD. A community police sample found that the victims and offenders were more likely to be younger, that more attacks occurred at night and outdoors, and that victims offered less resistance when compared with single offender rapes.

H. Cultural Considerations

The meaning of rape and the patient's response will be highly determined by the patient's cultural group and religious beliefs. The mental health clinician must understand the role of culture in treating rape victims, as failure to understand the cultural meaning of rape will impair the patient's progress. In many cultures, rape is considered to bring shame upon the woman and her family; she will be mistreated, blamed, or excluded from social events (e.g., socially outcast) or considered unworthy of marriage. When the clinician is not aware of the patient's culture and the cultural beliefs, attempting to correct these "misattributions" with the family or patient may result in more distress for the patient and may further preclude access to treatment.

I. Refugees

The world is estimated to have over 23 million refugees, with most displaced due to war, ethnic cleansing, religious conflicts, or political persecution. Since the time of antiquity, rape has been a sanctioned activity of the conqueror. Organized rape and torture were prominent in conflicts such as in Bosnia and Kosovo. Thus, refugees from war-torn areas of the world may be suffering not only from the trauma of war, displacement from their home, and the loss of friends and family, but they may have also suffered rape at the hands of the enemy. Whereas the community rapist may act to demean the victim, the rapist in war or political conflicts may also be asserting the "right" of the victor to rape and pillage, signifying their dominance and the powerlessness of the vanquished. Treatment approaches must attend to the multiple trauma experiences, issues of acculturation, and cross-cultural considerations.

J. Perpetrators

Rapists are a heterogeneous group. For most rapists, issues of control and aggression predominate. In the United States, the estimate is that 15% of forcible rapes are perpetrated by males under the age of 18; many of these individuals have a personal history of trauma or neglect and a history of committing other antisocial acts. One study found that 42% had suffered physical abuse, 39% were sexually abused, 26% suffered childhood neglect, and 63% were witness to severe domestic violence. Most rapists have aggressive and antisocial traits, and they show little empathy for their victims. Others may be socially inhibited and shy. Both groups may have underlying feelings of inadequacy with a desire to degrade, humiliate, or injure their victims. Estimates of the frequency of paraphilia among rapists vary widely, beginning with conservative estimates of 5%. Paraphilic rapists compose a subgroup of rapists who obtain sexual pleasure through the domination of an unwilling victim.

VI. Useful Contacts

Two useful contacts are the National Sexual Violence Resource Center, which can be reached by telephone at 877-739-3895; by fax at 717-909-0714; and by e-mail at *resources@nsvrc.org,* and the National Health Resource Center on Domestic Violence, which can be reached by telephone at 888-792-2873, by fax at 415-252-8991, and by website at *http://endabuse.org/programs/display.php3?DocID=41.*

ACKNOWLEDGMENT

The authors are indebted to Drs. Carol C. Nadelson, Malkah T. Notman, and Johanna Perlmutter for their earlier version of this chapter, which appeared in the second edition of this text.

ADDITIONAL READING

Acierno R, Resnick HS, Kilpatrick DG, et al. Risk factors for rape, physical assault, and posttraumatic stress disorder in women: examination of differential multivariate relationships. *J Anxiety Dis* 1999;13:541–563.

Brener ND, McMahon PM, Warren CW, et al. Forced sexual intercourse and associated health-risk behaviors among female college students in the United States. *J Consult Clin Psychol* 1999;67:252–259.

Breslau N, Chilcoat HD, Kessler RC, et al. Vulnerability to assaultive violence: further specification of the sex difference in post-traumatic stress disorder. *Psychol Med* 1999;29:813–821.

Brewin CR, Andrews B, Valentine JD. Meta-analysis of risk factors for posttraumatic stress disorder in trauma-exposed adults. *J Consult Clin Psychol* 2000;68:748–766.

Campbell R, Sefl T, Barnes HE, et al. Community services for rape survivors: enhancing psychological well-being or increasing trauma? *J Consult Clin Psychol* 1999;67:847–858.

Celano M, Hazzard A, Webb C, et al. Treatment of traumogenic beliefs among sexually abused girls and their mothers: an evaluation study. *J Abnorm Child Psychol* 1996;24:1–17.

Chemtob CM, Nakashima J, Carlson JG. Brief treatment for elementary school children with disaster-related PTSD: a field study. *J Clin Psychol* 2002;58:99-112.

Chemtob CM, Roitblat H, Hamada R, et al. A cognitive action theory of posttraumatic stress disorder. *J Anxiety Dis* 1988;2:253–275.

Cloitre M, Tardiff K, Marzuk PM, et al. Childhood abuse and subsequent sexual assault among female inpatients. *J Traumatic Stress* 1996;9:473–482.

Deblinger E, McLeer SV, Henry D. Cognitive-behavioral treatment for sexually abused children suffering post-traumatic stress: preliminary findings. *J Am Acad Child Adolesc Psychiatry* 1990;29:747–752.

Epstein JN, Saunders BE, Kilpatrick DG. Predicting PTSD in women with a history of childhood rape. *J Traumatic Stress* 1997;10:573–587.

Foa EB, Dancu CV, Hembree EA, et al. A comparison of exposure therapy, stress inoculation training, and their combination for reducing posttraumatic stress disorder in female assault victims. *J Consult Clin Psychol* 1999;67:194–200.

Foa EB, Hearst-Ikeda D, Perry KJ. Evaluation of a brief cognitive-behavioral program for the prevention of chronic PTSD in recent assault victims. *J Consult Clin Psychol* 1995;6:948–955.

Foa EB, Keane TM, Friedman MJ, eds. *Effective treatments for PTSD: practice guidelines from the International Society for Traumatic Stress Studies.* New York: Guilford Press, 2000.

Foa EB, Rothbaum BO. *Treating the trauma of rape: cognitive-behavioral therapy for PTSD.* New York: Guilford Press, 1998.

Gelpin E, Bonne OB, Peri T, et al. Treatment of recent trauma survivors with benzodiazepines: a prospective study. *J Clin Psychiatry* 1996;57:390–394.

Gilligan J. *Violence: our national epidemic.* New York: Putnam, 1996.

Hanson RF, Resnick HS, Saunders BE, et al. Factors related to the reporting of childhood rape. *Child Abuse Neglect* 1999;23:559–569.

Herman JL. Complex PTSD: a syndrome in survivors of prolonged and repeated trauma. *J Traumatic Stress* 1992;5:377–391.

Holmes MM, Resnick HS, Kilpatrick DG, et al. Rape-related pregnancy: estimates and descriptive characteristics from a national sample of women. *Am J Obstet Gynecol* 1996;175:320–324.

James B. *Treating traumatized children: new insights and creative interventions.* New York: Lexington Books, 1989.

Jenkins MA, Langlais PJ, Belis DA, et al. Attentional dysfunction associated with posttraumatic stress disorder among rape survivors. *Clin Neurol* 2000;14:7–12.

Kessler RC, Sonnega A, Bromet E, et al. Posttraumatic stress disorder in the national comorbidity survey. *Arch Gen Psychiatry* 1995;52:1048–1060.

Kilpatrick DG, Best CL, Saunders BE, et al. Rape in marriage and in dating relationships: how bad is it for mental health? *Ann N Y Acad Sci* 1988;528:335–344.

Kilpatrick DG, Edmunds CN, Seymour AK. *Rape in America: a report to the nation.* Arlington, VA: National Victim Center, 1992.

Krakow B, Germain A, Tandberg D, et al. Sleep breathing and sleep movement disorders masquerading as insomnia in sexual assault survivors. *Compr Psychiatry* 2000;41:49–56.

Ledray LE. SANE development and operation guide. *J Emerg Nurs* 1998;24:197–198.

March JS, Amaya-Jackson L, Murray MC, et al. Cognitive-behavioral psychotherapy for children and adolescents with posttraumatic stress disorder after a single-incident stressor. *J Am Acad Child Adolesc Psychiatry* 1998;37:585–593.

Marshall RD, Schneier FR, Flaaon BA, et al. An open trial of paroxetine in patients with noncombat-related, chronic posttraumatic stress disorder. *J Clin Psychopharmacol* 1998;18:10–18.

McCauley J, Deern DE, Kolodner K, et al. Clinical characteristics of women with a history of childhood abuse: unhealed wounds. *JAMA* 1997;277:1362–1368.

Nishith P, Mechanic MB, Resick PA. Prior interpersonal trauma: the contribution to current PTSD symptoms in female rape victims. *J Abnorm Psychol* 2000;109:20–25.

Osterman JE, Chemtob CM. Emergency intervention for acute traumatic stress. *Psychiatr Serv* 1999;50:738–739.

Otto MW, Penava SJ, Pollock PA, et al. Cognitive-behavioral and pharmacologic perspectives on the treatment of post-traumatic stress. In: Pollack MH, Otto MW, Rosenbaum JF, eds. *Challenges in psychiatric treatment: pharmacologic and psychosocial perspectives.* New York: Guilford Press, 1995:219–260.

Pearlstein T. Antidepressant treatment of posttraumatic stress disorder. *J Clin Psychiatry* 2000;61:40–43.

Raskind MA, Dobie DJ, Kanter ED, et al. The α_1-adrenergic receptor antagonist prazosin ameliorates combat trauma nightmares in veterans with posttraumatic stress disorder: a report of 4 cases. *J Clin Psychiatry* 2000;61:129–133.

Rentoul L, Appleboom N. Understanding the psychological impact of rape and serious sexual assault of men: a literature review. *J Psychiatr Ment Health Nurs* 1997;4:267–274.

Resick PA. *Cognitive processing therapy for rape victims: a treatment manual.* Newbury Park, CA: Sage Publications, 1992.

Resnick HR, Kilpatrick DG, Dansky BS, et al. Prevalence of civilian trauma and posttraumatic stress disorder in a representative national sample of women. *J Consult Clin Psychol* 1993;61:984–991.

Rickert VI, Weiman CM. Date rape among adolescents and young adults. *J Pediatr Adolesc Gynecol* 1998;11:167–175.

Roth S, Newman E, Pelcoitz D, et al. Complex PTSD in victims exposed to sexual and physical abuse: results from the DSM-IV field trial for posttraumatic stress disorder. *J Traumatic Stress* 1997;10:539–555.

Rothbaum BO. A controlled study of eye movement desensitization and reprocessing in the treatment of posttraumatic stress disordered sexual assault victims. *Bull Menninger Clin* 1977;61:317–334.

Rothbaum BO, Foa EB, Riggs D, et al. A prospective examination of post-traumatic stress disorder in rape victims. *J Traumatic Stress* 1992;5:455–457.

Rothbaum BO, Ninan PT, Thomas L. Sertraline in the treatment of rape victims with posttraumatic stress disorder. *J Traumatic Stress* 1996;9:865–871.

SANE manual and operation guide. Commonwealth of Massachusetts Executive Office, Health and Human Services and Department of Public Health Committee of Family and Community Health. Available at: http://www.sane-sart.com/SaneGuide/toc.asp. Accessed December 18, 2003.

Shaprio F. *Eye movement desensitization and reprocessing.* New York: Guilford Press, 1995.

Stein MB, Walker JR, Forde DR. Gender differences in susceptibility to posttraumatic stress disorder. *Behav Res Ther* 2000;38:619–628.

Taylor F, Raskind MA. The α_1-adrenergic antagonist prazosin improves sleep and nightmares in civilian trauma posttraumatic stress disorder. *J Clin Psychopharmacol* 2002;22:82–85.

Ullman SE. A comparison of gang and individual rape incidents. *Violence Victims* 1999;14:123–133.

van der Kolk BA. Physical and sexual abuse of adults. In: Kaplan HL, Sadock BJ, eds. *Comprehensive textbook of psychiatry,* 7th ed. New York: Lippincott Williams & Wilkins, 2000:2002–2008.

van der Kolk BA, Dreyfuss D, Michaels M, et al. Fluoxetine in posttraumatic stress disorder. *J Clin Psychiatry* 1994;55:517–522.

van der Kolk BA, McFarlane AC, Weisaeth L, eds. *Traumatic stress: the effects of overwhelming experience on mind, body and society.* New York: Guilford Press, 1996.

Veronen LJ, Kilpatrick DG. Stress inoculation training for rape victims. In: Meichenbaum D, Jaremko ME, eds. *Stress reduction and prevention.* New York: Plenum Press, 1983:341–374.

Wilson AE, Calhoun KS, Bernat JA. Risk recognition and trauma-related symptoms among sexually revictimized women. *J Consult Clin Psychol* 1999;67:705–710.

Yehuda R. Post-traumatic stress disorder. *N Engl J Med* 2002;346:108–114.

28. UNDERSTANDING AND ASSESSING PAIN AND PAIN SYNDROMES

Wayne A. Ury
Richard I. Shader

Pain is one of the most common symptoms from which patients suffer and for which relief is sought. Unfortunately, surveys of patients seen in primary care practices suggest that pain is underrecognized and often is inadequately treated. Most pain syndromes (i.e., possibly as high as 90%) can be diagnosed on the basis of a history and physical examination alone, and, with standard therapies, most acute and chronic cancer pain can be meaningfully alleviated; estimates suggest relief is possible for greater than 90% of patients with cancer-related pain. Although chronic pain remains a more elusive entity, recent improvements in pain management have made these syndromes more treatable and have reduced the likelihood of unwanted consequences from treatment.

Uncontrolled pain is a major public health problem that is only now beginning to be addressed formally by the medical community. It precludes a satisfactory quality of life by markedly interfering with the individual's activities of daily living and social interaction and by its impact on mood and psychologic functioning (e.g., increased risk of anxiety, depression, suicidal ideation). Back pain is the second leading cause of lost work days in the United States, with a cost to the economy and to workers suffering from this chronic medical problem. Seventy-five percent of patients with cancer and 50% of patients with human immunodeficiency virus suffer from moderate to severe, daily, chronic pain for a significant period of their illness. This has tremendous psychologic, social, and financial implications for the patient and his or her family. *Pain is even prevalent among well-functioning ambulatory patients; it compromises function in about one-half of the patients who experience it.*

Adequate assessment is the crucial first step in defining a treatment strategy for the patient with pain. The major goal of an assessment strategy is to use the most appropriate diagnostic and therapeutic approaches to define the cause of the pain and to direct its treatment. Advances in the understanding of the pathophysiology of pain, coupled with the availability of validated pain measurement tools, facilitate such an assessment. Identification and categorization of a wide range of distinct yet characteristic pain syndromes provide the clinical basis for choosing specific therapeutic strategies.

Advances in knowledge about pain need more integration into daily clinical practice. More importantly, pain should be viewed as a common symptom that can be detected by screening high-risk populations, such as cancer, acquired immunodeficiency syndrome (AIDS), and diabetic patients. Because many illnesses are accompanied by at least some amount of pain, clinicians should also consider pain detection and relief as an integral part of every patient's treatment plan. In general, pain should be managed in parallel and in concert with treatments aimed at disease eradication or containment.

I. Epidemiology

Pain is a major part of most acute and chronic illnesses. For example, approximately 50% of AIDS patients suffer from daily pain that is moderate to severe in nature. Almost 30% of adult diabetic patients suffer from pain due to diabetic neuropathy, foot ulcers, or recurrent cellulitis. Regrettably, recent research has found that approximately 40% of conscious patients are in moderate to severe pain during the last 10 days of life and that greater than 60% of postoperative patients are in moderate to severe pain during the first 72 hours after surgery.

Currently, the most informative epidemiology of pain syndromes is found in the oncology literature. It illustrates how pain is an underrecognized and poorly treated component of medical illness, even though pain is commonly known to be of high prevalence and to be a cause of great suffering. Prevalence data indicate that, currently, about 17 million people are living with cancer worldwide.

Numerous studies have demonstrated that the prevalence of pain increases with the progression of disease and that the intensity, type, and location of pain varies according to the primary site of cancer, the extent of disease, the rate of progression, and the treatments used. In one American survey of 1,308 oncology outpatients, 67% reported recent pain and 36% reported pain severe enough to impair function. Another study reported pain in 63% of 246 randomly selected inpatients and outpatients undergoing active treatment for prostate, colon, breast, or ovarian cancers; pain intensity was rated moderate to severe by 43% of respondents. Surveys of patients admitted to palliative care or hospice services suggest that pain is inadequately relieved in one-half to 80% of patients at the time of intake. In a French survey, 69% of the cancer patients rated their worst pain to be at a level that impaired their ability to function. Although these reports highlight cancer pain as a major problem affecting quality of life, pain is still poorly addressed by most clinicians.

II. Definitions and Categories of the Types of Pain

The International Association for the Study of Pain defines pain as "an unpleasant sensory and emotional experience associated with actual or potential tissue damage or described in terms of such damage." Pain is always subjective; each patient's description of pain will be different. Moreover, no definitive way exists for distinguishing pain occurring in the absence of tissue damage from pain resulting from damaged tissue.

However, simple and practical tools (e.g., visual analog scales) provide a means by which the severity of pain can be serially assessed. The combination of objective and subjective data can be used by the clinician to make a presumptive diagnosis, to develop an initial treatment plan, and to assess the response to treatment. Evaluating and treating pain is a clinical skill that requires both clinical acumen and up-to-date factual knowledge. Most importantly, it relies on a trusting ongoing relationship between the patient and care provider.

The general focus of diagnosis should be to understand the pathophysiologic process that underlies the pain, to assess the quality of the pain (e.g., description, temporal nature), and to gauge the severity of the pain. Although assessing the underlying cause of the pain may be impossible and even though, in some cases, the etiology of the pain does not determine the treatment approach, more often than not, without an adequate investigation and understanding of the underlying pathophysiologic process, pain relief may be inadequate and unsustainable. A review of 100 consecutive cancer patients with pain found that 61% had undiagnosed etiologies that had important treatment implications. Therefore, providing **morphine** to a patient with severe pain before a thorough workup makes the achievement of long-term relief less likely.

A. Types of Pain

Numerous ways of categorizing the different types of pain exist. These categories have practical value because they capture the multidimensional aspects of pain. They also can be confusing because they overlap with each other, and their descriptors can have different meaning and treatment implications in different patients. In general, pain can be classified based on its temporal nature (acute vs. chronic), intensity (mild, moderate, or severe), or physiologic basis (inflammatory, neuropathic, traumatic, postsurgical, cancer pain). However, the patients' subjective descriptions of the pain and how it affects their emotional, social, physical, and occupational functioning can often be the most important factor in understanding it and in determining a treatment plan.

B. Temporal Pattern

Pain may be defined on a temporal basis. That cancer patients have both acute and chronic pain is well recognized. Most surgical pain is of an acute (and severe) nature. Most arthritic pain is chronic, although it may be severe.

1. **Acute pain**. Acute pain is characterized by a well-defined temporal pattern of pain onset that is generally associated with subjective and objective physical signs and hyperactivity of the autonomic nervous system. Acute pain is usually self-limited, and it responds to analgesic drug ther-

apy and treatment of its precipitating cause. For acute muscle pain, applications of heat or cold may be beneficial. Acute pain can be further subdivided into subacute and intermittent or episodic types. **Subacute** pain describes pain that comes on over several days, often with increasing intensity, and it represents a pattern of progressive pain symptomatology. **Episodic** pain refers to pain that occurs during confined periods of time on a regular or irregular basis.

2. **Chronic pain**. Chronic pain is defined as pain that persists for more than 2 months, often with a less well-defined temporal onset. Adaptation of the autonomic nervous system occurs, and patients with chronic pain usually lack the objective signs common to the patient with acute pain. Chronic pain is associated with significant changes in personality, lifestyle, and functional ability. Such patients require a management approach that encompasses not only the treatment of the cause of pain but also attention to the complications that may have ensued in their functional status, social lives, and personalities as a result.

3. **Breakthrough and baseline pain**. Baseline pain is defined as that pain reported by patients as the average pain intensity experienced for 12 hours or more during a 24-hour period. Breakthrough pain is characterized by a transient increase in pain to greater than moderate intensity that occurs on a baseline pain of moderate intensity or less. In a study of 70 adult cancer inpatients, 65% reported breakthrough pain. Most breakthrough pain is usually thought to be associated with a known malignant cause; in one study, however, only one-fifth of these reports was associated temporally with tumor therapy and 4% were unrelated to either the cancer or its treatment.

C. **Intensity of Pain**

Pain may also be defined on the basis of intensity, and an extensive literature on the use of words to describe pain intensity is found. However, limitations to a unidimensional concept of pain described solely in terms of pain intensity is recognized. Specific categorical scales of pain intensity, in which patients are asked to describe their pain as mild, moderate, severe, or excruciating, have been used.

Visual analog scales have also been used. Numerical scales that ask patients to rate their pain as a number between 1 ("no pain") and 10 ("worst possible pain") are often commonly used. These different scales to capture a patient's experience of pain have their limitations, but they are part of a series of validated instruments that include a measure of pain intensity as one of the components of the pain experience to be defined. In one French study of 605 patients across all institutions (cancer centers, university hospitals, state hospitals, private clinics, and one home care setting), patients consistently rated their pain as being more severe than their doctors did, indicating that French physicians underestimate the severity of their patients' cancer pain.

D. **Neurophysiologic Classification of Pain**

Neurophysiologic classifications of different forms of pain can be helpful in understanding the physiologic or neuroanatomic basis of pain and can therefore help in defining a well-targeted treatment plan. Unfortunately, these classifications can also be confusing, and they can actually result in a failure to consider the other aspects of pain assessment, such as pain severity. Therefore, although considering the pathophysiology of a patient's pain is always important, the temporal nature, the severity, and the patient's subjective description need to also be factored into the assessment.

Pain can be caused by injury to a tissue, a peripheral nerve or nerve root, or the central nervous system. The two major modulators of pain are inflammation and neuronal activity. Therefore, the presence (or absence) of inflammation and neuronal damage or activity need to be considered in every patient's assessment. Inflammation can occur as a result of trauma, surgery, autoimmune and rheumatologic disorders, space-occupying lesions, infection, and tissue damage or destruction (by tumors). Examples of neuronal activity and damage that can cause pain include neuropathies, thalamic stroke or injuries causing afferent neuronal activity, radiculopathies and root compression, and nerve roots that were cut during a surgical procedure.

1. **Inflammation-mediated pain.** When injury to a tissue or organ happens, an "inflammatory response" occurs to protect and to repair the injured site(s). This response is what causes the sensation of pain. Prostaglandins, interleukins, tissue necrosis factors, and other molecules are the modulators that are the chemical basis of this type of pain. Inflammatory pain is generally described as throbbing, pressure-like, and achy.

   Nonsteroidal antiinflammatory drugs (NSAIDs) and, to some degree, **acetaminophen** reduce these effects by inhibiting the release and activity of prostaglandins and other modulators. Therefore, in general, whenever evidence for tissue injury is found, these agents should be considered. When inflammatory pain becomes moderate or severe, short-acting opioids may be needed to decrease the perception of pain by affecting the neurons by which the pain sensation is transmitted from the peripheral tissue to the brain.

2. **Neuropathic pain.** This type of pain results from damage to a nerve root or peripheral nerve. It is commonly seen in patients with human immunodeficiency virus (human immunodeficiency virus neuropathy and iatrogenic neuropathies secondary to protease inhibitors), diabetes mellitus (diabetic neuropathy), and obesity (sciatica). It is described as a burning or electrical sensation, and it can coexist with a loss of sensation. Although the basis of this type of pain is poorly understood, tricyclic antidepressants (TCAs) (e.g., **amitriptyline**) and certain anticonvulsants (e.g., **carbamazepine, gabapentin, valproic acid**) are effective.

III. **Principles of Clinical Assessment**

As noted, most pain can be diagnosed by history and physical examination alone. However, if a diagnosis remains unclear, a pain relief workup to diagnose the etiology of the problem should be initiated immediately in parallel to the initiation of pain treatment. Certain general principles should be considered when evaluating all patients who complain of pain (Table 28.1). Lack of attention to these general principles is a major cause for misdiagnosis of the specific pain syndrome.

TABLE 28.1. PRINCIPLES OF PAIN ASSESSMENT

Believe the patient's assessment of pain.
Take a careful history of the pain complaint to place it temporally in the patient's medical history.
Assess the characteristics of each pain, including its site, its pattern of referral, its aggravating and relieving factors, and its impact on the activities of daily living and quality of life.
Clarify the temporal aspects of the pain as follows: acute, subacute, chronic, baseline, intermittent, breakthrough, or incident.
List and prioritize each pain complaint.
Evaluate the response to previous and current pain (analgesic) and other therapies (e.g., chemotherapy, antimicrobials).
Evaluate the psychologic state of the patient.
Ask if the patient has a past history of alcohol or drug dependence.
Perform a careful medical and neurologic examination.
Order and personally review the appropriate diagnostic procedures.
Treat the patient's pain to facilitate the necessary workup.
Design the diagnostic and therapeutic approach to suit the individual.
Provide continuity of care from evaluation to treatment to ensure patient compliance and to reduce patient anxiety.
Reassess the patient's response to pain therapy at regular intervals.

The most important guiding principle in pain assessment (and treatment) is to *always believe the patient.* Clinicians have been shown to have a tendency to minimize or dispute a patient's rating of pain severity. This can result in inadequate assessment and treatment.

That the clinician and patient design a diagnostic and therapeutic approach that suits the individual needs and style of each patient is also of great importance. The evaluation of the patient must also be closely allied to the patient's level of function, ability to participate in a diagnostic workup, and willingness to undergo the necessary diagnostic approaches; to objective evidence that treatment approaches may be beneficial; and to life expectancy. Careful judgment should be used in choosing the diagnostic approaches. Only those tests that will have a direct impact on the choice of the therapeutic strategy should be employed. The random use of diagnostic procedures in this group of patients is inappropriate, and it may have an adverse effect on the quality of life for such patients. Open discussion with the patient about the need for assessment and the therapeutic options is critical as this will provide the necessary dialogue that will allow the patient to be part of the decision-making process. In some patients, diagnostic procedures, such as myelography or magnetic resonance imaging, are inappropriate because they simply confirm the existence of disease for which no safe treatments are available.

A. **Role of the Patient's History in the Assessment of Pain**

Critical to the management of the patient with pain is the establishment of a trusting relationship with the physician. The complaint of pain is a symptom, not a diagnosis. Remembering that the diagnosis of the specific pain syndrome and a complete understanding of the psychologic state of the patient is not always made on the initial evaluation is important. In fact, several weeks may be required to define its nature because of the lack of radiologic or pathologic verification. Numerous examples point out the limitations of diagnostic procedures in providing "proof" of the validity of patients' complaints.

A comprehensive evaluation involves taking a careful history; performing a detailed medical, neurologic, and psychologic evaluation; developing a series of diagnosis-related hypotheses; and ordering the appropriate diagnostic studies. The history should include the patient's description of (a) the site of the pain, (b) the quality of the pain, (c) any exacerbating and relieving factors, (d) its temporal pattern, (e) its exact onset, (f) the associated symptoms and signs, (g) its interference with activities of daily living, (h) its impact on the patient's emotional state, and (i) any response(s) to previous and current analgesic therapies. Multiple pain complaints are common in patients with advanced disease. Prioritizing them before pain treatment is initiated is usually helpful.

B. **Evaluation of the Emotional State of the Patient**

Psychologic factors have been shown to play a significant role in accounting for the differences in pain experiences in patients with cancer and other serious illnesses. Therefore, classifying the patient's current level of anxiety and depression and learning whether episodes were experienced before pain onset are imperative. Information on how the patient handled previous episodes of pain may provide insight into whether a pattern of chronic illness behavior is present. Because patients have their own unique understanding of the meaning of pain to them, having each patient elaborate this meaning is useful. Always keeping in mind the idea that complaints of physical pain can often be a way of expressing emotional pain or conflict is important.

C. **Relationship Between Anxiety and Depressive Disorders and Pain Complaints**

Depression, anxiety, social isolation, and poor adherence to other prescribed therapies have all been shown to result from undiagnosed, untreated, or inadequately treated pain. Depression disorders occur in as many as 25% of cancer patients. Although the development of depression in cancer patients has been shown to be independent of the degree and/or severity of pain, other studies in cancer and noncancer populations have shown that depressed patients have a greater perception of pain, that they are more severely affected, and that they are less responsive to pain treatment. Treatment of depression (see Chapter 18) or anxiety (see Chapter 14) has been shown to reduce patients' perceptions of their pain and to improve their responsiveness to pain treatment.

Unrelieved or escalating pain can be a reason for suicide (see Chapter 17) and for requests for physician-assisted suicide in patients with debilitating chronic or terminal illness. Therefore, special attention should be given to complete pain relief and regular reassessment. The physician needs to be available and to respond rapidly to worsening pain. To assess patients' capabilities of asking for help when their pain worsens, asking them to define what they would do if the pain were to become intractable or intolerable and if they ever have suicidal thoughts or a pact with a family member is helpful.

D. Addictive Disorders and Pain

The potential for **alcohol** and drug abuse, especially in those patients with a previous history of addiction, to occur as a result of treatment is a common concern among clinicians. However, good evidence exists that shows that this concern is probably only warranted in those patients with a past or current history of drug or alcohol addiction.

Surveys of cancer patients show that most are fearful of becoming addicted and that they would actually prefer not to use opioids for pain relief. Studies of patient-controlled anesthesia have shown that, with the exception of patients with addiction, patients will tend to underuse their pain medication unless they are strongly encouraged by staff to use it. Even though a limited population for whom patient-controlled anesthesia opioid use may be problematic does exist, those jurisdictions (usually states) that permit it have special regulations to govern its use. Clinicians need to understand and to follow any regulations and policies governing the prescription of opioids and other pain remedies in their practice locale.

Patients with a history of addiction have an ethical right to pain relief and the same treatment options as nonaddicted patients. Unfortunately, as a result of the prevailing negative attitudes about drug addiction, patients with a history of premorbid addiction are at high risk for poor assessment and treatment of their pain. Their complaints are often ignored or discounted, and treatments that are necessary for relief, such as opioids, are avoided. In addition to being aware of this tendency among clinicians, the clinician must also realize that, if a patient with a history of addiction does not get adequate pain relief, he or she may turn to illicit drugs or **alcohol**. In patients who have a history of addiction or in situations where the clinician has a strong suspicion of active illicit drug use, a clinician (usually a psychiatrist) with expertise in addiction should be consulted. Making these patients aware of these concerns and perhaps requiring participation in a drug treatment program as a prerequisite for treatment with opioids is also important.

E. Stress-Aggravated Pain Syndromes

Several pain syndromes do exist in which depression, anxiety, and stress (see Chapters 14 and 18) clearly play a causal role in the development of symptoms and their severity. These include disorders or syndromes, such as fibromyalgia, irritable bowel disorder, and atypical chest pain. In addition, keeping in mind that chest pain, chronic abdominal pain, and headaches are classic ways in which depression and anxiety present themselves in the primary care setting is important. In fact, approximately 20% of patients with major depressive episodes have been shown to have chronic complaints of headaches. In those patients in whom pain is integral to their generalized anxiety disorder or major depressive episode, treatment of the primary psychiatric illness will usually result in a resolution of the pain complaints.

Although the pathophysiologic basis of these syndromes remains unclear, treatment of any underlying depression and anxiety with antidepressants or cognitive-behavior psychotherapy has been shown to be of benefit. TCAs, at dosages used to treat major depressive disorder, have been shown to be effective in decreasing the number and severity of pain complaints, in improving functional status, and in improving sleep. Although benzodiazepines can be of short-term benefit in relieving anxiety, increasing a patient's pain perception threshold, and decreasing back and muscle tension, they should be used for brief periods of time, preferably in conjunction with antidepressant treatment or psychotherapy.

F. **"Psychosomatic" Pain Syndromes**

In addition, some patients suffer from somatoform illnesses in which pain is either the primary or major complaint. These include somatoform disorder, which was formerly called psychogenic pain syndrome, hypochondriasis, and conversion disorders. Although an in-depth discussion of these syndromes is beyond the scope of this chapter, one guiding principle is clear—*these generally are diagnoses of exclusion.* Before they can be invoked as the cause of pain, the possibility of a medical or neurologic etiology, an addictive disorder, an affective disorder, or an anxiety disorder needs to be ruled out. Because differentiating these is quite complex, a psychiatrist with expertise in consultation liaison psychiatry should be consulted.

Interestingly, some data suggest that greater than 90% of patients with four or more pain complaints per visit with their primary care physician for which no medical or neurologic etiology can be found meet criteria for major depressive disorder or dysthymic disorder. Another finding is that, in greater than 90% of these patients, most or all of the pain complaints resolved with TCA treatment. Therefore, an empirical trial of a TCA, the class of antidepressants with the most support in the literature, or of another type of antidepressant at the standard dosages used to treat major depressive disorder should be considered.

G. **Physical and Neurologic Examinations**

These examinations usually provide the data necessary to corroborate the history. A thorough examination also allows the clinician to inspect the patient visually, to palpate the site of pain, and to look for the associated physical and neurologic signs that might help to define the nature of the pain complaint. A more definitive treatment approach can then be initiated.

Realizing that, even in some patients with severe pain, minimal or no physical or neurologic findings may be found during the initial examination is important. In these instances, treatment that provides pain relief should be instituted immediately; then a thorough diagnostic workup is initiated. Frequent reassessments may help in establishing the diagnosis, as well as the patient's response to treatment and the need for continued care.

H. **Diagnostic Studies in Pain Assessment**

Ordering and personally reviewing the appropriate diagnostic studies as soon as possible is important. Often, starting empirical treatment of the pain is also imperative so that short-term pain relief and a path to eradicating or altering the underlying cause of the pain can both occur as soon as possible. For example, if a patient with metastatic lung cancer complaining of severe leg pain and chest pain is admitted to the emergency room, while the clinician is trying to elucidate the cause(s) of this patient's pain, a high potency oral or intravenous (i.v.) opioid should be started. Treating the pain as soon as possible will also help to facilitate the appropriate workup because the patient will be more relaxed and will be more able to tolerate the necessary workups and procedures.

Although rapid relief of the pain should always be the first goal in caring for a patient in pain, of importance is not losing sight of the need to understand the etiology of the pain so that the underlying cause can be treated. A reasonable workup should be initiated the day the patient presents with a new pain complaint to confirm the clinical diagnosis and to define the site and extent of the underlying cause of the pain. As a general principle, one should consider an approach to a diagnostic workup for pain that uses imaging tests, nuclear medicine technologies, and laboratory studies. This comprehensive strategy may not always be helpful. Doing unnecessary tests is not only expensive, but this also can reinforce illness behaviors and patienthood in those with hypochondriasis. Only tests that have a direct bearing on the treatment plan should be ordered.

Providing specific guidelines for the diagnostic workup for each of the different types and locations of pain is beyond the scope of this chapter. However, using the patient with cancer and pain complaints as an archetype for considering the approach to deciding on a diagnostic workup for pain, in general, computed tomography and magnetic resonance imaging represent the most useful diagnostic procedures. Although plain radiographic films are useful screening procedures, they should not be used to overrule a clinical diagnosis if they are negative. Evaluation of the extent of metastatic disease may help to discern the relationship of the pain complaint to possible recurrent disease; for example, the postmastectomy pain syndrome that occurs secondary to the interruption of the intercostobrachial nerve is not causally associated with recurrent disease.

IV. Principles of Treatment

Probably the two most crucial tenets of treating pain are the following: **always believe that the patient's pain is real,** and **be optimistic that the pain can be alleviated** when it is appropriately treated. *The fact that the overwhelming majority of causes and presentations of pain are treatable is possibly one of the best kept secrets in clinical practice.* Not knowing this and accepting pain can be an insurmountable obstacle to good pain management; when clinicians do not believe they can treat a problem, they may set lower standards or not even try at all, especially if they harbor negative attitudes about the patient or the treatment. Unfortunately, this is most strikingly seen in patients with acute or chronic severe pain, many of whom suffer from cancer. They do not receive opioids when their use is indicated, because of their doctors' attitudes about pain, medicinal opioids as illicit drugs, or the patients who may need this care (e.g., patients with a history of addiction or psychiatric patients).

That patients not believe that their pain is their fault is important; no suggestion should be made that they should have sought treatment sooner or that they should have used more appropriate or effective treatments. For patients to try home or folk remedies, over-the-counter drugs, or herbal or other alternative remedies (e.g., acupuncture) before seeking traditional help is not uncommon. Additionally, clinicians need to prioritize for each patient the use of treatments to eliminate or to modify any underlying disease process, to reduce pain transmission, or to dampen pain awareness or receptivity.

A. Approaches to Management

When deciding how to treat a patient's pain, current symptomatology and any current and past medical conditions must be considered. The most important aspects of a patient's pain that determine the treatment approach are (a) its severity; (b) its underlying pathophysiology (i.e., inflammatory, neuropathic); (c) its temporal nature (acute versus chronic); (d) its effects on physical, psychologic, and occupational function; and (e) any physical examination findings. These factors need to be considered in the context of the underlying disease process that is causing or is associated with the pain (e.g., cancer, appendicitis) and the patient's current and past medical history (e.g., AIDS, systemic lupus erythematosus). The nature of the pain and the patient's medical history are only part of the equation; the clinician also needs to consider the patient's personality and style in approaching illness, his or her past experiences with pain, and the current emotional state.

Although addressing specific syndromes (e.g., fibromyalgia, AIDS neuropathy) is beyond the scope of this chapter, providing an overview of the approach to the patient in pain; how elements of the pain history, medical history, and psychologic factors are used in determining treatment; the core principles of the neuropharmacology of pain treatment; and how these can be realistically applied in the clinical setting is possible.

Pain Relief Ladder

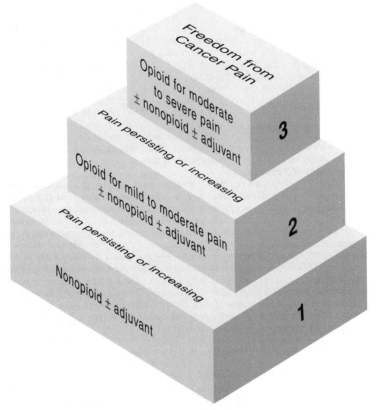

FIG. 28.1. The World Health Organization three-step cancer pain treatment ladder.

B. Determinants of Management

1. **Severity of pain**. In 1990, the World Health Organization adopted the concept of the step-wise ladder approach (Fig. 28.1) to rating pain severity and to providing treatments that would be appropriate to the patient's degree of pain. Based on an extensive body of research in pain assessment and care, the "ladder" was developed to provide objective assessment and standardized treatment approaches. The conferees also clearly opined that opioids are necessary for the treatment of severe pain; they also concurred that opioids are likely to be needed for treating "moderate" levels of pain in some patients. However, now a consensus is seen among pain experts that, independent of other medical or patient factors, for "mild" pain (based on visual analog scale self-assessment scores ranging from 0 to 3), an NSAID or **acetaminophen** (Table 28.2) is indicated. For "moderate" pain, a higher dose of an NSAID or a combination (Table 28.3) of an NSAID and an opioid—either a lower potency opioid (e.g., **codeine, oxycodone**) or a low dosage (but an equivalent amount of **morphine** equivalents; Table 28.4) of a higher potency opioid—is indicated. In terms of **morphine** equivalents, in a population of patients having severe pain,

TABLE 28.2. NONSTEROIDAL ANTIINFLAMMATORY DRUGS AND ACETAMINOPHEN ORAL DOSING FOR CHILDREN OR ADULTS WEIGHING MORE THAN 50 KILOGRAMS

NSAID	Oral dosing (mg)
Acetaminophen	500–650 q4h
	975 q6h
Aspirin	650 q4h
	975 q6h
Carprofen	100 t.i.d.
Diflunisal	500 q12h
Etodolac	200–400 q6–8h
Fenoprofen	300–800 q6h
Ibuprofen	400–600 q6h
Ketoprofen	25–60 q6–8h
Ketorolac tromethamine	10 q4–6h (max = 40/d)
	30 q6h (i.m.) (for no more than 5 d)
Meclofenamate	50–100 q6h
Mefenamic acid	250 q6h
Naproxen	250–275 q6–8h

Abbreviations: i.m., intramuscular; NSAID, NonSteroidal AntiInflammatory Drug; t.i.d., three times a day.

adequate relief will generally require more equivalents than should be needed for a patient with moderate pain. However, the clinician should remember that considerable individual variation is common. "Severe" pain deserves a higher potency opioid at a higher number of **morphine** equivalents than would be given for moderate levels of pain and, when the patient can tolerate it, an NSAID.

Almost contemporaneously with the publication of the World Health Organization ladder, the "additive effect" concept was introduced (i.e., combining an opioid and an NSAID when treating moderate to severe pain lowers the potential risk of side effects and toxicity from one or both

TABLE 28.3. SOME OPIOID AND NONOPIOID COMBINATION AGENTS

Opioid	Nonopioid(s)
Codeine	Acetaminophen
Dihydrocodeine	Acetaminophen, caffeine
Dihydrocodeine	Acetylsalicylic acid, caffeine
Hydrocodone	Acetaminophen
Hydrocodone	Ibuprofen
Oxycodone	Acetaminophen[a]
Oxycodone	Acetylsalicylic acid
Pentazocine	Acetaminophen[b]
Propoxyphene	Acetaminophen
Propoxyphene	Acetylsalicylic acid, caffeine
Tramadol	Acetaminophen

[a]Tylox contains sulfites; Percocet 2.5/325 does not.
[b]Talacen contains sulfites.

TABLE 28.4. APPROXIMATE EQUIPOTENT DOSING IN CHILDREN AND ADULTS WEIGHING MORE THAN 50 KILOGRAMS FOR SELECTED OPIOIDS

Agent	Oral Route	Parenteral Route (in mg)
Morphine	30 mg q3–4h (all day)	10 q3–4h
Morphine (controlled release)	90–120 mg q12h	—
Hydromorphone	7.5 mg q3–4h	1.5 q3–4h
Levorphanol	4 mg q6–8h	2 q6–8h
Meperidine	300 mg q2–3h	100 q2–3h
Methadone	20 mg q6–24h	10 q6–8h
Oxymorphone	—	1 q3–4h
Codeine (with acetaminophen)	180–200 mg q3–4h	130 q3–4h
Hydrocodone (with ibuprofen or acetaminophen)	30 mg q3–4h	—
Oxycodone (with aspirin or acetaminophen)	30 mg q3–4h	—

drugs). In general, the use of an opioid combined with an NSAID is accepted practice in the early phases of treatment of moderate to severe pain. However, an expanding literature on geriatric populations supports avoiding NSAIDs, with the exception of **acetaminophen**, when NSAIDs are needed (a) for chronic pain relief, regardless of the degree of pain; (b) in the treatment of acute pain when high doses would be needed; or, (c) when based on history, the patient is at high risk for renal failure or gastrointestinal (GI) bleeding. The most significant toxicities in both long-term and short-term use of NSAIDs in elderly patients are renal failure and GI hemorrhage. Whether cyclooxygenase-2 (COX-2) inhibitors significantly reduce the risk of GI bleeding in the elderly or in patients with a past history of GI hemorrhage is still unresolved.

2. **Pathophysiology of pain.** Understanding the underlying causes and the subjective nature of the pain are critical to developing an effective treatment plan. To try to understand what is causing the pain is always necessary; if the underlying etiology can be treated, the likelihood of a more complete and longer term relief is greater. Again, this involves a thorough history and physical examination and possibly imaging and laboratory studies. For patients in whom a space-occupying lesion, trauma causing tissue or nerve damage, an abscess, or nerve compression exists, surgery, a nerve block, or some other procedure (e.g., corticosteroids to reduce edema) is likely necessary to bring relief.

Until an appropriate procedure can be performed, medication should be used to provide temporary relief. One commonly held belief is that, when such procedures are needed, pain medication should not be given because medication may "mask" any pain signaling a worsening of the patient's condition (e.g., a ruptured appendix in a patient awaiting appendectomy). No objective literature exists supporting this belief. In fact, randomized double-blind trials have shown that patients with severe acute abdominal pain awaiting surgery and given i.v. **morphine** have better outcomes that those given a placebo.

In addition to understanding the pathophysiology or disease process that is causing the pain, determining if the pain is primarily related to inflammation, a problem in the peripheral or central nervous system, or some combination of the two is also necessary. In general, an inflammatory process calls for the use of an NSAID or a corticosteroid. Pain that is severe or that is related to a neuronal process requires an opioid. In situations in which pain is due to a neuropathic process (e.g., peripheral

neuropathies, reflex sympathetic dystrophy, nerve damage), certain TCAs or selected anticonvulsants (e.g., **gabapentin**) are likely to be beneficial.
3. **Temporal nature of pain**. Chronic pain requires a clearly delineated treatment plan that focuses on accurate diagnosis and goals of treatment. Although the same could be said about acute pain treatment, an approach that works to maximize physical; psychologic; social; and, if possible, occupational functioning and that respects the patient's views of treatment is most likely to be successful. Patients who suffer from chronic pain can benefit from the following:

- Consultation with a pain specialist to address diagnostic issues and therapeutic options (for some patients ongoing care with that specialist may be indicated);
- Psychologic care (e.g., antidepressants or anxiolytics for any depression or anxiety, individual psychotherapy addressing issues of chronic illness, support groups);
- Physical therapy to maximize physical functioning;
- Occupational therapy to address the activities of daily living and to overcome disability;
- The expertise of a palliative care team for terminal disease. In some patients, their ongoing and severe pain may require surgery or a nerve blockade to bring relief.

Unfortunately, the acute versus chronic dichotomization remains a source of controversy. Acute pain is seen by some clinicians as being deserving of more aggressive management, whereas chronic pain is often approached as untreatable and as related to emotional problems or "weakness." As has been noted, chronic pain is often comorbid with depression or anxiety, and, when chronic pain is effectively treated, depressive and anxiety symptoms improve. Although this is a correlational finding, many clinicians believe that such results indicate that some of the psychiatric symptoms are triggered by or are maintained by pain.

Concerns about the possibility of addiction with chronic opioid use have led some clinics to adopt an "opioid-free" policy; opioid-containing medications are not allowed. No clear evidence exists to support the idea that the length of opioid use leads to a higher risk of addiction. This view may be the result of confusion about the concepts of **tolerance, physical or physiologic dependence**, and **addiction** (see below).

Although some patients may require "maintenance" opioids and the dosages needed to relieve pain will likely increase over time, this is the result of a normal physiologic process (i.e., **tolerance**). This is important because only patients with a history of addiction appear to be at risk for addiction. For the patient at risk for addiction or for one who is currently using illicit drugs, an addiction treatment program should be a mandated part of the pain treatment plan when opioids are to be used. Opioids should never be excluded as a treatment option when they are likely to work. The physiologic and psychologic concepts related to opioid treatment and addiction are discussed below (see section IV.B.6). *Remember that the first goal, whether with acute or chronic pain treatment, is the alleviation of the patient's pain in as rapid a manner as possible.*
4. **Physical examination findings**. Unfortunately, physical examination findings are an unreliable indicator of the presence (or absence) of or the severity of pain. Patients can have acute severe pain or debilitating chronic pain with either no or minimal physical examination findings. This is best exemplified by ischemic bowel syndrome; in these patients, the pain complaints frequently are out of proportion to the physical examination findings. The presence of physical findings may help to guide treatment; in general, their absence should not. Clarifying and resolving a physical examination finding should not be a primary goal of treatment unless its treatment will promptly relieve the patient's pain.

5. **Physical and psychologic functioning**. Improving a patient's functioning should be at the core of any pain treatment plan. Determining the patient's current level of function and the appropriate goals of treatment is often a complex multidisciplinary task. Physicians; nurses; occupational and physical therapists; other allied health professionals; and, most importantly, patients and their families need to work together to develop a realistic treatment plan that considers the patients' views as central to any plan. This can be particularly important for certain cognitive tasks. When high opioid doses interfere with the performance or completion of these tasks, a patient may want to lower the dosage even when knowing greater pain is likely. Clinicians should facilitate this when requested to do so.

6. **Concerns About Dependence, Tolerance, and Addiction**. As a result of physiologic adaptation, **physical** or **physiologic dependence** often develops in patients who take opioids for greater than 2 to 4 weeks. If the opioid they are taking is not tapered when the time comes to discontinue it, a characteristic withdrawal syndrome may develop when the opioid is abruptly stopped; this is the **morphine or heroin** abstinence syndrome described in Chapter 10. As a result of increases and changes in affected opioid receptors, **tolerance** occurs, and, over time, increasing dosages of opioids are needed to maintain the same level of analgesia. Both dependence and tolerance are normal physiologic processes; neither *per se* is indicative of addiction. Opioid requirements are quite variable among individuals, and they are not directly related to a patient's weight, size, or age. Therefore, the rate at which physical dependence or tolerance develops is not predictable. Some patients may require increases in their total daily dosage that range from 5% to 25% every 2 to 14 days; others can remain on the same maintenance dosage for years.

By contrast, **addiction** is an abnormal pattern of behavior that is based on a belief that a drug will produce a desired euphoria or some other wanted physical or psychologic state. The addicted person believes that the drug is essential. Addicted individuals crave the drug, and they will use any means to obtain it, including endangering themselves and others. Continued use leads to social, psychologic, family, occupational, or physical problems. Interestingly, addiction can be present with or without the development of physical dependence, although, in general, increasing dosages are sought to achieve the initial euphoria.

As was noted above, only addiction-prone persons have a meaningful likelihood of becoming addicted to opioids that are taken therapeutically for pain relief. One prospective study followed approximately 14,000 patients who received opioids and found that, among patients with no prior history of addiction, the risk of addiction was 0.4% when opioids were taken for the relief of acute pain. Among those in remission from opioid addiction, about 30% relapsed (i.e., they returned to opioid misuse).

Patients sometimes develop tolerance to an opioid dose after as little as 5 to 7 days. After a short time, they may complain of inadequate pain relief, anxiety, irritability, or even withdrawal symptoms. They will request and sometimes demand that their dosage is increased or will come to the doctor's office saying they ran out of medication because they needed rescue doses or that they used a family member's pain medicine or alcohol for relief. When their pain is relieved, they do not seek the drug; they function normally and display no other signs of addiction. This pattern is called "pseudo-addiction." It is a recognized behavior pattern that understandably results from the development of tolerance.

C. **Specific Pharmacologic Treatments**

1. **Overview**. Understanding that the pathophysiology of the disease process is causing the patient's pain can be a key element to a successful pharmacologic treatment plan. A basic step is determining whether the pain is primarily inflammatory in origin, a problem in the periph-

eral or central nervous system, or some combination of these two. In general, an inflammatory process calls for the use of an NSAID. As was noted earlier, severe pain or pain related to a neuronal process usually requires an opioid.

To treat any pain-related process other than tissue damage or inflammation, neuronal activity needs to be modified. In most patients with severe pain and in a number of patients with moderate pain, an opioid or some combination of medicines (e.g., a benzodiazepine, an anticonvulsant) is needed to decrease the patient's level of pain perception adequately and, as a result, their experienced level of pain. These medications modulate the activity of μ opioid receptors and the release of endogenous opioids. Opioids, and to some extent dopamine, act in the cortex and on some subcortical structures to alter pain perception. In neuropathic pain (e.g., peripheral neuropathies, reflex sympathetic dystrophy, nerve damage), selected TCAs or anticonvulsants are indicated. Most treatment plans for moderate to severe pain involve the consideration of inflammatory and neuronal processes and therefore combination therapy.

2. **NSAIDs**. NSAIDs include selective COX-2 inhibitors (e.g., celecoxib, rofecoxib, valdecoxib), **acetaminophen**, and standard or traditional antiinflammatory agents (Table 28.2). These agents all provide pain relief through their actions on prostaglandins and other modulators of tissue inflammation. Because **acetaminophen**'s direct effect on prostaglandins is not typical of the other NSAIDs and its effects on inflammation is considerably lower, some clinicians consider it separately.

   a. **Indications**. In general, these drugs are indicated (a) for a mild to moderate level of acute or chronic pain (e.g., mild rheumatic or osteoarthritic pain, mild lower back pain) with use as a single agent, (b) in acute pain with a significant component of tissue inflammation (e.g., a sprained ankle that is swollen, tendinitis), (c) in combination with opioids for the treatment of moderate to severe acute or chronic pain (e.g., pain due to a lung tumor, a fractured ankle), or (d) for antipyretic activity (e.g., fever from infection or tumor).

      Although NSAIDs are generally similar in their effectiveness, differences that may play a significant role in choosing among them do exist. In commonly prescribed dosages, **acetaminophen** is slightly less effective as an antipyretic and in reducing direct tissue inflammation, yet it has considerably less GI and renal toxicity. Other NSAIDs and selective COX-2 inhibitors are essentially identical in short-term and longer term treatment efficacy, but, in patients who require these drugs chronically, the selective COX-2 inhibitors may have a lower risk for gastritis or GI hemorrhage. Despite some remaining degree of controversy over the costs and benefits, selective COX-2 inhibitors are in greater demand than ever. This may be partly because "new" interventions are sometimes helpful in patients with chronic pain. Because the risk of GI hemorrhage is low when the exposure to NSAIDs is short-term, the additional costs of selective COX-2 inhibitors may not be justified for acute pain treatment.

   b. **Acetaminophen**. Acetaminophen has been studied in both acute and chronic pain treatment and in many different patient populations. It is effective as a first-line agent for mild to moderate acute and chronic pain and as a second drug for use in combination with an opioid for moderate to severe pain. In both acute and chronic use, it carries a significantly lower risk of GI hemorrhage, other bleeding problems, or renal insufficiency and renal failure compared with standard NSAIDs. As such, it should probably be tried first. In addition, unlike standard NSAIDs, it is not an established cause of hypertension, urticaria, GI reflux, or gastritis.

      (1) **Metabolism. Acetaminophen** is primarily metabolized by the liver. It should be prescribed at lower dosages or avoided alto-

gether in patients with significant liver disease or in those with lower **glutathione** stores available for phase 2 conjugation (e.g., diabetes mellitus, significant **alcohol** consumption). Because some elderly persons may have reduced hepatic oxidative or conjugative capacities, initial dosing with two-thirds of the standard adult dosage should be considered. Although **acetaminophen** is a useful alternative to NSAIDs in patients who have impaired creatinine clearance or renal function, NSAIDs are not necessarily an alternative to acetaminophen in patients with impaired liver function because of the potential risk of bleeding (decreased hepatic production of clotting factor).

   (2) Contraindications. In a patient with adequate liver function, **acetaminophen** is a safe and effective treatment. However, when used in excessively high doses or in the setting of heavy **alcohol** use, even for short "binge" periods, it can result in irreversible liver failure and death. If either of these situations is suspected, the patient should be brought to an emergency room immediately. After an overdose of 15 pills, if a patient is not given *N*-acetly cysteine within approximately 4 hours, a significant number of patients will develop irreversible hepatic damage and perhaps failure. Liver transplantation may be necessary (see Chapter 3).

 c. Standard NSAIDs and selective COX-2 inhibitors. These are quite comparable in efficacy. They are both effective for inflammation, the relief of mild to moderate pain, and the potentiation of the actions of an opioid in moderate to severe pain. However, these agents generally have a higher percentage of patients who will develop some or serious side effects. As was noted, in patients who require these drugs chronically and in those who are at high risk of GI bleeding, the selective COX-2 inhibitors have a slightly lower risk of GI discomfort, gastritis, or hemorrhage. If they carry less risk of GI hemorrhage with short-term use in those who are not at high risk for GI hemorrhage (e.g., no concomitant use of high-dose corticosteroids) is not clear.

   Both classes of NSAIDs carry a significantly greater number of side effects and toxicity than does **acetaminophen**. The major side effects of NSAIDs and COX-2 inhibitors are GI hemorrhage, other bleeding problems, gastritis or gastroesophageal reflux disease (GERD), urticaria, hypertension, and renal insufficiency and renal failure. As a result, in cases of both acute and chronic pain, **acetaminophen** should be tried first. However, for the development of sudden inflammation (e.g., a twisted ankle) or as an antipyretic (e.g., for higher fevers, tumor-related fever), these drugs are superior to **acetaminophen**.

   (1) Metabolism. NSAIDs and COX-2 inhibitors rely on both hepatic and renal metabolism. The hepatic cytochromes (see Chapter 29) that metabolize these drugs can easily be affected by interactions with other drug classes, thus resulting in either a longer or shorter duration of action. Because some elderly persons may have reduced hepatic oxidative or conjugative capacities, initial dosing with two-thirds of the standard adult dosage should be considered. **Acetaminophen** is a useful alternative in patients who have impaired creatinine clearance or renal function.

   (2) Contraindications. This class of medications should, in general, be avoided in patients with significant active hepatic or renal disease, but each case needs to be carefully evaluated. In patients who have a history of recurrent GI hemorrhage or other bleeding problems, NSAIDs and COX-2 inhibitors should be stopped, if at all possible, and chronic opioid and other alternatives for pain relief should be considered in consultation with a pain specialist.

 3. Opioids. Opioids are the current mainstay of severe pain management, and they are needed in certain cases of moderate level pain. Unfortunately, as a result of a variety of misconceptions about their medicinal use, they are underused or are used ineffectively. This is unfortunate because opioids are effective and they have a wide therapeutic index. When they are used appropriately and side effects are anticipated and treated, most patients with moderate to severe acute pain obtain relief from these medications.

    a. Mechanism of action. Systemically administered opioids act in a variety of ways by binding to central opioid receptors[1]. A decrease in the level of pain perception occurs; this is a central action—the pain perception threshold is raised to a higher level. Independent of their direct effect on pain perception, opioids also decrease anxiety and reduce the sympathetic outflow that some patients experience with severe pain. Like endogenous opioids, some opioids produce a sense of euphoria that may counteract some of the depressive effects of pain. This euphoria is sustained for only a few days after the initiation of treatment; opioids are not a useful treatment for depressive symptoms, even in patients suffering from chronic pain.

    b. Indications. Opioids are the principal treatment for severe pain; they may also be needed for certain patients with moderate levels of pain. Although they are generally used in combination with an NSAID, opioids may be used alone when NSAID use poses a significant risk of side effects. They are also indicated for use in chronic pain when the long-term use of an NSAID for mild to moderate pain would pose a significant risk of GI bleeding, hypertension, or renal failure. In 2000, the American Geriatrics Society recommended that elderly patients who require long-term pain medication should be given an opioid, rather than an NSAID, to reduce the likelihood of these complications. The American Geriatrics Society recommendation is recent, and opioid use in chronic pain management remains a controversial area.

    c. Metabolism. Opioids rely on hepatic and renal clearance for their metabolism and elimination. Because any central nervous system active drug's effect is also determined by receptor activity in the central nervous system, the brain also plays an important role, especially in the length of the intended effect of the drug and in central nervous system-related side effects (e.g., sedation, nausea, myoclonus). Patients with impaired cognition, dementia, and delirium are at the greatest risk of central nervous system-related side effects. Patients with impaired renal function are at the greatest risk for myoclonus. In both groups, the patient's starting dosage should be approximately two-thirds of that of other adult patients. These patients should also be frequently assessed for side effects.

    d. How to prescribe opioids. Opioids are prescribed based on a set of pharmacologic equivalents that uses **morphine sulfate** as its standard, the half-life of the particular agent, and the route of administration. As a general rule, opioids should be administered by an oral or i.v. route, because intramuscular and subcutaneous administration are painful and their absorption is variable. Intravenous routes have a more rapid onset and shorter duration of action. Therefore, for patients with acute severe pain or for patients who develop breakthrough pain, an i.v. route is preferable. Because no "first-pass" effect is seen in patients who receive opioids parenterally, the same quantity will be more potent when given as a parenteral dose than is an oral dose of the same drug. In general, the parenteral dose of an opioid is one-third of the oral dose.

---

[1]Although the actions of opioids are mainly central, some peripheral action may also occur, as is well demonstrated by the fact that, when administered locally (i.e., into a knee joint), binding to putative μ opioid receptors in the periphery produces pain relief.

For the treatment of acute pain, 10 mg of **morphine** i.v. every 4 hours (or its equivalent) is recommended as a starting dose. The patient should then be reassessed in approximately 30 minutes and should be given additional medication based on the reduction of the patient's objective pain rating, with zero pain as the goal of treatment. Each additional administration should be given as a "rescue dose" every 2 hours i.v. until pain relief is achieved. The total dosage required over the first 24-hour period should then be tallied and divided into a standing dosage regimen. Even after the first 24 hours (and throughout the treatment course for patients with serious progressive or chronic illness), rescue medication should be available, and its use should then be added to the standing 24-hour dosage.

Once pain relief has been achieved, the patient's medication should be adjusted to the most convenient dosing regimen for that individual whenever possible. In general, this means long-acting oral forms of opioids (e.g., MS Contin or Avinza[2], **methadone**, Oxy Contin, **fentanyl**). The **fentanyl** subcutaneous patch or the "lollypop," which is absorbed through the buccal mucosa, provides an alternative to oral medication for those who cannot swallow oral medication. Likewise, liquid **morphine** (e.g., Roxinol) can be given to those who cannot swallow pills.

All patients who are started on an opioid and who have a functional GI tract should be started on a bowel regimen (e.g., motility agents and increased dietary fiber[3]) to prevent constipation. In addition, they should be advised to increase their intake of fluids. Because constipation will occur throughout the use of an opioid, this medication should be continued until the opioid is stopped.

  e. **Hydroxyzine.** Some clinicians prescribe oral **hydroxyzine** (500 to 1,000 mg) to potentiate the analgesic effects of **morphine sulfate** and to reduce any **morphine**-induced urticaria.

  f. **Physiologic dependence and tolerance** (also see section IV.B.6). Patients who take opioids for greater than 2 to 4 weeks will probably develop physiologic dependence, meaning that withdrawal symptoms and signs will develop if their opioid is suddenly stopped. Tolerance occurs when, as a result of the up-regulation of opioid receptors, increasing dosages of opioids are needed to achieve or to maintain the same intended effect. Both are normal physiologic processes, and neither is indicative of addiction.

  As noted earlier, patients may develop tolerance after only 5 to 7 days at a certain dosage level. Opioid requirements are quite variable among individuals, and they are not clearly related to a patient's weight, size, or age. The rate at which physiologic dependence or tolerance develops is not predictable. Some patients may require increases in their total daily dosage ranging from 5% to 25% every 2 to 14 days, whereas others can remain on the same maintenance dosage for years. No therapeutic ceiling exists for opioids[4]; daily dosages of as high as 35,000 mg have been reported.

  g. **Side effects and their treatment**
     (1) **Respiratory depression** results from the effects of opioids on the medullary respiratory center. Aside from addiction, this is

---

[2]Avinza is a once-daily extended-release capsule formulation of morphine sulfate (30, 60, 90, 120 mg). Opening these capsules and sprinkling the combination of immediate-release and extended-release components onto soft foods (e.g., applesauce) is possible. ***Of importance is noting the fact that this formulation contains fumaric acid, which may cause renal toxicity, especially when dosing exceeds 1,600 mg per day.***

[3]Generally well-tolerated sources of fiber include fruit juices (with pulp), raw fruits (with skins and seeds), raw vegetables, whole-grain cereals and breads, canned prunes or apricots, nuts, and dried figs and dates. Gas-producing foods should be avoided (e.g., beans, cabbage), even though they may be high in fiber.

[4]Because of its fumaric acid ingredient, the Avinza formulation of morphine sulfate has a maximum dose of 1,600 mg per day.

probably the most feared side effect among many clinicians. Clinical experience suggests that this fear is unfounded; respiratory depression is an extremely rare occurrence (less than 0.025% of patients), and fear of it probably results in the undermedicating of many patients with acute pain.

Defined as a respiratory rate of less than 8 breaths per minute, this side effect appears to be limited to opioid-naive patients who have significant lung or central nervous system disease and then only during the first dosage. After a patient has received one dose with no significant decrease in respiratory rate or two doses when the respiratory rate is 12 or greater, no risk of future occurrence is present. Confusion about this danger probably occurs because of the potentially fatal accidental respiratory depression that happens in tolerant heroin addicts who mistakenly use an extremely high dose of concentrated heroin.

Naloxone, a short-acting opioid antagonist, should only be used when the respiratory rate goes below 6 per minute, when it becomes irregular or agonal, when an overdose is suspected, or when the respiratory depression is accompanied by oversedation or unresponsiveness. This is because the use of **naloxone** can precipitate severe withdrawal symptoms and the worsening of pain control. In most patients, if one dose of the medication is withheld and then the dosage of opioid is decreased, the episode will resolve and will not recur. In situations where respiratory depression has been documented, the dosage should be increased more slowly than it would normally be.

(2) **Constipation** is the most common opioid side effect (greater than 40%); it can occur at any point in treatment, and it is independent of the route of administration. Constipation results from the actions of opioids at μ receptors in the gut. It is best prevented by recommending the following when opioid use is initiated: starting a motility agent; advising an increase in the daily intake of fluids by 25%, unless contraindications to doing so are present; and increasing fiber intake.

Clinicians should inquire about constipation at each visit. When patients report constipation, they should be advised to increase physical activity and fluid intake and to start using a daily stool softener (e.g., **docusate sodium**), and they should have the dose of their motility agent increased by 50% or should start a stronger one (e.g., **magnesium citrate**, **lactulose**). Constipation *per se* should not be a reason for decreasing the dosage of the opioid or for the use of **naloxone**. Rather, it calls for more aggressive management of the constipation while still providing adequate analgesia.

(3) **Nausea** occurs in 5% to 10% of patients during the first 24 to 96 hours of treatment, independent of any that is related to constipation. It is generally self-limited, and it can usually be treated with supportive treatment (e.g., hydration, light diet). When medication is necessary, the short-term use of **haloperidol**, 1 mg twice daily, or **lorazepam**, 0.5 mg twice daily, is usually effective.

(4) **Myoclonus** is a syndrome of uncontrollable sustained clonic jerking movements throughout the extremities and facial muscles that occurs as the result of an excess of the opioid metabolite 6-mercaptopurine. Myoclonus is quite rare, and it usually occurs in patients who are seriously ill or who have impaired renal function. Treatment involves lowering the dose of opioid or widening the time interval between doses, i.v. hydration, or, when needed, low doses of benzodiazepines. When myoclonus occurs, consultation with a pain specialist is recommended.

(5) **Sedation** can occur when an opioid is first started, when rapid dosage escalations are made, when hepatic or renal metabolism is impaired, or when the patient becomes more ill. The most common occurrence of sedation is seen during the first 72 hours; it is usually self-limited. When sedation extends beyond this initial period, discussions between clinician and patient should take place regarding the benefits of pain relief and balancing them with the side effect of sedation to find an approach consistent with the patient's life-style. The elderly are at greater risk for excess sedation, and their dosage increments should be slower, if possible, than those seen with younger adults.

When pain persists and it is severe, extremely high doses of opioids are sometimes needed for relief. In some cases, the required high doses may cause stupor or unconsciousness as a side effect ("double effect"). In patients for whom the intended goal of treatment is pain relief, rather than sedation, hastened death, or euthanasia, the ethical principle of double effect provides for continuing this dosage, but only with the patient's or surrogate's consent.

h. **Pain treatment in patients with addiction and those at risk for relapse**. As was noted above, opioids are frequently underused or are ineffectively used because of a variety of misconceptions about their medicinal use. Probably the biggest roadblock to their use is a concern about causing addiction. This largely results from the negative attitudes of many people in society toward addicts, in which medicinal opioid use is incorrectly equated with illicit narcotic use. Because of this, fears of triggering addiction during medicinal use, even in those with no prior history of addiction or misuse of drugs, abound. These fears need to be overcome by more education and training in medical school and residency and by further research that addresses these obstacles. Unfortunately, the recent upsurge in the illicit use and theft of the long-acting oral opioid Oxy Contin has increased the public's negative attitudes toward more liberal availability of medicinal opioids.

Tolerance *per se* occurs when, as a result of the up-regulation of opioid receptors, increasing dosages of opioids are needed over time to achieve the same intended effect. Both are normal physiologic processes, and neither is indicative of addiction. As opposed to those with tolerance, addicts seek greater dosages to achieve a greater sense of euphoria or "high." Patients who are drug seeking will often go to several different providers so they can obtain an ample supply, will lie about lost prescriptions, and will often return for refills before the expected date.

(1) **Distinguishing addiction from tolerance**. Some patients are quite demanding and irritable when they need medication to avoid the symptoms of withdrawal or because they are in greater pain as a result of the development of tolerance. However, once they receive the proper dosage of opioid to relieve their pain, these behaviors resolve. Patients who are not suffering from addiction will also not crave the drug nor exhibit dangerous behaviors to obtain it. In addition, no evidence of impairment is observed in social, psychologic, family, occupational, or physical functioning as a result of its use.

In an interesting set of studies looking at whether patients would try to give themselves extra doses of morphine when patient-controlled anesthesia is used for severe pain relief, no patients (i.e., those with no prior history of addiction or without traits associated with addiction) had any pattern of extra use nor did they exhibit any drug-seeking behavior. Although this research is limited, it seems to support the view that the risk of unanticipated addiction is quite low and that it should not cause a clinician to avoid its use in patients who lack a prior history of addiction.

(2) **Treatment approach for patients with a history of addiction and those at risk of relapse**. Patients with a history of addiction or who are currently using illicit drugs or alcohol deserve the same right to pain relief as those who are not suffering from addiction. They also need to be involved in a treatment program to manage their addiction or prevent a relapse. Making treatment of the addiction a condition for prescribing opioids to such persons is reasonable; however, withholding opioids because of the clinician's concerns about addiction is not reasonable when they are needed.

The dangers of escalating illicit drug use and relapse are quite real. As was noted previously, some studies have shown relapse rates of about 30% in at-risk persons, whereas other studies have found that 10% to 20% of patients using heroin before pain treatment increased their use of heroin shortly after starting pain treatment.

A workable approach to the treatment of addiction is referral to a drug and alcohol treatment program that allows its clients to take pain medication. This may actually be quite problematic because many programs do now allow continued use, and many local alcoholics and narcotics anonymous groups are adamantly opposed to members using medicinal opioids or psychotropic medication. Even with a successful referral, regular contact between the clinician managing the pain and the addiction treatment program is of importance.

4. **Selected anticonvulsants and TCAs**. Further discussion of the use of these agents is beyond the scope of this chapter, which is focused on the generalist clinician. Discussion with a pain specialist or clinic should be considered for more information about the longer term use of these agents.

D. **Nonpharmacologic Treatments for Chronic Pain**
Although no single approach to the nonpharmacologic treatment of chronic pain has received universal acceptance, some general principles and approaches appear central to those that enjoy some degree of acceptance, especially in multidisciplinary pain clinic settings. Most clinicians agree that nonpharmacologic treatments do not work when the pain intensity is already quite high. Among the approaches that may be considered as an adjunct to medication for moderate to severe pain are biofeedback (using electromyography or digital skin temperature); hypnosis (see Chapter 23); acupuncture, which is thought by many to work through release of endogenous opioids; diversionary activities or distraction; improved physical conditioning and exercise; meditation; and relaxation techniques (see Chapter 14). These and other techniques alone or in combination with medication can be part of effective self-management strategies.

V. **Barriers to Pain Assessment and Adequate Pain Management**
Lack of knowledge about pain assessment methodology is one of the common barriers associated with inadequate pain treatment. Physicians, patients, and the public, through a series of well-validated surveys, have defined the numerous barriers that interfere with adequate cancer pain management. These barriers have been categorized broadly as patient related, physician related, and institution related.

The **patient-related barriers** include (a) a reluctance to report pain, (b) a reluctance to follow treatment recommendations, (c) fears of tolerance and addiction, (d) concerns about side effects, (e) beliefs that pain is an inevitable consequence and that it must be accepted, (f) fears of disease progression, (g) fears of injections, and (h) culture-specific ideas about the causes and meanings of pain.

Closely allied to these patient-related obstacles are **physician-related barriers**. One study reported that when patients rated their pain as moderate to severe, oncology fellows failed to appreciate the severity of the problem in 73% of their patients. In two studies, the discrepancy between patient and physician evaluation of the severity of the problem was a major predictor of inadequate relief. Knowledge deficits in cancer pain assessment and treatment are the norm more than the exception. Several studies have revealed an extremely low correlation between self-evaluation of clinical skills in pain therapy and the correct responses to clinical vignettes.

Institutional barriers include the lack of a language of pain and the failure to use validated pain measurement tools in clinical practice. The lack of time committed to pain as a priority, the lack of economic resources committed to its treatment, and the serious legal restrictions to drug prescribing and drug availability add further impediments to adequate pain treatment. These impediments have been widely discussed in the literature. When these barriers are found, specific programs need to be instituted to provide the framework for change.

VI. **Additional Help**

Help for referrals or patient support may be found by contacting the American Academy of Pain Management (209-533-9744; *http://www.aapainmanage.org/*), the American Pain Foundation (888-615-7246; *http://www.painfoundation.org/*), or the American Chronic Pain Association (916-632-0922; *http://www.theacpa.org/*).

ADDITIONAL READING

Averbuch M, Katzper M. Gender and the placebo analgesic effect in acute pain. *Clin Pharm Ther* 2001;70:287–291.

Beecher HK. The powerful placebo. *JAMA* 1955;159:1602–1606.

Bressler LR, Geraci MC, Schatz BS. Misperceptions and inadequate pain management in cancer patients. *Ann Pharmacother* 1993;25:1225–1230.

Caldwell JR, Rapaport RJ, Davis JC, et al. Efficacy and safety of a once-daily morphine formulation in chronic, moderate-to-severe osteoarthritis pain: results from a randomized, placebo-controlled, double-blind trial and an open-label extension trial. *J Pain Sympt Manage* 2002;23:278–291.

Cherny N, Portenoy R. The management of cancer pain. *CA Cancer J Clin* 1994; 44:263–303.

Cleeland C. Documenting barriers to cancer pain management. In: Chapman C, Foley K, eds. *Current and emerging issues in cancer pain.* New York: Raven Press, 1993:321–330.

Cleeland C, Gonin R, Hatfield A, et al. Pain and its treatment in outpatients with metastatic cancer. *N Engl J Med* 1994;30:592–596.

Eliot L, Butler J, Devane J, et al. Pharmacokinetic evaluation of a sprinkle-dose regimen of a once-daily, extended-release morphine formulation. *Clin Ther* 2002;24:260–268.

Foley K. Competent care for the dying instead of physician-assisted suicide. *N Engl J Med* 1997;336:54–58.

Ingham J, Foley K. Pain and the barriers to its relief at the end of life: a lesson for improving end of life health care. *Hospice J* 1998;13:89–100.

Jacox A, Carr D, Payne R. *Management of cancer pain.* Clinical practice guidelines. Rockville, MD: Agency for Health Care Policy and Research, 1994.

McCarberg BH, Barkin RL. Long-acting opioids for chronic pain: pharmacotherapeutic opportunities to enhance compliance, quality of life, and analgesia. *Am J Therap* 2001;8:181–186.

Portenoy R, Thaler H, Kornblith A. Symptom prevalence, characteristics and distress in a cancer population. *Qual Life Res* 1994;2:183–189.

Sees KL, Clark HW. Opioid use in the treatment of chronic pain: assessment of addiction. *J Pain Sympt Manage* 1993;8:257–264.

Von Roenn J, Cleeland C, Gronin R, et al. Physician attitudes and practice in cancer pain management. A survey from the Eastern Cooperative Oncology Group. *Ann Intern Med* 1993;119:121–126.

29. DRUG INTERACTIONS IN PSYCHOPHARMACOLOGY[1]

Karthik Venkatakrishnan
Richard I. Shader
Lisa L. von Moltke
David J. Greenblatt

A clinically significant drug interaction occurs when the therapeutic or toxic effects of a medication are altered by coadministration with another drug. Likely possibilities include diminished efficacy or enhanced efficacy or toxicity. Conceptually, to think of these interactions as happening between an inhibiting or inducing agent, which one can think of as the "**perpetrator**," and the affected agent, which one can think of as the "**victim**," can be helpful (Fig. 29.1). Drug interactions are particularly notable when the victim drug has a relatively narrow therapeutic index (e.g., tricyclic antidepressants [TCAs], **lithium**, mood-stabilizing anticonvulsants). Some interactions are predictable, and they are easily understood because they involve the action of two or more separate agents working through different receptors or different sites on the same receptor to enhance the same pharmacodynamic (see below) outcome (e.g., increased central nervous system [CNS] depression when a sedative-hypnotic agent, such as **diazepam**, is taken with **alcohol**). Some are easily understood pharmacokinetically (e.g., when two drugs are substrates for the same catabolic enzyme and compete for it). Others are unpredictable; these are discovered by chance or through large-scale epidemiologic studies. An example of the latter is the potentiation of oral anticoagulants by the sedative-hypnotic **chloral hydrate**. Regrettably, unexpected interactions may sometimes result in serious or fatal drug toxicity.

I. **Classification of Drug–Drug Interactions: A Mechanistic Perspective**
Drug interactions may be categorized as **pharmacodynamic** (i.e., additive, antagonistic, or synergistic effects at the level of mechanism of action at the target or effect site) or **pharmacokinetic** (i.e., modulation of the time course or magnitude of drug concentrations in body compartments and thus of drug action at the effect or target site). Drug antagonism can occur when one drug prevents another from reaching or acting at its receptor or binding site. A classic example of such an interaction is that between the TCAs and the antihypertensive agent **guanethidine**. The mechanism of action of TCAs partly involves the inhibition of neurotransmitter reuptake at the noradrenergic synapse. The site of action of **guanethidine** is the presynaptic adrenergic neuron where it works as a "substitute or false neurotransmitter" and depletes catecholamine-containing vesicles of their native neurotransmitter, thereby producing an antihypertensive effect. **Guanethidine** reaches its site of action by active transport into the neuron, a process mediated by the same transporter that is responsible for norepinephrine reuptake. In patients receiving TCAs, the function of this transporter is blocked by the antidepressant. As a result, **guanethidine** cannot reach its site of action, making it ineffective as an antihypertensive agent.
Pharmacokinetic interactions can result from a variety of mechanisms, including the modulation of hepatic drug biotransformation, renal clearance, drug transport, distribution, and plasma protein binding. One drug may alter the bioavailability of another by changing its dissolution characteristics, altering the ambient pH, causing variations in gastrointestinal motility, inhibiting presystemic extraction at the level of the small intestine or liver, or modulating drug transport in the intestine. Some drugs are excreted in significant amounts

---

[1]This chapter is deliberately long. This decision was made to address the relatively sparse background that many students and clinicians have about drug metabolism and drug interactions.

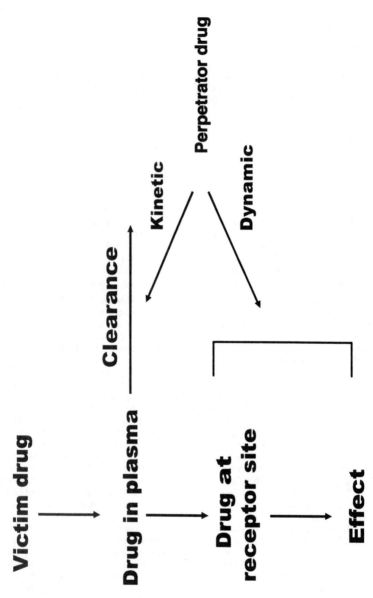

FIG. 29.1. A model for drug interactions.

by the kidney, and their excretion may be modified by agents that alter glomerular filtration, tubular function, or urinary pH. For example, **thiazide diuretics** increase the elimination of **sodium** and inhibit the renal clearance of **lithium**; coadministration may result in **lithium** toxicity, unless compensatory dosage reductions of **lithium** are made.

Many pharmacokinetic drug interactions result from the modulation of drug biotransformation or metabolism. The liver is the major site of drug metabolism, with the small intestine playing a secondary, yet important, role in the oral clearance of certain therapeutic agents. A number of psychotropic drugs can inhibit or induce hepatic drug metabolizing enzymes, thereby impairing or enhancing, respectively, the liver's ability to detoxify coadministered drugs. Metabolic drug–drug interactions in psychopharmacology can occur in two ways. First, the metabolic clearance of the psychotropic agent may be altered by another coadministered psychotropic or nonpsychotropic agent. Second, the metabolic clearance of a nonpsychotropic agent may be altered by a psychotropic agent. Several examples of both kinds of interactions have been noted in the clinical literature, and representative examples follow. For example, the detoxification of the TCA **nortriptyline** requires hepatic biotransformation via hydroxylation, a reaction catalyzed by the hepatic microsomal enzyme cytochrome P-450 (CYP) 2D6 (see section II). The antifungal agent **terbinafine** is a potent inhibitor of CYP 2D6. Consider a patient receiving long-term **terbinafine** for onychomycosis. Initiation of antidepressant treatment in this patient with usual therapeutic doses of **nortriptyline** may result in **nortriptyline**-related toxicity because **nortriptyline** concentrations in the plasma, and hence at the sites of pharmacologic or toxicologic action (e.g., brain and heart, respectively), can increase beyond the upper limit of the therapeutic range due to impaired hepatic clearance. In the above example, modulation of the clearance of a psychotropic agent by a coadministered drug belonging to an unrelated therapeutic category is evident. The reverse is illustrated in the interaction between the antimalarial prodrug **proguanil** and the selective serotonin reuptake inhibitor (SSRI) antidepressant **fluvoxamine**, a potent inhibitor of CYP 2C19. **Proguanil** actions require hepatic biotransformation to its active metabolite **cycloguanil**, a step mediated by CYP 2C19. As a result, **proguanil**'s antimalarial efficacy may be compromised in a patient receiving **fluvoxamine** through its impairment of CYP 2C19-mediated metabolite formation.

During the last few decades, a dramatic increase has occurred in the understanding of the molecular biology and biochemistry of the CYP enzymes, enabling a better understanding and improved prediction of metabolic drug–drug interactions in psychopharmacology. Although the widespread use of SSRIs has greatly improved the prognosis of the depressed patient, it has also become evident that the SSRIs constitute a group of drugs with a high risk of drug interactions as a result of CYP inhibition. Thus, a large fraction of drug interactions in psychopharmacology is mediated by metabolic mechanisms, especially at the level of the CYP enzymes. The following discussion of human CYP enzymes and their interactions with psychopharmacologics will hopefully not only allow the psychiatrist to be aware of the reported interactions (e.g., in a package insert or a computerized drug interaction program) but also will provide a mechanistic basis that will allow their management and the forecasting of unidentified interactions.

II. Human Cytochrome P-450 Isozymes and Psychopharmacologic Agents

CYP enzymes are estimated to account for the biotransformation of approximately 60% of the commonly prescribed drugs in the United States. Although the human drug-metabolizing CYPs are expressed in several tissues, they are concentrated in the smooth endoplasmic reticulum of the zone III hepatocytes in the liver, with lower levels of expression in the intestine, lungs, kidneys, and brain. The multiple CYP enzymes are classified into families, subfamilies, and isoforms based on a systematic nomenclature. The major human drug-metabolizing CYPs belong to families 1, 2, and 3, with the specific isoforms of interest to drug interactions in psychopharmacology being 1A2, 2B6, 2C9, 2C19, 2D6, and 3A4.

CYP 1A2 is the primary enzyme responsible for the human hepatic metabolism of **phenacetin, tacrine, caffeine,** and **theophylline,** and it also plays a role in the metabolism of **clozapine** and **imipramine.** Clinically significant CYP 1A2 inhibitors include the SSRI antidepressant **fluvoxamine,** the antihelminthic agent **thiabendazole,** and the fluoroquinolone antibiotics **ciprofloxacin** and **enoxacin.**

CYP B6 is the sole mediator of the hydroxylation of the antidepressant **bupropion,** and it contributes significantly to the metabolism of the anticonvulsant **S-mephenytoin,** the barbiturate **S-mephobarbital,** the alkylating anticancer agent **cyclophosphamide,** and the intravenous anesthetic **propofol.** CYP 2B6 activity is inhibited by the SSRI antidepressants **fluvoxamine, sertraline,** and **paroxetine** and by **norfluoxetine,** the active metabolite of **fluoxetine,** based on *in vitro* studies. Based on *in vitro* studies, the antiretroviral agents **ritonavir** and **efavirenz** are also potent CYP 2B6 inhibitors.

CYP 2C8 plays a major role in the biotransformation of the antineoplastic agents **paclitaxel** and *all trans*-**retinoic acid.** This enzyme is also partially responsible for the metabolism of the nonbenzodiazepine (BZ) hypnotic **zopiclone,** based on *in vitro* studies. The clinical implications of CYP 2C8-mediated drug metabolism remain to be understood, and insufficient information is available on the clinical consequences of inhibition or induction of this enzyme.

CYP 2C9 is the primary enzyme responsible for the metabolism of the oral hypoglycemic agent **tolbutamide,** the anticoagulant **S-warfarin,** the anticonvulsant **phenytoin,** the antihypertensive agent **losartan,** and several nonsteroidal antiinflammatory drugs. Clinically significant CYP 2C9 inhibitors include **fluoxetine** and **fluvoxamine,** the sulfonamide antimicrobials **sulfamethoxazole** and **sulfinpyrazone,** and the azole antifungal agents **miconazole** and **fluconazole.** Clinically significant inducers of CYP 2C9 include **barbiturates, carbamazepine,** and **rifampin.**

CYP 2C19 is polymorphically expressed, and it contributes significantly to the clearance of the monoamine oxidase inhibitor (MAOI) **moclobemide,** the BZ **diazepam,** the antiulcer drug **omeprazole,** the antimalarial agent **proguanil,** and the antidepressants **citalopram** and **amitriptyline.** Clinically significant CYP 2C19 inhibitors include **fluvoxamine, omeprazole, fluconazole,** and the antithrombotic agent **ticlopidine.** The genetic polymorphisms associated with this isoform result in a poor metabolizer phenotype at a frequency of less than 5% in whites and at a greater frequency of 12% to 20% in Asian populations.

CYP 2D6 is partly or entirely responsible for the metabolism of a variety of psychopharmacologic and cardiovascular drugs, including **thioridazine, perphenazine, desipramine, nortriptyline, paroxetine, venlafaxine, codeine, metoprolol, encainide, flecainide, propafenone, propofol,** and **mexiletine.** Clinically significant CYP 2D6 inhibitors include **fluoxetine** and **paroxetine;** the conventional antipsychotic agents **haloperidol, thioridazine, chlorpromazine,** and **perphenazine;** the allylamine antifungal agent **terbinafine;** the antithrombotic drug **ticlopidine;** the antiretroviral agent **ritonavir;** and the antiarrhythmic agent **quinidine.** CYP 2D6 is polymorphically expressed with a frequency of poor metabolizers of approximately 5% to 10% in the white population. Table 29.1 lists some substrates and inhibitors for CYP 2D6.

CYP 3A4 is the most abundant CYP enzyme in both the human liver and small intestine. Most oxidatively biotransformed therapeutic agents are metabolized at least in part by this enzyme. Examples of drugs that are primarily metabolized by CYP 3A4 include immunosuppressants, such as **cyclosporin A** and **tacrolimus;** sedative-hypnotic agents, such as **midazolam, triazolam,** and **alprazolam;** antidepressants, such as **trazodone** and **nefazodone;** the conventional antipsychotic agent **haloperidol;** calcium channel blockers such as **nifedipine, felodipine,** and **diltiazem;** antiarrhythmic agents, such as **amiodarone, quinidine,** and **lidocaine;** antiinfective agents, such as **erythromycin, quinine, ritonavir, saquinavir,** and **amprenavir;** antineoplastic agents, such as **etoposide, ifosfamide, tamoxifen,** and **vinblastine;** synthetic opioids, such as **fen-**

TABLE 29.1. SELECTED EXAMPLES OF CYTOCHROME P-450 2D6 SUBSTRATES AND INHIBITORS

Substrates	Inhibitors
Desipramine	Quinidine
Nortriptyline	Fluoxetine/norfluoxetine
Venlafaxine	Paroxetine
Codeine	Terbinafine
Tramadol	Perphenazine
β-Adrenergic receptor	Ticlopidine
antagonists (many)	
Antiarrhythmic agents (many)	
Dextromethorphan	

tanyl, **alfentanil**, and **sufentanil**; and the nonsedating antihistaminic agents **terfenadine**, **loratadine**, and **astemizole**. Table 29.2 lists some substrates for CYP 3A.

Examples of clinically significant CYP 3A4 inhibitors include the macrolide antibiotic **erythromycin**, the azole antifungal agents **ketoconazole** and **itraconazole**, the antiretroviral drug **ritonavir**, the calcium channel blocking agent **diltiazem**, the progestin **gestodene**, and the active metabolite of fluoxetine **norfluoxetine**. Inducers of CYP 3A4 include **rifampin, dexamethasone, phenytoin, carbamazepine, phenobarbital, ritonavir,** and **nevirapine**, as well as the herbal antidepressant **St. John's wort**. Table 29.3 lists some inhibitors and inducers of CYP 3A.

The various CYP enzymes have distinct yet overlapping substrate specificities. Thus, in many cases, multiple enzymes can mediate the metabolism of a single drug. The consequence of CYP inhibition for a "pure" substrate of a single CYP isoform will be different from that for a drug that can be metabolized by multiple enzymes. This is evident upon examination of the drug interactions of the sedative-hypnotic agents **triazolam** and **zolpidem** with the CYP 3A4-inhibitory antifungal agent **ketoconazole**. **Triazolam** is a "pure" CYP 3A4 substrate; **zolpidem** is metabolized by multiple CYP isoforms, including CYP 3A4. Coadministration of **ketoconazole** with **triazolam** results in a clinically significant interaction due to a greater than 90% inhibition of **triazolam** clearance. The pharmacodynamic consequences of this interaction can be profound, and they manifest as enhanced CNS depression and prolonged sleep time when compared with the short-lived hypnotic effects of **triazolam** taken by itself. On the other hand, coadministration of **zolpidem** with **ketoconazole** results in

TABLE 29.2. SELECTED EXAMPLES OF CYTOCHROME P-450 3A SUBSTRATES

Benzodiazepines (short half-life)	HMG-CoA reductase
Buspirone	inhibitors (statins)
Trazodone	Zolpidem
Nefazodone	Amitriptyline
Cyclosporin	Imipramine
Calcium channel blockers	Sertraline
Quinidine	Citalopram
HIV protease inhibitors	Diazepam
Sildenafil	Clozapine

Abbreviations: HIV, human immunodeficiency virus; HMG-CoA, β-hydroxy-β-methylglutaryl-coenzyme A.

TABLE 29.3. SELECTED EXAMPLES OF CYTOCHROME P-450 3A INHIBITORS AND INDUCERS

	Inhibitors	
Higher risk	**Moderate risk**	**Inducers**
Ketoconazole	Fluconazole	Rifampin
Itraconazole	Fluvoxamine	Barbiturates
Nefazodone	Fluoxetine	Carbamazepine
Ritonavir (acute use)	Calcium channel blockers	Ritonavir (chronic use)
Erythromycin	Grapefruit juice	Nevirapine
Clarithromycin	Other HIV protease inhibitors	St. John's wort
	Delavirdine	
	Cimetidine	

Abbreviation: HIV; human immunodeficiency virus.

only a 40% decrement in **zolpidem's** oral clearance. This is because CYP 3A4 accounts only for 40% to 60% of **zolpidem's** catabolism. CYPs 2C9 and 1A2 also metabolize **zolpidem** and can thus compensate when CYP 3A4 is inhibited. Thus, an understanding of the relative contributions of CYP enzymes mediating the biotransformation of a drug is useful for predicting the magnitude and clinical consequences of an interaction resulting from metabolic inhibition.

Although the inhibition of a CYP isoform that plays a relatively minor role in the overall metabolism of a drug is generally clinically unimportant, the consequences of induction of such relatively minor contributors should not be overlooked. This is because, when induced, the relative contribution of low-affinity CYP isoforms will increase due to increased hepatic enzyme content, which can result in an acceleration of overall drug clearance.

Another important consideration in predicting the outcome of a metabolic drug interaction is the pharmacokinetic properties of the victim drug. This can be explained by considering the interactions between the BZs **triazolam** or **alprazolam** and the CYP 3A4 inhibitor **ketoconazole**. As was discussed above, the clinical consequences of the inhibition of **triazolam** clearance by **ketoconazole** are significant; the interaction results in a large increase in the peak plasma concentration that is attained after an oral dose of **triazolam**, as well as an exaggerated pharmacodynamic response to the drug. On the other hand, the consequences of metabolic inhibition by **ketoconazole** on **alprazolam**, another "pure" CYP 3A4 substrate, pharmacokinetics and pharmacodynamics are much more modest; a significant prolongation of its elimination half-life is seen, coupled with an insignificant increase in its peak plasma concentrations. **Alprazolam** is a poorly extracted drug having high oral bioavailability. Conversely, **triazolam** undergoes extensive presystemic extraction by CYP 3A4-mediated metabolism both in the liver and the small intestine. Thus, inhibition of metabolism of **triazolam** will result in a large increase in peak plasma concentrations after an oral dose and in enhanced pharmacodynamic activity. On the contrary, the predominant effect of metabolic inhibition for a poorly extracted victim drug will be a prolongation of the elimination half-life, which is less likely to affect the pharmacodynamic effects after single doses.

Worth emphasizing is that, although CYPs are the most important drug metabolizing enzymes in humans and are generally the focus of drug interaction mechanisms, other non-CYP enzymes (e.g., glucuronosyl transferases, N-acetyltransferase, epoxide hydrolase) are also important for some psychopharmacologic agents. For example, **lorazepam** undergoes glucuronidation that can be inhibited by the uricosuric agent **probenecid**, resulting in a decrease in **lorazepam** clearance. Acetylation steps involve the enzyme N-acetyltransferase.

This enzyme reveals a genetic polymorphism; that is, a single gene yields two or more alleles, and the least common allele is present in at least 1% of the population. "Slow" acetylator status is found in approximately one-half of white and African-American cohorts. Some Oriental and Eskimo cohorts contain about 10% and 5% slow acetylators, respectively. The most common slow allele that is found in whites is not present in Japanese cohorts. The metabolism of **phenelzine** involves an acetylation step. **Carbamazepine** undergoes CYP 3A4-mediated oxidation to a toxic epoxide metabolite that undergoes hydrolysis by epoxide hydrolase to yield a nontoxic diol metabolite. **Valproic acid** (VPA) can inhibit epoxide hydrolase, and coadministration with **carbamazepine** can result in neurotoxicity due to elevated levels of **carbamazepine epoxide**.

In addition to metabolic biotransformation, other processes that influence the pharmacokinetics of a drug include protein binding and drug transport. Modulation of active (i.e., energy-dependent) drug transport by P-glycoprotein is being increasingly recognized as a mechanism of drug–drug interactions. P-glycoprotein is an important molecular determinant of the oral bioavailability, tissue distribution, and the clearance of several therapeutically used drugs (e.g., **cyclosporin, digoxin, anthracycline antineoplastic agents, vinca alkaloids, opioids, human immunodeficiency virus [HIV] protease inhibitors**). Fortunately, most commonly used prescription psychotropic agents are not clinically important P-glycoprotein substrates. In fact, avid P-glycoprotein substrates are generally excluded from the CNS due to the barrier function of this transporter in the blood–brain barrier. Interestingly though, the over-the-counter herbal antidepressant **St. John's wort** is a clinically significant inducer of P-glycoprotein; studies demonstrate a decrease in the oral bioavailability and plasma concentrations of P-glycoprotein substrates, such as **digoxin, indinavir**, and **cyclosporin**, when they are coadministered with this herbal preparation. (*Note:* The net cyclosporin effect is mediated additionally via the induction of CYP 3A4.)

III. **Overview of Drug Interactions With Psychopharmacologic Agents**

Valuable data on drug interactions have been developed in the last several decades. Misinformation has also been published and perpetuated. Interactions are sometimes suspected on the basis of clinical observation of one or two cases. Unfortunately, when these appear in the medical literature as case reports, many readers and drug-interaction databases interpret them as depicting established fact. Systematic study often reveals such apparent interactions to be coincidental or spurious. Animal studies are another potential source of misinformation. Drug interactions that are strikingly evident in animal investigations may have no clinical relevance. Finally, biochemical or pharmacokinetic theory may predict certain interactions. Regrettably, these theoretical or *in vitro* interactions may be depicted as fact, even when clinical experience does not substantiate them. Uncritical interpretation of case reports, animal studies, *in vitro* data, or theoretical models can generate and perpetuate "facts" that are not really facts.

In the remainder of this chapter, a limited overview of drug interactions relevant to clinical psychopharmacology is presented. Every effort has been made to evaluate the strength of the evidence and to cull out published speculation. Examples of representative agents are presented. For some classes of agents, the interaction may generalize to the whole class. For others, the interaction may be specific to the noted drugs. This chapter is intended to raise clinicians' awareness of drug interactions; it cannot substitute for reading current product labeling on a specific medication or for consulting an up-to-date drug interaction text or computer program. Each major grouping of psychopharmacologic agents is presented separately.

A. **Conventional Antipsychotic Agents (Neuroleptics)**

These classes of agents (e.g., phenothiazines, butyrophenones) generally have a wide therapeutic index, so an alteration in their own metabolism is rarely a clinical problem in either their reducing efficacy or producing toxicity. However, given the understandable trend toward using the lowest possible doses of these agents, any interaction that further lowers a drug's concentration could have clinical significance. Some antipsychotic agents affect the metabolism of other drugs (e.g., TCAs, **phenytoin**), and some of these interactions have important clinical implications. Most significant interactions reflect toxicity as a consequence of pharmacodynamic interactions. However, recent *in vitro* studies indicate that **perphenazine** and **thioridazine** and, to a lesser extent, **chlorpromazine** and **haloperidol** are clinically significant CYP 2D6 inhibitors and that they can produce decrements in the clearance of drugs that are in large part metabolized by this enzyme.

1. **Anticholinergic agents.** Anticholinergic antiparkinsonian agents (e.g., **benztropine, biperiden, trihexyphenidyl**) are commonly given with antipsychotic agents to reduce the extrapyramidal effects of the latter (see Chapter 20). When they are used with the so-called low potency antipsychotic agents (e.g., **chlorpromazine, thioridazine**), additive anticholinergic effects may lead to toxicity (e.g., delirium, paralytic ileus). Whether anticholinergic agents affect the efficacy of antipsychotic agents remains unresolved; most studies suggest that they do not.

2. **Mood-stabilizing anticonvulsant agents. Carbamazepine** induces microsomal enzymes, and it may lead to lower systemic levels of antipsychotic medications. This may result in clinical deterioration, but the consequences are highly variable depending on the doses of the specific antipsychotic agent, whether it has active or toxic metabolites, the disorder(s) being treated, and other concurrent drug therapies. **VPA** may inhibit the metabolism of **chlorpromazine** but not that of **haloperidol**. **Chlorpromazine** may inhibit the metabolism of **phenytoin**. **Prochlorperazine** and **thioridazine** may similarly interact with **phenytoin**, but often no change in metabolism is seen with these combinations. **Haloperidol** does not affect **phenytoin** levels; **phenytoin**, however, may reduce **haloperidol** or **clozapine** levels. Antipsychotic agents (e.g., **loxapine**) may lower the seizure threshold and may antagonize the actions of **phenytoin**.

3. **Antidepressants.** TCAs increase the plasma levels of some antipsychotic drugs. **Imipramine** and **nortriptyline** increase **chlorpromazine** levels. **Fluoxetine** impairs **haloperidol** metabolism; it likely interferes with the metabolism of other antipsychotic agents as well, because oxidative metabolism is characteristic for this group. **Fluoxetine** may have indirect additive or synergistic effects in reducing dopamine activity, which may lead to extrapyramidal symptoms. When **perphenazine** is combined with **paroxetine**, an increase in **perphenazine** plasma levels and CNS side effects, including extrapyramidal effects, can occur. Both **fluoxetine** and **paroxetine** are potent CYP 2D6 inhibitors, explaining at least in part their interactions with a number of conventional antipsychotic agents. Bupropion as an inhibitor of CYP 2D6 also has the potential to inhibit the clearance of agents, such as **haloperidol** and **thioridazine**.

   Haloperidol, thiothixene, chlorpromazine, perphenazine, and **fluoxetine** inhibit the metabolism of **imipramine, desipramine**, and **nortriptyline. Thioridazine** increases **desipramine** levels. These effects are mediated via the inhibition of CYP 2D6-mediated metabolism of the TCAs. Increased levels of many TCAs may lead to anticholinergic problems (e.g., constipation, paralytic ileus) or cardiac toxicity (e.g., prolonged PR or QTc intervals); monitoring of electrocardiograms is strongly advised.

4. **Antihypertensives.** The two major types of interactions of clinical concern between antipsychotic agents and antihypertensives are those that cause delirium (see Chapter 4) and those with an enhanced or blocked hypotensive effect, depending on the specific antihypertensive agent. **Captopril** and perhaps other angiotensin-converting enzyme inhibitors, **propranolol**, and **methyldopa** may have enhanced hypotensive effects when they are coadministered with **chlorpromazine**. Although this ef-

fect seems predictable from **chlorpromazine's** strong α_1-adrenergic receptor antagonist properties, even **haloperidol** may interact with **propranolol** to produce serious hypotensive episodes. **Atenolol,** a drug that is predominantly cleared renally, may be a useful alternative to **propanolol** and **metoprolol** when CYP 2D6-inhibitory antipsychotic agents, such as **thioridazine** or **perphenazine,** are used. **Chlorpromazine** coadministration with **methyldopa** may be associated with both hypotension and hypertension. The antihypertensive effect of **guanethidine** may be reduced by the concomitant use of **chlorpromazine,** because the latter inhibits noradrenergic reuptake. The antagonism is weaker with or **thiothixene;** it does not occur, however, with **molindone. Bethanidine, debrisoquin,** and **guanadrel** are similar to **guanethidine** in their mechanisms of action, and they would be expected to interact with antipsychotic agents in a similar manner.

5. **Benzodiazepines.** The most serious interaction between BZs and antipsychotic agents causes respiratory depression that may occur when **clozapine** is concurrently used with a BZ. Other antipsychotic agents do not appear to present problems when they are given together with BZs, and combinations are frequently used. Patients taking **alprazolam** with **fluphenazine or haloperidol** may have higher antipsychotic agent blood levels. When additional sedation is required, adding a BZ is often preferable to using higher doses of antipsychotic agents.

6. **Lithium.** Encephalopathic syndromes characterized by lethargy, fever, confusion, extrapyramidal symptoms, and cerebellar dysfunction have been reported when **lithium** is coprescribed with some antipsychotic agents. Although most of these reports have involved a **haloperidol–lithium** combination, similar reports are found with **thioridazine, perphenazine,** and **thiothixene.** The greater reporting frequency for the **haloperidol–lithium** interaction likely reflects the greater clinical use of this combination. Many believe that these reports reflect patients with idiosyncratic manifestations of **lithium** toxicity (i.e., these are not true drug interactions). Nevertheless, caution should be used when prescribing these combinations, even though most patients tolerate them well.

7. **Antiretroviral agents.** The coadministration of the HIV-1 protease inhibitor **ritonavir** and **pimozide** is contraindicated. This interaction may involve the inhibition of drug transport, as well as the inhibition of CYP 3A4. **Ritonavir** also is a potent inhibitor of CYP 2D6, and it may thus impair the clearance of **perphenazine, risperidone,** and **thioridazine.**

8. **Antiarrhythmic agents.** The clearance of **propafenone** and **encainide** is CYP 2D6 mediated. Coadministration with **thioridazine** or **perphenazine** can potentially result in the impairment of clearance.

9. **Other medications.** Antacids, **cimetidine,** and antidiarrheals may impair the absorption of some antipsychotic agents. **Cimetidine** may impair the metabolism of **clozapine** and may lead to toxicity. **Buspirone** may increase **haloperidol** levels. When **alcohol** is ingested during the use of some antipsychotic agents, it may enhance sedation. **Alcohol** use may also worsen extrapyramidal symptoms. The coadministration of **amantadine** and **thioridazine** can worsen the tremor in elderly patients with Parkinson disease. However, whether **amantadine** combined with other antipsychotic agents produces a similar response is not known. **Erythromycin** and **clarithromycin** impair the metabolism of **pimozide** via the inhibition of CYP 3A4, resulting in cardiac toxicity (e.g., bradycardia); thus, coadministration is contraindicated. **Ketoconazole** has been shown to reduce the clearance of **quetiapine. Azithromycin**

may be a safe alternative macrolide antibiotic because it does not inhibit CYP activity.

B. Atypical (novel) antipsychotic agents. Unlike the conventional antipsychotic agents, several of which are inhibitors of CYP 2D6, the atypical agents **clozapine, olanzapine, quetiapine,** and **ziprasidone** do not perpetrate drug interactions as CYP inhibitors.

1. **Clozapine** is associated with a significant risk for agranulocytosis, the mechanism of which remains unclear. Therefore, **clozapine** should not be used with other agents having a known potential to suppress marrow function (i.e., a potential pharmacodynamic interaction). In addition, the oxidation metabolism of **clozapine,** which is mediated by multiple CYP isoforms, including 2C19, 3A4, 1A2, and 2D6, is impaired by the coadministration of any SSRIs that inhibit these CYPs. The most notable of these is **fluvoxamine.** The resulting increase in serum concentrations of **clozapine** may increase the likelihood of **clozapine**'s unwanted effects. (*Note:* Although many of these unwanted effects are concentration dependent, concentration *per se* is not.) Such combinations should be approached with caution, and patients may require close monitoring.

2. **Olanzapine's** metabolism is mediated by CYPs 1A2 and 2D6, flavin-containing monooxygenase 3, and glucuronidation. Because of the contribution of CYP 1A2 to the metabolism of both olanzapine and clozapine, the clearance of these two agents is higher—and, therefore, the steady-state concentrations are lower—in smokers. Even so, routine dosage adjustments are not usually recommended.

3. **Quetiapine** undergoes hepatic clearance that is largely mediated by CYP 3A4. Coadministration of CYP 3A4 inhibitors can therefore result in impaired clearance and elevated concentrations, as has been shown with the CYP 3A-inhibiting azole antifungal agent **ketoconazole.** CYP 3A inducers may exert the reverse effect. Increased amounts of **quetiapine** may be required for patients taking this along with **phenytoin** or other CYP 3A inducers (e.g., **carbamazepine,** barbiturates, **rifampin,** glucocorticoids). Coadministration with **thioridazine** produces an approximately 70% increase in the apparent oral clearance of **quetiapine** and an associated decrease in the steady-state concentrations of **quetiapine.** The mechanism of this interaction is unclear because **thioridazine** has not been shown to produce clinically significant induction of CYP 3A in humans.

4. **Ziprasidone's** clearance is mediated by CYP 3A4 and by the non-CYP cytosolic enzyme aldehyde oxidase[2]. Two-thirds of ziprasidone's clearance in humans is mediated by aldehyde oxidase, whereas the remaining one-third is mediated largely by CYP 3A4. Thus, the magnitude of any pharmacokinetic interaction resulting from CYP 3A4 inhibition or induction should be small. No clinically significant inhibitors or inducers of aldehyde oxidase have been identified at the present time. Based on this and published findings to date, **ziprasidone** is not expected to be a victim of clinically significant drug interaction resulting from CYP inhibition or induction, although **carbamazepine** may cause a small increase in **ziprasidone** clearance. However, because of the infrequent but potentially life-threatening significance of QTc interval prolongation (see Chapter 20), **ziprasidone** should not be used with other agents known to have this effect, and it should be used with caution and close monitoring when combined with potent CYP 3A inhibitors.

5. **Aripiprazole's** literature is too limited at this time to comment on its drug interaction liability.

---

[2]Aldehyde oxidase is a molybdenum-containing cytosolic redox enzyme that catalyzes the oxidation of azaheterocyclic compounds, such as zaleplon and famciclovir, and the reduction of zonisamide. Menadione, a vitamin K analogue, is an *in vitro* antagonist.

C. Monamine Oxidase Inhibitors

All MAOIs currently marketed in the United States (e.g., **phenelzine, tranylcypromine, isocarboxazid, selegiline**), when they are used in dosages that are effective in depression, are nonselective inhibitors of the enzymes monoamine oxidase A and B. (*Note:* **Selegiline** becomes nonselective at dosages of greater than 10 mg per day.) This effect has to be considered when these agents are coadministered with other medications that affect biogenic amine metabolism.

Although most clinicians immediately associate monoamine oxidase inhibition with antidepressant agents, remembering that other compounds have potent inhibitory actions on monoamine oxidase is important (e.g., the cancer chemotherapy agent **procarbazine**, the antihypertensive agent **pargyline**, the antibiotic **linezolid**).

1. **Antidepressants**. The combined use of any MAOI with another type of antidepressant should either be avoided or should be prescribed only with caution and careful monitoring in patients refractory to more conventional approaches. Some combinations are more likely to be problematic than others, and some patients are more susceptible to harmful complications. Unfortunately, which will cause this cannot always be determined in advance. When an interaction does occur, it usually involves some combination of central excitation, restlessness, rigidity, hyperpyrexia, respiratory depression, coma, or cardiovascular shock. Death may ensue. This unfortunate clinical outcome is most often a form of serotonin syndrome. Therefore, antidepressants with strong or selective proserotonergic activity are of special concern. These include **fluoxetine, sertraline, paroxetine, fluvoxamine,** and **clomipramine**, as well as some other TCAs. One exception in this category may be **trazodone**; some reports have suggested that concurrent use with **phenelzine** is safe. Combinations of **amitriptyline** with **tranylcypromine** or **phenelzine** and of **trimipramine** with **phenelzine** or **isocarboxazid** have also been used safely. That **nortriptyline**, in modest dosages, can also be used safely in combination with MAOIs seems probable. Some of the most serious interactions have involved **clomipramine** or **imipramine**; combinations of MAOIs with these two TCAs are best avoided. Some clinicians also avoid the use of MAOIs with **desipramine**.

Combinations of **moclobemide** with **nortriptyline** or **desipramine** may result in impaired clearance of these antidepressants and in toxicity because studies of **sparteine** and **dextromethorphan** metabolism in healthy volunteers have shown **moclobemide** to be a CYP 2D6 inhibitor.

Although the safety of selected combinations seems reasonably clear, any greater efficacy for combination therapy has not been established. Despite this, some clinical experience supports cautious trials of appropriate combinations in patients refractory to other treatment regimens. When combination oral therapy is chosen, initiating both medications at the same time and at lower than usual dosages is safest. Another possible role for combination therapy is to provide sedation with, for example, low doses of **trazodone** or **trimipramine** for patients on MAOIs who are having difficulty with sleep-onset insomnia. No data on the use of **mirtazapine** for this adjunctive role could be located.

2. **Antihypertensive agents**. **Reserpine**, when it is administered with an MAOI, may result in autonomic arousal, delirium, agitation, or hypertension. The antihypertensive action of **guanethidine**, and possibly also of **clonidine**, may be blocked when it is given with an MAOI. Some clinicians recommend avoiding **propranolol** altogether or using only low doses of the drug to prevent hypertensive reactions in patients also taking an MAOI. The hypotensive action of thiazide diuretics may be

potentiated by MAOIs. One case report suggests that hallucinosis may be seen with **pargyline**, an MAOI used in the treatment of hypertension, and **methyldopa**; however, some patients tolerate this combination without difficulty. Nonetheless, in animal models, a central excitatory syndrome occurs with this combination.

3. **Antipsychotic agents. Droperidol** may potentiate hypotension in patients taking an MAOI. (*Note:* **Droperidol** is not available in some countries because of its association with lengthened QTc intervals.) **Chlorpromazine** and other antipsychotic agents may block the pressor response to **tyramine** in patients taking MAOIs.

4. **Sedative-hypnotics**
   a. **Barbiturates.** MAOIs may enhance and prolong barbiturate sedation and other barbiturate effects due to an inhibition of metabolism of the barbiturate.
   b. **Benzodiazepines and other hypnotic agents binding to the benzodiazepine receptor.** Chorea has been reported in one patient and edema in two others. Given the widespread clinical use of these combinations, concomitant use seems unlikely to be problematic.
   c. **Buspirone.** Elevated blood pressure has been reported in a few patients already receiving MAOIs when **buspirone** was started in them; other monitored patients have not shown blood-pressure changes while taking **buspirone** and MAOIs. Nevertheless, conservative clinical practice should include periodic blood-pressure monitoring. The package insert for **buspirone** recommends that it not be given with MAOIs.
   d. **Alcohol. Pargyline** may cause a **disulfiram**-like reaction when **alcohol** is coingested. **Tyramine**-free alcoholic beverages probably do not interact with other MAOIs.
   e. **Ginseng. Ginseng**, which is found in many herbal health remedies, may cause insomnia, headache, tremor, and even hypomania when it is ingested by patients taking MAOIs.
   f. **Hypoglycemic agents.** An enhanced hypoglycemic response may occur in patients taking MAOIs and **insulin** or oral hypoglycemics.
   g. **Opioids.** Two types of interactions may occur between opioids and MAOIs. The first is a syndrome characterized by hypotension or, less commonly, hypertension; excitement; sweating; rigidity; and hyper-reflexia that can progress to hyperthermia, coma, and death. This syndrome may occur after **meperidine** or **dextromethorphan** (or a structurally close analogue) is administered to patients who are taking an MAOI. *These opioid analgesics should be avoided in patients receiving MAOIs.*
      The second type of interaction is the potentiation of opioid effects. Some clinicians recommend one-fifth to one-half of the typical opioid dose when analgesia is accomplished with **fentanyl**, **morphine**, or **codeine**. However, the latter agents do not appear to cause the dangerous interactions noted with **meperidine**-like agents.
   h. **Succinylcholine. Phenelzine** may reduce pseudocholinesterase levels; prolonged apnea after **succinylcholine** administration has been reported in one **phenelzine**-treated patient. In general, **mivacurium** or **rapacuronium** can be safely substituted for **succinylcholine** (see Chapter 24).
   i. **Sympathomimetic amines.** Direct-acting sympathomimetic amines, such as **epinephrine**, **norepinephrine**, and **isoproterenol**, may have enhanced pressor effects when they are administered to patients taking MAOIs; hypertensive crises may occur. Hypertensive reactions and crises are more common, however, after the use of indirect-acting sympathomimetics (e.g., dextroamphetamine, ephedrine, phenylpropanolamine, pseudoephedrine, reserpine, tyramine) in patients taking MAOIs. **Levodopa** (**L-dopa**) should also be avoided.

D. Tricyclic Antidepressants and Other Heterocyclic or Atypical Antidepressants

1. **Analgesics.** Proserotonergic antidepressants (e.g., **amitriptyline, imipramine, trazodone**) are sometimes prescribed to relieve migraine headaches and temporomandibular joint pain or to treat a variety of other chronic pain syndromes. In these and other conditions, they may be coadministered with opioid analgesics. Animal studies and clinical experience suggest that antidepressants may enhance opioid analgesia. Some evidence implies that proserotonergic antidepressants may be the most effective; **desipramine**, however, potentiates **morphine** analgesia in some animal models.

2. **Anesthetic agents.** Halothane and **pancuronium** may induce cardiac arrhythmias in patients on antidepressants that have anticholinergic properties (e.g., **amitriptyline**).

3. **Anticoagulants.** A single case report describes a 30% reduction in prothrombin time in a patient taking **trazodone** and warfarin.

4. **Antihypertensive agents.** The antihypertensive effects of **guanethidine, bethanidine,** and **debrisoquin** are blocked by antidepressants that inhibit the presynaptic transporter of **norepinephrine** (see above). Virtually all available TCAs have this action to some degree; **doxepin** and **trimipramine** are the weakest. Newer antidepressants, such as **fluoxetine, sertraline, paroxetine, nefazodone, bupropion,** and **trazodone**, have even weaker norepinephrine-transporter blocking properties, and they thus should not antagonize the antihypertensive action of **guanethidine** or its related compounds. **Venlafaxine** has norepinephrine-transporter blocking properties.

   As an inhibitor of CYP 2D6, **bupropion** could increase the hypotensive effects of β-adrenergic receptor antagonists, such as **metoprolol**.

   The antihypertensive action of **clonidine** also may be blocked by some antidepressants. **Desipramine, imipramine,** and **amitriptyline** reverse the antihypertensive effects of **clonidine** in humans, and animal studies suggest other TCAs act similarly. **Bupropion** does not interact with **clonidine**.

5. **Barbiturates.** Barbiturates induce hepatic microsomal enzymes and enhance the metabolism of oxidatively metabolized antidepressants.

6. **Carbamazepine.** A growing number of reports note that **carbamazepine** may induce the metabolism of **imipramine, desipramine, nortriptyline,** and **bupropion**. As with the barbiturates, **carbamazepine** is likely to induce the metabolism of all oxidatively metabolized antidepressants. Additive or synergistic cardiotoxicity has also been reported. Some evidence from animal studies and one case report suggests that **imipramine** and **desipramine** may inhibit **carbamazepine** metabolism, thus leading to **carbamazepine toxicity**, as levels of the 10,11-epoxide metabolite of **carbamazepine** are elevated. Although some authorities caution against combining **carbamazepine** and MAOIs, clinical experience suggests that the combination of **phenelzine** or **tranylcypromine** with **carbamazepine** is safe and that it does not affect **carbamazepine** blood levels.

7. **Cimetidine. Cimetidine** impairs the metabolism of **desipramine, doxepin, amitriptyline, nortriptyline,** and other oxidatively metabolized antidepressants; **ranitidine** and **famotidine** do not.

8. **Digoxin. Trazodone** may elevate **digoxin** levels.

9. **Disulfiram.** This drug inhibits the metabolism of **imipramine, desipramine,** and other oxidatively metabolized antidepressants. Delirium has been reported with the combination of **disulfiram** and **amitriptyline**. It has been suggested to potentiate the effects of **amitriptyline** by an unknown mechanism.

10. **Estrogens.** Women on long-term low-dose **estrogen**-containing oral contraceptive treatment and those on estrogen replacement may have a

decreased clearance of **imipramine**. This can lead to toxicity unless appropriate dosage reductions are made.

11. **Alcohol.** With the exception of the selective serotonin reuptake inhibiting antidepressants (see section III.E) and **bupropion**, antidepressants enhance the sedative and psychomotor effects of alcohol. Acute alcohol consumption inhibits the metabolism of most antidepressants; chronic alcohol use, in the absence of cirrhosis, leads to enhanced drug metabolism.

12. **Levodopa.** The anticholinergic properties of TCAs may impair the absorption of L-dopa. Whether this occurs with **paroxetine** is not known.

13. **Triiodothyronine (T₃).** T_3 augmentation of antidepressants may be useful in some treatment-refractory depressions, particularly in women.

14. **Methylphenidate.** Methylphenidate may inhibit the metabolism of **imipramine** and other antidepressants having a CYP 2D6-mediated pathway. In some patients with treatment-refractory depressions, the addition of a stimulant, such as **methylphenidate** or **pemoline**, may be beneficial.

15. **Phenytoin.** Some reports suggest that **imipramine, nortriptyline,** and **trazodone** may increase **phenytoin** levels.

16. **Reserpine.** Reserpine has been used to potentiate antidepressant response, and it may be associated with a greater propensity for medication-induced switching into mania. Significant adverse effects may be associated with these combinations.

17. **Antiarrhythmic agents. Bupropion,** through its inhibition of CYP 2D6, can increase concentrations of type 1C antiarrhythmic agents, such as **propafenone** and **flecainide.**

18. **Sulfonylureas.** Hypoglycemia has been reported when sulfonylureas have been administered with **doxepin** and **nortriptyline.** This likely could occur with other TCAs.

19. **Sympathomimetic amines.** The effects of direct-acting sympathomimetic amines may be enhanced in patients taking antidepressants. As long as intravenous administration is avoided, this rarely presents clinical problems. Pressor effects of indirect-acting sympathomimetics (**ephedrine, pseudoephedrine, tyramine,** and others) may be antagonized by the TCAs, **venlafaxine, mirtazapine,** and **maprotiline,** because norepinephrine reuptake is reduced or blocked.

20. **Antiretroviral agents.** The HIV-1 protease inhibitor **ritonavir** is a potent CYP 2D6 inhibitor, and it produces an extremely large mean increase in the area under the curve of **desipramine.** An interaction with **nortriptyline** is also highly likely because of the similar mechanism of clearance (CYP 2D6 mediated). Clinically significant interactions with the tertiary amines **imipramine** and **amitriptyline** are also likely due to the broad-spectrum CYP inhibitory effects of **ritonavir** and the inhibition of downstream metabolism of the demethylated active metabolites of these drugs. CYP 2D6 is the primary molecular determinant of the clearance (via O-demethylation) of the serotonin and norepinephrine reuptake inhibitor antidepressant **venlafaxine,** and thus **ritonavir** can be expected to impair its clearance. **Nefazodone** and **trazodone** are CYP 3A4 substrates based on *in vitro* studies, and **ritonavir** is a highly potent CYP 3A4 inhibitor. (*Note: The net effect of* **ritonavir** *on CYP 3A4 substrates is difficult to predict because* **ritonavir** *produces concurrent inhibition and induction of this enzyme.*) The exact nature of the interaction will depend on the dose of treatment with **ritonavir** and the time of ingestion before the addition of the CYP 3A4 substrate.

21. **Antifungal agents.** The allylamine antifungal agent **terbinafine** is a potent inhibitor of CYP 2D6 based on *in vitro* and *in vivo* studies. Case reports of **nortriptyline** toxicity and elevated plasma concentrations in **terbinafine**-treated patients are available. A clinically significant interaction with **desipramine** is also likely, given the importance of CYP 2D6 to **desipramine** clearance. The CYP 3A4-inhibitory antifungal

agent **ketoconazole** inhibits **reboxetine** clearance, which is reflected as a 1.5-fold prolongation of the elimination half-life of single dose **reboxetine**. An increase in steady-state **reboxetine** concentrations is thus predicted to result from CYP 3A4 inhibition. **Ketoconazole** and **itraconazole** may impair the clearance of **trazodone** and **nefazodone**, given the importance of CYP 3A4 in their metabolism.

E. **Specific Serotonin Reuptake Inhibiting Antidepressants**
The SSRI antidepressants **fluoxetine, fluvoxamine, sertraline, paroxetine**, and **citalopram** are all CYP enzyme inhibitors with varying specificities and potencies toward the multiple isoforms. **Citalopram** is the only SSRI without any clinically significant CYP inhibitory activity, and thus it is superior to the other agents from a drug interaction perspective. CYP 3A4 is inhibited by **norfluoxetine**, the active metabolite of **fluoxetine**. Given the high plasma concentrations of **norfluoxetine** that are attained during multiple-dose administration of **fluoxetine**, significant drug interactions occur between **fluoxetine** and CYP 3A4 substrates. Because of the long half-life of **norfluoxetine** (7 to 15 days), a significant risk of interaction exists for weeks after cessation of **fluoxetine** therapy. Thus, the inhibitory effects of **fluoxetine** take a sustained interval to reach maximum effect, and they persist for an extended period of time. **Fluoxetine** and **paroxetine** are potent CYP 2D6 inhibitors. **Sertraline** and **desmethylsertraline** are weak CYP 2D6 inhibitors. **Fluoxetine** and **fluvoxamine** inhibit CYP 2C9, and clinically significant interactions are likely with CYP 2C9 substrate drugs with a narrow therapeutic index, such as **phenytoin** or **warfarin**, necessitating an adjustment of dosage and emphasizing the importance of therapeutic drug monitoring in patients receiving these drug combinations. The same is true for sertraline as well, although it is a much weaker CYP 2C9 inhibitor and interactions with CYP 2C9 substrates are less likely and are probably variable. **Paroxetine, sertraline, fluvoxamine**, and **norfluoxetine** are all inhibitors of CYP 2B6 activity *in vitro,* and they can potentially impair the clearance of the antidepressant and antismoking agent **bupropion**. **Fluvoxamine** is a potent inhibitor of CYP 1A2 and CYP 2C19 and a less potent, yet clinically significant, inhibitor of CYPs 2C9 and 3A4.

1. **Antidepressants**. **Fluoxetine** inhibits the metabolism of all TCAs to varying degrees. Concomitant administration of **fluoxetine** and **desipramine**, for example, may lead to a 10-fold reduction in clearance as a result of CYP 2D6 inhibition and to 4-fold prolongation of the elimination half-life. When **imipramine** and **fluoxetine** are coadministered, clearance may be reduced fourfold. The effects on imipramine and **amitriptyline** clearance are of a smaller magnitude because multiple CYP isoforms metabolize these tertiary amine TCAs, and CYP 2D6 and 3A4, the main targets of **fluoxetine** and **norfluoxetine**, respectively, only partially contribute to their metabolic clearance. Nevertheless, the interactions are clinically meaningful because of the inhibition of the downstream metabolism of the pharmacologically active N-demethylated metabolites of the TCA by the SSRI.

Fluoxetine impairs **bupropion** clearance. If this interaction is not considered, the coadministration of **fluoxetine** and **bupropion** may result in a clinical syndrome resembling stimulant-induced psychosis or a **bupropion**-induced lowering of seizure threshold, even at doses of **bupropion** below 400 mg per day. This is explained at least in part by the **norfluoxetine**-mediated inhibition of CYP 2B6, the major molecular determinant of bupropion clearance in humans. Similar interactions of the CYP 2B6-inhibitory SSRIs **paroxetine, sertraline**, and **fluvoxamine** with bupropion can be predicted based on *in vitro* studies. The addition of **bupropion** to patients receiving SSRI antidepressants is not uncommon. Such combination treatments may potentially increase the risk of **bupropion**-related seizures, and an appropriate dosage adjustment may be necessary.

Combination therapy with TCAs and **fluoxetine** is sometimes tried to improve response rates in refractory depression, to reverse tolerance to **fluoxetine's** antidepressant response, or to induce hypnotic effects in patients with insomnia as a prominent symptom of depression or secondary to **fluoxetine**. **Trazodone** may be used for hypnotic effects in patients receiving **fluoxetine**, and the potential inhibition of CYP 3A4-mediated metabolism of **trazodone** by **norfluoxetine** may need to be considered.

2. **Antipsychotic agents.** Fluoxetine may impair the metabolism of some antipsychotic agents, resulting in elevated serum levels of the latter. Because of the wide therapeutic index of antipsychotic agents, this is usually not of clinical significance. In some cases, however, enhanced dopaminergic activity may lead to extrapyramidal symptoms, some of which may be due to a pharmacodynamic interaction.

3. **Barbiturates and benzodiazepines.** Concomitant administration of **fluoxetine** may impair the metabolism of barbiturates and triazolobenzodiazepines, thus enhancing their sedative and psychomotor effects. The effect on barbiturates is CYP 2D6 mediated; the triazolobenzodiazepine effect is CYP 3A4 mediated. Inhibition of the clearance of **triazolam, alprazolam, estazolam,** and **midazolam** by **fluoxetine** is mainly explained by the potent CYP 3A4-inhibitory effects of **norfluoxetine**. **Fluvoxamine** decreases the clearance of intravenous **midazolam** by 33%. The effects on oral **midazolam** are expected to be greater given the large contribution of the small intestine in the presystemic extraction of oral **midazolam**.

4. **Buspirone.** The antianxiety effect of **buspirone** may be reversed by **fluoxetine**. One uncontrolled study suggested that **buspirone** may augment **fluoxetine's** effects in obsessive-compulsive disorder; this was not confirmed by a subsequent controlled trial. **Fluvoxamine** was shown to produce a small decrease in buspirone clearance in a controlled study with healthy volunteers. Although the interaction may be minor from a pharmacokinetic standpoint, a pharmacodynamic interaction is possible when combining any proserotonergic agent with an SSRI.

5. **Mood-stabilizing anticonvulsants.** Elevated levels of **carbamazepine** and toxicity have resulted with concurrent **fluoxetine** administration. Increases in **VPA** blood levels without clinical consequences have also been reported.

6. **Cyproheptadine.** Cyproheptadine, when used to treat anorgasmia in patients taking **fluoxetine**, may antagonize the antidepressant and anorectic effects of **fluoxetine**.

7. **Alcohol.** Fluoxetine does not affect the psychomotor performance, subjective effects, or metabolism of **alcohol**. Similarly, other SSRIs do not appear to affect or to be affected by **alcohol**. Some studies suggest that SSRI use may decrease *ad libitum* **alcohol** intake in both animals and humans.

8. **Lithium.** Lithium may augment the antidepressant response to **fluoxetine**, but a potential for toxicity also exists. **Fluvoxamine** may produce seizures and hyperpyrexia when combined with **lithium**. This may be a form of serotonin syndrome, in which case it could occur when **lithium** and any SSRI are combined.

9. **L-Tryptophan.** The combination of L-**tryptophan** and **fluoxetine, sertraline,** or **paroxetine** may result in toxicity when high doses are administered. Symptoms of agitation, restlessness, insomnia, aggressive behavior, headaches, chills, nausea, abdominal cramps, and diarrhea have been reported. This may be a variant of a **serotonin syndrome.**

10. **Opioids.** Fluoxetine may potentiate the analgesic effects of opioids in animal models of pain, but clinical experience with the combination is limited. The analgesic and narcotic effects of codeine can be expected to

be diminished in patients receiving antidepressant therapy with **fluox-etine** or **paroxetine** due to the inhibition of the CYP 2D6-mediated O-demethylation process that produces the pharmacologically active metabolite morphine. Whether **bupropion** would also inhibit the bio-transformation of **codeine** to **morphine** has not been established. The synthetic opioids **fentanyl, sufentanil, alfentanil**, and **methadone** are all primarily metabolized by CYP 3A4. The apparent oral clearance of these agents may be impaired by **fluoxetine** due to the inhibition of CYP 3A4 by **norfluoxetine**. In principle, the pharmacokinetics of in-travenous **fentanyl** and **sufentanil** should not be affected by **fluoxe-tine** because of their high extraction ratio, which makes their clearance flow dependent.

11. **Calcium channel blocking agents**. Three patients in whom concur-rent use of **fluoxetine** and calcium channel blocking agents led to un-wanted effects have been described; these effects were presumed to be secondary to increased concentrations of calcium channel blocking agents. **Verapamil** was associated with edema in one patient and with an increase in headaches in another. **Nifedipine** was associated with nausea and flushing in the third patient. These interactions are most likely explained by the inhibition of CYP 3A4-mediated clearance of these calcium channel blocking agents by **norfluoxetine**. To minimize the risk of an interaction, **paroxetine, sertraline**, or **citalopram** may be suitable alternatives for patients receiving calcium channel blocking agents.

12. **Antiarrhythmic agents**. The clearance of **propafenone** and **en-cainide** is CYP 2D6 mediated. Coadministration with **fluoxetine** or **paroxetine** can result in the impairment of clearance. Because **propafenone's** major metabolite 5-hydroxy propafenone is pharmaco-logically active, the predominant effect of clearance impairment is en-hanced β-adrenergic receptor antagonism, a side effect of **propafenone** that is not shared by the metabolite. **Fluvoxamine** coadministration results in an approximately 40% decrement in the clearance of **quini-dine**, a CYP 3A4 substrate, which is consistent with the moderate inhi-bition of CYP 3A4 by this SSRI.

13. **β-Adrenergic receptor antagonists**. The clearance of **metoprolol** is CYP 2D6 mediated. **Paroxetine** is a potent inhibitor of **metoprolol** metabolism *in vitro*, and it produces an 83% decrement in oral **meto-prolol** clearance and enhanced pharmacodynamic effects as measured by reductions in exercise heart rate and exercise systolic blood pressure. Case reports of severe bradycardia when metoprolol was coadministered with **fluoxetine** are available and are consistent with the *in vitro* data. Dosage reductions of **metoprolol** may be required when it is coadmin-istered with **paroxetine** or **fluoxetine**. **Fluvoxamine** is reported to in-crease the plasma concentrations and effects of **propranolol**, an effect that is probably explained by the inhibition of CYP 1A2.

14. **Tacrine**. **Fluvoxamine** (100 mg per day) causes an 88% decrease in the apparent oral clearance of **tacrine**, and it may potentially modu-late the hepatotoxicity of **tacrine**, depending on the relative contribu-tion of **tacrine** and its reactive metabolites to this toxicity. This interaction results from potent CYP 1A2 inhibition by **fluvoxamine**. The prevalence of tacrine use has diminished since the introduction of other agents for Alzheimer disease that are not CYP 1A2 substrates (see Chapter 5).

15. **Melatonin**. **Fluvoxamine** is a clinically significant inhibitor of **mela-tonin** clearance, and plasma **melatonin** levels are increased upon coad-ministration. The interaction is characterized by a large increase in the peak plasma melatonin concentrations without an alteration of the elim-ination half-life; it is explained by the inhibition of CYP 1A2-mediated metabolism of **melatonin**.

F. Lithium

Because **lithium** is not metabolized by the liver, enzyme induction and inhibition have no relevance for the understanding of **lithium's** drug interactions. Renal excretion is primarily responsible for lithium clearance; drugs that affect renal function, especially sodium reabsorption, may have clinically important effects on **lithium** levels. The therapeutic index of lithium is narrow; small increments in therapeutic **lithium** levels may lead to toxicity. Pharmacodynamic interactions may also be important in **lithium** therapy, and some CNS toxicity (e.g., confusion, memory loss, fever, seizures) may occur with **haloperidol** and **lithium** in the absence of elevated serum **lithium** levels (intracellular levels may be elevated as reflected by increased red blood cell concentrations; see Chapters 19 and 20).

1. **Aminophylline** and **theophylline**. These increase **lithium** excretion, and they have been used to treat **lithium** toxicity, although osmotic diuretics, intravenous **sodium bicarbonate**, and dialysis are preferred for serious **lithium** intoxication (see Chapter 3). Patients with pulmonary diseases who take **lithium** together with these drugs should have **lithium** levels monitored and the dosage increased when necessary.

2. **Antimicrobials**. Several antimicrobials (e.g., **spectinomycin, tetracycline, metronidazole**) have been associated with increased **lithium** levels in case reports. The interactions have not been systematically studied in humans. In animal studies, **lithium** clearance was not affected by **tetracycline, ampicillin,** or metronidazole.

3. **Antidepressants. Lithium** may potentiate the therapeutic effects of MAOIs, TCAs, atypical antidepressants, and SSRIs. As with many drug combinations that enhance the response, a risk of increased toxicity is also seen. Caution should also be exercised when the combination is used to treat depressed bipolar patients because **lithium** may not provide prophylaxis against the ability of antidepressants to increase cycling.

4. **Antihypertensive agents**. See section III.F.11 for a review of the diuretics. Angiotensin-converting enzyme inhibitors may elevate serum **lithium** levels and thus may lead to toxicity. The glomerular filtration rate in some patients taking lithium may depend on angiotensin II, thus putting these patients at risk for lithium toxicity. **Enalapril, captopril,** and any related agents should be used with caution in **lithium**-treated patients. Alternative antihypertensive medications are preferable.

   In patients taking **lithium, methyldopa** may cause a toxic syndrome that is characterized by confusion, tremors, slurred speech, blurred vision, sedation, and dysphoria. It may occur even in the presence of therapeutic **lithium** levels.

   Patients with bipolar disorder have smaller decrements in blood pressure when they are given **clonidine** while taking **lithium**, compared with patients taking **clonidine** alone.

   β-Adrenergic receptor antagonists and **prazosin** do not appear to interact with **lithium**. They may be the preferred antihypertensive agents for patients taking **lithium**.

5. **Antiinflammatory agents**. Increased **lithium** levels and toxicity have been reported when patients taking **lithium** have also taken **indomethacin, diclofenac, clomethacin, phenylbutazone,** or **ibuprofen. Aspirin** and **sulindac** do not elevate serum **lithium** levels.

6. **Antipsychotic agents** (see section III.A.6).

7. **Antithyroid agents. Lithium** enhances the action of thyroid-suppressing agents, such as **methimazole** and **carbimazole**; it has been used as an adjunct to radioactive iodine in the treatment of thyrotoxicosis. Lithium use may expose or aggravate hypothyroidism in patients with Hashimoto (autoimmune) hypothyroidism.

8. **Benzodiazepines**. A single case report describes hypothermia (30°C [86°F]) and a comatose state with reduced reflexes, dilated pupils, hypo-

tension, bradycardia, and absent piloerector response that were produced by the combination of **lithium** and **diazepam**. No subsequent reports have appeared; this may best be understood as an idiosyncratic reaction. In another report, steady-state serum **lithium** concentrations were increased by 3% when **alprazolam** was given concurrently, a change that was clinically insignificant.

The combination of **lithium** with a BZ (e.g., **clonazepam, lorazepam**) is a common practice to control agitation in bipolar patients in the acute stages of mania. Based on the extensive clinical use of these combinations, BZs appear to be a safe and useful adjunct to **lithium** therapy. Animal studies do suggest the possibility of an interaction between **lithium** and BZs, although the relevance of these results to clinical practice is not apparent. For example, some studies have shown decreases in BZ receptor density in the rat frontal cortex after 4 weeks of **lithium** administration.

9. **Digitalis glycosides.** In a single case report, the combination of **lithium** and **digoxin** resulted in confusion and nodal bradycardia alternating with atrial fibrillation in the presence of therapeutic lithium levels. Some clinicians believe that, with proper clinical monitoring, the combination can be used safely.

10. **Disulfiram.** Rats have increased mortality when **disulfiram** and **lithium** are administered concurrently, but no clinically significant interactions have been reported in humans.

11. **Diuretics.** Diuretics are generally divided into the following seven classes: osmotic diuretics, carbonic anhydrase inhibitors, thiazide diuretics, loop diuretics, aldosterone antagonists, potassium-sparing diuretics, and methylxanthines. Osmotic diuretics, such as urea, and carbonic anhydrase inhibitors, such as **acetazolamide**, increase lithium excretion. The thiazides consist of the thiazide diuretics plus other agents that are chemically dissimilar yet work through similar mechanisms of action (e.g., the sulfonamide derivatives **chlorthalidone, quinethazone, metolazone, methyclothiazide,** and **indapamide**). All agents in this class impair the excretion of **lithium**, and many case reports of severe toxicity have appeared that describe patients in whom appropriate decreases in **lithium** dosage were not made. Most case reports suggest that symptom onset occurs rapidly, within 2 to 10 days after adding the diuretic and **lithium**. With a 25 mg daily dose of **hydroflumethiazide** or a 2.5 mg daily dose of **bendrofluazide**, an average reduction in renal lithium clearance of 24% occurred; some patients showed no change. Other studies with **chlorothiazide** report average reductions in lithium clearance of 40%, 58%, and 68%, for daily **chlorothiazide** doses of 500, 750, and 1,000 mg, respectively. Therefore, a reduction of approximately 40% in the **lithium** dose may be required when a daily dose of 500 mg **chlorothiazide** is coadministered. Similarly, a 35% increase in the mean serum **lithium** level was found in normal volunteers taking 900 mg **lithium carbonate** and 50 mg of **hydrochlorothiazide** daily. Most clinicians reduce the **lithium** dosage by approximately 50% when this combination is used. In addition to the treatment of hypertension in bipolar patients, the benzothiadiazides are sometimes used to treat **lithium**-induced diabetes insipidus.

Loop diuretics, such as **furosemide** and **bumatanide**, have been associated with **lithium** toxicity in case reports, but carefully designed studies have not demonstrated a clinically significant effect. One study found an 11% decrease in **lithium** clearance after single doses of 40 or 80 mg of **furosemide**. In another study, 40 mg of **furosemide** added to **lithium carbonate** (900 mg per day) resulted in no significant change in the serum **lithium** levels in five of six volunteers; in the sixth volunteer, however, the level increased from 0.44 to 0.72 mEq per L, coincident with her premenstrual period. The consequences of the addition of

furosemide to **lithium** appear to be less predictable than those for the addition of thiazides. In part, this may reflect differences in usage—**furosemide** is often used in single doses, whereas thiazides are more often used chronically, and **potassium to lithium** alterations may be less critical. Frequent serum monitoring is required when the combination is used.

Ethacrynic acid does not have a clinically significant effect on **lithium** clearance. Single doses of the aldosterone antagonist **spirono-lactone** do not have a clinically important effect on lithium clearance; daily doses of 100 mg per day, however, may cause increases in serum **lithium** concentration.

The **potassium**-sparing diuretics **triamterene** and **amiloride** have not been extensively studied in combination with **lithium**. One case report with **triamterene** describes an elevation in the lithium level from 0.65 to 0.95 mEq per L. In a study of the effects of **amiloride** on **lithium**-induced polyuria, the mean **lithium** levels did not change significantly, although one patient had an increase from 0.8 to 2 mEq per L. When **potassium**-sparing diuretics lead to large volume contractions and reduced glomerular filtration, they appear possibly to reduce **lithium** clearance. As was discussed earlier, methylxanthines, such as **aminophylline**, **theophyline**, and **caffeine**, may increase **lithium** clearance and may thereby lower the serum levels.

12. **Alcohol**. **Lithium** may block the **alcohol**-induced subjective "high," may decrease the desire to continue drinking, and may reduce the cognitive dysfunction associated with intoxication. **Lithium**, however, is not an effective agent to treat **alcohol** withdrawal; its role in promoting abstinence after the withdrawal period is uncertain.

13. **Anticonvulsants (e.g., phenytoin, carbamazepine, and VPA)**. The combination of **lithium** and **phenytoin** may produce a toxic state that is characterized by coarse tremor, drowsiness, ataxia, gastrointestinal symptoms, and coma. In two of three reported cases, **lithium** levels were within the therapeutic range. Preexisting brain injury or damage may predispose a patient to this toxic interaction. In most cases, these drugs can be coadministered safely, as long as close supervision and monitoring occur.

    Carbamazepine is often coadministered with **lithium** in refractory bipolar patients (see Chapter 19). Although occasional reports of additive toxicity are seen, these are rare and they are thought by some to reflect too rapid dosage increases of **carbamazepine**. Both drugs reduce thyroid activity, which should be monitored during combination therapy. **Lithium** may obscure **carbamazepine**-induced decreases in leukocytes and neutrophils; this outcome is **not** prophylactic against **carbamazepine**-induced myelosuppression. **Carbamazepine** has an antidiuretic effect; this, however, is not an effective treatment for **lithium**-induced diabetes insipidus. **Lithium** may reduce the hyponatremia caused by **carbamazepine**. **VPA** added to **lithium** may improve the response in some patients with refractory bipolar disorder.

14. **Electroconvulsive therapy (ECT) and anesthesia** (see also Chapter 24). When patients taking **lithium** must undergo general anesthesia for surgery or ECT, the potential for several drug interactions exists. **Methoxyflurane**, an inhalational anesthetic, should be avoided because it can cause renal toxicity. Because renal excretion is the major mechanism of **lithium** elimination, the two agents are rarely used together.

    Some clinicians recommend that barbiturate dosages are reduced or that their use be avoided in patients taking **lithium** based on animal data that demonstrate increased barbiturate sleeping times in lithium-treated mice. This appears to be an acute effect of **lithium** that is not seen during chronic treatment in mice; no interactions in humans have been reported. In another animal study, one strain of rat became oliguric with decreased renal clearance after the use of **amobarbital** anesthesia. **Ketamine**, an injectable anesthetic agent that produces dissociative anesthesia, should be avoided in patients taking **lithium** because it may prolong seizure duration during ECT.

With respect to ECT, an initial case report suggested that delayed recovery from anesthesia could occur after ECT in patients taking **lithium**. A subsequent retrospective chart review in 17 patients who had a total of 78 treatments indicated that **lithium** use did not prolong anesthesia duration. Further complicating the issue of **lithium** and ECT are reports that patients may be more likely to develop greater memory loss, confusion, and atypical neurologic findings if they are receiving lithium while being treated with ECT.

The use of certain neuromuscular blocking agents must be avoided in patients taking **lithium**. One report describes a woman taking **lithium** who required an emergency cesarean section. Anesthesia was induced by **pancuronium, thiopental**, and **succinylcholine**. Postoperatively, apnea requiring mechanical ventilation occurred for a 4-hour period. In another case, a woman receiving **lithium** required an elective thoracotomy; anesthesia was induced by **thiamylal, succinylcholine**, and **pancuronium bromide**. Reversal of her neuromuscular blockade required **atropine** and **neostigmine**.

A number of animal studies support an interaction between **lithium** and neuromuscular blocking agents. Several studies indicate that **lithium** prolongs the duration of the blockade produced by **succinylcholine, decamethonium**, or **pancuronium**. These data, taken together with the case reports of surgical complications, suggest that **lithium** should be avoided during elective anesthesia.

G. Benzodiazepines and Nonbenzodiazepine γ-Aminobutyric Acid-A Receptor Agonists

1. **Aminophylline, theophylline**, and **caffeine**. These may antagonize the action of **diazepam, lorazepam**, and probably all BZs. This interaction may be secondary to reduced γ-aminobutyric acid (GABA) transmission by competition at the BZ receptor site or by effects at the adenosine receptor.

2. **Anesthetic agents**. Case reports have suggested that **diazepam** can increase the magnitude of the neuromuscular blockade produced by **gallamine** and that it can decrease that of **succinylcholine**. Other reports have not supported these findings. **Midazolam** does not affect the neuromuscular blockade produced by **succinylcholine** or **pancuronium**. The intravenous anesthetic agent **propofol** acts synergistically with the BZs when this combination is used in the induction of general anesthesia. The mechanism of this interaction is the apparent increased affinity of **propofol** to GABA$_A$ receptors in the presence of the BZ agonists.

3. **Antacids**. The transformation of **clorazepate** to **desmethyldiazepam** is dependent on gastric pH, and concomitant administration of an antacid may reduce the rate and amount of **desmethyldiazepam** that is formed. In chronic dosing of **clorazepate**, however, steady-state levels are not significantly affected by antacids. Antacids may also reduce the rate, but not the extent, of **diazepam** or **chlordiazepoxide** absorption. When single doses of BZs are administered with antacids, the subjective relief of anxiety may be delayed.

4. **Anticonvulsants**. VPA may increase the unbound fraction of **diazepam** twofold due to the displacement of **diazepam** from plasma albumin, theoretically causing a temporary increase in BZ effects. However, no evidence exists to indicate that a clinically important interaction occurs *in vivo*. Some reports suggest **VPA** may also inhibit **diazepam** metabolism. **VPA** does not affect **clonazepam** metabolism, although case reports of oversedation and the appearance of absence seizures with the combination do exist.

Several reports have indicated that **diazepam** may increase **phenytoin** levels; the opposite effect has also been reported. **Chlordiazepoxide** and **clonazepam** may also increase **phenytoin** serum levels. Clearance of **diazepam, clonazepam, and oxazepam** and possibly of other BZs may be enhanced by **phenytoin**.

Carbamazepine induces the metabolism of **clonazepam** and **alprazolam** and probably of other oxidatively metabolized BZs. **Tiagabine** does not alter **triazolam** pharmacokinetics or pharmacodynamics.

5. **Antituberculosis agents. Isoniazid** decreases the clearance of **diazepam, triazolam**, and probably all BZs metabolized by demethylation or hydroxylation. **Rifampin** is an enzyme inducer that increases the clearance of **diazepam, triazolam**, and **midazolam** and probably that of all other oxidatively metabolized BZs. **Triazolam** may be ineffective in patients taking **rifampin**; **temazepam** may be a useful alternative. The clearance of the imidazopyridine BZ receptor agonist **zolpidem** is also induced by **rifampin**, leading to a considerable reduction in hypnotic effect.

6. **Barbiturates.** These have additive sedative effects when they are given with BZs; they may also induce the metabolism of BZs.

7. **Cigarette (tobacco) smoking.** Although a retrospective study indicated that the sedative effect of **diazepam** was reduced in smokers, carefully designed studies have found no difference in the metabolism of **chlordiazepoxide, lorazepam**, or **triazolam** between smokers and nonsmokers. The half-life of **estazolam** is lower in smokers compared with nonsmokers. Most, but not all, studies have found no difference in **diazepam** metabolism in smokers versus nonsmokers. Conflicting reports exist concerning **clorazepate**. That any interaction between BZs and cigarette smoking would present clinical problems is unlikely. Curiously, **nicotine patches** contain a product warning for an interaction between **nicotine** and **oxazepam**, the basis for which is not obvious—especially since the patches are free of the inhaled aryl hydrocarbons that were presumed to account for any of the interactions observed between cigarette smoking and oxidatively metabolized BZs.

8. **Clozapine.** See section III.B.

9. **Digoxin.** A small increase in the **digoxin** half-life and increased serum levels of **digoxin** may occur in the presence of **diazepam**. One case report describes an increase in **digoxin** levels with **alprazolam**, but a larger study found no interaction.

10. **Disulfiram.** Disulfiram impairs the metabolism of **chlordiazepoxide and diazepam** and probably of other BZs metabolized by **demethylation** or hydroxylation. It does not affect the metabolism of **lorazepam** or **oxazepam**.

11. **Alcohol.** The combination of **alcohol** and BZs enhances sedation, respiratory depression, and psychomotor impairment. Some studies suggest that **temazepam** may produce a less intense interaction with **alcohol**. The pharmacokinetic interactions between **alcohol** and the BZs are complex, and studies are contradictory, depending in part on whether single (inhibiting) or chronic (inducing) **alcohol** ingestion is involved and on the BZ's metabolic pathway.

12. **Histamine (H_2) receptor antagonists. Cimetidine** impairs the metabolism of **chlordiazepoxide; diazepam; dealkylflurazepam**, the active metabolite of **flurazepam; alprazolam**; and **triazolam**. Evidence for an interaction with **midazolam** is contradictory. **Cimetidine** does not alter the metabolism of **oxazepam, lorazepam**, or **temazepam**, although **lorazepam** absorption may be increased in the presence of **cimetidine**. In patients who require therapy with BZs and H_2 blockers, **famotidine** or **ranitidine** may be more suitable. When **cimetidine** is used, BZs that primarily undergo glucuronidation (e.g., **lorazepam**) may be less likely to produce a clinically significant

interaction. An interesting and as yet unexplained interaction is the reduction in the clearance of **triazolam** by **ranitidine**.

13. **Heparin.** In healthy nonfasting subjects, **heparin** can cause a rise in the free fraction of **diazepam, chlordiazepoxide,** and **oxazepam** but not in **lorazepam.** In principle, this would not present clinical problems because the increased BZ effects would be transient.

14. **Levodopa.** Anecdotal reports suggest that BZs may decrease the antiparkinsonian effects of L-dopa.

15. **Oral contraceptives.** Oral contraceptives containing **ethinyl estradiol** reduce the clearance of both **diazepam** and **chlordiazepoxide.** In one study of women receiving oral contraceptives, the mean clearances of **triazolam** and **alprazolam** were not altered; however, the half-life of **alprazolam** was increased by 29%. Data for BZs metabolized by glucuronidation (e.g., **lorazepam, oxazepam, temazepam**) are contradictory; the reasons for this are not yet established.

16. **Tricyclic antidepressants. Imipramine** plasma levels may increase during concurrent **alprazolam** treatment. The effects on other antidepressants are unknown.

17. **Propranolol and other β-adrenergic receptor antagonists. Propranolol** may reduce the clearance of **diazepam** but not that of **alprazolam** or **lorazepam. Metoprolol** may also impair **diazepam** clearance, but **atenolol** does not. In general, BZs metabolized by N-demethylation or N-dealkylation (e.g., **diazepam, flurazepam**) are most likely to interact with β-adrenergic receptor antagonists.

18. **Calcium channel blockers.** The coadministration of the CYP 3A4 inhibitors **mibefradil, verapamil,** and **diltiazem** with **triazolam** or **midazolam** is contraindicated. Large increases in plasma concentrations and CNS depressive effects have been demonstrated, and interactions of a smaller magnitude may occur with alprazolam as well.

19. **Antibiotics. Erythromycin** and **clarithromycin** inhibit the CYP 3A4-mediated metabolism of triazolam, alprazolam, and midazolam. Coadministration results in decreased BZ clearance and increased CNS depression. Interactions with flunitrazepam are also likely based on *in vitro* studies. **Azithromycin** does not inhibit CYP 3A4, and it may be a suitable alternative. When **erythromycin** or **clarithromycin** is used, BZs that primarily undergo glucuronidation (e.g., **lorazepam**) may be less likely to produce a clinically significant interaction.

20. **Antiretroviral agents.** The HIV-1 protease **ritonavir** is a highly potent inhibitor of CYP 3A4, the primary enzyme that mediates the clearance of the oxidatively metabolized BZs **triazolam, alprazolam,** and **midazolam.** Short-term low dose **ritonavir** inhibits **triazolam** and **alprazolam** clearance to a clinically significant extent. However, long-term treatment with **ritonavir** for 10 days did not significantly alter **alprazolam** clearance. This is because **ritonavir** treatment results in an acute inhibitory effect, while continued or chronic treatment causes an induction of CYP 3A4. Concurrent inhibition and induction of CYP 3A4 makes the prediction of the outcome of a drug interaction difficult. If a patient is on long-term **ritonavir** and a BZ is added, the net effect may be difficult to predict because the net effects of induction and inhibition may balance out, resulting in a minor interaction. If, however, antiretroviral treatment with **ritonavir** is initiated in a patient receiving a BZ, such as **triazolam** or **alprazolam,** the acute effects of inhibition of CYP 3A4 will produce a clinically significant increase in the plasma concentrations of the BZ and thus increased CNS depression. Based on *in vitro* studies, the HIV-1 protease inhibitor **nelfinavir** is also a CYP 3A4 inhibitor, and coadministration with **triazolam** or **midazolam** is contraindicated.

21. **Antifungal agents.** The azole antifungal agents **ketoconazole, itraconazole,** and **voriconazole** are potent CYP 3A4 inhibitors, and they

impair the clearance of **triazolam, alprazolam,** and **midazolam.** *In vitro* studies predict clinically significant effects on **flunitrazepam** clearance as well. Coadministration of **ketoconazole, itraconazole,** or **voriconazole** with these BZs results in greatly enhanced CNS depression, and thus it is contraindicated. In patients taking these antifungal agents, **temazepam** may be chosen as a hypnotic in place of **triazolam.** In patients taking **triazolam, alprazolam,** or **midazolam, terbinafine,** rather than **itraconazole,** may be chosen for the treatment of dermatophytic infections. Although **fluconazole** is a less potent inhibitor of CYP 3A4, it does produce a significant impairment of **triazolam** and **midazolam** clearance, and coadministration requires a dose reduction of the BZ. The clearance of **zolpidem** is impaired by only 40% by **ketoconazole,** and the interaction with **itraconazole** and **fluconazole** is clinically unimportant. **Itraconazole** does not produce a clinically significant interaction with **zopiclone.**

    22. Selective serotonin reuptake inhibitors. See section III.E.3.

H. Carbamazepine

    Carbamazepine has several properties that predispose it to drug interactions. It is an inducer of the cytochrome P-450 system, and it is subject to autoinduction. **Carbamazepine** metabolism is exclusively hepatic; it can be affected by other drugs that induce or impair hepatic metabolism. It also has an active metabolite, **carbamazepine-10,11-epoxide.** Any evaluation of drug interactions must take into account the effects on both the parent compound and this potentially more toxic metabolite.

    1. Anesthetic and neuromuscular blocking agents. One case report describes tachyarrhythmias after **halothane** anesthesia in an 8-year-old girl receiving **carbamazepine.** Recovery from the neuromuscular blocking effects of **pancuronium** and **vocuronium** is faster in patients taking **carbamazepine.**

    2. Antianxiety agents. See section III.G.4.

    3. Antimicrobial agents. Erythromycin and **triacetyloleandomycin** inhibit the metabolism of **carbamazepine.** Macrolide antibiotics, with the exception of **azithromycin,** should be used with caution in patients taking **carbamazepine.** Clearance of the tetracyclic antibiotic **doxycycline** is enhanced with concurrent **carbamazepine** treatment. Apparently, **carbamazepine** has no effect on the metabolism of **tetracycline, methacycline, oxytetracycline, demeclocycline,** or **chlortetracycline.** However, **demeclocycline** and other tetracyclines inhibit antidiuretic hormone-sensitive adenylate cyclase activity, and they may reduce the hyponatremia that is sometimes produced by **carbamazepine.** No data are found concerning an interaction between **carbamazepine** and **minocycline,** a tetracyclic antibiotic that is partially metabolized in the liver. **Carbamazepine** metabolism is impaired with the coadministration of **isoniazid;** cases of neurotoxicity have been reported.

    4. Anticoagulants. The metabolism of **warfarin** is increased, and its anticoagulant effect is reduced in the presence of **carbamazepine.** Frequent monitoring of prothrombin times is necessary when **carbamazepine** is added to or withdrawn from a therapeutic regimen.

    5. Other anticonvulsants. VPA impairs the metabolism of the epoxide metabolite of **carbamazepine** by inhibiting the enzyme epoxide hydrolase. It also displaces **carbamazepine** from plasma proteins. Neurotoxicity may result from this combination, and plasma levels may not appear to be elevated if the epoxide level is not separately analyzed and reported. **Carbamazepine** lowers the levels of **VPA** and increases the levels of its 2-propyl-4-pentanoic acid metabolite, which is hepatotoxic and teratogenic. Despite potential problems, this drug combination is widely and usually safely used in the treatment of epilepsy.

Phenytoin induces the metabolism of **carbamazepine** and, to a lesser extent, of its epoxide metabolite. The effects of **carbamazepine** on **phenytoin** levels are variable. One case report describes sinoatrial block in an elderly woman taking the combination, thus suggesting an increased risk of cardiotoxicity with concurrent use.

Carbamazepine does not alter **phenobarbital** levels, but **phenobarbital** does induce the metabolism of **carbamazepine** and, to a lesser extent, of the epoxide. **Carbamazepine** reduces **primidone** levels while increasing the level of its metabolite **phenobarbital**. **Primidone** decreases **carbamazepine** levels.

Population pharmacokinetic studies indicate that **tiagabine** clearance is 60% greater in patients taking **carbamazepine**, whether with or without other enzyme-inducing antiepileptic drugs. This is most likely explained by the induction of CYP 3A4. **Tiagabine** does not affect the steady-state plasma concentrations of **carbamazepine** or its epoxide metabolite in patients with epilepsy.

6. **Antidepressants. Carbamazepine** induces the metabolism of **imipramine, desipramine, nortriptyline, and bupropion** and perhaps that of other antidepressants. Additive or synergistic cardiotoxicity has also been reported. Some evidence from both animal studies and one case report suggests that **imipramine** and **desipramine** may inhibit **carbamazepine** metabolism, leading to toxicity. Increased **carbamazepine** blood levels and clinical toxicity have been noted with the concurrent use of **fluoxetine**.

Although some authorities caution against the combination of **carbamazepine** and MAOI antidepressants, clinical experience suggests that the combination of **phenelzine** or **tranylcypromine** with carbamazepine is safe and that it does not alter **carbamazepine** plasma levels.

7. **Calcium channel blocking agents. Diltiazem** and **verapamil**, but not **nifedipine** or **nimodipine**, inhibit the metabolism of **carbamazepine**, which may lead to increased levels and possible neurotoxicity.

8. **Cyclosporine. Carbamazepine** induces the metabolism of **cyclosporine**; it may reduce its clinical effectiveness when dosage adjustments are not made.

9. **Digoxin.** Bradycardia has been reported with the combination of **digoxin** and **carbamazepine**. In addition, anecdotal evidence suggests that carbamazepine may reduce **digoxin** levels and that **digoxin** may increase **carbamazepine levels**; this is not well established.

10. **Danazol. Danazol**, a synthetic androgen used in the treatment of fibrocystic breast disease and endometriosis, impairs the clearance of **carbamazepine**; it may lead to toxicity.

11. **Glucocorticoids. Carbamazepine** induces the metabolism of **dexamethasone, prednisolone**, and **methylprednisolone**. It has also been associated with false-positive **dexamethasone** suppression tests, probably from the increased metabolism of **dexamethasone** or from direct effects on the hypothalamic-pituitary-adrenal axis.

12. **Histamine receptor antagonists. Cimetidine** may cause transient increases in **carbamazepine** levels, but these usually are not clinically significant. **Ranitidine** does not interact with **carbamazepine; famotidine** also probably does not.

13. **Lithium.** See section III.F.13.

14. **Opioids. Carbamazepine** may induce the metabolism of **methadone** and may reduce its levels enough to lead to mild withdrawal symptoms. **Propoxyphene** and **dextropropoxyphene** may inhibit the metabolism of **carbamazepine**, leading to increased levels and neurotoxicity. **Carbamazepine** has been used to potentiate the analgesic effects of **hydromorphone** in pain syndromes. Higher doses than usual are required to maintain **fentanyl** anesthesia in patients taking **carbamazepine**.

15. **Oral contraceptives. Carbamazepine** may be associated with breakthrough bleeding and pregnancy in women taking oral contraceptives. Proposed mechanisms of the interaction are the increased metabolism of **ethinyl estradiol** and **levonorgestrel** or an increase in the binding globulins for the sex hormones. A larger than typical dose of **ethinyl estradiol** may be required. Some authorities recommend starting the treatment with a preparation containing 50 g of **ethinyl estradiol** and then increasing this when breakthrough bleeding occurs.

16. **Theophylline. Carbamazepine** may induce the metabolism of **theophylline**, leading to subtherapeutic levels and the exacerbation of asthma symptoms.

17. **Conventional antipsychotic agents.** See section III.A.2.

I. **Valproic Acid**

The metabolism of **VPA** occurs via glucuronidation and β-oxidation to yield 2-E **VPA**, 3-hydroxy VPA, and 3-keto VPA. Thus, CYP inhibitors do not affect **VPA** clearance. Other anticonvulsants, such as **phenytoin, carbamazepine**, and **phenobarbital**, can induce **VPA** metabolism. Patients on **VPA** monotherapy will generally have longer half-lives than will those receiving polytherapy with other anticonvulsants.

1. **Antacids.** An aluminum hydroxide-magnesium hydroxide antacid was found to increase the extent of absorption of a single 500 mg dose of **VPA**. The clinical significance of this finding is unknown, but antacids are often administered with **VPA** to counter its gastrointestinal effects.

2. **Antidepressants.** Increases in the **VPA** elimination half-life were seen after doses of 100 mg per day of **amitriptyline** for 3 weeks. The clearance and the extent of absorption, however, were not affected. The clinical significance of this interaction is not known. Increases in **VPA** blood levels that were without clinical consequences have been observed with the concurrent use of **fluoxetine**.

3. **Antipsychotic agents. Chlorpromazine**, but not **haloperidol**, may be associated with increases in the steady-state levels of **VPA** when it is coadministered. **Chlorpromazine** may inhibit the metabolism of **VPA** (see section III.A).

4. **Aspirin.** The steady-state free fraction of **VPA** may increase from 12% to 43% during concurrent **aspirin** administration. **Aspirin** may displace **VPA** from protein-binding sites. **Aspirin** decreases **VPA** clearance by the inhibition of β-oxidation. The dosage of **VPA** may need to be reduced when aspirin is added.

5. **Carbamazepine.** See section III.H.5.

6. **Clonazepam and diazepam.** See section III.G.4.

7. **Ethosuximide.** VPA inhibits the metabolism of ethosuximide. Dosage reduction is necessary and plasma concentration monitoring of both drugs is desirable when this combination is used.

8. **Barbiturates.** VPA impairs **phenobarbital** metabolism; decreased clearance and the prolonged elimination half-life of phenobarbital in the presence of VPA have been consistently demonstrated. Without an appropriate adjustment of the phenobarbital dose, this combination can result in increased CNS depression. The combination may also result in lowered VPA levels due to phenobarbital-mediated enzyme induction. Dosage adjustments based on careful monitoring of serum concentrations are necessary. Data with **primidone** and VPA are contradictory. **Mephobarbital** may also decrease the serum levels of VPA. The unbound fraction of **thiopental** may be increased in patients taking VPA. This could enhance its anesthetic effects, but the clinical significance of this interaction is unknown.

9. **Phenytoin.** VPA inhibits the metabolism of **phenytoin** and displaces it from its protein-binding sites. Some reports have indicated that, when **VPA** is added to **phenytoin**, total serum phenytoin levels decline whereas the free fraction increases. The magnitude of this change is

highly variable, and some studies actually report declines in both measures. In most cases the interaction will not result in serious problems, although toxicity characterized by delirium and increased seizure frequency has been observed. The susceptible patient appears to be one who has high levels of **phenytoin** before the introduction of **VPA**; the transient increase in unbound **phenytoin** leads to toxicity.

10. **Felbamate.** The coadministration of **VPA** and **felbamate** (1,200 to 2,400 mg per day) produces up to a 50% increase in peak plasma concentrations of **VPA**. Use of this combination generally requires a reduction in the dose of **VPA**.

11. **Zidovudine.** VPA (250 or 500 mg every 8 hours) has been shown to decrease **zidovudine** clearance by 38% without altering its elimination half-life in HIV-seropositive patients.

12. **Rifampin.** Treatment with 600-mg daily doses of **rifampin** for 5 days resulted in a 40% increase in the apparent oral clearance of VPA. Patients taking **rifampin** may need an adjustment of their VPA dose.

13. **Other interactions.** VPA displaces **warfarin** and **tolbutamide** from plasma proteins, although the clinical significance of this effect is not known.

J. **Central Nervous System Stimulants, Especially Agents Used in the Treatment of Attention Deficit Hyperactivity Disorder (see Chapter 22)**

A decreased seizure threshold has been reported in patients receiving **pemoline** concomitantly with antiepileptic medications. **Insulin** requirements in diabetes mellitus may be altered in association with the use of **methamphetamine** and the concomitant dietary regimen. Methamphetamine may decrease the hypotensive effect of **guanethidine**. Methamphetamine should not be used concurrently with **MAOIs**. Literature reports suggest that methamphetamines may be associated with significant elevation of plasma corticosteroids. This should be considered if the determination of plasma corticosteroid levels is desired in a patient taking methamphetamine. The combination of methamphetamine with **ethanol** results in increased cardiac work, which may produce cardiac toxicity.

K. **Buspirone**

Buspirone has a high presystemic extraction, making it particularly susceptible to metabolic drug interactions. Buspirone clearance is significantly impaired and plasma concentrations are elevated upon coadministration with CYP 3A4 inhibitory drugs, such as the calcium channel blockers **diltiazem** and **verapamil**, the azole antifungal agent **itraconazole**, and the macrolide antibiotic **erythromycin**. These interactions are also characterized by increasing the pharmacodynamic effects of **buspirone**. **Rifampin** treatment causes a significant induction of buspirone clearance, and the pharmacodynamic effects are reduced. Induction by **phenytoin** and carbamazepine is also likely, and this requires investigation.

IV. **Herbals and Natural Products**

A. **St. John's Wort**

The over-the-counter herbal antidepressant **St. John's wort** is associated with a high risk of pharmacokinetic drug interactions that stem from the modulation of CYP-mediated metabolism and P-glycoprotein–mediated transport of coadministered substrates of these proteins. Some of the constituents of St. John's wort (e.g., hyperforin, I3,II8-biapigenin, and hypericin) are all highly potent inhibitors of CYP 3A4—with submicromolar inhibition constants—*in vitro*. No *in vivo* evidence indicates that St. John's wort is a CYP 3A4 inhibitor. Furthermore, potent inhibition of CYPs 2C9, 2D6, and 1A2 has also been described in *in vitro* experiments. In contrast to the results of these *in vitro* studies performed in liver microsomal systems that do not support the biosynthesis of the metabolic enzymes, other *in vitro* studies using human hepatocytes have described the induction of CYP 3A4 by St. John's wort, an effect that is mediated by the activation of the pregnane X receptor. Thus, although St. John's wort is an inhibitor of CYP activity *in vitro*, its inductive effects, which are generally observable only after multiple dose administration of the herbal, form the basis of several clinically important interactions with CYP 3A substrates, such as **cyclosporin** and **oral contraceptive agents**. Such drug combinations result in subtherapeutic plasma concentrations of the CYP 3A substrate with the potential consequences of transplant rejection (**cyclosporin**) or ineffective contraception (oral contraceptives). In addition to its effect on CYP 3A substrates, St. John's wort also decreases the plasma concentrations of **digoxin**, probably via induction of P-glycoprotein, an efflux transporter in the small intestine; thus, it potentially reduces the absorption of P-glycoprotein substrates, such as **cyclosporin** and **digoxin**. In addition, tannic acid present in St. John's wort may inhibit the absorption of **iron**.

B. Grapefruit Juice

Certain furanocoumarin constituents of grapefruit juice are potent irreversible inhibitors of CYP 3A4. Intake of grapefruit juice results in an increase in oral bioavailability of some CYP 3A substrates, with a decrease in the apparent oral clearance. However, intravenous clearance is generally unaffected, demonstrating that the effect of grapefruit juice is to inhibit the CYP 3A-mediated metabolism in the small intestine, without affecting hepatic drug extraction. Several psychopharmacologic agents, such as the oxidatively metabolized BZs **triazolam** and **alprazolam**, and antidepressants, such as **trazodone** and **nefazodone**, are metabolized almost entirely by CYP 3A4, and they are also administered by the oral route. Clinically significant interactions with grapefruit juice have been described for **triazolam**, a CYP 3A substrate with high presystemic extraction. Interactions with drugs, like **alprazolam**, with low to moderate extraction ratios are less significant.

V. Additional Information

Many medical facilities and pharmacies maintain and use drug interaction software programs. Many clinicians have similar programs on their personal computers or personal digital assistants (PDAs). Although they provide useful information and they are a good starting place, many of the programs are not up to date, and many include interactions from case reports in the literature where causality has not been established. Useful information is available on the following websites:

http://medicine.iupui.edu/flockhart/
http://www.gentest.com/human_p450_database/srchh450.asp
http://www.drugdigest.org/DD/
http://www.healthatoz.com/Atoz/Jsp/drugdb/drugSearch.jsp
http://drugsearch.doctorsnetaccess.com/
http://www.personalmd.com/drugdatabase.shtml
http://www.mhc.com/Cytochromes/

ADDITIONAL READING

Blackwell B. Monoamine oxidase inhibitor interactions with other drugs. *J Clin Psychopharmacol* 1991;11:55–59.

Ciraulo DA, Shader RI. Fluoxetine drug-drug interactions. I. Antidepressants and antipsychotics. *J Clin Psychopharmacol* 1990;10:48–50.

Ciraulo DA, Shader RI. Fluoxetine drug-drug interactions. II. *J Clin Psychopharmacol* 1990;10:213–217.

Ciraulo DA, Shader RI, Greenblatt DJ, Creelman W, eds. *Drug interactions in psychiatry*. Baltimore: Williams & Wilkins, 1989.

Goff DC, Baldessarini RJ. Drug interactions with antipsychotic agents. *J Clin Psychopharmacol* 1993;13:55–70.

Greenblatt DJ, Patki KC, von Moltke LL, et al. Drug interactions with grapefruit juice: an update. *J Clin Psychopharmacol* 2001;21:357–359.

Greenblatt DJ, von Moltke LL. Sedative-hypnotic and anxiolytic agents. In: Levy RH, Thummel KE, Trager WF, et al., eds. *Metabolic drug interactions*. Philadelphia: Lippincott Williams & Wilkins, 2000:259–270.

Greenblatt DJ, von Moltke LL, Harmatz JS, et al. Human cytochromes and some newer antidepressants: kinetics, metabolism, and drug interactions. *J Clin Psychopharmacol* 1999;19:23S–35S.

Hansten PD, Horn JR. *Drug interactions*, 6th ed. Philadelphia: Lea & Febiger, 1989.

Johnson FN, ed. *Lithium combination treatment*. Basel, Switzerland: Karger, 1987.

Ketter TA, Post RM, Worthington K. Principles of clinically important drug interactions with carbamazepine. Part I. *J Clin Psychopharmacol* 1991;11:198–203.

Ketter TA, Post RM, Worthington K. Principles of clinically important drug interactions with carbamazepine. Part II. *J Clin Psychopharmacol* 1991;11:306–313.

Ragheb M. The clinical significance of lithium-nonsteroidal antiinflammatory drug interactions. *J Clin Psychopharmacol* 1990;10:350–354.

Shinn AF, ed. *Evaluations of drug interactions*. New York: Macmillan, 1988.

Small JG, Milstein V. Lithium interactions: lithium and electroconvulsive treatment. *J Clin Psychopharmacol* 1990;10:346–349.

Spina E, Pisani F, Perucca E. Clinically significant pharmacokinetic drug interactions with carbamazepine. *Clin Pharmacokinet* 1996;31:198–214.

Sproule BA, Naranjo CA, Bremner KE, et al. Selective serotonin reuptake inhibitors and CNS drug interactions: a critical review of the evidence. *Clin Pharmacokinet* 1997;33:454–471.

Venkatakrishnan K, von Moltke LL, Greenblatt DJ. Effects of the antifungal agents on oxidative drug metabolism in humans: clinical relevance. *Clin Pharmacokinet* 2000;38:111–180.

Venkatakrishnan K, von Moltke LL, Greenblatt DJ. Human drug metabolism and the cytochromes P450: application and relevance of in vitro models. *J Clin Pharmacol* 2001;41:1149–1179.

von Moltke LL, Greenblatt DJ. Drug transporters in psychopharmacology—are they important? *J Clin Psychopharmacol* 2000;20:291–294.

Yuan R, Flockhart DA, Balian JD. Pharmacokinetic and pharmacodynamic consequences of metabolism-based drug interactions with alprazolam, midazolam, and triazolam. *J Clin Pharmacol* 1999;39:1109–1125.

APPENDICES

I. USE OF APPROVED DRUGS FOR UNLABELED INDICATIONS

Richard I. Shader

In many instances, physicians prescribe medication for indications other than those covered by United States Food and Drug Administration (FDA)-approved labeling (e.g., carbamazepine for mood disorders). Similarly, dosages or routes of administration (e.g., intravenous haloperidol for intensive care unit or cardiac care unit agitation or psychosis) may exceed or may differ from those covered by FDA-approved labeling, or they may not be mentioned in it. Nevertheless, these actions by physicians are an appropriate part of responsible patient care. Risk management considerations suggest that several steps should be taken by the physician when such deviations from labeling are necessary. First, the physician should document in the patient's record that he or she is aware that a variation from labeling is being undertaken, and he or she should record the reasons for doing so. Relevant supportive literature references should be given. Consultations, if any, with other knowledgeable colleagues or specialists should be recorded. Whenever a treatment is undertaken that specifically is cautioned against in the labeling, a supporting note from a knowledgeable colleague or specialist is an especially important step (e.g., if a monoamine oxidase inhibitor is combined with a tricyclic antidepressant).

The actual FDA position on labeling (*FDA Drug Bulletin,* April 1982) is clearly supportive of appropriate patient care. It is as follows:

> The appropriateness or the legality of prescribing approved drugs for uses not included in their official labeling is sometimes a cause of concern and confusion among practitioners.
>
> Under the Federal Food, Drug, and Cosmetic (FD&C) Act, a drug approved for marketing may be labeled, promoted, and advertised by the manufacturer only for those uses for which the drug's safety and effectiveness have been established and which FDA has approved. These are commonly referred to as "approved uses." This means that adequate and well-controlled clinical trials have documented these uses, and the results of the trials have been reviewed and approved by FDA.
>
> The FD&C Act does not, however, limit the manner in which a physician may use an approved drug. Once a product has been approved for marketing, a physician may prescribe it for uses or in treatment regimens or patient populations that are not included in approved labeling. Such "unapproved" or, more precisely, "unlabeled" uses may be appropriate and rational in certain circumstances and may, in fact, reflect approaches to drug therapy that have been extensively reported in medical literature.
>
> The term "unapproved uses" is, to some extent, misleading. It includes a variety of situations ranging from unstudied to thoroughly investigated drug uses. Valid new uses for drugs already on the market are often first discovered through serendipitous observations and therapeutic innovations, subsequently confirmed by well-planned and executed clinical investigations. Before such advances can be added to the approved labeling, however, data substantiating the effectiveness of a new use or regimen must be submitted by the manufacturer to FDA for evaluation. This may take time and, without the initiative of the drug manufacturer whose product is involved, may never occur. For that reason, accepted medical practice often includes drug use that is not reflected in approved drug labeling.
>
> With respect to its role in medical practice, the package insert is informational only. FDA tries to assure that prescription drug information in the package insert accurately and fully reflects the data on safety and effectiveness on which drug approval is based.

II. HERBAL REMEDIES, OVER-THE-COUNTER DRUGS, AND THE FOOD AND DRUG ADMINISTRATION: A PERSPECTIVE

Richard I. Shader

In 1972, the United States Food and Drug Administration embarked on its congressionally mandated task of evaluating the safety and efficacy of nonprescription drugs, also known as over-the-counter drugs or OTCs. Seventeen panels were formed, and, over the next 18 years, many herbal remedies were included among the compounds reviewed. When the panel reports were released in 1990, those OTCs reviewed were placed into the following three categories: I, safe and effective; II, unsafe or ineffective; and III, insufficient evidence to reach conclusions. No original work was commenced to inform these categories. Instead, conclusions were based on industry-supplied data or outside sources.

For many herbals and botanicals, data were lacking or were, at best, scant, and most of these agents were automatically classified in categories II or III. Examples of drugs that were listed in category I include the laxative psyllium seed or plantago and the topical analgesic red pepper or capsicum. Selected herbals are currently being studied in the United States. Germany's Commission E has conducted some research, and some agents are being considered by other countries. In recent years, safety issues have appeared about a number of compounds that were assumed to be safe based on their records of extensive exposure. However, two recent revelations reinforce the idea that all agents should be studied systematically (i.e., hepatic toxicity currently linked to the sedative-hypnotic kava-kava; drug interactions resulting from the antidepressant St. John's wort, based on its induction of CYP 3A4 and of the membrane transporter protein P-glycoprotein).

III. A PROTOTYPICAL OUTLINE OF THE MENTAL STATUS EXAMINATION

Richard I. Shader

I. **Demography, Appearance, Behavior, and Attitude**
   A. Appearance and Level of Consciousness
   B. Motor Status and Behavior
   C. Interpersonal Behavior and Attitude
II. **The Chief Complaint**
III. **Characteristics of Speech (Talk)**
   A. Descriptors
      1. Volume, tone, and quality
      2. Articulation and enunciation
      3. Rate and coherence
      4. Initiation
   B. Patterns and Styles
      1. Loose associations
      2. Word salad
      3. Blocking
      4. Circumstantiality
      5. Tangentiality
      6. Perseveration
      7. Flight of ideas
      8. Mutism
IV. **Cognitive Status**
   A. Attention and Concentration
   B. Orientation
   C. Memory
   D. Language and Communication Ability
   E. Judgment and Abstraction
      1. Reasoning
      2. Similarities and differences
      3. Proverb interpretation
V. **Content of Thought**
   A. Delusions
   B. Hallucinations
   C. Other Forms of Disordered Thought
VI. **Affect and Mood**
   A. Affect
   B. Mood
VII. **Insight**

IV. A TECHNIQUE FOR PROMOTING THE RELAXATION RESPONSE[1]

Richard I. Shader

I. **Basic Elements**
   A. A quiet environment
   B. A comfortable posture
   C. A mental device (a meaningful word or phrase)
   D. A passive attitude
II. **Instructions**
   A. Sit in a comfortable position in a quiet environment.
   B. Close your eyes.
   C. Deeply relax all your muscles, beginning at your feet and progressing up to your face (i.e., feet, calves, thighs, lower torso, chest, shoulders, neck, hands). Allow them to remain relaxed.
   D. Breathe through your nose. Become aware of your breathing. While breathing out, say silently to yourself the word "one" ("won") or some other word or short phrase that is meaningful to you (i.e., breathe in, breathe out, saying "won"; breathe in, breathe out, saying "won").
   E. Continue this way for 20 minutes. You may open your eyes periodically to check the time, but do not use an alarm. Do this once or twice daily and not within 2 hours after any meal.
   F. Sit quietly for a few minutes, first with your eyes shut and then with them open, when you finish each 20-minute exercise.
   G. The goal is a passive attitude. Deep relaxation will not always occur, and distracting thoughts will come into your mind. When you become conscious of them, ignore them and sustain the breathing exercise.

---

[1]Adapted from Benson H. *The relaxation response*. New York: Morrow, 1975; and Benson H, Beary JF, Carol MP. The relaxation response. *Psychiatry* 1974;37:37–46, with permission.

V. THE MINI-MENTAL STATE EXAMINATION

The Mini-Mental State Examination (MMSE) takes, on average, 5 to 10 minutes to complete. More time may be needed for the highly distractible or hard of hearing patient. The major value of the MMSE is that it may reveal deficits in a patient who, with a more casual and less systematic testing approach, might seem unimpaired. The MMSE is effective in avoiding the false-positive diagnosis of organic mental disorder (OMD) in hospitalized patients (specificity, 82%); it also has good sensitivity (i.e., 87% of actual OMD inpatients may be detected). See also Appendix VI.

TABLE V.1. MINI-MENTAL STATE EXAMINATION

	Maximum Score[a]
Orientation	
Ask about the date first and then about the season, and so on.	
What is the (year), (season), (month), (day of month), and (day of week)?	5
Ask about the hospital or building first and then about the other aspects of location.	
Where are we (e.g., [floor], [building], [town], [state], [country])?	5
Registration	
Tester names three unrelated objects, then asks patient to repeat them.[b]	3
Attention and calculation	
Serial 7s (five successive subtractions of 7 are scored, beginning with 7 from 100 [i.e., 93, 86, 79, 72, 65]). Stop after five subtractions.	5
Alternatively, patient is asked to spell "world" backward.	
Recall	
What were the three objects learned earlier?	3
Language and praxis	
Tester points to a pencil and a wristwatch and asks patient to name them.	2
Patient is asked to do the following:	
Repeat "No ifs, ands, or buts."	1
Follow the three-stage verbal command "Take this piece of paper in your right hand, fold it in half, and then put it on the floor."	3
Follow the printed command "Close your eyes."	1
Make up and write a short sentence.	1
Copy this design (two interlocking pentagons).	1
Maximum total score	30

[a]One point is given for each correct response. Total scores < 24 generally suggest dementia or delirium. Seven to 12 errors suggest mild to moderate impairment, and >12 errors suggest severe impairment.
[b]If the patient scores < 3 on the first trial, the tester repeats the objects (up to six times) until the patient learns them in preparation for recall testing.
Adapted from Folstein MF, Folstein S, McHugh PR. Mini-mental state: a practical method of grading cognitive state of patients for the clinician. *J Psychiatr Res* 1975;12:189–198, with permission. See also Nelson A, Fogel BS, Faust D. Bedside cognitive screening instruments: a critical assessment. *J Nerv Ment Dis* 1986;174:73–83; and Anthony JC, LeResche L, Niaz U. Limits of the "mini-mental state" as a screening test for dementia and delirium among hospital patients. *Psychol Med* 1982;12:397–408, with permission.

VI. THE SHORT PORTABLE MENTAL STATUS QUESTIONNAIRE

Similar in many respects to the Mini-Mental State Examination (MMSE) that appears in Appendix V, the Short Portable Mental Status Questionnaire (SPMSQ)[1] differs slightly in that it adjusts the scoring to take the patient's level of education into account. The SPMSQ also omits the visuomotor copying and reading tasks of the MMSE. The SPMSQ is highly effective in avoiding the false-positive diagnosis of organic mental disorders (OMD) (specificity of greater than 95%), but it does not have powerful sensitivity (i.e., less than 60% of actual OMD patients may be detected).

QUESTIONS OR TASKS

1. What is today's date (month or day of the year or month, respectively)?
2. What day of the week is it?
3. What is the name of this place?
4. What is your telephone number (or, if the patient does not have a telephone, your home address)?
5. How old are you now?
6. In what year were you born (month and day of the year and month, respectively)?
7. Who is the current President of the United States?
8. Who was the President just before this one?
9. What was your mother's maiden name?
10. Subtract 3 from 20 and keep subtracting all the way to zero.

SCORING

One point is given for each correct response.

0–2 errors: Normal
3–4 errors: Mild impairment
5–7 errors: Moderate impairment
8–10 errors: Severe impairment

Allow scores to range one error higher if subject had no grade school education. Allow one fewer error if the subject had education beyond high school.

---

[1] Adapted from Pfeiffer E. A short portable mental status questionnaire for the assessment of organic brain deficits in elderly patients. *J Am Geriatr Soc* 1975;22:433–441, with permission. See also Fillenbaum G. Comparison of two brief tests of organic brain impairment, the MSQ and the Short Portable MSQ. *J Am Geriatr Soc* 1980;28:381–384, with permission.

VII. ALGORITHMS FOR PSYCHOPHARMACOLOGY

David N. Osser
Robert D. Patterson

I. **Algorithms Attempt to Capture the Thought Processes of Experts as They Determine the Best Approaches to Specific Clinical Situations**
Evidence-supported algorithms are a distillation of the scientific basis for practice. Many organizations and individuals produce them. This appendix is a list of psychopharmacology algorithms and practice guidelines that contain algorithmic sequences.

A. **Evaluating Algorithm Quality**
Algorithm quality may be evaluated in a number of ways.

1. **Is the algorithm up to date?** Algorithms get out of date quickly as new medications are marketed, as new uses of older medications are discovered, and as new studies establish more clearly the role of existing medications. The best algorithms are frequently updated. For example, the authors of this appendix maintain their algorithms on the Internet (*http://www.mhc.com/Algorithms/*) and update them when mandated by important new developments. The Texas Medication Algorithm Project also updates its algorithms periodically and posts these changes on the Internet (*http://www.mhmr.state.tx.us/centraloffice/medicaldirector/ TMAP.html*). One journal (*Primary Psychiatry*) has published an annually updated issue that is devoted to psychiatric algorithms.

2. **Has the algorithm been peer reviewed?** Publication in a major journal ensures this.

3. **Are there reasons to suspect bias?** Algorithms developed under grants from pharmaceutical firms should be carefully examined by the potential user. For example, sometimes experts are brought together in a "closed symposium" in a resort area, served delicious meals, and paid an "honorarium." There, they may produce a consensus guideline or algorithm, which is subsequently published in a "supplement" to a journal. Of importance is taking into account that these supplements, as well as the symposia that they chronicle, are usually paid for by pharmaceutical firms. The articles in supplements often do not undergo external peer review the way that articles in the journal that the supplements resemble do. The introductory texts of algorithms produced in this way should be carefully inspected to see if intensive peer review has in fact occurred. The content should be evaluated to see if these algorithm quality standards have been met. Not surprisingly, sponsored algorithms often strongly endorse the sponsor's product, and they generally downplay the clinical importance of or even neglect to mention other products that have evidence of usefulness for the indications described. They may underplay or may omit discussion of the side effects of the endorsed products even when a substantial evidence basis for concern exists. For example, the "consensus" may be that selective serotonin reuptake inhibitors are first line for a particular indication, but no discussion may be included of the very high incidence of sexual dysfunction with selective serotonin reuptake inhibitors and of how that might influence the consideration of alternative medications.

4. **Does the algorithm incorporate evidence of safety, as well as of efficacy or effectiveness?** The algorithm's decision points should consider efficacy as suggested in controlled empirical studies, as well as effectiveness in the real world, as determined by outcome studies and expert opinion. Side-effect risks should be strongly considered in the se-

lection of drugs at each step in the algorithm. The evidence basis for proposed differences in safety should be made explicit. Sometimes, use of, with the patient's informed consent, a medication with less evidence of efficacy but a more benign side-effect profile is preferable to that of a medication with stronger evidence of efficacy but more problematic side effects. Similarly, clinicians can be confused about what the practice implications are when the United States Food and Drug Administration has approved a medication for a particular indication. This means that the medication has been found effective and reasonably safe to use, but it does not mean that the medication should always be used at the top of the algorithm for that indication when another drug might be safer.

5. **Do the decision points contain primary recommendations and appropriate options?** The algorithms should offer several options at each step, whenever possible, to account for individual patient susceptibilities and concerns about side effects.

6. **Are any differences from other algorithms or the opinions of other experts discussed?** Algorithm authors ideally should acknowledge when other published algorithms or prominent experts have reached different conclusions. An examination of the evidence behind the disagreements and an attempt to resolve the differences should be included. If the evidence does not permit a clear preference, the alternative recommendations should be offered as options. An example of a difference would be in the sequence of medications recommended before the use of **clozapine** in patients with schizophrenia. Some algorithms recommend trials of one new-generation atypical antipsychotic and one conventional neuroleptic as the minimum requirements for a trial of **clozapine**. Others suggest two atypicals and one conventional and then **clozapine**. Yet another recommends trying three currently available atypicals (e.g., **olanzapine, quetiapine, risperidone**) plus one conventional before considering **clozapine** the treatment of choice. At the present time, the authors of this appendix prefer trying two atypicals (i.e., **risperidone, olanzapine**) and one conventional agent before using **clozapine**, particularly because the effectiveness of **quetiapine** in treatment-resistant cases is uncertain and routinely requiring patients to endure four therapeutic trials before having the opportunity to consider **clozapine** seems unnecessary. **Clozapine** is still the most powerful option for patients with an unsatisfactory response to other antipsychotics, despite its many side effects. **Ziprasidone** and **aripiprazole** were recently introduced. Whether they may substitute for the above options or should be added to the pre-**clozapine** sequence of treatments is not clear as yet.

7. **How completely does the algorithm cover possible clinical scenarios?** Algorithms are ideally expected to provide an appropriate end point for every possible clinical situation—either a recommendation, which sometimes may be limited to a statement that insufficient evidence exists to warrant specific suggestions, or an acknowledgment that a particular situation is beyond the scope of the algorithm. In expert system terminology, the latter is described as "failing gracefully," in contrast to giving a wrong recommendation. Wrong recommendations can occur if the algorithm writers have never considered the particular clinical situation.

II. Good Algorithms Are Helpers, Not Dictators

Consultation with a high quality algorithm is a way to determine what the available evidence and expert opinion suggest might be the best practice for a typical patient. The clinician may use this information as a starting point in the process of deciding what would be best for the individual patient at hand. If a deviation from the algorithm's recommendation seems appropriate, the reasoning should be clear to the physician. Explaining this reasoning to the patient and documenting it in the medical record are prudent.

III. Selected Algorithm Papers

The following algorithms are arranged by diagnosis and are listed chronologically by date of publication, starting with the most recent. General references and collections of brief algorithms are in separate lists at the end. Because of the rapidly changing nature of psychopharmacology practice, only algorithms published since 1997 are included. The authors intend to maintain an updated list of algorithms on their website at *http://www.mhc.com/Algorithms/*.

A. Schizophrenia

Osser DN, Sigadel R. Short-term inpatient pharmacotherapy of schizophrenia. *Harvard Rev Psychiatry* 2001;9:89–104. Latest update at *http://www.mhc.com/Algorithms/*.

Expert Consensus Guideline Series. Treatment of schizophrenia. *J Clin Psychiatry* 1999;60:3–80.

Osser DN, Zarate CA Jr. Consultant for the pharmacotherapy of schizophrenia. *Psychiatr Ann* 1999;29:252–267. Latest update at *http://www.mhc.com/Algorithms/*.

Miller AL, Chiles JA, Chiles JK, et al. The Texas Medication Algorithm Project (TMAP) schizophrenia algorithms. *J Clin Psychiatry* 1999;60:649–657. Latest update at *http://www.mhmr.state.tx.us/centraloffice/medicaldirector/TMAP.html*.

Working Group for the Canadian Psychiatric Association and the Canadian Alliance for Research on Schizophrenia. Canadian clinical practice guidelines for the treatment of schizophrenia. *Can J Psychiatry* 1998;43:25S–40S.

B. Depression

Crismon ML, Trivedi M, Pigott TA, et al. The Texas Medication Algorithm Project: report of the Texas consensus conference panel on medication treatment of major depressive disorder. *J Clin Psychiatry* 1999;60:142–156. Latest update at *http://www.mhmr.state.tx.us/centraloffice/medicaldirector/TMAP.html*.

DeBattista C, Solvaason B, Nelson C, et al. Major depression and its subtypes. In: Fawcett J, Stein DJ, Jobson KO, eds. *Textbook of treatment algorithms in psychopharmacology*. New York: John Wiley & Sons, 1999:38–57.

Osser DN, Patterson RD. Algorithms for the pharmacotherapy of depression, part one (unipolar, dysthymia), part two (psychotic, treatment-refractory, comorbid). *Directions in Psychiatry* 1998;18:303–333. Latest update at *http://www.mhc.com/Algorithms/*.

C. Bipolar Depression

Sachs GS, Printz DJ, Kahn DA, et al. The expert consensus guideline series: medication treatment of bipolar disorder 2000. *Postgrad Med Special Rep* 2000;Spec No:1–104.

Dantzler A, Osser DN. Algorithms for the pharmacotherapy of acute depression in patients with bipolar disorder. *Psychiatr Ann* 1999;29:270–284. Latest update at *http://www.mhc.com/Algorithms/*.

Dennehy EB, Suppes T. Medication algorithms for bipolar disorder. *J Pract Psychiatry Behav Health* 1999;5:142–152. Latest update at *http://www.mhmr.state.tx.us/centraloffice/medicaldirector/TMAP.html*.

Goodwin GM, Bourgeois ML, Conti L, et al. Treatment of bipolar depressive mood disorders: algorithms for pharmacotherapy. *Int J Psychiatry Clin Pract* 1997;1:S9–S12.

D. Bipolar Mania

Sachs GS, Printz DJ, Kahn DA, et al. The expert consensus guideline series: medication treatment of bipolar disorder 2000. *Postgrad Med Special Rep* 2000;Spec No:1–104.

Dennehy EB, Suppes T. Medication algorithms for bipolar disorder. *J Pract Psychiatry Behav Health* 1999;5:142–152. Latest update at *http://www.mhmr.state.tx.us/centraloffice/medicaldirector/TMAP.html*.

Bauer MS, Callahan AM, Chowdary J, et al. Clinical practice guidelines for bipolar disorder from the Department of Veterans Affairs. *J Clin Psychiatry* 1999;60:9–21.

Post RM, Denicoff KD, Frye MA, et al. Algorithms for bipolar mania. In: Rush AJ, ed. *Mood disorders: systematic medication management.* Basel, Switzerland: Karger, 1997:114–145.

Kusumaker V, Yatham LN, Haslam DR, et al. The treatment of bipolar disorder: review of the literature, guidelines, and options. Treatment of mania, mixed state, and rapid cycling. *Can J Psychiatry* 1997;42:79S–86S.

E. Panic Disorder

Coplan JD, Gorman JM. Panic disorder. In: Fawcett J, Stein DJ, Jobson KO, eds. *Textbook of treatment algorithms in psychopharmacology.* New York: John Wiley & Sons, 1999:88–98.

Osser DN, Renner JA Jr, Bayog R. Algorithms for the pharmacotherapy of anxiety disorders in patients with chemical abuse and dependence. *Psychiatr Ann* 1999;29:285–301. Latest update at *http://www.mhc.com/Algorithms/.*

Rosenbaum JF, Pollack MH, Friedman SJ. The pharmacotherapy of panic disorder. In: Rosenbaum JF, Pollack MH, eds. *Panic disorder and its treatment.* New York: Marcel Dekker, 1998:153–180.

F. Posttraumatic Stress Disorder

Alarcon RD, Glover S, Boyer W, et al. Proposing an algorithm for the pharmacological treatment of posttraumatic stress disorder. *Ann Clin Psychiatry* 2000;12:239–246.

Expert Consensus Guideline Series. Treatment of posttraumatic stress disorder. *J Clin Psychiatry* 1999;60:1–76.

Osser DN, Renner JA Jr, Bayog R. Algorithms for the pharmacotherapy of anxiety disorders in patients with chemical abuse and dependence. *Psychiatr Ann* 1999;29:285–301. Latest update at *http://www.mhc.com/Algorithms/.*

G. Social Anxiety Disorder (Social Phobia)

Sutherland SM, Davidson JR. Social phobia. In: Fawcett J, Stein DJ, Jobson KO, eds. *Textbook of treatment algorithms in psychopharmacology.* New York: John Wiley & Sons, 1999:107–118.

Osser DN, Renner JA Jr, Bayog R. Algorithms for the pharmacotherapy of anxiety disorders in patients with chemical abuse and dependence. *Psychiatr Ann* 1999;29:285–301. Latest update at *http://www.mhc.com/Algorithms/.*

Marshall RD, Schneier FR. An algorithm for the pharmacotherapy of social phobia. *Psychiatr Ann* 1996;26:210–216.

H. Obsessive-Compulsive Disorder

Greist JH, Jefferson JW. Pharmacotherapy for obsessive-compulsive disorder. *Br J Psychiatry* 1998;173:64–70.

Francis A, Docherty JP, Kahn DA. Treatment of obsessive-compulsive disorder: the Expert Consensus Guideline series. *J Clin Psychiatry* 1997; 58:11–27.

I. Generalized Anxiety Disorder

Osser DN, Renner JA Jr, Bayog R. Algorithms for the pharmacotherapy of anxiety disorders in patients with chemical abuse and dependence. *Psychiatr Ann* 1999;29:285–301. Latest update at *http://www.mhc.com/Algorithms/.*

J. Body Dysmorphic Disorder

Phillips KA. Pharmacotherapy of body dysmorphic disorder: a review of empirical evidence and a proposed treatment algorithm. *Psychiatr Clin North Am Ann Drug Ther* 2000;7:59–82.

K. Agitation in the Patient With Dementia

Kahn DA, Alexopoulos GS, Silver JM, et al. Treatment of agitation in elderly persons with dementia: a summary of the Expert Consensus Guidelines. *J Pract Psychiatry Behav Health* 1998;4:265–276.

Colenda CC. Managing agitated dementia patients: a decision analysis approach. *J Pract Psychiatry Behav Health* 1997;3:156–164.

L. Personality Disorders

Soloff PH. Psychopharmacology of borderline personality disorder. *Psychiatr Clin North Am* 2000;23:169–192.

Soloff PH. Algorithms for pharmacological treatment of personality dimensions: symptom-specific treatment for cognitive-perceptual, affective, and impulsive-behavioral dysregulation. *Bull Menninger Clin* 1998;62:195–214.

M. Attention Deficit Hyperactivity Disorder

Bhandary AN, Fernandez F, Gregory RJ, et al. Pharmacotherapy in adults with ADHD. *Psychiatr Ann* 1997;27:545–555.

N. Child and Adolescent Psychopharmacology

Emslie GJ, Mayes TL, Hughes CW. Updates in the pharmacologic treatment of childhood depression. *Psychiatr Clin North Am Ann Drug Ther* 2000;7: 235–256.

Martin A, Kaufman J, Charney D. Pharmacotherapy of early-onset depression: update and new directions. *Child Adolesc Psychiatr Clin North Am* 2000;9:135–157.

Birmaher B, Brent D, Heydl P. Childhood-onset depressive disorders. In: Fawcett J, Stein DJ, Jobson KO, eds. *Textbook of treatment algorithms in psychopharmacology*. New York: John Wiley & Sons, 1999:135–163.

Davanzo PA. Mood stabilizers in the treatment of juvenile bipolar disorder: advances and controversies. *Child Adolesc Psychiatr Clin North Am* 2000; 9:159–182.

Pliszka SR, Greenhill LL, Crismon ML, et al. The Texas children's medication algorithm project: report of the Texas Consensus Conference Panel on medication treatment of childhood attention-deficit/hyperactivity disorder, part I. Part II. Tactics. *J Am Acad Child Adolesc Psychiatry* 2000; 39:908–927.

O. General Articles on the Theory and Practice of Constructing Algorithms

Trivedi M, Rush AJ, Crismon ML, et al. Treatment guidelines and algorithms. *Psychiatr Clin North Am Ann Drug Ther* 2000;7:1–22.

Patterson RD. The Harvard psychopharmacology algorithm project. *Psychiatr Ann* 1999;29:248–250.

Hartley DS III. The language of algorithms. In: Fawcett J, Stein DJ, Jobson KO, eds. *Textbook of treatment algorithms in psychopharmacology*. New York: John Wiley & Sons, 1999:15–31.

Gilbert DA, Altshuler KZ, Rago WV, et al. Texas medication algorithm project: definitions, rationale, and methods to develop medication algorithms. *J Clin Psychiatry* 1998;59:345–351.

Jobson KO. International Psychopharmacology Algorithm Project: algorithms in psychopharmacology. *Int J Psychiatry Clin Pract* 1997;1:S3–S8.

Colenda CC. Managing agitated dementia patients: a decision analysis approach. *J Pract Psychiatry Behav Health* 1997;3:156–164.

P. Other References of Interest on Algorithms and Guidelines

Waddell C. So much research evidence, so little dissemination and uptake. *Evidence-Based Mental Health* 2001;4:3–5.

Stein DJ, Seedat S, Niehaus D, et al. Psychiatric algorithms for primary care, part I and part II. *Primary Psychiatry* 2000;7:45–69, 35–68. *This collection of algorithms addresses many clinical problems seen by primary care physicians. These algorithms are updated annually.*

Geyman JP, Deyo RA, Ramsey SD. *Evidence-based clinical practice: concepts and approaches.* Boston, MA: Butterworth-Heinemann, 2000.

Shore MF. Algorithms and the quality of care. *Psychiatr Ann* 1999;29:315–316.

Cabana MD, Rand CS, Powe NR, et al. Why don't physicians follow clinical practice guidelines? A framework for improvement. *JAMA* 1999;282: 1458–1465.

Rush AJ, Crismon ML, Toprac MG, et al. Implementing guidelines and systems of care: experiences with the Texas Medication Algorithm Project (TMAP). *J Pract Psychiatry Behav Health* 1999;5:75–86.

Montgomery SA. Algorithms—a European perspective. In: Fawcett J, Stein DJ, Jobson KO, eds. *Textbook of treatment algorithms in psychopharmacology*. New York: John Wiley & Sons, 1999:1–6.

Trivedi MH, DeBattista C, Fawcett L, et al. Developing treatment algorithms for unipolar depression in cyberspace: International Psychopharmacology Algorithm Project. *Psychopharmacol Bull* 1998;34:355–359.

Sato M, Higuchi T, Yamawaki S. Proposals for the rational selection of drugs in the treatment of schizophrenia and mood disorders [in Japan]. *Psychiatry Clin Neurosci* 1999;53:S1–S82. *Algorithms are from the Proceedings of International Meeting on Japan Psychopharmacology Algorithms.*

Janicak PG, Davis JM, Preskorn SH, et al. *Principles and practice of psychopharmacotherapy,* 3rd ed. Philadelphia: Lippincott Williams & Wilkins, 2001. *This textbook has algorithm-like "strategies" throughout the text.*

SUBJECT INDEX

SUBJECT INDEX

Note: Page numbers followed by *f* indicate figures; those followed by *t* indicate tables.